医学词根手册

A Dictionary of Medical Roots

主编 于斌 李鹏
副主编 崔纪芳 张捷 刘蕊
编委 梁嘉钰 付轩 林映希

天津出版传媒集团
天津科学技术出版社

图书在版编目（CIP）数据

医学词根手册 / 于斌，李鹏主编. -- 天津 ：天津科学技术出版社，2025. 8. -- ISBN 978-7-5742-3260-0

I. R

中国国家版本馆 CIP 数据核字第 2025XM0056 号

医学词根手册

YIXUE CIGEN SHOUCE

责任编辑：张　卓

责任印制：兰　毅

出　　版：天津出版传媒集团 / 天津科学技术出版社

地　　址：天津市西康路 35 号

邮　　编：300051

电　　话：（022）23332400

网　　址：www.tjkjcbs.com.cn

发　　行：新华书店经销

印　　刷：北京捷迅佳彩印刷有限公司

开本 889×1194　1/48　印张 19.5　字数 400 000

2025 年 8 月第 1 版第 1 次印刷

定价：128.00元

序

作为深耕医学教育领域多年的践行者，我们时常感慨医学术语犹如精密的密码，精准编织着国际医学交流的网络，却也因源自古希腊语、拉丁语的独特脉络，成为横亘在无数学子与国际医学前沿间的挑战。威普爱生教育作为国内专注涉外医学培训领域的先锋力量，始终以搭建中外医学教育与实践互通桥梁为使命，在助力学子跨越国际医学门槛的历程中，我们无比清楚：突破医学术语关，不仅是知识的跨越，更是中国医学与世界对话的关键钥匙。

《医学词根手册》的诞生，恰如迷雾中的灯塔。主编于斌及团队以深厚积淀凝练350余个核心词根，巧妙拆解临床医学术语的密码，让复杂术语变得条理清晰。这不仅是学习方式的革新，更蕴含着深远的社会价值 —— 它赋予医学生挑战海外医师执照的底气，让科研工作者能更高效地研读SCI文献、在顶尖期刊迸发思想火花；它推动中国医学科研成果以更专业的姿态走向世界，助力中国从医学领域的参与者成长为规则制定者。

能够见证这部手册的问世，威普爱生教育与有荣焉。手册涵盖临床医学核心词根，结合实用例证，将晦涩术语转化为可掌握的知识单元，无论是医学生、科研人员还是医学从业者，皆能从中汲取力量。它不仅是一本工具手册，更是攀登国际医学高峰的阶梯。

我们诚心推荐《医学词根手册》，愿它成为万千医学追光者手中的利器，照亮他们在国际医学天地中驰骋的道路，也让中国医学在世界舞台，因这清晰的“术语之声”而愈发璀璨，真正成为国际医学规则的有力构建者！

威普爱生教育CEO 胡玉华

前 言

英语的医学术语往往听起来令人生畏，甚至让那些以英语为母语的人，也常常望而却步。我当年在英国做医生的时候，一个重要的技能就是要用病人听得懂的语言去和他们交流。那么，既然连普通的英国人都听不懂这些词汇，作为医学从业者，我们为什么非要学习并使用它们呢？其实答案很简单，因为这些医学术语有非常明确的定义，而普通的英语在描述医学概念的时候，词义往往没有那么清晰。我们都知道，写英文论文非常注重用词的多样性，以便让整篇文章看起来没有那么枯燥。但通过使用近义词来获得的语言多样性，只局限在形容词和动词，而不能用于名词。医学术语作为名词，其近义词往往代表不同的概念，而一旦在文章中使用不同的专业术语名词，往往会导致其描述对象发生偏移。

于是，使用医学术语便成了一个在医学学习和交流过程中无法逃避的环节。这些术语往往来自古希腊语和拉丁语，因此很多以英语为母语的人也不知晓它们的意思，这无疑又增加了这些词汇的神秘性和专业性。但即使这样，世界上绝大部分国家，不论他们的母语是什么，往往都使用相同的词汇体系来学习医学并进行交流。在过去几十年，我国已经在很多领域深度参与了国际合作，并在诸多领域处于世界领先水平。而医学之所以还没有和世界深度接轨，这些专业术语是一个重要的壁垒。

医学术语之所以仍然能在全世界范围内被使用，除了它的高精准性之外，另外一个原因就是它远没有我们想象的那么难以掌握。这是因为，医学术语中的大部分词汇都是由词根构成的。我总结了将近 400 个词根，几乎涵盖了临床医学相关学科的大部分词汇。我希望，通过阅读这本手册，读者能够在看到一个新的医学术语时，首先想到的是它能否被拆分以获得词根，因为记忆词根的工作量要远小于记忆每一个由词根构成的医学术语。我国的大学英语四、六级考试，往往要求学生掌握 4000 ～ 6000 个单词，而我们只需要付出考四六级的十分之一的努力，就可以掌握几乎所有的医学术语。

拥有无障碍阅读医学术语的能力，能够丰富医学生的人生选择。它会让我们有足够的信心去考取海外医师执照，获得海外工作经验。它也可以大幅提升我们阅读 SCI 文章的速度，同时增加对其理解的深度。从 2023 年开始，我国学者发表的 SCI 文章总数就已经超过了美国，成为世界第一。未来，我们需要做的是更多地在顶尖国际期刊发表文章。在很多情况下，我们投稿失败，并不是因为我们的数据不够好，而往往是因为我们由于语言的限制，不能基于现有数据写出有深度的文章。而能够理解和使用好这些医学术语，无疑会给我们的科研数据锦上添花，让我们的科研成果能更多地被同行引用。使用专业术语撰写的临床指南，也更可能被其他国家的医院使用，让我们真正成为医学规则的制定者。

本书 A–G 部分由副主编崔纪芳编写、翻译；H–M 部分由副主编张捷编写，主编于斌翻译；N–R 部分由主编李鹏编写、翻译；S–Z 部分由副主编刘蕊编写，主编李鹏翻译。主编于斌负责全书整理与校对。

目 录

A

B

C

D

E

F

G

H

I

J

K

L

M

N

O

P

R

S

T

U

V

X

Z

a-（没有）

aplasia 发育不全

词根 a-（没有）+ -plasia（生长）
例句 Bone marrow aplasia can lead to severe anemia. 骨髓发育不全可能导致严重贫血。

agnosia 失认症

词根 a-（没有）+ -gnosia（识别能力）
例句 Agnosia is the inability to recognize objects. 失认症指识别物体的能力丧失。

anemia 贫血

词根 a-（没有）+ -emia（血症）
例句 Iron deficiency anemia is common in women. 缺铁性贫血在女性中很常见。

atrophy 萎缩

词根 a-（没有）+ -trophy（营养生长）
例句 Muscle atrophy occurs after prolonged immobility. 长期不活动会导致肌肉萎缩。

aphasia 失语症

词根 a-（没有）+ -phasia（言语）
例句 Aphasia is a common symptom after a stroke. 失语症是中风后的常见症状。

asepsis 无菌状态

词根 a-（没有）+ -sepsis（感染）
例句 Surgical asepsis is crucial for preventing infections. 手术无

菌状态对预防感染至关重要。

anorexia 食欲缺乏

词根 a-（没有）+ -orexia（食欲）

例句 Anorexia can be a symptom of various medical conditions. 食欲缺乏可能是多种疾病的症状。

apnea 呼吸暂停

词根 a-（没有）+ -pnea（呼吸）

例句 Sleep apnea can lead to poor sleep quality. 睡眠呼吸暂停会导致睡眠质量下降。

amnesia 失忆症

词根 a-（没有）+ -mnesia（记忆）

例句 Traumatic brain injuries may cause amnesia. 创伤性脑损伤可能导致失忆症。

asthenia 无力

词根 a-（没有）+ -sthenia（力量）

例句 Chronic fatigue syndrome can lead to asthenia. 慢性疲劳综合征可能导致无力。

acanth-（棘状的）

acanthocyte 棘形红细胞

词根 acanth-（棘状）+ -cyte（细胞）

例句 Acanthocytes are seen in patients with liver disease. 棘形红细胞可见于肝病患者。

acanthosis 棘皮症

词根 acanth-（棘状）+ -osis（病态）

例句 Acanthosis nigricans is associated with insulin resistance. 黑棘皮病与胰岛素抵抗有关。

acantholysis 棘融解

词根 acanth-（棘状）+ -lysis（分解）

例句 Acantholysis is seen in autoimmune skin diseases. 棘融解可见于自身免疫性皮肤病。

acanthoma 棘状细胞瘤

词根 acanth-（棘状）+ -oma（肿瘤）

例句 Acanthomas are benign skin tumors. 棘状细胞瘤是一种良性皮肤肿瘤。

acanthopelvis 棘状骨盆

词根 acanth-（棘状）+ pelvis（骨盆）

例句 Acanthopelvis is a rare pelvic abnormality. 棘状骨盆是一种罕见的骨盆异常。

acanthion 棘点

词根 acanth-（棘状）+ -ion（小体）

例句 The acanthion is an anatomical landmark on the skull. 棘点是颅骨上的一个解剖标志。

acanthocheilonema 棘唇线虫

词根 acanth-（棘状）+ cheilo-（唇）+ nema（线虫）

例句 Acanthocheilonema is a parasitic nematode. 棘唇线虫是一种寄生线虫。

acanthocyte anemia 棘形细胞贫血

词根 acanth-（棘状）+ -cyte（细胞）+ anemia（贫血）

例句 Acanthocyte anemia is seen in severe liver disease. 棘形细胞贫血可见于严重的肝病。

acanthodermatitis 棘状皮炎

词根 acanth-（棘状）+ dermat-（皮肤）+ -itis（炎症）

例句 Acanthodermatitis causes thickened and scaly skin. 棘状皮炎

会导致皮肤增厚和脱屑。

acanthocytosis 棘形红细胞增多

词根 acanth-（棘状）+ -cytosis（细胞增多）

例句 Acanthocytosis is associated with neuroacanthocytosis syndromes. 棘形红细胞增多与神经棘红细胞增多症有关。

acro-（末端）

acromegaly 肢端肥大症

词根 acro-（末端）+ -megaly（增大）

例句 Acromegaly is caused by excessive growth hormone production. 肢端肥大症是由生长激素分泌过多引起的。

acroparesthesia 末端感觉异常

词根 acro-（末端）+ -paresthesia（感觉异常）

例句 Acroparesthesia is common in patients with carpal tunnel syndrome. 末端感觉异常在腕管综合征患者中很常见。

acrocyanosis 末端发绀

词根 acro-（末端）+ cyan-（青紫色）+ -osis（病态）

例句 Acrocyanosis is a condition where the fingers and toes turn blue due to poor circulation. 末端发绀是由循环不良导致手指和脚趾发蓝的情况。

acrodynia 肢端痛

词根 acro-（末端）+ -dynia（疼痛）

例句 Acrodynia was historically associated with mercury poisoning. 肢端痛在历史上与汞中毒有关。

acromion 肩峰

词根 acro-（末端）+ -mion（结构）

例句 The acromion is a bony projection on the scapula. 肩峰是肩

胛骨上的一个骨性突起。

acrophobia 恐高症

词根 acro-（高处 / 建筑的末端）+ -phobia（恐惧）

例句 People with acrophobia feel anxious when looking down from heights. 恐高症患者从高处向下看时会感到焦虑。

acroarthritis 肢端关节炎

词根 acro-（末端）+ arthr-（关节）+ -itis（炎症）

例句 Acroarthritis affects the small joints of the hands and feet. 肢端关节炎影响手部和脚部的小关节。

acrocephaly 尖头畸形

词根 acro-（末端）+ cephal-（头部）+ -y（状态）

例句 Acrocephaly results from premature fusion of skull sutures. 尖头畸形是由颅缝过早闭合引起的。

acromioclavicular joint 肩锁关节

词根 acro-（末端）+ myo-（肌肉）+ clavicular（锁骨）

例句 The acromioclavicular joint connects the clavicle and the scapula. 肩锁关节连接锁骨和肩胛骨。

acroosteolysis 末端骨溶解

词根 acro-（末端）+ osteo-（骨）+ -lysis（溶解）

例句 Acroosteolysis is a condition characterized by bone resorption in the fingers and toes. 末端骨溶解是一种手指和脚趾发生骨吸收的病症。

actino-（放射的）

actinomycosis 放线菌病

词根 actino-（放射）+ myco-（真菌）+ -osis（病态）

例句 Actinomycosis is a chronic bacterial infection that forms abscesses. 放线菌病是一种形成脓肿的慢性细菌感染。

actinodermatitis 放射性皮炎

词根 actino-（放射）+ dermat-（皮肤）+ -itis（炎症）

例句 Actinodermatitis can result from prolonged exposure to radiation. 放射性皮炎可能是长时间接触辐射引起的。

actinotherapy 放射治疗

词根 actino-（放射）+ -therapy（治疗）

例句 Actinotherapy is used in cancer treatment. 放射治疗用于癌症治疗。

actinomycete 放射菌

词根 actino-（放射）+ -mycete（真菌）

例句 Actinomycetes are commonly found in soil and are known for their ability to produce antibiotics. 放射菌常见于土壤中，且以其能够产生抗生素而闻名。

actinograph 放射计

词根 actino-（放射）+ -graph（记录仪）

例句 An actinograph measures the intensity of radiation. 放射计用于测量辐射强度。

actinocyte 放射细胞

词根 actino-（放射）+ -cyte（细胞）

例句 Actinocytes play a role in certain immune responses. 放射细胞在某些免疫反应中起作用。

actinodermosis 放射性皮肤病

词根 actino-（放射）+ derm-（皮肤）+ -osis（病态）

例句 Actinodermosis is a chronic condition caused by radiation exposure. 放射性皮肤病是由辐射暴露引起的一种慢性病。

actinomorphic 放射对称的

词根 actino-（放射）+ morph-（形态）+ -ic（形容词后缀）
例句 Certain flowers exhibit actinomorphic symmetry. 某些花具有放射对称性。

actinoscopy 放射检查

词根 actino-（放射）+ -scopy（检查）
例句 Actinoscopy is used in radiological diagnostics. 放射检查用于放射学诊断。

actinotoxicity 放射毒性

词根 actino-（放射）+ toxic（毒性）+ -ity（状态）
例句 Actinotoxicity refers to cellular damage caused by radiation. 放射毒性指由辐射引起的细胞损伤。

USMLE Step 1　样题

A premature (pre-) child is born in respiratory (re-; spir-) distress and is emergently intubated (tub-). Synthetic pulmonary surfactant (surf-; act-) is administered with no improvement in pulmonary function. After conducting a detailed physical examination, the pediatrician believes that this child's condition is related to a failure of the embryonic pleuroperitoneal (pleuro-; peritone-) folds to form and close. What physical examination finding would support the most likely diagnosis in this child?

(A) Bowel sounds in the left lower lung zone

(B) Continuous cardiac murmur

(C) Marked splenomegaly (spleno-; mega-)

(D) Midline deviation of the trachea

中文翻译

一个早产儿出生时出现呼吸窘迫，接受紧急插管治疗。给予合成肺表面活性物质后，其肺功能并未改善。在进行详细的体格检查后，儿科医生认为该患儿的病情与胚胎期胸腹膜襞未能形成和闭合有关。下列哪项体格检查发现最能支持该患儿的病情诊断？

(A) 在左下肺区听到肠鸣音
(B) 持续性心脏杂音
(C) 明显脾肿大
(D) 气管向中线偏移

题目和答案中出现的词根

pre-：在……之前
re-：反复
spir-：呼吸
tub-：管
surf-：表面的
act-：作用的
pleuro-：胸膜的
peritone-：腹膜的
spleno-：脾脏的
mega-：大

adeno-（腺体）

adenopathy 腺病

词根 adeno-（腺体）+ -pathy（病态）

例句 Swollen lymph nodes are a common sign of adenopathy. 淋巴结肿大是腺病的常见症状。

adenoma 腺瘤

词根 adeno-（腺体）+ -oma（肿瘤）

例句 Adenomas are usually benign but may require monitoring. 腺瘤通常是良性的，但可能需要监测。

adenitis 腺炎

词根 adeno-（腺体）+ -itis（炎症）

例句 Adenitis can cause pain and swelling in the affected area. 腺炎可能会导致受影响区域的疼痛和肿胀。

adenocarcinoma 腺癌

词根 adeno-（腺体）+ carcinoma（癌）

例句 Lung adenocarcinoma is one of the most common types of lung cancer. 肺腺癌是十分常见的肺癌类型之一。

adenohypophysis 腺垂体

词根 adeno-（腺体）+ hypophysis（垂体）

例句 The adenohypophysis secretes important hormones like growth hormone. 腺垂体分泌生长激素等重要激素。

adenoidectomy 腺样体切除术

词根 adeno-（腺体）+ -ectomy（切除术）

例句 Children with chronic infections may need an adenoidectomy.

患有慢性感染的儿童可能需要接受腺样体切除术。

adenogenesis 腺生成

词根 adeno-（腺体）+ -genesis（生长）

例句 Adenogenesis is crucial for glandular tissue development. 腺生成对于腺体组织的发育至关重要。

adenopathy (lymphadenopathy) 淋巴腺病

词根 adeno-（腺体）+ -pathy（病态）

例句 Lymphadenopathy often accompanies infections. 淋巴腺病常伴有感染。

adenomyosis 腺肌病

词根 adeno-（腺体）+ myo-（肌肉）+ -osis（病态）

例句 Adenomyosis can cause severe menstrual cramps. 腺肌病可能引起严重的痛经。

adenectomy 腺体切除术

词根 adeno-（腺体）+ -ectomy（切除术）

例句 An adenectomy is performed to remove abnormal glandular tissue. 腺体切除术用于去除异常腺体组织。

adjuv-（辅）

adjuvant therapy 辅助治疗

词根 adjuv-（辅）+ -ant（形容词后缀）

例句 Adjuvant therapy is often used after primary cancer treatment. 辅助治疗通常在癌症主要治疗手段之后采用。

adjuvant chemotherapy 辅助化疗

词根 adjuv-（辅）+ chemotherapy（化疗）

例句 Adjuvant chemotherapy helps reduce cancer recurrence. 辅助化疗有助于降低癌症复发的风险。

adjuvant immunotherapy 辅助免疫治疗

词根 adjuv-（辅）+ immunotherapy（免疫治疗）

例句 Adjuvant immunotherapy boosts the body’s immune response. 辅助免疫治疗增强人体免疫反应。

adjuvant radiation therapy 辅助放射治疗

词根 adjuv-（辅）+ radiation（放射）+ therapy（治疗）

例句 Adjuvant radiation therapy is given after surgery. 辅助放射治疗在手术后进行。

adjuvant vaccine 辅助疫苗

词根 adjuv-（辅）+ vaccine（疫苗）

例句 Some vaccines contain adjuvants to enhance immune response. 一些疫苗含有佐剂以增强免疫反应。

adjuvant medication 辅助药物

词根 adjuv-（辅）+ medication（药物）

例句 Adjuvant medications can help manage chronic pain. 辅助药物有助于缓解慢性疼痛。

adjuvanticity 辅助性

词根 adjuv-（辅）+ -ticity（性质）

例句 The adjuvanticity of a compound determines its immune-boosting effect. 一种化合物的辅助性决定了其免疫增强效果。

adjuvant analgesia 辅助镇痛

词根 adjuv-（辅）+ analgesia（镇痛）

例句 Adjuvant analgesia is used alongside opioids for pain relief. 辅助镇痛药与阿片类药物一起使用以缓解疼痛。

adjuvant therapy for autoimmune disease 自身免疫病的辅助治疗

词根 adjuv-（辅）+ therapy（治疗）

例句 Adjuvant therapy helps control autoimmune disorders. 辅助治疗有助于控制自身免疫疾病。

adjuvant endocrine therapy 辅助内分泌治疗

词根 adjuv-（辅）+ endocrine（内分泌）+ therapy（治疗）

例句 Adjuvant endocrine therapy is common in breast cancer treatment. 辅助内分泌治疗在乳腺癌治疗中很常见。

aero-（气的）

aerosol 气溶胶

词根 aero-（空气）+ -sol（溶解）

例句 An aerosol is a suspension of fine particles or droplets in air, often used in inhalation therapy for respiratory conditions. 气溶胶是空气中的细小颗粒或液滴的悬浮物，通常用于呼吸系统疾病的吸入治疗。

aeroembolism 气体栓塞

词根 aero-（空气）+ embolism（栓塞）

例句 Aeroembolism occurs when air bubbles enter the bloodstream, potentially causing blockages in blood vessels. 气体栓塞是指气泡进入血流，可能导致血管堵塞。

aerobic 有氧的

词根 aero-（空气）+ -bic（生活）

例句 Aerobic exercises are physical activities that improve cardiovascular health by increasing oxygen intake. 有氧运动是通过增加氧气摄入来改善心血管健康的体育活动。

anaerobic 无氧的

词根 an-（无）+ aero-（空气）+ -bic（生活）

例句 Anaerobic bacteria thrive in environments without oxygen

and can cause infections such as abscesses. 厌氧细菌在没有氧气的环境中繁殖，并可引起脓肿等感染症状。

aeroallergy 空气过敏

词根 aero-（空气）+ allergy（过敏）
例句 Aeroallergy refers to allergic reactions triggered by airborne allergens, such as pollen or dust. 空气过敏是指由空气中的过敏原（如花粉或尘土）引发的过敏反应。

aerophagia 吞气症

词根 aero-（空气）+ phagia（吞咽）
例句 Aerophagia is a condition where a person swallows air excessively, which can lead to bloating and discomfort. 吞气症是一种过度吞咽空气的状况，可能导致腹胀和不适。

aerotherapy 空气疗法

词根 aero-（空气）+ therapy（治疗）
例句 Aerotherapy is the use of air or oxygen as a therapeutic treatment, often used for respiratory conditions. 空气疗法以空气或氧气作为治疗手段，常用于呼吸系统疾病。

aerosinusitis 气窦炎

词根 aero-（空气）+ sinusitis（窦炎）
例句 Aerosinusitis is inflammation of the sinuses caused by changes in air pressure, often seen in divers or frequent flyers. 气窦炎是由气压变化引起的窦腔炎症，常见于潜水员或频繁乘飞机者。

aerospace medicine 航空医学

词根 aero-（空气）+ space（空间）+ medicine（医学）
例句 Aerospace medicine focuses on the health and medical issues of astronauts and pilots, dealing with the challenges of air and space travel. 航空医学专注于宇航员和飞行员的健康和医疗问题，应对与航空和太空旅行相关的挑战。

aerobiology 空气生物学

词根 aero-（空气）+ bio-（生物）+ -logy（学科）

例句 Aerobiology is the study of biological particles, such as pollen, bacteria, and viruses, in the air. 空气生物学是研究空气中生物颗粒（如花粉、细菌和病毒）的学科。

aerophilous 嗜气的

词根 aero-（空气）+ philous（喜爱的）

例句 Aerophilous organisms thrive in oxygen-rich environments, such as those found in the lungs or airways. 嗜气生物在富含氧气的环境中生长繁殖，如肺部或呼吸道中。

-agon（结合）

antagonist 拮抗剂

词根 anti-（反对）+ -agon（结合）

例句 Beta-blockers act as antagonists to adrenaline. β 受体阻滞剂为肾上腺素的拮抗剂。

agonist 激动剂

词根 -agon（结合）

例句 Morphine is an opioid agonist that relieves pain. 吗啡是一种阿片类激动剂，可缓解疼痛。

coagonist 协同激动剂

词根 co-（共同）+ -agon（结合）

例句 GLP-1 coagonists are used in diabetes treatment. GLP-1 协同激动剂用于糖尿病治疗。

antagonism 拮抗作用

词根 anti-（反对）+ -agon（结合）

例句 The antagonism between insulin and glucagon regulates blood sugar levels. 胰岛素和胰高血糖素之间的拮抗作用调节血糖水平。

glucagon 胰高血糖素

词根 gluc-（糖）+ -agon（结合）
例句 Glucagon is a hormone that increases blood sugar levels by stimulating the liver to release glucose. 胰高血糖素是一种激素，通过刺激肝脏释放葡萄糖来提高血糖水平。

-algia（疼痛）

neuralgia 神经痛

词根 neur-（神经）+ -algia（疼痛）
例句 Trigeminal neuralgia causes severe facial pain. 三叉神经痛会引起剧烈的面部疼痛。

myalgia 肌痛

词根 myo-（肌肉）+ -algia（疼痛）
例句 Influenza often causes myalgia and fatigue. 流感通常会引起肌肉疼痛和疲劳。

arthralgia 关节痛

词根 arthr-（关节）+ -algia（疼痛）
例句 Patients with rheumatoid arthritis experience chronic arthralgia. 类风湿关节炎患者会经历慢性关节痛。

fibromyalgia 纤维肌痛综合征

词根 fibro-（纤维）+ myo-（肌肉）+ -algia（疼痛）
例句 Fibromyalgia is characterized by widespread musculoskeletal pain. 纤维肌痛综合征的特征是广泛的肌肉骨骼疼痛。

gastralgia 胃痛

词根 gastro-（胃）+ -algia（疼痛）

例句 Gastralgia can be a symptom of gastritis. 胃痛可能是胃炎的症状。

odontalgia 牙痛

词根 odont-（牙齿）+ -algia（疼痛）
例句 Odontalgia is commonly caused by dental cavities. 牙痛通常由龋齿引起。

cephalalgia 头痛

词根 cephal-（头部）+ -algia（疼痛）
例句 Migraines are a type of cephalalgia. 偏头痛是一种头痛类型。

otalgia 耳痛

词根 oto-（耳）+ -algia（疼痛）
例句 Middle ear infections often cause otalgia. 中耳感染通常会引起耳痛。

coxalgia 髋关节痛

词根 cox-（髋）+ -algia（疼痛）
例句 Coxalgia can result from osteoarthritis. 髋关节痛可能由骨关节炎引起。

thoracalgia 胸痛

词根 thorac-（胸）+ -algia（疼痛）
例句 Thoracalgia may be a symptom of pleurisy. 胸痛可能是胸膜炎的症状。

-alis（与……有关的）

renalis 肾脏的

词根 ren-（肾）+ -alis（与……有关的）
例句 The renalis arteries supply blood to the kidneys. 肾动脉为肾脏提供血液。

pulmonalis 肺的

词根 pulmon-（肺）+ -alis（与……有关的）

例句 The pulmonary artery carries deoxygenated blood to lungs. 肺动脉将缺氧血输送到肺部。

facialis 面部的

词根 faci-（面部）+ -alis（与……有关的）

例句 Facial nerve paralysis affects expressions. 面神经麻痹会影响面部表情。

brachialis 肱的

词根 brachi-（肱；臂）+ -alis（与……有关的）

例句 The brachialis muscle assists in elbow flexion. 肱肌帮助肘关节屈曲。

carotidalis 颈动脉的

词根 carotid-（颈动脉）+ -alis（与……有关的）

例句 The carotid artery supplies blood to the brain. 颈动脉向大脑供血。

spinalis 脊柱的

词根 spin-（脊柱）+ -alis（与……有关的）

例句 The spinalis muscle is part of the erector spinae group. 脊柱肌是竖脊肌群的一部分。

cerebralis 大脑的

词根 cerebr-（大脑）+ -alis（与……有关的）

例句 The cerebralis arteries supply the brain with oxygen. 大脑动脉为大脑供氧。

ulnaris 尺骨的

词根 uln-（尺骨）+ -aris（与……有关的）

例句 The ulnaris artery runs along the forearm. 尺动脉沿着前臂

走行。

radialis 桡骨的

词根 radi-（桡骨）+ -alis（与……有关的）

例句 The radialis artery is commonly used to check the pulse. 桡动脉常用于测量脉搏。

temporalis 颞部的

词根 tempor-（颞部）+ -alis（与……有关的）

例句 The temporalis muscle helps in jaw movement. 颞肌有助于下颌运动。

USMLE Step 1 样题

A 72-year-old African-American man undergoes hip surgery. On his third hospital day, he develops chest pain, tachycardia (tachy-; -cardia), dyspnea (dys-; -pnea), and a low-grade fever. The man goes into cardiac arrest and efforts to resuscitate (re-; suscit-) him are unsuccessful. On autopsy a massive pulmonary embolus is discovered. Which of the following would most likely predispose the patient to this event?

(A) Factor VIII deficiency

(B) Low serum homocysteine (homo-) levels

(C) Mutation in the factor V gene

(D) Overproduction of protein C

(E) Von Willebrand factor deficiency

中文翻译

一名 72 岁的非洲裔美国男性接受了髋关节手术。在他住院的第 3 天，他出现了胸痛、心动过速、呼吸困难和低热。该男子发生了心搏骤停，抢救未能成功。尸检发现其存在大面积肺栓塞。以下哪项因素最可能为该患者发病的诱因？

(A) 凝血因子 Ⅷ 缺乏
(B) 血清同型半胱氨酸水平低
(C) 凝血因子 V 基因突变
(D) 蛋白 C 过量生产
(E) 冯 • 维尔布兰因子缺乏

题目和答案中出现的词根

tachy-：快速的
-cardia：心脏的（这里指心跳）
dys-：困难的；疼痛的；错误的
-pnea：呼吸
re-：重新；反复
-suscit：站起
homo-：同的

allo-（其他的；异体的）

allotransplantation 异体移植

词根 allo-（其他的）+ transplantation（移植）
例句 Allotransplantation is commonly performed in organ transplants. 异体移植在器官移植中很常见。

allogeneic 同种异体的

词根 allo-（其他的）+ -geneic（基因相关）

例句 Allogeneic bone marrow transplantation is used to treat leukemia. 同种异体骨髓移植用于治疗白血病。

allograft 同种异体移植物

词根 allo-（其他的）+ -graft（移植物）

例句 An allograft is a tissue transplant from another person. 同种异体移植物是来自他人的组织移植。

alloantibody 同种抗体

词根 allo-（其他的）+ antibody（抗体）

例句 Alloantibodies can cause complications in blood transfusions. 同种抗体可能在输血过程中引起并发症。

alloimmune response 同种免疫反应

词根 allo-（其他的）+ immune（免疫）

例句 Alloimmune responses can lead to transplant rejection. 同种免疫反应可能导致移植排斥。

allopathy 对抗疗法

词根 allo-（其他的）+ -pathy（治疗方法）

例句 Allopathy is a system of medicine that uses drugs to counteract diseases. 对抗疗法是一种利用药物来抵抗疾病的医学体系。

allosteric regulation 变构调节

词根 allo-（其他的）+ -steric（空间构型）

例句 Allosteric regulation plays a role in enzyme activity. 变构调节在酶活性中起重要作用。

allodynia 异痛症

词根 allo-（其他的）+ -dynia（疼痛）

例句 Patients with fibromyalgia often experience allodynia. 纤维肌痛综合征患者经常会出现异痛症。

allozyme 同种异构酶

词根 allo-（其他的）+ -zyme（酶）

例句 Allozymes are variants of enzymes found within a species. 同种异构酶是某一物种内存在的不同酶变体。

alloderm 异体皮肤移植

词根 allo-（其他的）+ derm（皮肤）

例句 Alloderm is used in reconstructive surgery. 异体皮肤移植用于整形外科手术。

USMLE Step 2 样题

A 64-year-old man presents with diarrhea (dia-; -rrhea) and intermittent (inter-; mitt-) abdominal cramps for the last six weeks. He also reports poor appetite and fatigue, and has lost 12 pounds over this time period. His past medical history is significant for hypertension (hyper-; -tension) and chronic low back pain. He has intermittent (inter-; mitt-) right knee swelling and tenderness that responds to ibuprofen. His temperature is 37.3°C (99.1°F), blood pressure is 142/84 mmHg, pulse is 98/min, and respirations (re-; spir-; -ation) are 16/min. Physical examination reveals tenderness in the left lower quadrant without rebound (re-) or guarding. Digital rectal examination is positive for occult blood. His blood work shows:

WBC 14,600 mm^3

Hemoglobin (hemo-; -globin) 9.6 mg/dL

Hematocrit (hemato-; -crit) 30%

Platelets (plate-; -lets) 214,000 mm^3

Erythrocyte (eryth-;-cyte) Sedimentation Rate 126 mm/hr

Flexible sigmoidoscopy (sigmoid-; -scopy) reveals erythematous (eryth-; -matous) friable mucosa extending from the rectum to the sigmoid colon. Small shallow ulcers are also seen. Which of the following is the most likely finding on biopsy of the affected areas?

(A) Epithelial (epi-) necrosis

(B) Fibrinous pseudomembranes (peuso-)

(C) Neutrophilic (neutro-; -phil) cryptitis (cryp-; -itis)

(D) Sheets of malignant cells

(E) Small vessel vasculitis (vascu-; -itis)

中文翻译

一名64岁的男性，近6周以来出现腹泻和间歇性腹部绞痛。他还自述食欲差和疲劳，且在此期间体重减轻了约5.4 kg。他既往有高血压和慢性腰痛病史，右膝间歇性肿胀和压痛，用布洛芬治疗有效。他的体温为37.3℃，血压为142/84 mmHg，脉搏98次/分钟，呼吸16次/分钟。

体格检查显示左下腹压痛，无反跳痛或肌紧张。数字直肠指检发现隐血阳性。血液检查结果如下：

白细胞 14,600 /mm^3

血红蛋白 9.6 mg/dL

血细胞比容 30%

血小板 214,000 /mm^3

红细胞沉降率（ESR）126 mm/hr

乙状结肠镜检查显示从直肠到乙状结肠的黏膜发红、易碎，同时可见小的浅表性溃疡。以下哪一项是受累区域活检最可能发现的病理改变？

(A) 上皮坏死

(B) 纤维素性假膜

(C) 中性粒细胞浸润隐窝炎（中性粒细胞性隐窝炎）

(D) 恶性细胞成片分布

(E) 小血管血管炎

题目和答案中出现的词根

inter-：在……之间

mitt-：时间区间（表示间歇性的）

dia-：通过

-rrhea：流出

hyper-：高

-tension：张力；压力

re-：重新

hemo-：血

-globin：球蛋白

hemato-：血

-crit：分离法（血液分离法指代红细胞比容，即血清和红细胞的分离）

plate-：板状的

-lets：小

eryth-：红色

-cyte：细胞

sigmoid-：乙状的

-scopy：镜

-matous：病理状态的

epi-: 在……上（或旁）

peuso-：假的

neutro-：中性的

-phil：嗜

cryp-：隐的

-itis：炎症

vascu-：血管的

ambly-（暗；弱）

amblyopia 弱视

词根 ambly-（弱）+ -opia（视力）

例句 Amblyopia is often referred to as “lazy eye”. 弱视通常被称为“懒惰眼”。

amblyacousia 听力减退

词根 ambly-（弱）+ acousia（听觉）

例句 Amblyacousia is a common symptom of aging. 听力减退是衰老的常见表现。

amblychromatic 染色较淡的

词根 ambly-（弱）+ chromatic（颜色）

例句 Amblychromatic cells stain lightly under a microscope. 弱色性细胞在显微镜下染色较浅。

amblyopic strabismus 弱视性斜视

词根 ambly-（弱）+ -opic（视力）+ strabismus（斜视）

例句 Children with amblyopic strabismus require early intervention. 儿童的弱视性斜视需要早期干预。

amblyoscope 弱视镜

词根 ambly-（弱）+ -scope（观察仪器）

例句 An amblyoscope is used to assess binocular vision. 弱视镜用于评估双眼视觉。

amblyesthesia 感觉迟钝

词根 ambly-（弱）+ -esthesia（感觉）
例句 Amblyesthesia can result from nerve damage. 感觉迟钝可能是由神经损伤引起的。

amblylogia 言语迟缓

词根 ambly-（弱）+ logia（言语）
例句 Amblylogia is seen in children with developmental delays. 言语迟缓在发育迟缓的儿童中常见。

amin-（氨）

amino acid 氨基酸

词根 amin-（氨）+ acid（酸）
例句 Amino acids are the building blocks of proteins. 氨基酸是蛋白质的基本组成单位。

aminotransferase 氨基转移酶

词根 amin-（氨）+ transferase（转移酶）
例句 Elevated aminotransferase levels indicate liver damage. 氨基转移酶升高表明肝脏受损。

amine 胺类化合物

词根 amin-（氨）
例句 Amines are important in neurotransmitter synthesis. 胺类化合物在神经递质合成中起重要作用。

aminuria 尿氨症

词根 amin-（氨）+ -uria（尿）
例句 Aminuria is observed in metabolic disorders. 尿氨症可见于

代谢性疾病。

aminobenzoic acid 氨基苯甲酸

词根 amin-（氨）+ benzoic acid（苯甲酸）
例句 Aminobenzoic acid is used in sunscreen formulations. 氨基苯甲酸用于防晒霜配方中。

aminoglycoside 氨基糖苷类抗生素

词根 amin-（氨）+ glycoside（糖苷）
例句 Aminoglycosides are effective against gram-negative bacteria. 氨基糖苷类抗生素对革兰阴性菌有效。

aminopeptidase 氨肽酶

词根 amin-（氨）+ peptidase（肽酶）
例句 Aminopeptidase plays a role in protein metabolism. 氨肽酶在蛋白质代谢中起作用。

aminoderivative 氨基衍生物

词根 amin-（氨）+ derivative（衍生物）
例句 Aminoderivatives are widely used in pharmaceuticals. 氨基衍生物广泛用于制药。

aminocaproic acid 氨基己酸

词根 amin-（氨）+ caproic acid（己酸）
例句 Aminocaproic acid helps control bleeding disorders. 氨基己酸有助于控制出血性疾病。

aminophenol 氨基酚

词根 amin-（氨）+ phenol（酚）
例句 Aminophenol derivatives are used in pain relievers. 氨基酚衍生物用于镇痛药物中。

amyelo-（脊髓的）

amyelencephalia 无脊髓脑畸形

词根 amyelo-（脊髓的）+ encephalia（脑）

例句 Amyelencephalia is a rare congenital disorder. 无脊髓脑畸形是一种罕见的先天性疾病。

amyelopathy 脊髓病变

词根 amyelo-（脊髓的）+ -pathy（病态）

例句 Amyelopathy can cause progressive neurological deficits. 脊髓病变可能导致进行性神经功能障碍。

amyelogenesis 脊髓发育不全

词根 amyelo-（脊髓的）+ -genesis（生长）

例句 Amyelogenesis affects fetal nervous system development. 脊髓发育不全影响胎儿神经系统的发育。

myelomalacia 脊髓软化症

词根 myelo-（脊髓的）+ -malacia（软化）

例句 Myelomalacia is often caused by spinal cord ischemia. 脊髓软化症通常由脊髓缺血引起。

amyelination 脊髓髓鞘形成不足

词根 amyelo-（脊髓的）+ -ination（过程）

例句 Amyelination defects are linked to multiple sclerosis. 脊髓髓鞘形成不足与多发性硬化症有关。

amyelotrophy 脊髓萎缩

词根 amyelo-（脊髓的）+ -trophy（生长）

例句 Amyelotrophy leads to progressive muscle weakness. 脊髓萎

缩导致进行性肌肉无力。

amyelosis 脊髓病

词根 amyelo-（脊髓的）+ -osis（病态）
例句 Amyelosis can be caused by severe spinal cord injuries. 脊髓病可能由严重的脊髓损伤引起。

amyelorrhagia 脊髓出血

词根 amyelo-（脊髓的）+ -rrhagia（出血）
例句 Amyelorrhagia requires immediate medical attention. 脊髓出血需要立即接受医疗救治。

amyelorrhea 脊髓液外漏

词根 amyelo-（脊髓的）+ -rrhea（流出）
例句 Amyelorrhea may occur after spinal surgery. 脊髓液外漏可能发生在脊柱手术后。

amyeloplastic 脊髓再生的

词根 amyelo-（脊髓的）+ -plastic（重塑的）
例句 Amyeloplastic therapies aim to repair spinal cord damage. 脊髓再生疗法旨在修复脊髓损伤。

ana-（反）

anaphylaxis 过敏性休克

词根 ana-（反）+ -phylaxis（保护）
例句 Anaphylaxis is a severe allergic reaction that requires immediate treatment. 过敏性休克是一种需要立即治疗的严重过敏反应。

analgesia 无痛

词根 ana-（反）+ -gesia（痛觉）
例句 Epidural anesthesia provides analgesia during childbirth. 硬膜外麻醉在分娩时提供无痛作用。

anaerobic 厌氧的

词根 ana-（反）+ -aerobic（需氧的）

例句 Anaerobic bacteria thrive in oxygen-free environments. 厌氧细菌在无氧环境中生长。

anamnestic response 回忆性免疫反应

词根 ana-（反）+ -mnestic（记忆）

例句 The anamnestic response enhances immunity upon re-exposure to a pathogen. 回忆性免疫反应在再次暴露于病原体时增强免疫力。

anacidity 无酸性

词根 ana-（反）+ -acidity（酸度）

例句 Anacidity is a condition where the stomach produces little to no acid. 无酸性是指胃几乎不产生酸的状态。

USMLE Step 2　样题

A 56-year-old woman with cirrhosis (cirrh-; -osis) presents with a 2-week history of increasing abdominal distension. She has mild encephalopathy (en-; cephal-; -pathy) and esophageal (eso-; phag-) varices without bleeding. Her cirrhosis is due to chronic hepatitis (hepat-; -itis) type B. She has a past history of ascites treated successfully with conservative management. She is currently on sodium, water and protein restriction, maximal doses of spironolactone and furosemide, and lactulose (lact-; -ulose). Temperature is 36.6°C (97.9°F). Blood pressure is 120/70 mmHg, pulse is 80/min, and respirations (re-; spir-; -ation) are 30/min. She has a flapping tremor and labored breathing. Abdominal examination shows marked abdominal distension. An X-ray film of the chest is unremarkable. Abdominal ultrasound shows peritoneal fluid and splenomegaly (spleno-; -mega), liver hyperechogenicity (hyper-; echo-) and nodularity (nodul-), and portal vein width of 16 mm; no masses are evident. Which of the following is the most appropriate next step in the management of this patient's ascites?

(A) Intravenous (intra-; -venous) furosemide therapy
(B) Tapping of some amount of ascitic fluid
(C) Peritoneojugular (peritone; jugul-) shunt
(D) Distal splenorenal (splen-; renal) shunt (selective shunt)
(E) Side-to-side portocaval (porto-; -caval) shun

中文翻译

一名 56 岁的女性肝硬化患者，出现了为期两周的腹胀加重。她有轻度脑病和无出血的食管静脉曲张。她的肝硬化由慢性乙型肝炎引起。她既往有腹水病史，并通过保守治疗缓解。她目前正在接受限钠、限水和限蛋白的饮食治疗，服用最大剂量的螺内酯和呋塞米，并使用乳果糖。

她的体温为 36.6℃，血压为 120/70 mmHg，脉搏 80 次 / 分钟，呼吸 30 次 / 分钟。查体发现扑翼样震颤和呼吸困难。腹部检查显示明显腹胀。胸部 X 线检查未见异常。腹部超声提示腹腔积液和脾肿大，肝脏呈高回声并可见结节，门静脉宽度为 16 mm，未见肿块。以下哪项是下一步最合适的腹水处理方式？

(A) 静脉注射呋塞米
(B) 抽取部分腹水
(C) 腹膜 - 颈静脉分流术

(D) 脾 - 肾远端选择性分流术

(E) 门 - 腔静脉旁路术

题目和答案中出现的词根

cirrh-：橘黄色（这里表示肝，因为肝病引起皮肤和黏膜的黄染）

-osis：病理状态（肝脏的病理状态，这里指肝硬化）

en-：内的

cephal-：脑

-pathy：病

eso-：内的

phag-：吞；吃

hepat-：肝脏的

-itis：炎症

lact-：乳的

-ulose：糖

spleno-：脾脏的

-mega：肥大

hyper-：高

echo-：回声

nodul-：结节

intra-：在……内

-venous：静脉的

peritone-：腹膜的

jugul-：颈部的

renal：肾脏的

porto-: 门的

-caval: 体的；腔的

aneurys-（血管异常膨胀）

aneurysm 动脉瘤

词根 aneurys-（血管异常膨胀）

例句 A ruptured aneurysm can lead to life-threatening bleeding. 破裂的动脉瘤可能导致危及生命的出血。

aneurysmectomy 动脉瘤切除术

词根 aneurys-（血管异常膨胀）+ -ectomy（切除术）

例句 An aneurysmectomy is performed to remove an abnormal artery bulge. 动脉瘤切除术用于去除异常的动脉膨胀部分。

aneurysmorrhaphy 动脉瘤修补术

词根 aneurys-（血管异常膨胀）+ -rrhaphy（缝合）

例句 Aneurysmorrhaphy involves suturing a weakened arterial wall. 动脉瘤修补术涉及缝合薄弱的动脉壁。

aneurysmoplasty 动脉瘤整形术

词根 aneurys-（血管异常膨胀）+ -plasty（整形术）

例句 Aneurysmoplasty can reinforce blood vessels to prevent rupture. 动脉瘤整形术可以强化血管以防止破裂。

aneurysmal dilation 动脉瘤扩张

词根 aneurys-（血管异常膨胀）+ -mal（异常）

例句 Aneurysmal dilation can be detected using ultrasound imaging. 动脉瘤扩张可以通过超声成像检测。

aneurysmal hemorrhage 动脉瘤性出血

词根 aneurys-（血管异常膨胀）+ hemorrhage（出血）

例句 An aneurysmal hemorrhage is a medical emergency. 动脉瘤性出血是一种医疗急症。

aneurysm stent graft 动脉瘤支架移植术

词根 aneurys-（血管异常膨胀）+ stent（支架）+ graft（移植）
例句 Aneurysm stent graft is used to reinforce a weakened artery wall. 动脉瘤支架移植术用于强化薄弱的动脉壁。

aneurysm coil embolization 动脉瘤线圈栓塞术

词根 aneurys-（血管异常膨胀）+ coil embolization（线圈栓塞）
例句 Coil embolization is a minimally invasive treatment for brain aneurysms. 线圈栓塞术是一种治疗脑动脉瘤的微创手术。

aneurysmal dissection 动脉瘤剥离

词根 aneurys-（血管异常膨胀）+ dissection（剥离）
例句 Aneurysmal dissection occurs when blood enters the arterial wall layers. 动脉瘤剥离发生在血液进入动脉壁层时。

angio-（血管）

angiology（血管学）

词根 angio-（血管）+ -logy（学科）
例句 Angiology focuses on diseases affecting blood vessels. 血管学研究影响血管的疾病。

angioplasty（血管成形术）

词根 angio-（血管）+ -plasty（成形术）
例句 Angioplasty is used to widen narrowed arteries. 血管成形术用于扩张狭窄的动脉。

angiogenesis（血管生成）

词根 angio-（血管）+ -genesis（生成）
例句 Angiogenesis plays a crucial role in wound healing. 血管生

成在伤口愈合过程中起关键作用。

angiopathy（血管病）

词根 angio-（血管）+ -pathy（病变）
例句 Diabetic angiopathy can lead to serious complications. 糖尿病血管病可导致严重的并发症。

angiogram（血管造影）

词根 angio-（血管）+ -gram（图像）
例句 An angiogram helps diagnose blocked arteries. 血管造影有助于诊断动脉阻塞。

angiography（血管造影术）

词根 angio-（血管）+ -graphy（影像）
例句 Coronary angiography helps detect heart blockages. 冠状动脉造影术有助于检测心血管阻塞。

angioedema（血管性水肿）

词根 angio-（血管）+ edema（肿胀）
例句 Angioedema can cause severe swelling of the face and throat. 血管性水肿可导致面部和喉咙严重肿胀。

angiitis（血管炎）

词根 angio-（血管）+ -itis（炎症）
例句 Angiitis can lead to severe vascular complications. 血管炎可能导致严重的血管并发症。

hemangioma（血管瘤）

词根 hem-（血液）+ angio-（血管）+ -oma（肿瘤）
例句 Hemangiomas are benign tumors made up of blood vessels. 血管瘤是一种由血管组成的良性肿瘤。

angiosarcoma（血管肉瘤）

词根 angio-（血管）+ sarcoma（肉瘤）

例句 Angiosarcoma is a rare and aggressive cancer. 血管肉瘤是一种罕见且侵袭性强的癌症。

lymphangioma（淋巴管瘤）

词根 lymph-（淋巴）+ angio-（血管）+ -oma（肿瘤）

例句 Lymphangioma is a rare malformation of the lymphatic system. 淋巴管瘤是一种罕见的淋巴系统畸形。

angiocarditis（心血管炎）

词根 angio-（血管）+ carditis（心脏炎症）

例句 Angiocarditis may develop due to bacterial infections. 心血管炎可能由细菌感染引起。

angiocardiography（心血管造影术）

词根 angio-（血管）+ cardio-（心脏）+ -graphy（影像）

例句 Angiocardiography is used to visualize heart vessels. 心血管造影术用于显示心脏血管的状况。

angiostenosis（血管狭窄）

词根 angio-（血管）+ stenosis（狭窄）

例句 Angiostenosis can restrict blood flow and cause ischemia. 血管狭窄可能限制血流并导致缺血。

angiosclerosis（血管硬化）

词根 angio-（血管）+ sclerosis（硬化）

例句 Angiosclerosis is common in patients with hypertension. 血管硬化在高血压患者中很常见。

angiomyolipoma（血管肌脂肪瘤）

词根 angio-（血管）+ myo-（肌肉）+ lipo-（脂肪）+ -oma（肿瘤）

例句 Angiomyolipoma is a benign tumor affecting the kidneys. 血管肌脂肪瘤是一种影响肾脏的良性肿瘤。

aniso-（大小不等的）

anisocoria 瞳孔大小不等

词根 aniso-（不等的）+ coria（瞳孔）

例句 Anisocoria can be a sign of neurological disorders or eye trauma. 瞳孔大小不等可能是神经系统疾病或眼部创伤的表现。

anisocytosis 红细胞大小不均

词根 aniso-（不等的）+ cytosis（细胞状态）

例句 Anisocytosis is commonly seen in anemia and other blood disorders. 红细胞大小不均通常出现在贫血和其他血液疾病中。

anisometropia 屈光参差

词根 aniso-（不等的）+ metropia（视力）

例句 Anisometropia can cause difficulties in binocular vision and depth perception. 屈光参差可能导致双眼视功能障碍和深度感知问题。

anisomelia 肢体不等长

词根 aniso-（不等的）+ melia（肢体）

例句 Severe anisomelia may require surgical correction to restore functional symmetry. 严重的肢体不等长可能需要手术矫正以恢复功能对称性。

anisotropy 各向异性

词根 aniso-（不等的）+ tropy（方向性）

例句 The anisotropy of bone tissue contributes to its mechanical properties. 骨组织的各向异性有助于形成其力学特性。

anisomastia 乳房大小不等

词根 aniso-（不等的）+ mastia（乳房）

例句 Anisomastia can be corrected through plastic surgery if it causes psychological distress. 如果乳房大小不等导致心理困扰，可以通过整形手术矫正。

anisophoria 眼位不等

词根 aniso-（不等的）+ phoria（眼位）
例句 Anisophoria may lead to visual discomfort and headaches. 眼位不等可能引起视觉不适和头痛。

anisokaryosis 细胞核大小不均

词根 aniso-（不等的）+ karyosis（核状态）
例句 Anisokaryosis is often an indicator of malignant cell transformation. 细胞核大小不均通常是恶性细胞变性的标志。

anisopoikilocytosis 红细胞形态和大小异常

词根 aniso-（不等的）+ poikilo-（多形的）+ cytosis（细胞状态）
例句 Anisopoikilocytosis is frequently observed in severe anemia cases. 红细胞形态和大小异常常见于严重贫血患者。

anisosthenia（肌力不均）

词根 aniso-（不等的）+ sthenia（肌力）
例句 Anisosthenia is a common symptom in neuromuscular disorders. 肌力不均是神经肌肉疾病的常见症状。

ankyl-（僵硬）

ankylosis 关节强直

词根 ankyl-（僵硬）+ -osis（病态）
例句 Ankylosis can result from severe arthritis. 关节强直可能是由严重的关节炎引起的。

ankylosing spondylitis 强直性脊柱炎

词根 ankyl-（僵硬）+ spondyl-（脊柱）+ -itis（炎症）

例句 Ankylosing spondylitis primarily affects the spine. 强直性脊柱炎主要影响脊柱。

ankylodactyly 指趾强直

词根 ankyl-（僵硬）+ dactyl-（手指；脚趾）

例句 Ankylodactyly is a congenital condition affecting finger mobility. 指趾强直是一种影响手指活动的先天性疾病。

ankylocheilia 唇强直

词根 ankyl-（僵硬）+ cheilia（唇部）

例句 Ankylocheilia can interfere with normal mouth function. 唇强直可能影响正常的口腔功能。

ankylopodia 足关节僵硬

词根 ankyl-（僵硬）+ pod-（足部）

例句 Ankylopodia can affect walking ability. 足关节僵硬可能影响行走能力。

ankyloblepharon 睑缘粘连

词根 ankyl-（僵硬）+ blepharon（眼睑）

例句 Ankyloblepharon is a rare eyelid disorder. 睑缘粘连是一种罕见的眼睑疾病。

ankyloglossa 舌系带过短

词根 ankyl-（僵硬）+ glossa（舌头）

例句 Ankyloglossa can cause speech difficulties in children. 舌系带过短可能导致儿童语言障碍。

ankyloglossia 舌系带粘连

词根 ankyl-（僵硬）+ glossia（舌头）

例句 Severe ankyloglossia may require surgical correction. 严重的舌系带粘连可能需要手术矫正。

ankylophobia 关节僵直恐惧症

词根 ankyl-（僵硬）+ -phobia（恐惧症）

例句 Ankylophobia is the fear of joint immobility. 关节僵直恐惧症是对关节活动受限的恐惧。

ano-（肛门）

anorectal 肛门直肠的

词根 ano-（肛门）+ rectal（直肠）

例句 Anorectal disorders include hemorrhoids and fissures. 肛门直肠疾病包括痔疮和肛裂。

anoplasty 肛门成形术

词根 ano-（肛门）+ -plasty（整形术）

例句 Anoplasty is performed to correct congenital anal defects. 肛门成形术用于矫正先天性肛门缺陷。

anoderm 肛门皮肤

词根 ano-（肛门）+ derm（皮肤）

例句 The anoderm is highly sensitive due to its rich nerve supply. 肛门皮肤因神经分布丰富而非常敏感。

anoscopy 肛门镜检查

词根 ano-（肛门）+ -scopy（检查）

例句 Anoscopy is used to diagnose hemorrhoids and anal fissures. 肛门镜检查用于诊断痔疮和肛裂。

anorexia 食欲缺乏

词根 ano-（肛门）+ -rexia（食欲）

例句 Anorexia is a common symptom in gastrointestinal disorders. 食欲缺乏是胃肠道疾病的常见症状。

anodynia 肛门疼痛

词根 ano-（肛门）+ -dynia（疼痛）

例句 Anodynia can be a symptom of anal fissures. 肛门疼痛可能是肛裂的症状。

anofistula 肛瘘

词根 ano-（肛门）+ fistula（瘘管）

例句 Anofistulas require surgical treatment. 肛瘘通常需要手术治疗。

anorectal abscess 肛周脓肿

词根 ano-（肛门）+ rectal（直肠）+ abscess（脓肿）

例句 Anorectal abscesses often result from bacterial infections. 肛周脓肿通常由细菌感染引起。

anoproctitis 肛门直肠炎

词根 ano-（肛门）+ proct-（直肠）+ -itis（炎症）

例句 Anoproctitis can cause pain and discomfort during bowel movements. 肛门直肠炎可能导致排便时疼痛和不适。

anococcygeal ligament 肛尾韧带

词根 ano-（肛门）+ coccygeal（尾骨的）+ ligament（韧带）

例句 The anococcygeal ligament connects the anus to the coccyx. 肛尾韧带连接肛门和尾骨。

anthrac-（炭的）

anthracosis 炭末沉着病

词根 anthrac-（炭）+ -osis（病态）

例句 Anthracosis is common in coal miners. 炭末沉着病在煤矿工人中很常见。

anthrax 炭疽病

词根 anthrac-（炭）

例句 Anthrax is caused by Bacillus anthracis. 炭疽病由炭疽杆菌引起。

anthracemia 血炭病

词根 anthrac-（炭）+ -emia（血症）

例句 Anthracemia occurs due to carbon particle accumulation in the blood. 血炭病是由血液中积累碳颗粒引起的。

anthracotoxic 炭毒性的

词根 anthrac-（炭）+ toxic（毒性）

例句 Prolonged exposure to anthracotoxic compounds can be harmful. 长期接触炭毒性化合物可能有害。

anthracoderma 炭黑皮肤病

词根 anthrac-（炭）+ derma（皮肤）

例句 Anthracoderma results from prolonged exposure to coal dust. 炭黑皮肤病是长期接触煤尘引起的。

anthracosilicosis 炭硅沉着病

词根 anthrac-（炭）+ silic-（硅）+ -osis（病态）

例句 Anthracosilicosis is a lung disease caused by inhaling coal and silica dust. 炭硅沉着病是一种由吸入煤尘和硅尘引起的肺病。

anthracolite 炭石化

词根 anthrac-（炭）+ -lite（石化）

例句 Anthracolite is formed under high pressure and temperature. 炭石化是在高温高压下形成的。

anthraconite 炭黑石

词根 anthrac-（炭）+ -ite（矿物）

例句 Anthraconite is used in industrial applications. 炭黑石用于工业应用。

anthracostatic 抗炭疽的

词根 anthrac-（炭）+ -static（抑制的）

例句 Anthracostatic agents help prevent anthrax infection. 抗炭疽剂有助于预防炭疽感染。

anti-（抗）

antibiotic 抗生素

词根 anti-（抗）+ biotic（生物的）

例句 Antibiotics are used to treat bacterial infections. 抗生素用于治疗细菌感染。

anticoagulant 抗凝剂

词根 anti-（抗）+ coagulant（凝血剂）

例句 Anticoagulants prevent blood clots in high-risk patients. 抗凝剂用于预防高危患者的血栓形成。

antiviral 抗病毒的

词根 anti-（抗）+ viral（病毒的）

例句 Antiviral drugs help manage infections like influenza. 抗病毒药物有助于治疗流感等感染。

antihypertensive 抗高血压的

词根 anti-（抗）+ hypertensive（高血压的）

例句 Antihypertensive medications lower blood pressure. 抗高血压药可降低血压。

antidepressant 抗抑郁药

词根 anti-（抗）+ depressant（抑郁的）

例句 Antidepressants are used to treat mood disorders. 抗抑郁药用于治疗情绪障碍。

antipyretic 退烧药

词根 anti-（抗）+ pyretic（发热的）

例句 Antipyretics help reduce fever in infections. 退烧药有助于降低感染引起的发热。

antifungal 抗真菌的

词根 anti-（抗）+ fungal（真菌的）

例句 Antifungal medications treat infections like athlete’s foot. 抗真菌药物用于治疗足癣等感染。

antiseptic 抗菌剂

词根 anti-（抗）+ septic（感染的）

例句 Antiseptics prevent infections in wounds. 抗菌剂可预防伤口感染。

antigen 抗原

词根 anti-（抗）+ -gen（产生）

例句 Antigens trigger immune responses in the body. 抗原能引发机体的免疫反应。

antitoxin 抗毒素

词根 anti-（抗）+ toxin（毒素）

例句 Antitoxins neutralize harmful bacterial toxins. 抗毒素可中和有害的细菌毒素。

LMCHK Part 1　样题

A 26-year-old woman presents to her general practitioner (GP) complaining of very heavy periods. Her cycle is regular and 21 days in length. Her periods last 8 days and she often has to change a pad or tampon every 30 to 40 minutes. There are frequently blood clots present. She does not experience intermenstrual (inter-;

mens-) or postcoital (post-; -coit) bleeding. Socially, she has 2 young children and feels her family is complete. She is a non-smoker. On examination, she has pale conjunctivae but is not symptomatic of anaemia (a-; -emia). Her haemoglobin (haem-; -globin) level is 109 g/L. What is the most appropriate management of this patient?

(A) Arrange transvaginal (trans-; vaginal) ultrasound (ultra-) scan

(B) Intrauterine (intra-; -uterine) system

(C) Mefenamic acid

(D) Tranexamic acid

(E) Combined oral contraceptive (contra-; ceptive) pill

中文翻译

一位 26 岁的女性向她的全科医生主诉月经量过多。她的月经周期正常，为 21 天。她的经期持续 8 天，经常需要每 30 到 40 分钟更换一次卫生巾或卫生棉条，且经血中常伴有血块。她没有月经间期或性交后出血。社会背景方面，她有两个年幼的孩子，自觉家庭美满。她不吸烟。查体显示其结膜苍白，但没有贫血症状。她的血红蛋白水平为 109 g/L。该患者最合适的治疗方法是什么？

(A) 经阴道超声检查

(B) 宫内系统

(C) 甲芬那酸

(D) 氨甲环酸

(E) 复方口服避孕药

题目和答案中出现的词根

inter-：在……之间

mens-：月的

post-：在……之后

-coit：性生活

a-：表示否定

-emia：血症

haem-：血的

-globin：球蛋白

trans-：跨；转

vaginal-：阴道的

ultra-：超

intra-：在……内

-uterine：子宫

contra-：反

-ceptive：获得

apo-（分离）

apoptosis 细胞凋亡

词根 apo-（分离）+ -ptosis（下垂；凋亡）

例句 Apoptosis is a natural process that removes damaged cells. 细胞凋亡是一种自然过程，用于清除受损细胞。

apocrine gland 顶浆分泌腺

词根 apo-（分离）+ -crine（分泌）

例句 Apocrine glands are found in the armpits and groin. 顶浆分泌腺位于腋窝和腹股沟。

aponeurosis 腱膜

词根 apo-（分离）+ -neurosis（神经或肌肉组织）

例句 The aponeurosis connects muscles to bones. 腱膜将肌肉连接至骨骼。

apomorphine 阿扑吗啡

词根 apo-（分离）+ morphine（吗啡）

例句 Apomorphine is used to treat Parkinson's disease. 阿扑吗啡用于治疗帕金森病。

apocarpous 离心皮的

词根 apo-（分离）+ carpous（果实）

例句 Some plants have apocarpous ovaries. 一些植物具有离心皮的子房。

apophyseal fracture 骨突骨折

词根 apo-（分离）+ -physeal（骨骼生长板）

例句 Apophyseal fractures are common in growing adolescents. 骨突骨折在处于发育期的青少年中很常见。

apoenzyme 脱辅酶

词根 apo-（分离）+ enzyme（酶）

例句 Apoenzymes require cofactors to become active. 脱辅酶需要辅因子才能激活。

apocrine sweat gland 顶泌汗腺

词根 apo-（分离）+ -crine（分泌）

例句 Apocrine sweat glands become active during puberty. 顶泌汗腺在青春期变得活跃。

apophysis 骨突

词根 apo-（分离）+ -physis（生长）

例句 The apophysis serves as an attachment site for muscles. 骨突

是肌肉附着的部位。

apomixis 无融合生殖

词根 apo-（分离）+ mixis（混合）

例句 Apomixis occurs in certain plants without fertilization. 无融合生殖发生在某些不需要受精的植物中。

aqua-（水的）

aqueous 含水的

词根 aqua-（水）+ -ous（形容词后缀）

例句 The aqueous solution contains dissolved salts. 该水溶液含有溶解的盐。

aquaphobia 恐水症

词根 aqua-（水）+ -phobia（恐惧）

例句 Aquaphobia is a common symptom of rabies infection. 恐水症是狂犬病感染的常见症状。

aqueous humor 房水

词根 aqua-（水）+ humor（液体）

例句 Aqueous humor maintains intraocular pressure in the eye. 房水维持眼内压的稳定。

aqueduct 脑导水管

词根 aqua-（水）+ duct（通道）

例句 The cerebral aqueduct connects the third and fourth ventricles. 脑导水管连接第三脑室和第四脑室。

aquatherapy 水疗法

词根 aqua-（水）+ therapy（治疗）

例句 Aquatherapy is beneficial for joint rehabilitation. 水疗法对关节康复有益。

aquaporin 水通道蛋白

词根 aqua-（水）+ porin（蛋白）

例句 Aquaporins regulate water transport across cell membranes. 水通道蛋白调节细胞膜内外的水分运输。

aquagenic urticaria 水源性荨麻疹

词根 aqua-（水）+ genic（引起的）+ urticaria（荨麻疹）

例句 Aquagenic urticaria causes skin rashes after water exposure. 水源性荨麻疹会导致皮肤在接触水后出现皮疹。

aquatic therapy 水中治疗

词根 aqua-（水）+ -tic（形容词后缀）+ therapy（治疗）

例句 Aquatic therapy is used for spinal cord injury rehabilitation. 水中治疗用于脊髓损伤康复。

aquadynia 水痛症

词根 aqua-（水）+ -dynia（疼痛）

例句 Aquadynia refers to pain triggered by water exposure. 水痛症指因接触水而引发的疼痛。

aquacapsulitis 湿性关节囊炎

词根 aqua-（水）+ capsulitis（关节囊炎）

例句 Aquacapsulitis can cause joint swelling due to fluid accumulation. 湿性关节囊炎可能因液体积聚而导致关节肿胀。

arachn-（蛛网状）

arachnoid mater 蛛网膜

词根 arachn-（蛛网状）+ -oid（类似）+ mater（脑膜）

例句 The arachnoid mater is one of the three layers of meninges. 蛛网膜是脑膜的三层结构之一。

arachnoiditis 蛛网膜炎

词根 arachn-（蛛网状）+ -itis（炎症）

例句 Arachnoiditis can cause severe chronic pain. 蛛网膜炎可导致严重的慢性疼痛。

arachnoid cyst 蛛网膜囊肿

词根 arachn-（蛛网状）+ -oid（类似）+ cyst（囊肿）

例句 Arachnoid cysts are fluid-filled sacs in the brain or spinal cord. 蛛网膜囊肿是大脑或脊髓中的充液囊。

arachnoid granulations 蛛网膜颗粒

词根 arachn-（蛛网状）+ granulations（颗粒）

例句 Arachnoid granulations help absorb cerebrospinal fluid. 蛛网膜颗粒有助于吸收脑脊液。

arachnoid hemorrhage 蛛网膜下腔出血

词根 arachn-（蛛网状）+ hemorrhage（出血）

例句 Arachnoid hemorrhage is a medical emergency. 蛛网膜下腔出血是一种医疗急症。

arachnoid space 蛛网膜下腔

词根 arachn-（蛛网状）+ space（空间）

例句 The arachnoid space contains cerebrospinal fluid. 蛛网膜下腔含有脑脊液。

arachnoid trabeculae 蛛网膜小梁

词根 arachn-（蛛网状）+ trabeculae（小梁）

例句 Arachnoid trabeculae provide structural support. 蛛网膜小梁提供结构支撑。

arachnoidea 蛛网膜组织

词根 arachn-（蛛网状）+ -idea（形态）

例句 Arachnoidea covers the brain and spinal cord. 蛛网膜组织覆

盖大脑和脊髓。

arachnoid villi 蛛网膜绒毛

词根 arachn-（蛛网状）+ villi（绒毛）

例句 Arachnoid villi aid in cerebrospinal fluid circulation. 蛛网膜绒毛有助于脑脊液循环。

arachnoidea syndrome 蛛网膜综合征

词根 arachn-（蛛网状）+ -idea（形态）+ syndrome（综合征）

例句 Arachnoidea syndrome can cause neurological deficits. 蛛网膜综合征可能导致神经功能缺陷。

archae-（古的）

archaebacteria 古细菌

词根 archae-（古的）+ bacteria（细菌）

例句 Archaebacteria thrive in extreme environments. 古细菌能在极端环境中生存。

archaeocyte 原始细胞

词根 archae-（古的）+ -cyte（细胞）

例句 Archaeocytes play a role in sponge regeneration. 原始细胞在海绵动物的再生过程中起作用。

archaeogenetics 古遗传学

词根 archae-（古的）+ genetics（遗传学）

例句 Archaeogenetics studies the DNA of ancient species. 古遗传学研究古代物种的 DNA。

archaeon 古生菌

词根 archae-（古的）+ -on（生物）

例句 Methanogens are a type of archaeon. 产甲烷菌是一种古生菌。

archaeal lipid 古生菌脂质

词根 archae-（古的）+ lipid（脂质）
例句 Archaeal lipids have unique chemical structures. 古生菌脂质具有独特的化学结构。

archaic reflex 原始反射

词根 archae-（古的）+ reflex（反射）
例句 The grasp reflex is an example of an archaic reflex. 抓握反射是原始反射的一个例子。

archaeoviral 古病毒的

词根 archae-（古的）+ viral（病毒的）
例句 Archaeoviral studies explore ancient viral evolution. 古病毒研究探索了病毒的远古演化。

archaeal genome 古生菌基因组

词根 archae-（古的）+ genome（基因组）
例句 The archaeal genome contains unique metabolic genes. 古生菌基因组包含独特的代谢基因。

archaezoa 古生原虫

词根 archae-（古的）+ zoa（动物）
例句 Archaezoa are primitive eukaryotic organisms. 古生原虫是原始的真核生物。

arche-（起始的）

menarche 初潮

词根 men-（月经）+ arche-（起始）
例句 Menarche typically occurs between ages 11 and 14. 初潮通常发生在 11 至 14 岁。

gonadarche 性腺发育期

词根 gonad-（性腺）+ arche-（起始）

例句 Gonadarche marks the beginning of puberty. 性腺发育期标志着青春期的开始。

thelarche 乳房发育初期

词根 thel-（乳房）+ arche-（起始）

例句 Thelarche is the first sign of puberty in females. 乳房发育初期是女性青春期的第一个标志。

adrenarche 肾上腺发育期

词根 adren-（肾上腺）+ arche-（起始）

例句 Adrenarche leads to increased production of androgens. 肾上腺发育期导致雄激素的增加。

ovarian archetype 卵巢原型

词根 ovarian（卵巢）+ arche-（起始）+ type（类型）

例句 The ovarian archetype is essential for reproductive health. 卵巢原型对生殖健康至关重要。

neuromenarche 神经性初潮

词根 neuro-（神经）+ men-（月经）+ arche-（起始）

例句 Neuromenarche is influenced by the hypothalamus. 神经性初潮受下丘脑的影响。

thelarche delay 乳房发育延迟

词根 thel-（乳房）+ arche-（起始）+ delay（延迟）

例句 Thelarche delay may indicate hormonal imbalance. 乳房发育延迟可能表明激素失衡。

archetypal development 原型发育

词根 arche-（起始）+ typal（类型）+ development（发育）

例句 Archetypal development is critical in embryogenesis. 原型发

育在胚胎发生过程中至关重要。

neuroarcheology 神经考古学

词根 neuro-（神经）+ arche-（起始）+ logy（学科）

例句 Neuroarcheology studies the evolution of brain function. 神经考古学研究大脑功能的进化。

archegenesis 原始发生

词根 arche-（起始）+ genesis（生长）

例句 Archegenesis refers to the early formation of life. 原始发生指生命的早期形成。

LMCHK Part 1 样题

A baby is born by an emergency caesarean section at 40 weeks, due to pathological cardiotocography (cardio-; toco-; -graphy). She appears normal at birth, with Apgar scores of 9 and 10 (1 and 5 minutes respectively). Soon after delivery, the midwife notes that the baby's respiratory (re-; spir-) rate is elevated (other observations are normal). Maternal antenatal (ante-; -natal) history is unremarkable and her observations were normal during labour. What is the most likely diagnosis?

(A) Pneumothorax (pneumo-; -thorax)

(B) Neonatal (neo-) pneumonia

(C) Tracheoesophageal (trach-; eso-; phag-) fistula (TOF)

(D) Transient tachypnoea (tachy-; -pnoea) of the newborn (TTN)

(E) Respiratory (re-; spir-) distress syndrome (RDS)

中文翻译

一名婴儿在足月（40 周）时因病理性胎心监护结果异常而紧急剖宫产出生。她出生时情况良好，阿普加评分为 9 分和 10 分（分别在出生后 1 分钟和 5 分钟时评估）。出生后不久，助产士注意到婴儿的呼吸频率增快（其余生命体征正常）。母亲孕期病史无明显异常，分娩过程中的各项观察指标也正常。最可能的诊断是什么？

(A) 气胸

(B) 新生儿肺炎

(C) 气管食管瘘（TOF）

(D) 新生儿暂时性呼吸急促（TTN）

(E) 呼吸窘迫综合征（RDS）

题目和答案中出现的词根

cardio-：心脏的

toco-：宫缩

-graphy：图像

re-：反复

spir：呼吸

ante-：在……之前

-natal：出生

pneumo-：肺的（气体）

-thorax：胸腔

neo-：新的

trachy-：快速的

eso-：内的

phag-：吃；吞

-pnoea：呼吸

arthro-（关节的）

arthritis 关节炎

词根 arthro-（关节的）+ -itis（炎症）

例句 Arthritis causes inflammation and pain in the joints. 关节炎引起关节的炎症和疼痛。

arthroplasty 关节成形术

词根 arthro-（关节的）+ -plasty（修复）

例句 Arthroplasty is a surgical procedure to replace a damaged joint. 关节成形术是用来替换受损关节的外科手术。

arthroscopy 关节镜检查

词根 arthro-（关节的）+ -scopy（检查）

例句 Arthroscopy allows surgeons to view the inside of a joint using a camera. 关节镜检查可使外科医生通过摄像头查看关节内部。

arthralgia 关节痛

词根 arthro-（关节的）+ algia（疼痛）

例句 Arthralgia can occur due to overuse or inflammatory conditions. 关节痛可能由过度使用或炎症性疾病引起。

arthrodesis 关节融合术

词根 arthro-（关节的）+ -desis（固定）

例句 Arthrodesis is performed to fuse a joint, typically in cases of severe arthritis. 关节融合术用于将关节融合，通常用于严重关节炎的病例。

arthrocentesis 关节穿刺

词根 arthro-（关节的）+ -centesis（穿刺）

例句 Arthrocentesis is used to remove fluid from a joint to reduce swelling. 关节穿刺用于抽取关节内积液以减轻肿胀。

arthropathy 关节病

词根 arthro-（关节的）+ -pathy（病态）

例句 Arthropathy is a general term for diseases affecting the joints. 关节病是指影响关节的疾病的总称。

arthrokinematics 关节运动学

词根 arthro-（关节的）+ kinematics（运动学）

例句 Arthrokinematics studies the movement of the bones within the joints. 关节运动学研究骨头在关节内的运动。

arthropod 节肢动物

词根 arthro-（关节的）+ pod（脚）

例句 Arthropods include insects, spiders, and crustaceans. 节肢动物包括昆虫、蜘蛛和甲壳类动物。

arthropathic 关节病的

词根 arthro-（关节的）+ -pathic（病态的）

例句 Arthropathic conditions can lead to reduced joint function. 关节病可能导致关节功能减退。

–ase（酶）

amylase 淀粉酶

词根 amyl-（淀粉）+ -ase（酶）

例句 Amylase breaks down starch into sugar. 淀粉酶将淀粉分解为糖。

lipase 脂肪酶

词根 lip-（脂肪）+ -ase（酶）

例句 Lipase helps digest dietary fats. 脂肪酶帮助消化膳食脂肪。

protease 蛋白酶

词根 prote-（蛋白质）+ -ase（酶）

例句 Protease is essential for protein digestion. 蛋白酶对蛋白质的消化至关重要。

lactase 乳糖酶

词根 lact-（乳糖）+ -ase（酶）

例句 Lactase deficiency leads to lactose intolerance. 乳糖酶缺乏会导致乳糖不耐受。

sucrase 蔗糖酶

词根 sucr-（蔗糖）+ -ase（酶）

例句 Sucrase converts sucrose into glucose and fructose. 蔗糖酶将蔗糖转化为葡萄糖和果糖。

DNase 脱氧核糖核酸酶（DNA 酶）

词根 DNA（脱氧核糖核酸）+ -ase（酶）

例句 DNase is used to degrade DNA in biological samples. DNA 酶用于降解生物样本中的 DNA。

RNase 核糖核酸酶（RNA 酶）

词根 RNA（核糖核酸）+ -ase（酶）

例句 RNase breaks down RNA molecules. RNA 酶降解 RNA 分子。

helicase 解旋酶

词根 helic-（螺旋）+ -ase（酶）

例句 Helicase unwinds DNA during replication. 解旋酶在复制过程中解开 DNA 双螺旋。

polymerase 聚合酶

词根 polymer-（聚合）+ -ase（酶）
例句 DNA polymerase synthesizes new DNA strands. DNA 聚合酶合成新的 DNA 链。

oxidase 氧化酶

词根 oxid-（氧化）+ -ase（酶）
例句 Oxidase enzymes are involved in oxidation reactions. 氧化酶参与氧化反应。

asthen-（无力）

myasthenia 肌无力

词根 my-（肌肉）+ asthen-（无力）
例句 Myasthenia gravis is an autoimmune disorder that causes muscle weakness. 重症肌无力是一种导致肌肉无力的自身免疫疾病。

neurasthenia 神经衰弱

词根 neur-（神经）+ asthen-（无力）
例句 Neurasthenia is characterized by chronic fatigue and anxiety. 神经衰弱的特征是慢性疲劳和焦虑。

asthenopia 视力疲劳

词根 asthen-（无力）+ opia（视力）
例句 Prolonged screen time can cause asthenopia. 长时间使用屏幕可能会导致视疲劳。

phlebasthenia 静脉无力

词根 phleb-（静脉）+ asthen-（无力）
例句 Phlebasthenia can lead to varicose veins. 静脉无力可能导致静脉曲张。

asthenic personality 无力性人格

词根 asthen-（无力）+ -ic（形容词后缀）

例句 People with an asthenic personality tend to be anxious and passive. 具有无力性人格的人往往焦虑且消极。

hysterical asthenia 歇斯底里性无力

词根 hyster-（子宫；情绪）+ asthen-（无力）

例句 Hysterical asthenia is often associated with psychological factors. 歇斯底里性无力通常与心理因素相关。

muscular asthenia 肌肉无力

词根 muscul-（肌肉）+ asthen-（无力）

例句 Muscular asthenia is common in elderly patients. 肌肉无力在老年患者中很常见。

neurocirculatory asthenia 神经循环无力

词根 neuro-（神经）+ circulatory（循环的）+ asthen-（无力）

例句 Neurocirculatory asthenia causes dizziness and fatigue. 神经循环无力会导致头晕和疲劳。

athero-（黏性的块）

atherosclerosis 动脉粥样硬化

词根 athero-（黏性的块）+ sclerosis（硬化）

例句 Atherosclerosis leads to the buildup of plaque in the arteries, restricting blood flow. 动脉粥样硬化导致动脉中形成斑块，限制血流。

atheroma 动脉粥样斑块

词根 athero-（黏性的块）+ -oma（肿瘤）

例句 An atheroma is a fatty deposit that can clog blood vessels. 动脉粥样斑块是一种脂肪沉积，可能会堵塞血管。

atherogenesis 动脉粥样硬化形成

词根 athero-（黏性的块）+ -genesis（生成）

例句 Atherogenesis is the process by which atherosclerotic plaques form in the arteries. 动脉粥样硬化生成是动脉粥样斑块在动脉中形成的过程。

atheromatosis 动脉粥样病

词根 athero-（黏性的块）+ -osis（病态）

例句 Atheromatosis is characterized by the widespread presence of atheromas in the arteries. 动脉粥样病以动脉中广泛存在动脉粥样斑块为特征。

atherogenic 动脉粥样硬化的

词根 athero-（黏性的块）+ -genic（产生的）

例句 Dietary factors such as high cholesterol intake are considered atherogenic. 高胆固醇摄入等饮食因素可引发动脉粥样硬化。

atheromatous plaque 动脉粥样斑块

词根 athero-（黏性的块）+ -matous（含有……的）

例句 Atheromatous plaques can lead to stroke and heart attacks. 动脉粥样斑块可能导致中风和心脏病发作。

atherogenesis 动脉粥样硬化形成

词根 athero-（黏性的块）+ -genesis（生成）

例句 Atherogenesis is a process in which fatty deposits accumulate in the arterial walls. 动脉粥样硬化形成是脂肪沉积物在动脉壁中累积的过程。

atherothrombotic 动脉粥样硬化性血栓形成的

词根 athero-（黏性的块）+ thrombo-（血栓）+ -tic（形容词后缀）

例句 Atherothrombotic events can block blood flow and result in heart failure. 动脉粥样硬化性血栓形成突发时，可阻塞血流，导致心力衰竭。

atherosclerotic 动脉粥样硬化的

词根 athero-（黏性的块）+ sclerotic（硬化的）

例句 Atherosclerotic changes in the arteries can increase the risk of heart disease. 动脉粥样硬化病变会增加患心脏病的风险。

-ation（将动词定格为静态名词）

inflammation 炎症

词根 inflamm-（点燃）+ -ation（动态定格）

例句 Chronic inflammation is linked to various diseases. 慢性炎症与多种疾病有关。

vaccination 疫苗接种

词根 vaccin-（疫苗）+ -ation（动态定格）

例句 Vaccination helps prevent infectious diseases. 疫苗接种有助于预防传染病。

circulation 循环

词根 circul-（循环）+ -ation（动态定格）

例句 Proper circulation is essential for cardiovascular health. 良好的血液循环对心血管健康至关重要。

respiration 呼吸

词根 respir-（呼吸）+ -ation（动态定格）

例句 Respiration provides oxygen to body tissues. 呼吸为身体组织提供氧气。

perspiration 出汗

词根 perspir-（排汗）+ -ation（动态定格）

例句 Perspiration helps regulate body temperature. 出汗有助于调节体温。

defecation 排便

词根 defec-（排泄）+ -ation（动态定格）

例句 Regular defecation is essential for digestive health. 规律排便对消化系统健康至关重要。

exhalation 呼气

词根 ex-（向外）+ hal-（呼吸）+ -ation（动态定格）

例句 Carbon dioxide is expelled during exhalation. 二氧化碳在呼气时被排出。

inhalation 吸气

词根 in-（向内）+ hal-（呼吸）+ -ation（动态定格）

例句 Oxygen enters the lungs during inhalation. 氧气在吸气时进入肺部。

coagulation 凝血

词根 coag-（凝固）+ -ation（动态定格）

例句 Platelets play a key role in blood coagulation. 血小板在凝血过程中起关键作用。

ossification 骨化

词根 oss-（骨）+ -ation（动态定格）

例句 Ossification is essential for bone growth. 骨化对于骨骼生长至关重要。

USMLE Step 1 样题

Atherosclerosis (athero-; scler-; -osis) is associated with numerous well-known risk factors, such as age, smoking, diabetes, hyperlipidemia (hyper-; lipid-; -emia), and a family history of atherosclerosis. LDL cholesterol is believed to be a key factor in the pathway through which hyperlipidemia causes atherosclerosis. What is most likely the first step in the pathogenesis (patho-; -genesis) of atherosclerosis caused by hyperlipidemia?

(A) Endothelial (endo-) dysfunction (dys-)

(B) Foam cell formation

(C) LDL cholesterol oxidation

(D) Monocyte (mono-; -cyte) activation

(E) Plaque formation

中文翻译

动脉粥样硬化与许多众所周知的危险因素相关，如年龄、吸烟、糖尿病、高脂血症和动脉粥样硬化家族史。低密度脂蛋白胆固醇（LDL 胆固醇）被认为是高脂血症引起动脉粥样硬化的关键因素。高脂血症引起动脉粥样硬化的发病机制中，最可能的第一步是什么？

(A) 内皮功能障碍

(B) 泡沫细胞形成

(C) LDL 胆固醇氧化

(D) 单核细胞活化

(E) 斑块形成

题目和答案中出现的词根

athero-：斑块

scler-：硬化

-osis：疾病状态

hyper-：高

lipid-：脂肪

-emia：血症

patho-：病理的

-genesis：产生

endo-：内

dys-：错误的；困难的；疼痛的

mono-：单个的

-cyte：细胞

aureus-/aureo-（金黄色）

staphylococcus aureus 金黄色葡萄球菌

词根 staphyl-（葡萄状）+ coccus（球菌）+ aureus（金黄色）

例句 Staphylococcus aureus can cause skin infections. 金黄色葡萄球菌可引起皮肤感染。

aureus pigment 金黄色色素

词根 aureus-（金黄色）+ pigment（色素）

例句 Aureus pigment gives certain bacteria their golden color. 金黄色色素使某些细菌呈现金黄色。

aureobacterium 金黄色杆菌属

词根 aureo-（金黄色）+ bacterium（细菌）

例句 Aureobacterium species are found in soil and water. 金黄色杆菌属存在于土壤和水中。

aureus syndrome 金黄色葡萄球菌综合征

词根 aureus-（金黄色）+ syndrome（综合征）

例句 Aureus syndrome includes symptoms of severe bacterial infection. 金黄色葡萄球菌综合征包括严重细菌感染的症状。

aureus dermatitis 金黄色皮炎

词根 aureus-（金黄色）+ dermatitis（皮炎）
例句 Aureus dermatitis is caused by staphylococcus aureus. 金黄色皮炎由金黄色葡萄球菌引起。

aureofungin 金黄色真菌素

词根 aureo-（金黄色）+ fungin（抗真菌药物）
例句 Aureofungin is used as an antifungal agent. 金黄色真菌素用作抗真菌药物。

aureomycin 金霉素

词根 aureo-（金黄色）+ mycin（抗生素）
例句 Aureomycin is an antibiotic used to treat bacterial infections. 金霉素是一种用于治疗细菌感染的抗生素。

aureotoxin 金黄色毒素

词根 aureo-（金黄色）+ toxin（毒素）
例句 Aureotoxin is a toxin produced by certain bacterial strains. 金黄色毒素是某些细菌菌株产生的毒素。

aureus otitis 金黄色葡萄球菌耳炎

词根 aureus-（金黄色）+ otitis（耳炎）
例句 Aureus otitis can cause severe ear infections. 金黄色葡萄球菌耳炎可导致严重的耳部感染。

aureus septicemia 金黄色败血症

词根 aureus-（金黄色）+ septicemia（败血症）
例句 Aureus septicemia requires urgent antibiotic treatment. 金黄色败血症需要紧急抗生素治疗。

USMLE Step 1 样题

A 25-year-old man presents with new-onset hemoptysis

(hemo-; -pty-; -sis) for the past 12 hours. The patient, who recently immigrated to the United States from Vietnam, has had fever and night sweats on a daily basis for the past four years. He has no other complaints and no past medical history. The patient is diagnosed with active tuberculosis (tubercul-; -osis) and sent home on an antimycobacterial (anti-; myco-; bacter-) regimen. One month later, the patient returns with new complaints of joint pain, photosensitivity (photo-), and a facial rash. Liver function tests are found to be elevated. Which of the following is the mechanism of action of the drug with the adverse effects described above?

(A) Disrupts the cell membrane's osmotic properties

(B) Inhibits arabinosyl transferases (-ase)

(C) Inhibits DNA-dependent RNA polymerase (poly-; -ase) encoded by the rpo gene

(D) Inhibits folic acid synthesis

(E) Inhibits synthesis of mycolic acids

中文翻译

一名25岁的男性在过去12小时内出现了新发咯血。他最近从越南移民到美国，过去4年中每天都有发热和夜间盗汗。他没有其他不适症状，也没有既往病史。他被诊断为活动性肺结核，并开始接受抗结核治疗方案。1个月后，患者复诊时新增关节疼痛、光敏感和面部皮疹症状，且肝功能检测显示升高。下列哪一种是与上述不良反应相关药物的作用机制？

(A) 破坏细胞膜的渗透性

(B) 抑制阿拉伯糖转移酶

(C) 抑制由 rpo 基因编码的 DNA 依赖性 RNA 聚合酶

(D) 抑制叶酸合成

(E) 抑制分枝菌酸的合成

题目和答案中出现的词根

hemo-：血

-pty-：吐

-sis：状态

tubercul-：结核的

-osis：病理状态

anti-：抗

myco-：真菌的

bacter-：细菌的

photo-：像；光

-ase：酶

poly-：多

auto-（自我）

autonomy 自主性

词根 auto-（自我）+ -nomy（法则）

例句 Autonomy in decision-making is a key principle in medical ethics. 决策中的自主性是医学伦理学中的一个关键原则。

autism 自闭症

词根 auto-（自我）+ -ism（状态）

例句 Autism spectrum disorders are characterized by challenges with social interaction. 自闭症谱系障碍以社交互动困难为特征。

autoimmune 自身免疫的

词根 auto-（自我）+ immune（免疫的）

例句 Autoimmune diseases occur when the immune system attacks the body's own tissues. 自身免疫性疾病发生在免疫系统攻击身体自身组织时。

autologous 自体的

词根 auto-（自我）+ -logous（相似的）

例句 Autologous stem cell transplantation uses patient's own cells for therapy. 自体干细胞移植使用患者自身的细胞进行治疗。

autopsy 尸检

词根 auto-（自我）+ -opsy（检查）

例句 An autopsy helps determine the cause of death in unclear cases. 尸检有助于在不明确的情况下确定死亡原因。

autocrat 独裁者

词根 auto-（自我）+ -crat（统治者）

例句 An autocrat in a healthcare setting may make unilateral decisions that impact patient care. 医疗环境中的独裁者可能做出影响患者护理的单方面决策。

autologous transplantation 自体移植

词根 auto-（自我）+ -logous（相似的）+ transplantation（移植）

例句 Autologous transplantation uses the patient's own tissue for a transplant. 自体移植使用患者自身的组织进行移植。

autointoxication 自体中毒

词根 auto-（自我）+ intoxication（中毒）

例句 Autointoxication occurs when the body accumulates toxins due to poor waste elimination. 自体中毒是指由于废物排泄不良，体内毒素积累的现象。

autoreactive 自我反应的

词根 auto-（自我）+ reactive（反应的）

例句 Autoreactive T cells are involved in autoimmune diseases. 自我反应性 T 细胞参与自身免疫性疾病的发生。

autolysis 自溶

词根 auto-（自我）+ -lysis（分解）

例句 Autolysis refers to the self-digestion of cells and tissues after death. 自溶指的是细胞和组织在死亡后自我消化的过程。

bacillus-（杆状）

bacillus 芽孢杆菌

词根 bacillus-（杆状）

例句 Bacillus is a type of bacteria that can cause infections like anthrax. 芽孢杆菌是一类可引发炭疽等感染的细菌。

bacilliform 杆状的

词根 bacilli-（杆状）+ form（形式）

例句 The bacilliform shape is characteristic of certain bacteria. 杆状形态是某些细菌的特征。

bacilluria 尿中杆菌

词根 bacillus-（杆状）+ -uria（尿症）

例句 Bacilluria refers to the presence of bacilli in the urine. 尿中杆菌是指尿液中存在芽孢杆菌。

bacillogenesis 芽孢形成

词根 bacillus-（杆状）+ -genesis（生成）

例句 Bacillogenesis is the process by which bacilli form spores. 芽孢形成是芽孢杆菌形成孢子的过程。

bacillary 芽孢杆菌的

词根 bacillus-（杆状）+ -ary（形容词后缀）

例句 Bacillary dysentery is caused by the ingestion of bacilli-contaminated food or water. 芽孢杆菌性痢疾由摄入受芽孢杆菌污染的食物或水引起。

Bacillus Calmette-Guérin（BCG）卡介苗

词根 bacillus-（杆状）

例句 Bacillus Calmette-Guérin（BCG）is a vaccine used to prevent tuberculosis. 卡介苗是预防结核病的疫苗。

bacillospore 芽孢杆菌孢子

词根 bacillus-（杆状）+ spore（孢子）

例句 Bacillospore formation allows the bacteria to survive extreme conditions. 芽孢杆菌孢子的形成使细菌能够在极端条件下生存。

bacillosis 芽孢病

词根 bacillus-（杆状）+ -osis（病态）

例句 Bacillosis is an infection caused by bacilli bacteria. 芽孢病是由芽孢杆菌引起的感染。

bacillitic 芽孢杆菌的

词根 bacilli-（杆状）+ -itic（形容词后缀）

例句 Bacillitic infections are caused by bacilli bacteria in the bloodstream. 芽孢杆菌性感染是由芽孢杆菌引起的血液感染。

baro-（压力）

barotrauma 气压伤

词根 baro-（压力）+ trauma（伤害）

例句 Barotrauma can occur when there is a sudden change in atmospheric pressure, such as during diving. 气压伤可能发生在大气压力发生剧烈变化时，如潜水过程中。

baroreceptor 压力感受器

词根 baro-（压力）+ receptor（感受器）

例句 Baroreceptors are responsible for sensing changes in blood pressure. 压力感受器负责感知血压变化。

baroclinic 气压梯度的

词根 baro-（压力）+ clinic-（倾斜）

例句 Baroclinic systems occur when air pressure and temperature gradients do not align. 气压梯度系统发生在气压和温度梯度不一致时。

baroreflex 压力反射

词根 baro-（压力）+ reflex（反射）
例句 The baroreflex helps maintain blood pressure homeostasis by adjusting heart rate and vessel diameter. 压力反射通过调整心率和血管直径来帮助维持血压的稳定。

barometric 气压的

词根 baro-（压力）+ metric（测量的）
例句 Barometric pressure can affect breathing, especially in patients with respiratory conditions. 气压可以影响呼吸，特别是对于患有呼吸系统疾病的患者。

barodontalgia 气压性牙痛

词根 baro-（压力）+ dental（牙齿的）+ algia（痛）
例句 Barodontalgia is a type of tooth pain that occurs due to changes in pressure, such as during flying. 气压性牙痛是一种由气压变化（如乘坐飞机时）引起的牙痛。

barosensitivity 气压敏感性

词根 baro-（压力）+ sensitivity（敏感性）
例句 Patients with barosensitivity may experience symptoms like headaches when exposed to rapid changes in pressure. 气压敏感的患者在经历快速气压变化时，可能会出现头痛等症状。

baroreceptor sensitivity 压力感受器敏感性

词根 baro-（压力）+ receptor（感受器）+ sensitivity（敏感性）
例句 Baroreceptor sensitivity can decrease with age, leading to issues in regulating blood pressure. 压力感受器敏感性随年龄增加可能下降，导致血压调节出现问题。

barocardiography 压力心电图

词根 baro-（压力）+ cardi-（心脏）+ -graphy（记录）

例句 Barocardiography is a diagnostic tool used to measure the effects of pressure on heart function. 压力心电图是一种用于测量压力对心脏功能影响的诊断工具。

bi-（两个）

bilateral 双侧的

词根 bi-（两个）+ lateral（侧面）

例句 Bilateral symptoms indicate that both sides of the body are affected. 双侧症状表明身体的两侧都受到了影响。

bicuspid 二尖瓣

词根 bi-（两个）+ cuspid（尖）

例句 The bicuspid valve is located between the left atrium and left ventricle of the heart. 二尖瓣位于心脏左心房和左心室之间。

bipolar 双极的

词根 bi-（两个）+ polar（极性）

例句 Bipolar disorder is characterized by extreme mood swings, ranging from depression to mania. 双相障碍的特征是极端的情绪波动，从抑郁到狂躁。

bifocal 双焦点的

词根 bi-（两个）+ focal（焦点）

例句 Bifocal lenses are designed to help people with both near-sightedness and far-sightedness. 双焦点镜片旨在帮助近视和远视患者。

biparietal 双顶的

词根 bi-（两个）+ parietal（顶骨的）

例句 The biparietal diameter measures the width of the fetal head during ultrasound. 双顶径是在超声检查中测量胎儿头部宽度的参数。

bifurcation 分叉

词根 bi-（两个）+ furcation（分开）

例句 The bifurcation of the trachea leads to the left and right bronchi. 气管分叉形成左支气管和右支气管。

binocular 双眼的

词根 bi-（两个）+ ocular（眼睛的）

例句 Binocular vision allows for depth perception and a wide field of view. 双眼视觉使人具备深度感知能力和广阔的视野。

biphasic 双相的

词根 bi-（两个）+ phasic（阶段的）

例句 Biphasic treatment refers to a medical intervention involving two different phases. 双相治疗指的是包含两个不同阶段的医学干预。

bivalve 双壳的

词根 bi-（两个）+ valve（瓣膜）

例句 Bivalve mollusks, such as clams and oysters, have two hinged shells. 双壳软体动物，如蛤蜊和牡蛎，具有两个铰链壳。

bifid（分裂的）

词根 bi-（两个）+ fid-（分开）

例句 Bifid spines are a condition in which the spine is split into two parts. 脊柱裂是一种脊柱分裂成两部分的病症。

bipolar disorder 双相障碍

词根 bi-（两个）+ polar（极性）

例句 Bipolar disorder involves extreme mood swings between depression and mania. 双相障碍表现为抑郁到狂躁之间的极端情绪

波动。

USMLE Step 1　样题

A 14-year-old girl is brought to the office by her mother because of a 3-month history of red bumps on her skin. The patient says the bumps are not itchy or painful but that she finds them embarrassing. She has no history of major medical illness and takes no medications. Her vital signs are within normal limits. Physical examination shows the findings in the photograph (-graph). Which of the following is the most likely diagnosis?

(A) Eczema

(B) Folliculitis (follicul-; -itis)

(C) Hidradenitis (hidr-; aden-; -itis)

(D) Keratosis pilaris (kerat-; -osis)

(E) Urticaria (Urtic-)

中文翻译

一名 14 岁的女孩在其母亲的陪同下前来就诊，主诉皮肤出现红色丘疹，已持续 3 个月。患者表示丘疹不痒也不痛，但她觉得它们很让人尴尬。她没有重大疾病史，也没有服用任何药物。她的生命体征正常。体格检查显示照片中的表现（照片省略）。以下哪项是最可能的诊断？

(A) 湿疹

(B) 毛囊炎

(C) 大汗腺炎

(D) 毛囊角化病

(E) 荨麻疹

题目和答案中出现的词根

-graph：图像

follicul-：滤泡

-itis：炎症

hidr-：汗

aden-：腺

-osis：病理状态

urtic-：荨麻

-blast（母细胞）

fibroblast 成纤维细胞

词根 fibro-（纤维）+ -blast（母细胞）

例句 Fibroblasts are responsible for producing collagen and extracellular matrix. 成纤维细胞负责产生胶原蛋白和细胞外基质。

osteoblast 骨母细胞

词根 oste-（骨）+ -blast（母细胞）

例句 Osteoblasts are the cells that form new bone tissue. 骨母细胞是形成新骨组织的细胞。

chondroblast 软骨母细胞

词根 chondro-（软骨）+ -blast（母细胞）

例句 Chondroblasts produce the extracellular matrix of cartilage. 软骨母细胞产生软骨的细胞外基质。

myoblast 肌母细胞

词根 myo-（肌肉）+ -blast（母细胞）

例句 Myoblasts fuse to form muscle fibers during muscle development. 肌母细胞在肌肉发育过程中融合形成肌纤维。

neuroblast 神经母细胞

词根 neuro-（神经）+ -blast（母细胞）

例句 Neuroblasts are precursors to neurons in the nervous system. 神经母细胞是神经系统中神经元的前体。

erythroblast 红细胞母细胞

词根 erythro-（红）+ -blast（母细胞）

例句 Erythroblasts mature into red blood cells in the bone marrow. 红细胞母细胞在骨髓中成熟为红细胞。

lymphoblast 淋巴母细胞

词根 lympho-（淋巴）+ -blast（母细胞）

例句 Lymphoblasts are immature cells that develop into lymphocytes. 淋巴母细胞是未成熟细胞，可发育为淋巴细胞。

hematoblast 血母细胞

词根 hemato-（血液）+ -blast（母细胞）

例句 Hematoblasts are stem cells that give rise to all blood cells. 血母细胞是产生所有血细胞的干细胞。

adipoblast 脂肪母细胞

词根 adipo-（脂肪）+ -blast（母细胞）

例句 Adipoblasts develop into adipocytes that store fat. 脂肪母细胞发育为存储脂肪的脂肪细胞。

USMLE Step 1 样题

A 32-year-old woman with type 1 diabetes mellitus has had progressive renal failure during the past 2 years. She has not yet started dialysis (dia-; -lysis). Examination shows no abnormalities (ab-). Her hemoglobin (hemo-; -globin) concentration is 9 g/dL, hematocrit (hemato-; -crit) is 28%, and mean corpuscular (corpus-) volume is 94 μm^3 . A blood smear shows normochromic (normo-; chrom-), normocytic (normo-; cyt-) cells. Which of the following is the most likely cause?

(A) Acute blood loss

(B) Chronic lymphocytic (lymph-; cyt-) leukemia (leuk-; -emia)

(C) Erythrocyte (erythro-; cyt-) enzyme deficiency

(D) Erythropoietin (erythro-; -poietin) deficiency

(E) Immunohemolysis (immuno-; hemo-; lysis)

(F) Microangiopathic (micro-; angio-; path-) hemolysis (hemo-; -lysis)

(G) Polycythemia (poly-; cyt-; -emia) vera

(H) Sickle cell disease

(I) Sideroblastic (sidero-; -blast) anemia

(J) β thalassemia (thalass-; -emia) trait

中文翻译

一名 32 岁的女性患有 1 型糖尿病，过去 2 年中肾功能逐渐衰竭，但尚未开始透析。检查结果未见异常。血红蛋白浓度为 9 g/dL，血细胞比容为 28%，平均红细胞体积为 94 μm^3。血涂片显示正常色素、正常细胞大小的红细胞。以下哪项是最可能的原因？

(A) 急性失血

(B) 慢性淋巴细胞白血病

(C) 红细胞酶缺乏

(D) 红细胞生成素缺乏

(E) 免疫溶血

(F) 微血管病变性溶血

(G) 真性红细胞增多症

(H) 镰状细胞病

(I) 铁粒幼细胞性贫血

(J) β 地中海贫血基因携带者

题目和答案中出现的词根

dia-：通过

-lysis：分解（通过分解，这里指代透析，即通过分解电解质来做体内外电解质置换）

ab-：否定

hemo-：血

-globin：球蛋白

-crit：分离法（血液分离法，指代红细胞比容，即血清和红细胞的分离）

corpus-：肉体的（这里指红细胞本体的）

normo-：正常的

chrom-：颜色（这里指红细胞颜色的深度）

cyt-：细胞（这里指细胞的大小）

lymph-：淋巴的

leuk-：白色的

-emia：血症

erythro-：红色的

-poietin：发生；生成

immuno- 免疫的

micro-：微小的

angio-：血管

path：病变的

poly-：多

sidero-：铁颗粒的

-blast：前体

thalass-：海洋的

blepharo-（眼睑的）

blepharitis 眼睑炎

词根 blepharo-（眼睑的）+ -itis（炎症）

例句 Blepharitis is an inflammation of the eyelids, often caused by bacterial infection. 眼睑炎是眼睑的炎症，通常由细菌感染引起。

blepharoplasty 眼睑成形术

词根 blepharo-（眼睑的）+ -plasty（修复）

例句 Blepharoplasty is a surgical procedure to correct eyelid deformities. 眼睑成形术是一种矫正眼睑畸形的外科手术。

blepharospasm 眼睑痉挛

词根 blepharo-（眼睑的）+ -spasm（痉挛）

例句 Blepharospasm causes involuntary twitching of the eyelid. 眼睑痉挛会导致眼睑的不自主抽搐。

blepharochalasis 眼睑松弛症

词根 blepharo-（眼睑的）+ -chalasis（松弛）

例句 Blepharochalasis is a condition where the skin of the eyelid becomes loose. 眼睑松弛症是一种眼睑皮肤变松的病症。

blepharoconjunctivitis 眼睑结膜炎

词根 blepharo-（眼睑的）+ conjunctiv-（结膜的）+ -itis（炎症）
例句 Blepharoconjunctivitis is an inflammation of the eyelids and the conjunctiva. 眼睑结膜炎是眼睑和结膜的炎症。

blepharomandibular 眼睑下颌的

词根 blepharo-（眼睑的）+ mandibular（下颌的）
例句 Blepharomandibular syndrome involves abnormal development of the eyelid and jaw. 眼睑下颌综合征包括眼睑和下颌的异常发育。

blepharopigmentation 眼睑色素沉着

词根 blepharo-（眼睑的）+ pigment（色素）
例句 Blepharopigmentation refers to the abnormal accumulation of pigment in the eyelid. 眼睑色素沉着是指眼睑中色素的异常积累。

blepharochalasia 眼睑松弛

词根 blepharo-（眼睑的）+ chalasia（松弛）
例句 Blepharochalasia can lead to excess skin on the eyelids. 眼睑松弛可能导致眼睑上的皮肤过多。

blepharorrhaphy 眼睑缝合术

词根 blepharo-（眼睑的）+ -rrhaphy（缝合）
例句 Blepharorrhaphy is a surgical procedure to repair the eyelid after injury. 眼睑缝合术是在眼睑受伤后进行修复的外科手术。

blepharostasis 眼睑固定症

词根 blepharo-（眼睑的）+ -stasis（静止）
例句 Blepharostasis is a condition where the eyelids do not move properly. 眼睑固定症是一种眼睑无法正常运动的病症。

-bolic（变化的过程）

metabolic 新陈代谢的

词根 meta-（变化）+ -bolic（变化的过程）

例句 Metabolic disorders can affect the body's ability to convert food into energy. 新陈代谢障碍可能影响身体将食物转化为能量的能力。

anabolic 合成代谢的

词根 ana-（上升）+ -bolic（变化的过程）

例句 Anabolic processes help build and repair tissues in the body. 合成代谢过程有助于在体内构建和修复组织。

catabolic 分解代谢的

词根 cata-（下降）+ -bolic（变化的过程）

例句 Catabolic reactions break down molecules into smaller units, releasing energy. 分解代谢反应将分子分解成更小的单位，释放能量。

amphibolic 两性代谢的

词根 amphi-（两性）+ -bolic（变化的过程）

例句 Amphibolic pathways serve both anabolic and catabolic functions. 两性代谢途径既服务于合成代谢，也服务于分解代谢功能。

exabolic 外源性代谢的

词根 exo-（外部）+ -bolic（变化的过程）

例句 Exabolic processes involve substances originating outside the body. 外源性代谢过程涉及来自体外的物质。

brady-（慢）

bradycardia 心动过缓

词根 brady-（慢）+ cardia（心脏）

例句 Bradycardia is a condition where the heart rate is slower than normal. 心动过缓是心率低于正常水平的病症。

bradykinin 缓激肽

词根 brady-（慢）+ kinin（激肽）

例句 Bradykinin is a peptide that causes blood vessels to dilate. 缓激肽是一种肽，能引起血管扩张。

bradyarrhythmia 缓慢心律失常

词根 brady-（慢）+ arrhythmia（心律失常）

例句 Bradyarrhythmia refers to abnormal heart rhythms that are slower than normal. 缓慢心律失常指的是心跳比正常情况下慢的异常心律。

bradyphasia 言语迟缓

词根 brady-（慢）+ phasia（言语）

例句 Bradyphasia involves a delay in the ability to speak or formulate words. 言语迟缓涉及说话或组织语言能力的延迟。

bradypsychia 心理迟缓

词根 brady-（慢）+ psychia（心理）

例句 Bradypsychia refers to a slowed thought process. 心理迟缓指的是思维过程的迟缓。

bradyphagia 吞咽迟缓

词根 brady-（慢）+ phagia（吞咽）

例句 Bradyphagia refers to slow or difficulty in swallowing. 吞咽

迟缓指的是吞咽过程的缓慢或困难。

bradythermia 低体温

词根 brady-（慢）+ thermia（体温）
例句 Bradythermia is characterized by an abnormally low body temperature. 低体温以异常低的体温为特征。

bradysonia 听力迟缓

词根 brady-（慢）+ sonia（听力）
例句 Bradysonia is the condition of delayed or slower hearing response. 听力迟缓是指听觉反应迟缓或缓慢的状态。

bradyspasm 缓慢痉挛

词根 brady-（慢）+ spasm（痉挛）
例句 Bradyspasm is a condition where muscle spasms occur at a slower rate. 缓慢痉挛是指肌肉痉挛发生的速度较慢。

bradyretina 视网膜迟缓

词根 brady-（慢）+ retina（视网膜）
例句 Bradyretina refers to a slow or delayed retinal response to light. 视网膜迟缓是指视网膜对光的反应较慢或延迟。

bronchio-（小支气管）

bronchiolitis 小支气管炎

词根 bronchio-（小支气管）+ -itis（炎症）
例句 Bronchiolitis is a common respiratory illness in young children, characterized by inflammation of the bronchioles. 小支气管炎是幼龄儿童常见的呼吸道疾病，特征是小支气管的炎症。

bronchiolitis obliterans 小支气管闭塞性病

词根 bronchio-（小支气管）+ obliterans（闭塞）
例句 Bronchiolitis obliterans is a condition where the small airways

become narrowed or obstructed. 小支气管闭塞性病是一种小气道变窄或堵塞的疾病。

bronchiogenic 小支气管源的

词根 bronchio-（小支气管）+ -genic（源的）

例句 Bronchiogenic carcinoma originates in the small bronchi and can spread to the lungs. 小支气管源性癌症起源于小支气管，并可能扩散到肺部。

bronchioplasty 支气管成形术

词根 bronchio-（小支气管）+ -plasty（修复）

例句 Bronchioplasty is a surgical procedure used to repair the bronchi after injury. 支气管成形术是一种修复受损支气管的外科手术。

bronchiolitis respiratoria 小支气管呼吸炎症

词根 bronchio-（小支气管）+ respiratoria（呼吸的）

例句 Bronchiolitis respiratoria causes difficulty breathing due to inflammation of the bronchioles. 小支气管呼吸炎症因小支气管发炎导致呼吸困难。

bronchiostenosis 支气管狭窄

词根 bronchio-（小支气管）+ -stenosis（狭窄）

例句 Bronchiostenosis is the narrowing of the bronchi due to inflammation or other conditions. 支气管狭窄是由于炎症或其他病症引起的支气管变窄。

bronchiogenic carcinoma 小支气管癌

词根 bronchio-（小支气管）+ -genic（源的）+ carcinoma（癌症）

例句 Bronchiogenic carcinoma can cause persistent coughing and shortness of breath. 小支气管癌可能导致持续咳嗽和呼吸急促。

bronchiology 支气管学

词根 bronchio-（小支气管）+ -ology（学科）

例句 Bronchiology is the study of the bronchi and related diseases. 支气管学是研究支气管及相关疾病的学科。

bronchiotomy 支气管切开术

词根 bronchio-（小支气管）+ -otomy（切开）
例句 A bronchiotomy is performed to relieve airway obstruction. 支气管切开术用于缓解气道阻塞。

bronchioscopy 支气管镜检查

词根 bronchio-（小支气管）+ -scopy（检查）
例句 Bronchioscopy is a procedure used to view the inside of the bronchi. 支气管镜检查是一种用于查看支气管内部的程序。

broncho-（支气管）

bronchoscopy 支气管镜检查

词根 broncho-（支气管）+ -scopy（检查）
例句 Bronchoscopy allows doctors to examine the airways for signs of infection or disease. 支气管镜检查可使医生检查气道中是否有感染或其他疾病的迹象。

bronchitis 支气管炎

词根 broncho-（支气管）+ -itis（炎症）
例句 Bronchitis is an inflammation of the bronchial tubes, often caused by a viral infection. 支气管炎是支气管的炎症，通常由病毒感染引起。

bronchospasm 支气管痉挛

词根 broncho-（支气管）+ spasm（痉挛）
例句 Bronchospasm is the sudden constriction of the bronchial muscles, leading to breathing difficulties. 支气管痉挛是指支气管肌肉突然收缩，导致呼吸困难。

bronchiectasis 支气管扩张症

词根 broncho-（支气管）+ -ectasis（扩张）

例句 Bronchiectasis is a condition where the bronchial tubes are permanently enlarged. 支气管扩张症是支气管永久性扩张的病症。

bronchography 支气管造影

词根 broncho-（支气管）+ -graphy（成像）

例句 Bronchography is an imaging technique used to view the bronchi and lungs. 支气管造影是一种成像技术，用于查看支气管和肺部。

bronchodilator 支气管扩张剂

词根 broncho-（支气管）+ dilator（扩张剂）

例句 Bronchodilators are used to relax and open the air passages in the lungs. 支气管扩张剂用于舒张肺部的气道。

bronchial asthma 支气管哮喘

词根 bronchial（支气管的）+ asthma（哮喘）

例句 Bronchial asthma is a condition that causes the bronchial tubes to narrow, making breathing difficult. 支气管哮喘是一种导致支气管狭窄，引发呼吸困难的病症。

bronchoplasty 支气管成形术

词根 broncho-（支气管）+ -plasty（修复）

例句 Bronchoplasty is a surgical procedure to repair damaged bronchial tubes. 支气管成形术是一种修复受损支气管的外科手术。

bronchogenic 支气管源的

词根 broncho-（支气管）+ -genic（产生的）

例句 Bronchogenic carcinoma is a type of lung cancer that originates in the bronchi. 支气管源性癌症是一种起源于支气管的肺癌类型。

USMLE Step 1 样题

A 32-year-old man comes to the office because of a 1-day history of cough productive of small amounts of blood and a 2-day history of shortness of breath and swelling of his ankles. He also has a 2-week history of progressive fatigue and episodes of dark urine. He has no history of major medical illness and takes no medications. His temperature is 37°C (98.6°F), pulse is 90/min, respirations (re-;spir-; -ation) are 18/min, and blood pressure is 175/110 mmHg. Pulse oximetry (oxi-; -metry) on room air shows an oxygen saturation of 91%. Diffuse inspiratory (in-; spir-; -ation) crackles are heard over all lung bases. There is 2+ pitting edema of both ankles. Results of laboratory studies are shown:

Hemoglobin (hemo-; -globin) 8.9 g/dL

Hematocrit (hemato-; -crit) 27%

Serum urea nitrogen 55 mg/dL

Creatinine (creat-) 2.9 mg/dL

Urine RBC 20–40/hpf

Urinalysis (urina-; -lysis) also shows some dysmorphic (dys-; morp-) RBCs and rare RBC casts. Examination of a kidney biopsy specimen shows crescentic (crescent-) glomerulonephritis (glomerulo-; nephr-; -itis) and linear deposition of IgG along the glomerular capillaries (capill-). This patient most likely has antibodies (anti-;-body) directed against which of the following antigens?

(A) Collagen

(B) Double-stranded DNA

(C) Nucleolar protein

(D) Phospholipid (phosph-; -lipid)

(E) Proteins in neutrophil (neutro-; -phil) cytoplasm (cyto-; -plasm)

中文翻译

一名 32 岁的男性因咳嗽 1 天并伴有少量咯血，呼吸急促和脚踝肿胀 2 天，前来就诊。他近 2 周来逐渐出现疲劳乏力，并伴有尿液颜色加深。他没有重大疾病史，也没有服用任何药物。他的体温为 37℃（98.6℉），脉搏为 90 次 / 分钟，呼吸为 18 次 / 分钟，血压为 175/110 mmHg。室内空气下的血氧饱和度为 91%。双肺底可闻及弥漫性的吸气性啰音。双侧脚踝有 2+ 级凹陷性水肿。实验室检查结果如下：

血红蛋白 8.9 g/dL

血细胞比容 27%

血清尿素氮 55 mg/dL

肌酐 2.9 mg/dL

尿液红细胞 20 ～ 40/ 高倍视野

尿液分析还显示存在畸形红细胞和稀有红细胞管型。肾活检样本检查显示新月体性肾小球肾炎，且 IgG 沿肾小球毛细血管线性沉积。该患者最可能针对以下哪种抗原产生抗体？

(A) 胶原

(B) 双链 DNA

(C) 核仁蛋白

(D) 磷脂

(E) 中性粒细胞细胞质中的蛋白质

题目和答案中出现的词根

re-：重新；反复

spir-：呼吸

-ation：表示动作的状态

oxi-：氧气的

-metry：测量

in-：向内（向内呼吸，表示吸气）

hemo-：血

-globin：球蛋白

hemato-：血

-crit：分离法

creat-：肉的

urina-：尿的

-lysis：分解（这里指尿液成分分解的检测）

dys-：困难的；异常的；错误的

morph-：形状

crescent-：新月的

glomerulo-：小球

nephr-：肾脏的

-itis：炎症

capill-：毛发

anti-：抗

-body：体

phosph-：磷

-lipid：脂

neurto-：中性的

-phil：嗜

cyto-：细胞的

-plasm：浆液（cytoplasm 是细胞内除了细胞核外的所有物质综合，包括细胞浆和细胞器；cytosol 特指细胞浆，即除去细胞核和细胞器的半胶体状液体）

burs-（关节减震囊的）

bursitis 滑囊炎

词根 burs-（关节减震囊的）+ -itis（炎症）
例句 Bursitis is the inflammation of the bursa, typically due to repetitive motion or pressure. 滑囊炎是滑囊的炎症，通常是由反复运动或压力引起的。

bursa 滑囊

词根 burs-（关节减震囊的）
例句 The bursa is a small, fluid-filled sac that helps reduce friction and cushion pressure points. 滑囊是一个小的充液囊，帮助减少摩擦并缓冲压力点。

bursoplasty 滑囊成形术

词根 burs-（关节减震囊的）+ -plasty（修复）
例句 Bursoplasty is a surgical procedure used to repair or remove an inflamed bursa. 滑囊成形术是一种修复或去除炎症滑囊的外科手术。

bursostatic 滑囊静态的

词根 burs-（关节减震囊的）+ -static（静态的）
例句 Bursostatic agents are used to reduce the inflammation and swelling of bursae in the body. 滑囊静态药物用于减少体内滑囊的炎症和肿胀。

bursectomy 滑囊切除术

词根 burs-（关节减震囊的）+ -ectomy（切除术）

例句 Bursectomy is the surgical removal of an inflamed bursa to relieve pain. 滑囊切除术是去除发炎滑囊的外科手术，用以缓解疼痛。

bursopathia 滑囊病

词根 burs-（关节减震囊的）+ -pathia（病）

例句 Bursopathia refers to a group of diseases affecting the bursae, often leading to inflammation and pain. 滑囊病是指影响滑囊的一组疾病，通常导致炎症和疼痛。

C

calc-（钙）

calcium 钙元素

词根 calc-（钙）+ -ium（元素）

例句 Calcium is an essential mineral for bone health and muscle function. 钙是维持骨骼健康和肌肉功能所必需的矿物质。

calcification 钙化

词根 calc-（钙）+ -ification（形成）

例句 Calcification occurs when calcium builds up in the body's tissues, leading to hardening. 钙化是钙在体内组织中积聚，导致硬化的过程。

calciprotein 钙结合蛋白

词根 calc-（钙）+ -protein（蛋白质）

例句 Calciprotein is a protein that binds calcium and is important in bone formation. 钙结合蛋白是一种结合钙的蛋白质，对于骨骼形成非常重要。

calcaneus 跟骨

词根 calc-（钙）+ -aneus（足跟的）

例句 The calcaneus is the bone that forms the heel of the foot. 跟骨是构成脚跟的骨骼。

hypocalcemia 低钙血症

词根 hypo-（低）+ calc-（钙）+ -emia（血液）

例句 Hypocalcemia is a condition characterized by low calcium levels in the blood. 低钙血症是血液中钙水平过低的病症。

hypercalcemia 高钙血症

词根 hyper-（过高）+ calc-（钙）+ -emia（血液）

例句 Hypercalcemia is a condition where calcium levels in the blood are abnormally high. 高钙血症是一种血液中钙水平异常升高的病症。

calciparine 钙帕林

词根 calc-（钙）+ -parine（类似物）

例句 Calciparine is a calcium salt used in certain medical treatments. 钙帕林是一种在某些治疗中使用的钙盐。

calcitriol 钙三醇

词根 calc-（钙）+ -triol（三醇）

例句 Calcitriol is the active form of vitamin D that helps regulate calcium levels in the body. 钙三醇是维生素 D 的活性形式，有助于调节体内的钙水平。

calcuim carbonate 碳酸钙

词根 calc-（钙）+ -carbonate（碳酸盐）

例句 Calcium carbonate is commonly used as a calcium supplement. 碳酸钙常用于补充钙。

calcified 钙化的

词根 calc-（钙）+ -ified（使……化）

例句 The arteries were calcified, which caused them to lose their flexibility. 动脉钙化，导致其失去弹性。

calva-（颅盖）

calvaria 颅盖

词根 calva-（颅盖）+ -ria（名词后缀）

例句 The calvaria is the upper part of the skull that protects the brain. 颅盖是保护大脑的颅骨上部。

calvarial 颅盖的

词根 calva-（颅盖）+ -ial（形容词后缀）
例句 The calvarial fracture was carefully treated with a surgical procedure. 颅盖骨折经过外科手术谨慎治疗。

calvarium 颅盖

词根 calva-（颅盖）+ -ium（名词后缀）
例句 The calvarium is the dome-like structure at the top of the skull. 颅盖是颅骨顶部像圆顶一样的结构。

calvectomy 颅盖切除术

词根 calva-（颅盖）+ -ectomy（切除术）
例句 Calvectomy is a surgical procedure to remove part of the calvaria. 颅盖切除术是切除部分颅盖的手术。

calvarial vault 颅盖拱顶

词根 calva-（颅盖）+ vault（拱顶）
例句 The calvarial vault refers to the domed portion of the skull that covers the brain. 颅盖拱顶指的是覆盖大脑的颅骨圆顶部分。

calvarial bone 颅盖

词根 calva-（颅盖）+ bone（骨）
例句 The calvarial bone plays a crucial role in protecting the brain from physical injury. 颅盖在保护大脑免受物理伤害方面起着关键作用。

calvans 颅盖

词根 calva-（颅盖）+ -ans（名词后缀）
例句 Calvans are skeletal structures within the skull that contribute to its formation. 颅盖是颅骨内构成其形态的骨骼结构。

subcalvaria 颅盖下的

词根 sub-（下）+ calva-（颅盖）+ -ial（形容词后缀）

例句 Subcalvarial infections occur beneath the calvaria and can affect the brain. 颅下感染发生在颅盖下，并可能影响大脑。

intracalvarial 颅盖内的

词根 intra-（内部）+ calva-（颅盖）+ -ial（形容词后缀）

例句 Intracalvarial pressure can increase due to head trauma or swelling. 由于头部创伤或肿胀，颅盖内的压力可能增加。

USMLE Step 1　样题

A 52-year-old woman comes to the office because of a 6-month history of intermittent (inter-; mitt-) headaches. Sometimes the pain improves when the patient lies down in a quiet room. Her temperature is 37.5°C (99.5°F), pulse is 86/min, respirations (re-; spir-; -ation) are 16/min, and blood pressure is 154/100 mmHg. The lungs are clear. Cardiac examination shows the point of maximal impulse displaced to the left and occasional skipped beats; there are no murmurs or rubs. There is no S3. Resting electrocardiography (electro-; cardio-; -grapy) shows left axis deviation with R waves greater than 30 mm in leads V5 through V6. Which of the following processes best explains the development of the left ventricular abnormalities in this patient?

(A) Excessive accumulation of glycogen

(B) Fibrosis of intraventricular (intra-; ventric-) conduction pathways

(C) Increased synthesis of contractile filaments

(D) Misfolding (mis-) and aggregation of cytoskeletal (cyto-) proteins

(E) Myocyte (myo-; -cyte) hyperplasia (hyper-; -plasia) as a result of induction of embryonic genes

中文翻译

一位 52 岁的女性因持续 6 个月的间歇性头痛前来就诊。患者有时在安静的房间里躺下后，头痛有所缓解。她的体温为 37.5°C（99.5°F），脉搏为 86 次 / 分钟，呼吸为 16 次 / 分钟，血压为 154/100 mmHg。肺部检查正常。心脏检查显示心尖搏动偏左，偶见漏搏；没有杂音或摩擦音。未闻及 S3 心音。静息心电图显示左轴偏移，V5 至 V6 导联 R 波振幅大于 30 mm。以下哪项机制最能解释此患者左心室的异常？

(A) 糖原过度积累

(B) 室内传导通路的纤维化

(C) 收缩丝的合成增加

(D) 细胞骨架蛋白的错误折叠和聚集

(E) 胚胎基因诱导导致的心肌细胞增生

题目和答案中出现的词根

inter-：在……之间

mitt-：时间区间

re-：重新；反复

spir-：呼吸

-ation：表示动作的状态

electro-：电的

cardio-：心脏的

-graphy：图像

intra-：在……内

ventric-：室的（这里指心室的）

mis-：错误的

cyto-：细胞的

myo-：肌肉

hyper-：高

-plasia：生长（指数量的增长，需要和 hypertrophy 区分，hypertrophy 指的是体积的增长）

campylo-（弯曲的）

campylobacter 弯曲菌

词根 campylo-（弯曲）+ -bacter（细菌）

例句 Campylobacter is a type of bacteria that can cause foodborne illnesses. 弯曲菌是一种能够引起食源性疾病的细菌。

campylomorph 弯曲形态

词根 campylo-（弯曲）+ -morph（形态）

例句 Campylomorph refers to organisms that have a curved or spiral shape. 弯曲形态是指具有弯曲或螺旋形状的生物。

campylous 弯曲的

词根 campylo-（弯曲）+ -ous（形容词后缀）

例句 Campylous bacteria are known for their characteristic spiral shape. 弯曲的细菌因其特有的螺旋形状而闻名。

campylography 弯曲图谱

词根 campylo-（弯曲）+ -graphy（记录；描写）

例句 Campylography is the process of recording the spiral shapes of certain microorganisms. 弯曲图谱记录某些微生物的螺旋形态。

campylocytic 弯曲细胞

词根 campylo-（弯曲）+ -cytic（细胞的）

例句 Campylocytic cells have a distinctive curved shape compared to other cell types. 弯曲细胞与其他细胞类型相比具有独特的弯曲形状。

campyloarthritis 弯曲性关节炎

词根 campylo-（弯曲）+ -arthritis（关节炎）

例句 Campyloarthritis is a type of joint inflammation associated with a curved infection. 弯曲性关节炎是一种与弯曲感染相关的关节炎类型。

campylothermophilic 耐热弯曲菌

词根 campylo-（弯曲）+ thermophilic（耐热的）

例句 Campylothermophilic bacteria thrive in hot environments and have a curved shape. 耐热弯曲菌在高温环境中生长良好，且呈弯曲形状。

campylotropism 弯曲趋性

词根 campylo-（弯曲）+ -tropism（趋向）

例句 Campylotropism is the movement of bacteria in response to their curved structure. 弯曲趋性是细菌对其弯曲结构做出反应的运动。

campylobacteriosis 弯曲菌病

词根 campylo-（弯曲）+ bacterio-（细菌）+ -osis（病态）

例句 Campylobacteriosis is an infection caused by the campylobacter bacteria. 弯曲菌病是由弯曲菌引起的感染。

campylocephalus 弯曲头部

词根 campylo-（弯曲）+ cephalus（头部）

例句 Campylocephalus refers to organisms with a curved head shape. 弯曲头部指的是生物具有弯曲的头部形状。

capn-（二氧化碳）

capnography 二氧化碳图谱

词根 capn-（二氧化碳）+ -graphy（记录；描写）

例句 Capnography is used to monitor the concentration of carbon dioxide in the exhaled air. 二氧化碳图谱用于监测呼气中的二氧化碳浓度。

capnometry 二氧化碳测量法

词根 capn-（二氧化碳）+ -metry（测量）

例句 Capnometry is the measurement of carbon dioxide levels during respiratory assessment. 二氧化碳测量法是在呼吸评估过程中测量二氧化碳水平。

capnocytophaga 二氧化碳嗜细胞菌

词根 capn-（二氧化碳）+ cytophaga（细胞食菌）

例句 Capnocytophaga is a genus of bacteria that thrive in the presence of carbon dioxide. 二氧化碳嗜细胞菌是一种在二氧化碳环境中繁殖的细菌属。

capnophilic 嗜二氧化碳细菌

词根 capn-（二氧化碳）+ -philic（喜好的）

例句 Capnophilic bacteria are microorganisms that thrive in high carbon dioxide environments. 嗜二氧化碳细菌是在高二氧化碳环境中繁殖的微生物。

capnology 二氧化碳学

词根 capn-（二氧化碳）+ -logy（学科）

例句 Capnology is the study of carbon dioxide levels in the body, particularly in relation to breathing. 二氧化碳学是研究体内二氧化碳水平及其与呼吸功能关联的学科。

hypercapnia 高碳酸血症

词根 hyper-（过度）+ capn-（二氧化碳）+ -ia（病态）

例句 Hypercapnia is a condition characterized by an excessive amount of carbon dioxide in the blood. 高碳酸血症是指血液中二氧化碳过多的病症。

hypocapnia 低碳酸血症

词根 hypo-（不足）+ capn-（二氧化碳）+ -ia（病态）

例句 Hypocapnia is a condition characterized by low levels of carbon dioxide in the blood. 低碳酸血症是指血液中二氧化碳水平低的病症。

capnometric 测量二氧化碳的

词根 capn-（二氧化碳）+ -metric（测量的）

例句 Capnometric devices are used to measure the carbon dioxide concentration during surgery. 二氧化碳测量设备用于在手术过程中测量二氧化碳浓度。

capnohemia 二氧化碳血症

词根 capn-（二氧化碳）+ -hemia（血液）

例句 Capnohemia is the presence of excessive carbon dioxide in the blood. 二氧化碳血症是指血液中二氧化碳过多的状态。

capnocytosis 二氧化碳细胞病

词根 capn-（二氧化碳）+ cytosis（细胞状态）

例句 Capnocytosis refers to the increased levels of carbon dioxide in the cells. 二氧化碳细胞病指的是细胞中二氧化碳浓度的增加。

carboxyl-（羧基）

carboxyl 羧基

词根 carboxyl-（羧基）

例句 The carboxyl group is a functional group found in many organic compounds. 羧基是许多有机化合物中存在的一个官能团。

carboxylation 羧基化

词根 carboxyl-（羧基）+ -ation（名词后缀）

例句 Carboxylation is the process of introducing a carboxyl group into a molecule. 羧基化是将羧基引入分子中的过程。

carboxylase 羧化酶

词根 carboxyl-（羧基）+ -ase（酶）

例句 Carboxylase is an enzyme that catalyzes the addition of a carboxyl group to a substrate. 羧化酶是一种催化羧基添加到底物上的酶。

carboxylic 羧基的

词根 carboxyl-（羧基）+ -ic（形容词后缀）

例句 Carboxylic acids are a group of organic acids that contain a carboxyl group. 羧酸是一类含有羧基的有机酸。

carboxylate 羧基化

词根 carboxyl-（羧基）+ -ate（动词后缀）

例句 The reaction causes the molecule to carboxylate, introducing a carboxyl group. 反应导致分子发生羧基化，引入一个羧基。

carboxymethylation 羧甲基化

词根 carboxyl-（羧基）+ methyl（甲基）

例句 Carboxymethylation is the process of attaching a carboxymethyl group to a molecule. 羧甲基化是将羧甲基团附加到分子上的过程。

carboxymethylcellulose 羧甲基纤维素

词根 carboxyl-（羧基）+ methyl（甲基）+ cellulose（纤维素）
例句 Carboxymethylcellulose is used as a thickening agent in the food industry. 羧甲基纤维素被用作食品加工中的增稠剂。

decarboxylation 脱羧化

词根 de-（去除）+ carboxyl-（羧基）+ -ation（动作或过程）
例句 Decarboxylation is the removal of a carboxyl group from a molecule, often releasing carbon dioxide. 脱羧化是去除分子中的羧基，通常伴随二氧化碳的释放。

carboxyhemoglobin 羧基血红蛋白

词根 carboxyl-（羧基）+ hemoglobin（血红蛋白）
例句 Carboxyhemoglobin forms when carbon monoxide binds to hemoglobin. 羧基血红蛋白是指一氧化碳与血红蛋白结合形成的产物。

monocarboxylate 单羧酸盐

词根 mono-（单一的）+ carboxylate（羧酸盐）
例句 Monocarboxylate is a molecule that contains only one carboxyl group. 单羧酸盐是一种只包含一个羧基的分子。

USMLE Step 1　样题

A 39-year-old man comes to the physician because of a 6-month history of progressive shortness of breath. He has had a cough productive of white sputum for 2 years. He smoked 1 pack of cigarettes daily for 16 years but quit 10 years ago. He is in mild respiratory (re-; spir-) distress with pursed lips and a barrel chest;

he is using the accessory muscles of respiration (re-; spir-; -ation). Breath sounds are distant and crackles are present in the lower lung fields bilaterally (bi-; lateral). Pulmonary (pulmon-) function tests show a decreased FEV1:FVC ratio, increased residual volume, and decreased diffusion capacity. An X-ray of the chest shows hyperinflation (hyper-; -inflation) and hypertranslucency (hyper-; trans-; luc) of the lower lobes of both lungs. Which of the following is the most likely diagnosis?

(A) Asthma

(B) Bronchiectasis (brochi-; -ectasis)

(C) Chronic pulmonary fibrosis

(D) Cystic fibrosis

(E) Emphysema (em-; phys-; -ema)

中文翻译

一名 39 岁男性因 6 个月来渐进性呼吸困难前来就诊。患者持续 2 年咳白色痰，既往有每日 1 包香烟、持续 16 年的吸烟史，但已于 10 年前戒烟。查体可见患者呈轻度呼吸窘迫状态，表现为撅唇呼吸及桶状胸，并动用辅助呼吸肌参与呼吸运动。双肺下野呼吸音减弱，双侧可闻及湿啰音。肺功能检查显示第 1 秒用力呼气量与用力肺活量比值降低、残气量增加、弥散功能下降。胸部 X 线片显示双肺下叶过度充气及透光度增高。以下哪项是最可能的诊断？

(A) 哮喘

(B) 支气管扩张症

(C) 慢性肺纤维化

(D) 囊性纤维化

(E) 肺气肿

题目和答案中出现的词根

re-：重新；反复

spir-：呼吸

bi-：双

-lateral：侧面

pulmon-：肺的

hyper-：高

-inflation：充气

trans-：跨；转

luc：光（这里指可以透过 X 线，在胸片显示为黑色）

bronchi-：支气管的

-ectasis：扩张

em-：在内的

phys-：气体

-ema：病态（气体在内的病态指的是肺气肿，“在内”指的是在肺泡内，但气体本来就在肺泡内，表现出病态的原因是肺泡融合引起气体在肺内蓄积过多）

carcino-（癌症的）

carcinoma 癌

词根 carcino-（癌症）+ -oma（肿瘤）

例句 Carcinoma is a type of cancer that starts in the epithelial cells, such as skin or organ linings. 癌是一种起源于上皮细胞的恶性肿

瘤，常见于皮肤或器官内表面等部位。

carcinogenesis 致癌作用

词根 carcino-（癌症）+ -genesis（产生）

例句 Carcinogenesis is the process by which normal cells are transformed into cancer cells. 致癌作用是正常细胞转变为癌细胞的过程。

carcinogenic 致癌的

词根 carcino-（癌症）+ -genic（产生的）

例句 Carcinogenic substances are chemicals or agents that can cause cancer in living tissues. 致癌物质是能够引发癌症的化学物质或因子。

carcinoma in situ 原位癌

词根 carcino-（癌症）+ -oma（肿瘤）+ in situ（原位）

例句 Carcinoma in situ refers to a cancerous growth that has not spread beyond the original site. 原位癌指的是一种未扩散到原位以外的癌性病变。

carcinomatosis 癌症广泛转移

词根 carcino-（癌症）+ -matosis（转移）

例句 Carcinomatosis occurs when cancer spreads throughout the body, often in the form of multiple tumors. 癌症广泛转移是指癌症扩散到全身，通常以多个肿瘤的形式出现。

carcinoembryonic antigen 癌胚抗原

词根 carcino-（癌症）+ embryonic（胚胎）+ antigen（抗原）

例句 Carcinoembryonic antigen（CEA）is a protein found in certain cancers and is used as a tumor marker in clinical tests. 癌胚抗原（CEA）是一种在某些癌症中发现的蛋白质，常用作临床测试中的肿瘤标志物。

carcinoid tumor 类癌肿瘤

词根 carcino-（癌症）+ -oid（类似的）+ tumor（肿瘤）

例句 A carcinoid tumor is a slow-growing cancer that often develops in the gastrointestinal system or lungs. 类癌肿瘤是一种生长缓慢的癌症，通常发生在胃肠系统或肺部。

carcinosarcoma 癌肉瘤

词根 carcino-（癌症）+ -sarcoma（肉瘤）

例句 Carcinosarcoma is a rare cancer that contains both carcinomatous and sarcomatous tissue components. 癌肉瘤是一种罕见的癌症，包含癌性和肉瘤性组织成分。

cardi-（心脏）

cardiology 心脏病学

词根 cardi-（心脏）+ -ology（学科）

例句 Cardiology is the branch of medicine that deals with the diagnosis and treatment of heart diseases. 心脏病学是研究心脏疾病的诊断和治疗的医学分支。

cardiovascular 心血管的

词根 cardi-（心脏）+ vascular（血管的）

例句 Cardiovascular diseases refer to conditions affecting the heart and blood vessels. 心血管疾病指的是影响心脏和血管的疾病。

cardiotonic 强心的

词根 cardi-（心脏）+ -tonic（增强的）

例句 Cardiotonic drugs are used to strengthen the heart's contraction force. 强心药用于增强心脏的收缩力。

cardiomegaly 心脏肥大

词根 cardi-（心脏）+ -megaly（肿大）

例句 Cardiomegaly is a condition where the heart becomes abnormally enlarged. 心脏肥大是一种心脏异常增大的病症。

cardiotoxic 有心脏毒性的

词根 cardi-（心脏）+ toxic（有毒的）

例句 Certain chemotherapy drugs can be cardiotoxic, leading to heart damage. 某些化疗药物可能具有心脏毒性，导致心脏损伤。

cardiopathy 心脏病

词根 cardi-（心脏）+ -pathy（病）

例句 Cardiopathy is a general term for heart diseases. 心脏病是指心脏疾病的总称。

cardiogenic 心源性的

词根 cardi-（心脏）+ -genic（产生的）

例句 Cardiogenic shock occurs when the heart is unable to pump sufficient blood to the organs. 心源性休克是指当心脏无法将足够的血液输送到器官时发生的情况。

cardioprotective 保护心脏的

词根 cardi-（心脏）+ protective（保护的）

例句 Certain medications have cardioprotective effects, reducing the risk of heart attack. 某些药物具有心脏保护作用，降低心脏病发作的风险。

cardiomyopathy 心肌病

词根 cardi-（心脏）+ myo-（肌肉）+ -pathy（病）

例句 Cardiomyopathy refers to diseases of the heart muscle that affect its function. 心肌病指的是影响心脏肌肉功能的心脏病。

electrocardiogram 心电图

词根 electro-（电）+ cardi-（心脏）+ -gram（记录）

例句 An electrocardiogram（ECG）is used to monitor the electrical activity of the heart. 心电图（ECG）用于监测心脏的电活动。

carp（o）-（腕）

carpal 腕骨

词根 carp-（腕）+ -al（形容词后缀）

例句 The carpal bones are a set of eight small bones that make up the wrist. 腕骨是一组由八块小骨组成的骨骼，构成了手腕。

carpitis 腕炎

词根 carp-（腕）+ -itis（炎症）

例句 Carpitis is an inflammation of the wrist joint. 腕炎是手腕关节的炎症。

carpalgia 腕痛

词根 carp-（腕）+ -algia（疼痛）

例句 Carpalgia is a condition characterized by wrist pain. 腕痛是一种以手腕疼痛为特征的病症。

carpectomy 腕切除术

词根 carp-（腕）+ -ectomy（切除术）

例句 Carpectomy is the surgical removal of part or all of the wrist joint. 腕切除术是手术切除部分或全部腕关节。

carpophalangeal 腕指关节

词根 carp-（腕）+ -phalangeal（指骨）

例句 The carpophalangeal joint is the joint between the wrist and the fingers. 腕指关节是手腕和手指之间的关节。

carpometacarpal 腕掌关节

词根 carp-（腕）+ -metacarpal（掌骨）

例句 The carpometacarpal joint connects the wrist with the palm of the hand. 腕掌关节连接手腕和手掌。

carpospasm 腕痉挛

词根 carp-（腕）+ -spasm（痉挛）

例句 Carpospasm refers to involuntary muscle contractions in the wrist. 腕痉挛是指手腕肌肉的不自主收缩。

carpography 腕图

词根 carp-（腕）+ -graphy（记录；描写）

例句 Carpography is the process of recording wrist movements. 腕图记录手腕运动。

carposcopy 腕镜检查

词根 carp-（腕）+ -scopy（检查）

例句 Carposcopy involves visual inspection of the wrist joint. 腕镜检查包括对手腕关节的视觉检查。

carpomalacia 腕骨软化症

词根 carp-（腕）+ -malacia（软化）

例句 Carpomalacia refers to the softening of the bones in the wrist. 腕骨软化症指的是手腕骨骼的软化。

cata-（向下；分解）

catabolism 分解代谢

词根 cata-（分解）+ -bolism（代谢）

例句 Catabolism is the process of breaking down molecules to release energy. 分解代谢是分解分子以释放能量的过程。

catatonic 紧张性的

词根 cata-（向下）+ tonic（紧张）

例句 Catatonic schizophrenia is a form of schizophrenia where the patient experiences immobility and stupor. 紧张性的精神分裂症是

一种精神分裂症类型，患者表现为运动不能和木僵状态。

catheter 导管

词根 cata-（向下）+ -ther（输送）

例句 A catheter is used to insert fluids into the body or drain them out. 导管用于向身体内输送液体或排出液体。

catacomb 地下墓穴

词根 cata-（向下）+ -comb（洞穴）

例句 The catacombs were used as burial places during ancient times. 这些地下墓穴在古代被用作墓地。

catalysis 催化

词根 cata-（分解）+ -lysis（分解）

例句 Catalysis is the process of increasing the rate of a chemical reaction by adding a substance. 催化是通过添加物质来加速化学反应速率的过程。

catalyst 催化剂

词根 cata-（分解）+ -lyst（促使者）

例句 A catalyst accelerates the chemical reactions without being consumed in the process. 催化剂在不被消耗的情况下加速化学反应。

catatonic state 昏迷状态

词根 cata-（向下）+ tonic（紧张）

例句 The patient was in a catatonic state, unresponsive to external stimuli. 患者处于昏迷状态，对外部刺激没有反应。

cataplexy 猝倒症

词根 cata-（向下）+ plex-（束缚）

例句 Cataplexy is the sudden loss of muscle strength triggered by strong emotions. 猝倒症是由强烈情绪引发的突发肌肉无力。

cavus-（弓；空）

cavum 腔

词根 cavus-（空）

例句 The cavum is a cavity or hollow space within the body, such as the ear canal. 腔是体内的一个空腔或空洞，如耳道。

cavitation 气蚀

词根 cavus-（空）+ -ation（动作或过程）

例句 Cavitation is the formation of cavities within a solid object or body. 气蚀是固体物体或身体内部形成空腔的过程。

cavum septi pellucidi 透明隔腔

词根 cavum-（空腔）+ septi（隔膜）+ pellucidi（透明的）

例句 The cavum septi pellucidi is a space in the brain between the two lateral ventricles. 透明隔腔是大脑中位于两侧脑室之间的空隙。

cavernous 海绵状的

词根 cavus-（空）+ -ous（形容词后缀）

例句 The cavernous sinus is a large vein located at the base of the skull. 海绵窦是位于颅底的大静脉。

cavus foot 高弓足

词根 cavus-（弓）+ foot（足）

例句 Cavus foot is a condition where the arch of the foot is excessively high. 高弓足是指足弓过高的足。

cavernoma 海绵状血管瘤

词根 cavern-（空）+ -oma（肿瘤）

例句 A cavernoma is a type of vascular tumor that forms a cavity in the brain or spinal cord. 海绵状血管瘤是一种血管肿瘤，形成脑部或脊髓中的空腔。

cavernicolous 穴居的

词根 cavern-（空）+ -icolous（居住的）

例句 Cavernicolous organisms live in caves or similar subterranean environments. 洞穴栖息生物生活在洞穴或类似的地下环境中。

cavum tympani 鼓室

词根 cavum-（空腔）+ tympani（鼓膜）

例句 The cavum tympani is the air-filled cavity in the middle ear. 鼓室是中耳中的充气腔。

cavum nasi 鼻腔

词根 cavum-（空腔）+ nasi（鼻）

例句 The cavum nasi refers to the nasal cavity, a hollow space inside the nose. 鼻腔是指鼻子的空腔，位于鼻内。

cavum mandibulae 下颌腔

词根 cavum-（空腔）+ mandibulae（下颌骨）

例句 The cavum mandibulae is the cavity within the mandible, or lower jawbone. 下颌腔是下颌骨内部的空腔。

USMLE Step 1　样题

A 34-year-old man comes to the office because of a 1-month history of diarrhea (dia-; -rrhea). He has a history of pheochromocytoma (pheo-; chrom-; cyt-; -oma) treated 2 years ago. His mother is being treated for a tumor of her parathyroid (para-; thyr-; -oid) gland. He has no other history of major medical illness and takes no medications. His temperature is 37.0°C (98.6°F), pulse is 84/min, respirations (re-; spir-; -ation) are 10/min, and blood pressure is 120/75 mmHg. Pulse oximetry (oxi-; -metry) on room air shows an oxygen saturation of 97%. Vital signs are within normal limits. Physical examination shows a 3-cm, palpable mass on the right side of the neck. A biopsy specimen of the mass shows a neuroendocrine (neuro-; endo-; -crine) neoplasm (neo-; -plasm) of parafollicular (para-; follicul-) cell origin. The most likely cause of the findings in this patient is a mutation in which of the following types of genes?

(A) Cell cycle regulation gene

(B) DNA mismatch (mis-) repair gene

(C) Metastasis (meta-; -statsis) suppressor gene

(D) Proto-oncogene (proto-; onco-; -gene)

(E) Tumor suppressor gene

中文翻译

一名 34 岁男性因持续 1 个月的腹泻就诊。他 2 年前曾患嗜铬细胞瘤并接受治疗。其母亲正在接受甲状旁腺肿瘤治疗。患者无其他重大疾病史，未服用任何药物。查体显示体温 37.0℃（98.6°F），脉搏 84 次 / 分，呼吸频率 10 次 / 分，血压 120/75 mmHg。室内空气下脉搏血氧仪显示血氧饱和度为 97%，生命体征均正常。体格检查发现右侧颈部可触及一 3 cm 肿块，肿块活检显示为滤泡旁细胞来源的神经内分泌肿瘤。该患者最可能的病因是以下哪类基因发生突变？

(A) 细胞周期调控基因

(B) DNA 错配修复基因

(C) 转移抑制基因

(D) 原癌基因

(E) 肿瘤抑制基因

题目和答案中出现的词根

dia-：通过（这里指通过肠道）

-rrhea：流出（通过肠道流出，指腹泻）

pheo-：深灰色（嗜铬细胞瘤细胞分泌的儿茶酚胺经过氧化在显微镜下呈深灰色）

chrom-：颜色

cyt-：细胞

-oma：瘤

para-：旁边

thyr-：盾

-oid：类似的（甲状腺的形状为类盾牌状）

re-：重新；反复

spir-：呼吸

-ation：表示动作的状态

oxi-：氧气的

-metry：测量仪

neuro-：神经的

endo-：内

-crine：分泌（这里指的是内分泌，即分泌入血。和它对应的外分泌，是分泌到体外，或者通向体外的解剖管道如胃肠道）

neo-：新的

-plasm：生长（新的生长，指肿瘤）

follicul-：滤泡

mis-：错误的

meta-：超过；在……后

-stasis：静止站立（超过静止站立的位置，表示转移）

proto-：原的（这里指被激活前的状态）

onco-：癌

-gene：基因

-cele（突出的结构）

hydrocele 水囊肿

词根 hydro-（水）+ -cele（突出的结构）

例句 A hydrocele is a fluid-filled sac around a testicle, causing swelling. 水囊肿是围绕睾丸的充液囊袋，导致肿胀。

meningocele 脑膜膨出

词根 meningo-（脑膜的）+ -cele（突出的结构）

例句 Meningocele occurs when the meninges protrude through an opening in the spine. 脑膜膨出是指脑膜通过脊柱的开口向外膨出的情况。

enterocele 肠膨出

词根 entero-（肠道）+ -cele（突出的结构）

例句 Enterocele is the protrusion of the small intestine into the pelvic cavity. 肠膨出是小肠膨出到盆腔的情况。

rectocele 直肠膨出

词根 recto-（直肠）+ -cele（突出的结构）

例句 Rectocele occurs when the wall of the rectum bulges into the vaginal area. 直肠膨出是指直肠壁膨出到阴道区域。

varicocele 精索静脉曲张

词根 varico-（静脉曲张）+ -cele（突出的结构）
例句 Varicocele refers to the enlargement of veins within the scrotum. 精索静脉曲张是指阴囊内静脉的肿胀。

centro-（中间）

centromere 着丝粒

词根 centro-（中间）+ -mere（部分）
例句 The centromere is the region of a chromosome where the sister chromatids are held together. 着丝粒是染色体上连接姐妹染色单体的区域。

centrosome 中心体

词根 centro-（中间）+ -some（体）
例句 The centrosome is the central body of a cell that organizes microtubules during cell division. 中心体是细胞的中央体，在细胞分裂过程中组织微管。

centropetal 向心的

词根 centro-（中间）+ -petal（向……的）
例句 Centropetal forces pull objects toward the center of a rotating body. 向心力是将物体拉向旋转体中心的力量。

centrosymmetric 中心对称的

词根 centro-（中间）+ -symmetric（对称的）
例句 The centrosymmetric molecule has symmetry about its central point. 中心对称分子围绕其中心点具有对称性。

centrocyte 中心细胞

词根 centro-（中间）+ -cyte（细胞）

例句 The centrocyte is a type of B cell that plays a role in immune responses. 中心细胞是参与免疫反应的 B 细胞类型。

centroblast 中心芽细胞

词根 centro-（中间）+ -blast（芽细胞）

例句 The centroblast is a rapidly proliferating B cell found in germinal centers during an immune response. 中心芽细胞是在免疫反应中出现在生发中心的快速增殖 B 细胞。

centrofugal 离心的

词根 centro-（中间）+ -fugal（远离的）

例句 Centrofugal nerve fibers carry impulses away from the central nervous system. 离心神经纤维将冲动从中枢神经系统传出。

centrosomal 中心体的

词根 centro-（中间）+ -somal（体的）

例句 Centrosomal proteins are involved in the organization of the microtubule network in cells. 中心体蛋白参与细胞中微管网络的组织。

centroplasm 中心质

词根 centro-（中间）+ -plasm（质）

例句 Centroplasm refers to the cytoplasm surrounding the centrosome in a cell. 中心质是细胞中围绕中心体的细胞质。

centromeric 着丝粒的

词根 centro-（中间）+ -meric（的）

例句 Centromeric regions are essential for proper chromosome segregation during cell division. 着丝粒区域对细胞分裂期间染色体的正常分离至关重要。

centrogenic 中间生成的

词根 centro-（中间）+ -genic（生成的）

例句 Centrogenic disorders are related to abnormalities in the central regions of chromosomes. 中心粒源性染色体病与染色体中央区域的异常有关。

centrocytosis 中心细胞增生

词根 centro-（中间）+ -cytosis（细胞增生）

例句 Centrocytosis refers to the increased number of centrocytes in the lymphoid tissue during an immune response. 中心细胞增生指的是在免疫反应期间淋巴组织中中心细胞数量的增加。

centronuclear 中心核的

词根 centro-（中间）+ -nuclear（核的）

例句 Centronuclear myopathy is a type of muscular dystrophy where the nuclei are abnormally located at the center of muscle fibers. 中心核型肌营养不良症是一种肌肉萎缩症，特征是肌肉纤维中的细胞核异常地位于中心。

centroplacental 中心胎盘的

词根 centro-（中间）+ -placental（胎盘的）

例句 Centroplacental structure refers to the central arrangement of tissues in certain placental mammals. 中心胎盘结构指的是某些胎盘哺乳动物胎盘组织呈中央排列。

centroblastic 中心芽细胞的

词根 centro-（中间）+ -blastic（芽细胞的）

例句 Centroblastic lymphoma is a type of cancer that affects centroblasts. 中心芽细胞淋巴瘤是一种影响中心芽细胞的癌症。

centrospheral 中心球的

词根 centro-（中间）+ -spheral（球的）

例句 Centrospheral cells are spherical cells found in the central regions of certain tissues. 中心球细胞是存在于某些组织中央区域的球形细胞。

centrocytolytic 中心细胞溶解的

词根 centro-（中间）+ -cytolytic（细胞溶解的）
例句 Centrocytolytic activity refers to the destruction of centrocytes in immune responses. 中心细胞溶解活性指的是在免疫反应中中心细胞的破坏。

centrolobular 中心小叶的

词根 centro-（中间）+ -lobular（小叶的）
例句 Centrolobular necrosis refers to the death of cells in the central part of the liver lobules. 中心小叶坏死是指肝小叶中央部分细胞的死亡。

cephal-（脑的）

cephalalgia 头痛

词根 cephal-（脑）+ -algia（疼痛）
例句 Cephalalgia is the medical term for headache. 头痛是指头部的疼痛。

cephalometry 头部测量

词根 cephal-（脑）+ -metry（测量）
例句 Cephalometry is the measurement of the dimensions of the head. 头部测量是测量头部的尺寸。

cephalopod 头足类动物

词根 cephal-（脑）+ -pod（足）
例句 Cephalopods are marine animals like squids and octopuses with well-developed brains. 头足类动物是像鱿鱼和章鱼这样的海洋动物，具有发达的大脑。

C

cephalic 头静脉

词根 cephal-（脑）+ -ic（形容词后缀）

例句 Cephalic veins are those that are located in the head and neck area. 头静脉是位于头部和颈部区域的静脉。

cephalothorax 头胸部

词根 cephal-（脑）+ thorax（胸部）

例句 The cephalothorax is the combined head and thorax in some arthropods, like spiders. 头胸部是一些节肢动物（如蜘蛛）中结合头部和胸部的区域。

cephalitis 脑炎

词根 cephal-（脑）+ -itis（炎症）

例句 Cephalitis is an inflammation of the brain, usually caused by infection. 脑炎是脑部的炎症，通常由感染引起。

cephalocentesis 脑穿刺术

词根 cephal-（脑）+ -centesis（穿刺）

例句 Cephalocentesis is a surgical procedure used to remove fluid from the brain. 脑穿刺术是一种用于从大脑中抽取液体的外科手术。

cephalospinal 脑脊液

词根 cephal-（脑）+ spinal（脊髓的）

例句 The cephalospinal fluid is the liquid that surrounds the brain and spinal cord. 脑脊液是环绕大脑和脊髓的液体。

cephalocervical 头颈部的

词根 cephal-（脑）+ cervical（颈部的）

例句 Cephalocervical disorders affect both the head and neck regions. 头颈疾病影响头部和颈部区域。

cephalosporin 头孢菌素

词根 cephal-（脑）+ -sporin（抗生素）

例句 Cephalosporins are a class of antibiotics used to treat bacterial infections. 头孢菌素是一类用于治疗细菌感染的抗生素。

-ception（感知）

perception 感知

词根 per-（通过）+ -ception（感知）

例句 Perception is the process of interpreting sensory information from the environment. 感知是解释来自环境的感觉信息的过程。

conception 怀孕；受孕

词根 con-（共同）+ -ception（感知）

例句 Conception occurs when a sperm fertilizes an egg. 受孕发生在精子与卵子结合的时刻。

misconception 误解

词根 mis-（错误）+ -ception（感知）

例句 A common misconception is that vaccines cause autism. 一个常见的误解是疫苗会导致自闭症。

deception 欺骗

词根 de-（去）+ -ception（感知）

例句 Deception involves misleading someone by altering their perception of reality. 欺骗是通过改变某人对现实的感知来误导他们。

preconception 怀孕前

词根 pre-（前）+ -ception（怀孕）

例句 It is important for women to receive proper preconception care to ensure a healthy pregnancy. 女性接受适当的怀孕前护理，对于确保健康妊娠至关重要。

-chalasia（松弛）

achalasia 贲门失弛缓症

词根 a-（没有）+ chalasia（松弛）

例句 Achalasia is a condition in which the lower esophagus does not relax properly, leading to difficulty swallowing. 贲门失弛缓症是一种下食管无法正常松弛，导致吞咽困难的病症。

chalasia of the cardia 贲门松弛

词根 chalasia（松弛）+ cardia（贲门）

例句 Chalasia of the cardia can lead to the regurgitation of stomach contents into the esophagus. 贲门松弛可能导致胃内容物回流到食管中。

esophageal chalasia 食管松弛症

词根 esophag-（食管的）+ chalasia（松弛）

例句 Esophageal chalasia refers to the abnormal relaxation of the lower esophageal sphincter. 食管松弛症是指下食管括约肌异常松弛的情况。

chalasia of the pylorus 幽门松弛症

词根 chalasia（松弛）+ pylorus（幽门）

例句 Chalasia of the pylorus can result in delayed gastric emptying. 幽门松弛症可能导致胃排空延迟。

myogenic chalasia 肌源性松弛症

词根 myo-（肌肉）+ -genic（源的）+ chalasia（松弛）

例句 Myogenic chalasia occurs when the muscles responsible for regulating certain openings are weak or defective. 肌源性松弛症发生在负责调节某些开口的肌肉虚弱或功能缺陷时。

cheil-（嘴唇）

cheilitis 唇炎

词根 cheil-（嘴唇）+ -itis（炎症）

例句 Cheilitis is the inflammation of the lips, often caused by infection or irritation. 唇炎是嘴唇的炎症，通常由感染或刺激引起。

cheiloplasty 唇成形术

词根 cheil-（嘴唇）+ -plasty（修复手术）

例句 Cheiloplasty is a surgical procedure to reconstruct or repair the lips. 唇成形术是用于重建或修复嘴唇的外科手术。

cheilosis 唇裂症

词根 cheil-（嘴唇）+ -osis（病态）

例句 Cheilosis is a condition characterized by cracks or sores at the corners of the mouth. 唇裂症是一种特征为嘴角裂缝或溃疡的病症。

cheilorrhaphy 唇缝合术

词根 cheil-（嘴唇）+ -rrhaphy（缝合）

例句 Cheilorrhaphy is the surgical repair or suturing of the lips. 唇缝合术是对嘴唇进行修复或缝合的外科手术。

cheilotomy 唇切开术

词根 cheil-（嘴唇）+ -otomy（切开）

例句 Cheilotomy involves the surgical incision of the lips. 唇切开术是指对唇部进行手术切开。

cheilomental 唇下角

词根 cheil-（嘴唇）+ mental（下巴）

例句 The cheilomental angle is the angle formed between the lower lip and the chin. 唇下角是下嘴唇与下巴之间形成的角度。

cheilostomatoplasty 唇口修复术

词根 cheil-（嘴唇）+ stomato-（口腔）+ -plasty（修复手术）
例句 Cheilostomatoplasty is a surgical procedure to repair both the lips and the oral cavity. 唇口修复术是同时修复嘴唇和口腔的外科手术。

cheilomalacia 唇软化症

词根 cheil-（嘴唇）+ -malacia（软化）
例句 Cheilomalacia refers to the softening of the lips, often seen in certain diseases. 唇软化症是指嘴唇的软化，常见于某些疾病中。

cheilorrhea 唇漏症

词根 cheil-（嘴唇）+ -rrhea（流出）
例句 Cheilorrhea is the excessive secretion or discharge from the lips. 唇漏症是指嘴唇的分泌物过多或流出。

cheilogen 唇生成

词根 cheil-（嘴唇）+ -gen（生成）
例句 Cheilogen is the term used to describe the formation of the lips during embryonic development. 唇生成是指在胚胎发育过程中嘴唇的形成。

chemo-（化学的）

chemotherapy 化学疗法

词根 chemo-（化学）+ therapy（治疗）
例句 Chemotherapy is a treatment that uses chemicals to kill or slow the growth of cancer cells. 化学疗法是一种使用化学物质杀死或减缓癌细胞生长的治疗方法。

chemoresistance 化疗抗药性

词根 chemo-（化学）+ resistance（抗性）

例句 Chemoresistance refers to the ability of cancer cells to resist the effects of chemotherapy drugs. 化疗抗药性指的是癌细胞抵抗化疗药物作用的能力。

chemoprevention 化学预防

词根 chemo-（化学）+ prevention（预防）

例句 Chemoprevention involves using chemical agents to reduce the risk of developing cancer. 化学预防是指使用化学药物降低患癌症的风险。

chemotherapeutic 化疗的

词根 chemo-（化学）+ therapeutic（治疗的）

例句 Chemotherapeutic agents are drugs used to treat cancer by targeting and killing cancer cells. 化疗药物是用于通过靶向并杀死癌细胞来治疗癌症的药物。

chemotaxis 趋化性

词根 chemo-（化学）+ taxis（移动）

例句 Chemotaxis refers to the movement of cells toward or away from certain chemicals, often seen in immune responses. 趋化性是指细胞朝向或远离某些化学物质的移动，通常出现在免疫反应中。

chemoresponse 化学反应

词根 chemo-（化学）+ response（反应）

例句 Chemoresponse refers to how well a cancer responds to chemotherapy treatment. 化学反应是指癌症对化疗的反应情况。

chemosensitivity 化疗敏感性

词根 chemo-（化学）+ sensitivity（敏感性）

例句 Chemosensitivity refers to the susceptibility of cancer cells to chemotherapy drugs. 化疗敏感性指的是癌细胞对化疗药物的易感性。

chemotactic factor 趋化因子

词根 chemo-（化学）+ tactic（方向）+ factor（因子）
例句 A chemotactic factor is a chemical substance that attracts cells, especially white blood cells, to areas of infection or injury. 趋化因子是吸引细胞（特别是白细胞）到感染或损伤区域的化学物质。

chemoprophylaxis 化学预防

词根 chemo-（化学）+ prophylaxis（预防）
例句 Chemoprophylaxis refers to the use of chemical agents to prevent disease, especially infections or cancer. 化学预防是指使用化学药物来预防疾病，特别是感染或癌症。

chemotrophic 化学营养的

词根 chemo-（化学）+ trophic（营养的）
例句 Chemotrophic bacteria derive energy from chemicals in their environment, rather than from sunlight. 化学营养的细菌从环境中的化学物质而非阳光中获取能量。

chemokine 趋化因子

词根 chemo-（化学）+ kinesis（运动）
例句 Chemokines are signaling proteins that induce the movement of immune cells to sites of infection or inflammation. 趋化因子是信号蛋白，诱导免疫细胞向感染或炎症部位移动。

chete-（毛发）

chetonychia 指甲毛发症

词根 chete-（毛发）+ onych-（指甲）

例句 Chetonychia refers to a condition where hair-like structures are found under the nails. 指甲毛发症是指在指甲下发现类似毛发的结构。

chetennopathy 毛发病

词根 chete-（毛发）+ -nopathy（病理）
例句 Chetennopathy is a disease that affects hair follicles, causing hair loss. 毛发病是一种影响毛囊的疾病，导致脱发。

chetenitis 毛囊炎

词根 chete-（毛发）+ -itis（炎症）
例句 Chetenitis is the inflammation of hair follicles, often caused by infection. 毛囊炎是毛囊的炎症，通常由感染引起。

cheteplasty 毛发修复术

词根 chete-（毛发）+ -plasty（修复手术）
例句 Cheteplasty is a procedure used to repair or restore damaged hair follicles. 毛发修复术是一种用于修复受损毛囊的手术。

chetectomy 毛发切除术

词根 chete-（毛发）+ -ectomy（切除术）
例句 Chetectomy is the surgical removal of hair follicles from certain parts of the body. 毛发切除术是从身体某些部位切除毛囊的外科手术。

trichetosis 毛发症

词根 tricho-（毛发）+ chete-（毛发）+ -osis（病态）
例句 Trichetosis refers to abnormal hair growth patterns on the skin. 毛发症是指皮肤毛发生长的异常。

chetoid 毛发状

词根 chete-（毛发）+ -oid（类似的）
例句 Chetoid refers to structures that resemble hair or hair follicles

in appearance. 毛发状指的是外观类似毛发或毛囊的结构。

chetenial 毛发的

词根 chete-（毛发）+ -ial（形容词后缀）
例句 The chetenial disorder affected the growth and texture of the hair. 毛发状病症影响了头发的生长和质地。

cheteoid 毛发状的

词根 chete-（毛发）+ -oid（类似的）
例句 Cheteoid conditions can cause irregularities in hair growth and distribution. 毛发状病症可能导致毛发生长和分布的不规则。

-chezia（大便）

dyschezia 排便困难

词根 dys-（异常）+ -chezia（大便）
例句 Dyschezia is a condition characterized by difficulty or pain during defecation. 排便困难症是一种以排便困难或疼痛为特征的病症。

hematochezia 鲜血便

词根 hemato-（血）+ -chezia（大便）
例句 Hematochezia refers to the passage of fresh blood through the rectum, often a sign of gastrointestinal bleeding. 鲜血便是指新鲜血液经直肠排出，通常是胃肠出血的迹象。

pseudochezia 假性排便 / 里急后重

词根 pseudo-（伪）+ -chezia（大便）
例句 Pseudochezia is the sensation of needing to defecate when the bowels are empty. 假性排便是指肠道空虚时仍然有排便的感觉。

proctochezia 肛门排便困难

词根 procto-（肛门）+ -chezia（大便）

例句 Proctochezia involves painful defecation from the anus, typically caused by hemorrhoids. 肛门排便困难通常是由痔疮引起的疼痛排便。

autochezia 自我排便

词根 auto-（自我）+ -chezia（大便）

例句 Autochezia refers to the act of self-administering treatment for constipation or other fecal disorders. 自我排便是指自我治疗便秘或其他排便障碍的行为。

diarrheochezia 腹泻排便

词根 diarrheo-（腹泻）+ -chezia（大便）

例句 Diarrheochezia involves the passage of loose, watery stools, often caused by infections. 腹泻是指排出松散、水样大便，通常由感染引起。

USMLE Step 1 样题

A 56-year-old man is brought to the emergency department by his wife 30 minutes after he had severe upper back pain and hoarseness before becoming comatose (coma-; -tose). He has hypertension (hyper-; -tension) treated with hydrochlorothiazide (hydro-; chloro-). His temperature is 37°C (98.6°F), pulse is 100/min, and blood pressure is 160/80 mmHg in the right arm and 100/60 mmHg in the left arm. Ophthalmologic (ophthalm-) examination shows ptosis and miosis of the left eye. There is anhidrosis (an-; hidr-; -osis) of the left side of the forehead (fore-), right hemiplegia (hemi-; -pleg), and a decreased left radial pulse. A chest X-ray shows a widened mediastinum (media-; stinum). Which of the following conditions is the most likely cause of these findings?

(A) Dissection of the aorta distal to the left subclavian (sub-; clav-) artery

(B) Dissection of the aorta extending into the left carotid (carot-) artery

(C) Dissection of the aorta extending into the left carotid artery and distal aortic arch

(D) Dissection of the proximal aorta extending into the right subclavian (sub-; clav-) artery

(E) Superior sulcus tumor

(F) Thrombus of the left carotid (carot-) artery

中文翻译

一名 56 岁男子因 30 分钟前出现剧烈上背痛和声音嘶哑，在其妻子陪同下被送至急诊科，随后陷入昏迷。该患者有高血压病史，长期服用氢氯噻嗪。查体显示体温 37℃（98.6℉），脉搏 100 次 / 分，右臂血压 160/80 mmHg，左臂血压 100/60 mmHg。眼科检查发现左眼睑下垂及瞳孔缩小。前额左侧无汗，右侧肢体偏瘫，左桡动脉搏动减弱。胸部 X 线片显示纵隔增宽。以下哪种情况是最可能的病因？

(A) 左锁骨下动脉远端主动脉夹层

(B) 主动脉夹层延伸至左颈动脉

(C) 主动脉夹层延伸至左颈动脉和远端主动脉弓

(D) 近端主动脉夹层延伸至右锁骨下动脉

(E) 上沟肿瘤

(F) 左颈动脉血栓

题目和答案中出现的词根

coma-：昏迷

-tose：表示一种病理状态，类似 -osis，但它是形容词词根，而 -osis 是名词词根。

hyper-：高

-tension：张力；压力

hydro-：氢

chloro-：氯

ophthalm-：眼睛的

an-：表示否定

hidr-：汗

-osis：病理状态

fore-：在……前

hemi-：半

-pleg：瘫痪

media-：中间的

stinum：站立（指代纵隔，因为它位于胸腔的中间）

sub-：在……下（在种类的下面，指的是亚类）

clav-：锁骨的

carot-：深睡

chloro-（氯）

chlorosis 萎黄病

词根 chloro-（氯）+ -osis（病态）

例句 Chlorosis is a condition where plants turn yellow due to a lack of chlorophyll, often due to excess chlorine. 萎黄病是植物因缺乏叶绿素而变黄的状况，通常由过量的氯导致。

chloride 氯化物

词根 chloro-（氯）+ -ide（化学物质）
例句 Sodium chloride is commonly known as table salt and is essential for body function. 氯化钠通常被称为食盐，对身体功能至关重要。

chlorophyll 叶绿素

词根 chloro-（氯）+ -phyll（叶）
例句 Chlorophyll is the green pigment in plants that absorbs light for photosynthesis. 叶绿素是植物中吸收光线进行光合作用的绿色色素。

chlorine 氯元素

词根 chloro-（氯）+ -ine（化学元素）
例句 Chlorine is a chemical element commonly used as a disinfectant. 氯是作为消毒剂广泛使用的化学元素。

chloracne 氯痤疮

词根 chloro-（氯）+ -acne（痤疮）
例句 Chloracne is a skin condition caused by exposure to chlorine or chlorinated compounds. 氯性痤疮是一种由接触氯或氯化合物引起的皮肤病。

chlorinated 含氯的

词根 chloro-（氯）+ -ated（化学处理）
例句 Chlorinated water is commonly used for sterilization in swimming pools. 氯化水常用于游泳池的消毒。

chlorohydrin 氯醇

词根 chloro-（氯）+ -hydrin（水合物）

例句 Chlorohydrins are a type of chemical compound that can be toxic to human health. 氯醇是一类化学化合物，可能对人类产生毒性。

chloroplegia 氯麻痹

词根 chloro-（氯）+ -plegia（麻痹）

例句 Chloroplegia is a rare condition in which the nerves become paralyzed due to exposure to chlorine. 氯麻痹是一种暴露于氯气导致神经麻痹的罕见病症。

chloroplast 叶绿体

词根 chloro-（氯）+ -plast（细胞质）

例句 Chloroplasts are the organelles in plant cells where photosynthesis occurs. 叶绿体是植物细胞中进行光合作用的细胞器。

chloramphenicol 氯霉素

词根 chloro-（氯）+ -amphenicol（抗生素）

例句 Chloramphenicol is an antibiotic used to treat a variety of infections. 氯霉素是一种用于治疗多种感染的抗生素。

USMLE Step 1 样题

A 32-year-old man comes to the office because of a 2-week history of fever and throat pain. He is 173 cm tall and weighs 63 kg; BMI is 21 kg/m^2 . His pulse is 110/min, respirations (re-; spir-; -ation) are 16/min, and blood pressure is 98/68 mmHg. Physical examination shows scattered 2- to 4-cm lymph nodes in the neck, axillae, and inguinal regions. There is a bilateral (bi-; -lateral) tonsillar exudate but no ulcerations. Results of laboratory studies are shown:

Hemoglobin (hemo-; -globin) 9.6 g/dL

Hematocrit (hemato-; -crit) 29%

Leukocyte (leuk-; cyt) count 1,500/mm^3

Platelet (plate-; -let) count 60,000/mm^3

A heterophile (hetero-; -phil) antibody (anti-; -body) test result is negative. Which of the following is the most likely diagnosis?

(A) Epstein-Barr virus infection

(B) Gonococcal (gon-; cocc-) pharyngitis (pharyn-; -itis)

(C) HIV infection

(D) Lymphogranuloma (lymph-; granul-; -oma) venereum infection

(E) Streptococcal (strepto-; cocc-) pharyngitis (pharyn-; -itis)

中文翻译

一名 32 岁男性因持续 2 周的发热和咽痛前来就诊。患者身高 173 cm，体重 63 kg，体质指数（BMI）为 21 kg/m^2。查体显示脉搏 110 次 / 分，呼吸频率 16 次 / 分，血压 98/68 mmHg。体格检查发现颈部、腋窝及腹股沟区域可见多个直径 2 ～ 4 cm 的散在淋巴结肿大。双侧扁桃体可见分泌物，但无溃疡形成。实验室检查结果如下：

血红蛋白 9.6 g/dL

血细胞比容 29%

白细胞计数 1,500/mm^3

血小板计数 60,000/mm^3

异嗜性抗体检测结果为阴性。以下哪项是最可能的诊断？

(A) Epstein-Barr 病毒感染

(B) 淋病性咽炎

(C) HIV 感染

(D) 性病淋巴肉芽肿感染

(E) 链球菌性咽炎

题目和答案中出现的词根

re-：重新；反复

spir-：呼吸

-ation：表示动作的状态

bi-：双

-lateral：侧

hemo-：血

-globin：球蛋白

hemato-：血

-crit：分离法

leuk-：白色的

cyt：细胞

plate-：板状的

-let：小的

hetero-：异的

-phil：嗜

anti：抗

-body：体

gon-：生殖的

cocc-：浆果状的

pharyn-：咽

-itis：炎症

lymph-：淋巴的

granul-：小颗粒

-oma：瘤

strepto-：链状的

cholangio-（胆管的）

cholangitis 胆管炎

词根 cholangio-（胆管）+ -itis（炎症）

例句 Cholangitis is an inflammation of the bile ducts, often caused by a bacterial infection. 胆管炎是胆管的炎症，通常由细菌感染引起。

cholangiogram 胆管造影

词根 cholangio-（胆管）+ -gram（记录）

例句 A cholangiogram is an X-ray image of the bile ducts, used to diagnose blockages. 胆管造影是胆管的X线检查，用于诊断堵塞。

cholangiopancreatography 胆胰管造影

词根 cholangio-（胆管）+ pancreato-（胰腺）+ -graphy（记录）

例句 Cholangiopancreatography is a technique used to visualize the bile and pancreatic ducts. 胆胰管造影是一种用于观察胆管和胰管的技术。

cholangiohepatitis 胆管肝炎

词根 cholangio-（胆管）+ hepat-（肝）+ -itis（炎症）

例句 Cholangiohepatitis refers to inflammation of both the bile ducts and the liver. 胆管肝炎是指胆管和肝脏的炎症。

cholangioscopy 胆管镜检查

词根 cholangio-（胆管）+ -scopy（检查）

例句 Cholangioscopy is a procedure used to examine the bile ducts using a fiber-optic scope. 胆管镜检查是一种使用光纤镜检查胆管

的方法。

cholangiocarcinoma 胆管癌

词根 cholangio-（胆管）+ carcin-（癌）+ -oma（肿瘤）
例句 Cholangiocarcinoma is a type of cancer that originates in the bile ducts. 胆管癌是一种源自胆管的癌症。

cholangiopathies 胆管病

词根 cholangio-（胆管）+ -pathy（病）
例句 Cholangiopathies refer to diseases that affect the bile ducts. 胆管病指的是影响胆管的疾病。

cholangiostomy 胆管造口术

词根 cholangio-（胆管）+ -stomy（造口术）
例句 Cholangiostomy is a surgical procedure where an opening is created in the bile duct for drainage. 胆管造口术是通过手术在胆管中创造一个开口以实现引流。

cholangioduodenostomy 胆管十二指肠造口术

词根 cholangio-（胆管）+ duodeno-（十二指肠）+ -stomy（造口术）
例句 Cholangioduodenostomy is a surgery that connects the bile duct to the duodenum. 胆管十二指肠造口术是一种将胆管与十二指肠连接的手术。

cholangiolithiasis 胆管结石

词根 cholangio-（胆管）+ -lithiasis（结石）
例句 Cholangiolithiasis refers to the presence of stones in the bile ducts. 胆管结石是指胆管中存在结石的病症。

chole-（胆的）

cholecystitis 胆囊炎

词根 chole-（胆）+ cyst-（囊）+ -itis（炎症）

例句 Cholecystitis is the inflammation of the gallbladder, often due to a gallstone blockage. 胆囊炎是胆囊的炎症，通常是由胆结石堵塞引起的。

cholestasis 胆汁淤积症

词根 chole-（胆）+ -stasis（停滞）

例句 Cholestasis is a condition where bile flow is impaired, leading to a build-up of bile in the liver. 胆汁淤积症是一种胆汁流动受阻，导致胆汁在肝脏内积聚的病症。

cholelithiasis 胆石症

词根 chole-（胆）+ lithiasis（结石）

例句 Cholelithiasis refers to the formation of gallstones in the gallbladder. 胆石症是指胆囊内形成胆结石。

cholecystectomy 胆囊切除术

词根 chole-（胆）+ cyst-（囊）+ -ectomy（切除术）

例句 Cholecystectomy is the surgical removal of the gallbladder. 胆囊切除术是切除胆囊的外科手术。

cholesterolemia 胆固醇血症

词根 chole-（胆）+ sterol（胆固醇）+ -emia（血液）

例句 Cholesterolemia is the presence of high levels of cholesterol in the blood. 胆固醇血症是指血液中胆固醇水平过高。

cholecystogram 胆囊造影

词根 chole-（胆）+ cyst-（囊）+ -gram（记录）

例句 A cholecystogram is an X-ray of the gallbladder used to detect gallstones. 胆囊造影是胆囊的 X 线检查，用于检测胆结石。

cholecystokinin 胆囊收缩素

词根 chole-（胆）+ cyst-（囊）+ -kinin（促使）

例句 Cholecystokinin is a hormone that stimulates the gallbladder to release bile. 胆囊收缩素是一种激素，刺激胆囊释放胆汁。

cholestyramine 考来烯胺

词根 chole-（胆）+ -styramine（类物质）

例句 Cholestyramine is a medication used to lower cholesterol levels. 考来烯胺是一种用于降低胆固醇水平的药物。

cholagogue 胆汁促排剂

词根 chole-（胆）+ -agogue（引导）

例句 Cholagogue is a substance that promotes the flow of bile from the liver. 胆汁促排剂是促进胆汁从肝脏分泌并流出的物质。

chondro-（软骨的）

chondrocyte 软骨细胞

词根 chondro-（软骨）+ -cyte（细胞）

例句 Chondrocytes are the cells found in cartilage tissue that maintain its matrix. 软骨细胞是存在于软骨组织中的细胞，负责维持其基质。

chondromalacia 软骨软化症

词根 chondro-（软骨）+ -malacia（软化）

例句 Chondromalacia refers to the softening or degeneration of cartilage, often affecting the knee. 软骨软化症指的是软骨的软化或退化，通常影响膝盖。

chondroplasty 软骨成形术

词根 chondro-（软骨）+ -plasty（修复手术）

例句 Chondroplasty is a surgical procedure used to repair damaged cartilage. 软骨成形术是一种用于修复受损软骨的外科手术。

chondrosarcoma 软骨肉瘤

词根 chondro-（软骨）+ sarcoma（肉瘤）

例句 Chondrosarcoma is a type of cancer that originates in the cartilage. 软骨肉瘤是一种起源于软骨的恶性肿瘤。

chondrogenesis 软骨生成

词根 chondro-（软骨）+ -genesis（生成）

例句 Chondrogenesis is the process by which cartilage is formed from mesenchymal cells. 软骨生成是间充质细胞分化形成软骨的过程。

chondrocostal 肋与肋软骨的

词根 chondro-（软骨）+ costal（肋骨的）

例句 Chondrocostal junctions refer to the areas where the cartilage meets the ribs. 软骨肋连接处是指软骨与肋骨连接的区域。

chondrodystrophy 软骨营养不良

词根 chondro-（软骨）+ -dystrophy（营养不良）

例句 Chondrodystrophy refers to disorders of cartilage development, often resulting in dwarfism. 软骨营养不良指的是软骨发育障碍，通常导致侏儒症。

chondritis 软骨炎

词根 chondro-（软骨）+ -itis（炎症）

例句 Chondritis is an inflammation of cartilage that can occur after an injury. 软骨炎是软骨的炎症，通常发生在受伤后。

chondrofibroma 软骨纤维瘤

词根 chondro-（软骨）+ fibro-（纤维）+ -oma（肿瘤）

例句 Chondrofibroma is a benign tumor that contains both cartilage and fibrous tissue. 软骨纤维瘤是一种良性肿瘤，含有软骨和纤维组织。

chondrectomy 软骨切除术

词根 chondro-（软骨）+ -ectomy（切除术）

例句 Chondrectomy is the surgical removal of cartilage tissue from the body. 软骨切除术是从体内切除软骨组织的手术。

chorio-（绒毛）

chorion（绒毛）

词根 chorio-（绒毛）

例句 The chorion is the outer membrane that surrounds the embryo in the early stages of development. 绒毛膜是胚胎早期发育阶段包裹胚胎的外层膜。

chorionic（绒毛的）

词根 chorio-（绒毛）+ -ic（形容词后缀）

例句 Chorionic villi are finger-like projections that form part of the placenta. 绒毛膜绒毛是形成一部分胎盘的指状突起。

chorionitis（绒毛膜炎）

词根 chorio-（绒毛）+ -itis（炎症）

例句 Chorionitis is the inflammation of the chorion, often occurring during infection. 绒毛膜炎是绒毛膜的炎症，通常在感染时发生。

choriocarcinoma（绒毛膜癌）

词根 chorio-（绒毛）+ carcin-（癌）+ -oma（肿瘤）

例句 Choriocarcinoma is a rare cancer that develops from trophoblastic tissue in the placenta. 绒毛膜癌是一种源于胎盘滋养层组织的罕见癌症。

chorionic villus sampling（绒毛膜取样）

词根 chorio-（绒毛）+ villus（绒毛）+ sampling（采样）

例句 Chorionic villus sampling is a prenatal test used to detect genetic abnormalities. 绒毛膜取样是一项用于检测遗传异常的产前测试。

chorioretinitis 绒毛膜视网膜

词根 chorio-（绒毛）+ retina（视网膜）+ -itis（炎症）
例句 Chorioretinitis is the inflammation of the choroid and retina of the eye. 绒毛膜视网膜炎是眼睛中脉络膜和视网膜的炎症。

choriocentesis 绒毛膜穿刺

词根 chorio-（绒毛）+ -centesis（穿刺）
例句 Choriocentesis is a prenatal diagnostic procedure used to sample chorionic tissue. 绒毛膜穿刺是一种用于取样绒毛膜组织的产前诊断方法。

choriocytic 绒毛膜细胞

词根 chorio-（绒毛）+ -cytic（细胞的）
例句 Choriocytic cells are the cells found in the chorion that form part of the placenta. 绒毛膜细胞是存在于绒毛膜中的细胞，构成胎盘的一部分。

choriogenesis 绒毛生成

词根 chorio-（绒毛）+ -genesis（生成）
例句 Choriogenesis is the process by which the chorion forms during pregnancy. 绒毛生成是妊娠过程中绒毛膜形成的过程。

chorioclonal 绒毛克隆的

词根 chorio-（绒毛）+ -clonal（克隆的）
例句 Chorioclonal antibodies are used in diagnostic tests to detect placental disorders. 绒毛克隆抗体用于检测胎盘疾病的诊断测试。

USMLE Step 1 样题

A 3-year-old boy is brought to the office because of a 2-day history of bulging of his left eye. He says his eye hurts. He has no history of major medical illness or recent trauma to the area, and he receives no medications. Vital signs are within normal limits. Physical examination shows exophthalmos (ex-; ophthalm-) of the left eye. MRI of the brain shows a 2-cm mass involving the ocular muscles of the left eye. A biopsy specimen of the mass shows malignant cells, some of which have striations. Which of the following is the most likely diagnosis?

(A) Neuroblastoma (neuro-; -blast; -oma)

(B) Pheochromocytoma (pheo-; chromo-; cyt-; -oma)

(C) Retinoblastoma (retino-; -blast; -oma)

(D) Rhabdomyosarcoma (rhabdo-; myo-; sarc-; -oma)

(E) Thyroid cancer

中文翻译

一名 3 岁男童因左眼突出 2 天就诊。患儿自述眼部疼痛，既往无重大疾病史，近期眼部区域未受外伤，且未服用任何药物。生命体征均正常。体格检查显示左眼眼球突出。头部磁共振成像显示左眼眼外肌存在一个 2 cm 的肿物。肿物活检结果显示存在恶性细胞，其中部分细胞可见条纹状结构。以下哪项是最可能的诊断？

(A) 神经母细胞瘤

(B) 嗜铬细胞瘤

(C) 视网膜母细胞瘤

(D) 横纹肌肉瘤

(E) 甲状腺癌

题目和答案中出现的词根

ex-：向外

ophthalm-：眼睛的

neuro-：神经的

-blast：前体

-oma：瘤

pheo-：深灰色

chromo-：颜色

cyt-：细胞

retino-：视网膜

rhabdo-：横条的

myo-：肌肉

sarc-：肉体的（这里泛指间质细胞发育的组织结构）

chrom-（染色；颜色）

chromosome 染色体

词根 chrom-（染色）+ -some（体）

例句 Chromosomes carry genetic information in the form of DNA. 染色体以 DNA 的形式携带遗传信息。

chromatin 染色质

词根 chrom-（染色）+ -atin（物质）

例句 Chromatin is a complex of DNA and proteins found in the nucleus. 染色质是存在于细胞核中的 DNA 和蛋白质的复合物。

chromatography 色谱法

词根 chrom-（颜色）+ -graphy（记录、描写）

例句 Chromatography is a technique used to separate mixtures based on color. 色谱法是一种根据颜色分离混合物的技术。

chromophore 色基

词根 chrom-（颜色）+ -phore（携带者）

例句 A chromophore is a molecule that absorbs light and gives color to a substance. 色基是吸收光并赋予物质颜色的分子。

chromic 含三价铬的

词根 chrom-（颜色）+ -ic（形容词后缀）

例句 Chromic acid is a strong oxidizing agent used in laboratory settings. 铬酸是一种强氧化剂，常用于实验室中。

chromocyte 色素细胞

词根 chrom-（颜色）+ -cyte（细胞）

例句 Chromocytes are cells that contain pigment or color. 色素细胞是含有色素或颜色的细胞。

hyperchromia 色素过多症

词根 hyper-（过度）+ chrom-（颜色）

例句 Hyperchromia refers to the excess of pigmentation in the skin. 色素过多症是指皮肤中的色素过量。

hypochromia 色素缺乏症

词根 hypo-（不足）+ chrom-（颜色）

例句 Hypochromia is a condition where the red blood cells have less color than normal. 色素缺乏症是一种红细胞比正常情况颜色浅的病症。

chromoblast 成色素细胞

词根 chrom-（颜色）+ -blast（芽、胚）

例句 Chromoblasts are cells that produce pigments in certain tissues. 成色素细胞是产生色素的细胞。

achromia 无色素症（色素缺乏）

词根 a-（无）+ chrom-（颜色）

例句 Achromia is a condition in which there is a complete absence of color. 无色素症是一种完全缺乏色素的病症。

chrono-（时间）

chronology 年表学

词根 chrono-（时间）+ -logy（学科）

例句 Chronology is the study of time and the sequence of events. 年表学是研究时间和事件顺序的学科。

chronotherapy 时间疗法

词根 chrono-（时间）+ -therapy（治疗）

例句 Chronotherapy is the use of timing to administer treatment in sync with the body's natural rhythms. 时间疗法是根据人体自然节律调整给药时间的治疗方法。

chronograph 计时器

词根 chrono-（时间）+ -graph（记录）

例句 A chronograph is a device used to measure and record time accurately. 计时器是一种用于精确测量和记录时间的设备。

chronicle 编年史

词根 chrono-（时间）+ -icle（小的）

例句 A chronicle is a detailed account or record of historical events in the order they occurred. 编年史是按事件发生顺序详细记载历史事件的记录。

chronometry 计时学

词根 chrono-（时间）+ -metry（测量）

例句 Chronometry is the science of measuring time accurately. 计

时学是精确测量时间的科学。

chronopathology 时序病理学

词根 chrono-（时间）+ patho-（疾病）+ -logy（学科）
例句 Chronopathology examines how the timing of diseases or conditions influences their development. 时序病理学研究疾病或病症的发生时间如何影响其发展。

chronically 长期地

词根 chrono-（时间）+ -ically（副词后缀）
例句 The patient was chronically ill, requiring ongoing medical attention. 患者长期生病，需要持续的医疗照护。

chronoscope 计时仪器

词根 chrono-（时间）+ -scope（仪器）
例句 A chronoscope is used to measure very precise intervals of time. 计时仪器用于测量非常精确的时间间隔。

chronobiology 生物时钟学

词根 chrono-（时间）+ bio-（生命）+ -logy（学科）
例句 Chronobiology is the study of biological rhythms and their effects on organisms. 生物时钟学是研究生物节律及其对生物体影响的学科。

cirrho-（黄色，即肝硬化引起的黄疸，代指硬化）

cirrhosis 肝硬化

词根 cirrho-（硬化）+ -osis（病态）
例句 Cirrhosis is a liver disease characterized by the replacement of liver tissue with scar tissue. 肝硬化是一种肝脏疾病，特征是肝组织被瘢痕组织替代。

cirrhotic 肝硬化性的

词根 cirrho-（硬化）+ -tic（形容词后缀）

例句 Cirrhotic liver failure occurs when the liver becomes severely damaged and no longer functions properly. 肝硬化性肝衰竭发生在肝脏严重受损并且无法维持正常功能时。

cirrhosis of the liver 肝硬化

词根 cirrho-（硬化）+ liver（肝脏）

例句 Cirrhosis of the liver is often caused by chronic alcohol abuse or viral infections like hepatitis. 肝硬化通常是由长期饮酒或如乙型肝炎等病毒感染引起的。

cirrhopathy 肝硬化病

词根 cirrho-（硬化）+ -pathy（病）

例句 Cirrhopathy refers to diseases related to liver cirrhosis and its complications. 肝硬化病指的是与肝硬化及其并发症相关的疾病。

cirrhotic syndrome 肝硬化综合征

词根 cirrho-（硬化）+ -tic（形容词后缀）+ syndrome（综合征）

例句 Cirrhotic syndrome refers to a group of symptoms that result from liver cirrhosis. 肝硬化综合征是指由肝硬化引起的一组症状。

cirrhosis-induced fibrosis 肝硬化引起的纤维化

词根 cirrho-（硬化）+ -osis（病态）+ fibrosis（纤维化）

例句 Cirrhosis-induced fibrosis can impair liver function by replacing healthy tissue with scar tissue. 肝硬化引起的纤维化会通过用瘢痕组织取代健康组织而损害肝功能。

cirrhostatic 抗肝硬化的

词根 cirrho-（硬化）+ -static（静止的）

例句 Cirrhostatic agents are drugs that inhibit the progression of cirrhosis. 抗肝硬化药物是抑制肝硬化进展的药物。

cirrhosis-related ascites 肝硬化相关腹水

词根 cirrho-（硬化）+ ascites（腹水）

例句 Cirrhosis-related ascites occurs when the liver cannot produce enough albumin, leading to fluid accumulation in the abdomen. 肝硬化相关腹水发生在肝脏无法产生足够白蛋白时，导致腹部液体积聚。

cirrhosis-associated hepatocellular carcinoma 肝硬化相关肝细胞癌

词根 cirrho-（硬化）+ -osis（病态）+ hepatocellular（肝细胞的）+ carcinoma（癌症）

例句 Cirrhosis-associated hepatocellular carcinoma is a common type of liver cancer in individuals with cirrhosis. 肝硬化相关肝细胞癌是肝硬化患者中常见的一种肝癌类型。

cirrhosis of the gallbladder 胆囊肝硬化

词根 cirrho-（硬化）+ gallbladder（胆囊）

例句 Cirrhosis of the gallbladder is a rare condition that can affect bile flow and digestion. 胆囊肝硬化是一种罕见的疾病，可能会影响胆汁排出和消化功能。

clostr-（梭状）

clostridium 梭状芽孢杆菌

词根 clostr-（梭状）

例句 Clostridium is a genus of bacteria, many of which are pathogenic and can cause severe infections. 梭状芽孢杆菌是一个细菌属，其中许多是致病的，能够引起严重的感染。

clostridial 梭状芽孢杆菌的

词根 clostr-（梭状）+ -ial（形容词后缀）

例句 Clostridial infections are caused by bacteria from the genus Clostridium. 梭状芽孢杆菌感染是由梭状芽孢杆菌属的细菌引起的。

clostridiolysin 梭状芽孢杆菌溶解素

词根 clostr-（梭状）+ lyso-（溶解）+ -in（蛋白质）

例句 Clostridiolysin is a toxin produced by clostridium bacteria that causes cell destruction. 梭状芽孢杆菌溶解素是由梭状芽孢杆菌产生的一种毒素，能够引起细胞破坏。

clostridiosis 梭状芽孢杆菌病

词根 clostr-（梭状）+ -iosis（病态）

例句 Clostridiosis is an infection caused by clostridium bacteria, often affecting the digestive system. 梭状芽孢杆菌病是由梭状芽孢杆菌引起的感染，通常影响消化系统。

clostridial myonecrosis 梭状芽孢杆菌性肌肉坏死

词根 clostr-（梭状）+ myo-（肌肉）+ necrosis（坏死）

例句 Clostridial myonecrosis, also known as gas gangrene, is a life-threatening infection caused by clostridium bacteria. 梭状芽孢杆菌性肌肉坏死，也称为气性坏疽，是由梭状芽孢杆菌引起的一种危及生命的感染。

clostridium tetani 破伤风梭状芽孢杆菌

词根 clostr-（梭状）+ tetani（破伤风）

例句 Clostridium tetani is the bacterium responsible for causing tetanus. 破伤风梭状芽孢杆菌是引起破伤风的细菌。

clostridium botulinum 肉毒梭状芽孢杆菌

词根 clostr-（梭状）+ botulinum（肉毒毒素）

例句 Clostridium botulinum produces a potent neurotoxin that can cause botulism. 肉毒梭状芽孢杆菌产生一种强效的神经毒素，能够引起肉毒中毒。

clostridial enterotoxin 梭状芽孢杆菌肠毒素

词根 clostr-（梭状）+ entero-（肠道）+ toxin（毒素）
例句 Clostridial enterotoxin is a toxin produced by Clostridium species that affects the intestines. 梭状芽孢杆菌肠毒素是梭状芽孢杆菌产生的一种毒素，影响肠道。

clostridium difficile 艰难梭状芽孢杆菌

词根 clostr-（梭状）+ difficile（困难的）
例句 Clostridium difficile is a bacterium that can cause severe colitis, especially after antibiotic treatment. 艰难梭状芽孢杆菌是一种细菌，能够引起严重的结肠炎，特别是在抗生素治疗后。

clostridium perfringens 产气梭状芽孢杆菌

词根 clostr-（梭状）+ perfringens（渗透的）
例句 Clostridium perfringens is known for causing gas gangrene and food poisoning. 产气梭状芽孢杆菌以引起气性坏疽和食物中毒而著名。

co-（共）

coexist 共存

词根 co-（共）+ exist（存在）
例句 Different species of animals can coexist in the same habitat. 不同物种的动物可以在同一栖息地共存。

cooperation 合作

词根 co-（共）+ oper-（工作）+ -ation（动作）
例句 Cooperation between healthcare providers is essential for effective patient care. 医疗服务提供者之间的合作对于有效的病患

护理至关重要。

coagulation 凝血

词根 co-（共）+ agul-（凝固）+ -ation（动作）

例句 Coagulation is the process by which blood changes from a liquid to a gel, stopping bleeding. 凝血是血液从液态转变为凝胶状并阻止出血的过程。

coenzyme 辅酶

词根 co-（共）+ enzyme（酶）

例句 Coenzymes are non-protein molecules that assist enzymes in catalyzing reactions. 辅酶是帮助酶催化反应的非蛋白分子。

collaborate 合作

词根 co-（共）+ labor（工作）

例句 The researchers decided to collaborate on the new project to share their expertise. 研究人员决定在新项目上进行合作，以共享他们的专业知识。

cohesion 凝聚力

词根 co-（共）+ hes-（黏附）

例句 Cohesion refers to the force that holds molecules of the same substance together. 凝聚力指的是将相同物质的分子黏在一起的力。

coagulate 凝固

词根 co-（共）+ agul-（凝固）

例句 The blood began to coagulate and form a clot to stop the bleeding. 血液开始凝固，形成血块以止血。

USMLE Step 1 样题

A previously healthy 52-year-old woman comes to the physician because of a 2-month history of fatigue, constipation (con-; stip-; -ation), and frequent urination (urin-; -ation). Her temperature is 37.1℃ (98.8°F), pulse is 80/min, respirations (re-; spir-; -ation) are 14/min, and blood pressure is 140/90mmHg. Diffuse crackles are heard bilaterally (bi-; lateral). Her serum calcium concentration is 11.1 mg/dL, and serum parathyroid (para-; thyr-; -oid) hormone concentration is decreased. A chest X-ray shows bilateral (bi-; lateral) hilar lymphadenopathy (lymph-; adeno-; -pathy) and interstitial (inter-; stit-) infiltrates. Which of the following is the most likely cause of this patient's hypercalcemia (hyper-; calc-; -emia)?

(A) Calcitriol (calc-; tri-; -ol) production by activated macrophages (macro-; phage)

(B) Local resorption (re-; sorpt-) of bone by metastases (meta-; -stasis)

(C) Parathyroid (para-; thyr-; -oid) hormone-related peptide secretion

(D) Secretion of parathyroid (para-; thyr-; -oid) hormone

(E) Secretion of thyroid (thyr-; -oid) -stimulating hormone

中文翻译

一名此前健康的 52 岁女性因过去两个月感到疲劳、便秘和尿频而就医。她的体温为 37.1℃（98.8°F），脉搏 80 次 / 分钟，呼吸 14 次 / 分钟，血压 140/90 mmHg。双肺可闻及弥漫性湿啰音。她的血清钙浓度为 11.1 mg/dL，血清甲状旁腺激素浓度降低。胸部 X 线片显示双侧肺门淋巴结肿大及间质性浸润。以下哪项是该患者高钙血症最可能的原因？

(A) 活化巨噬细胞产生钙三醇

(B) 转移灶引起的局部骨吸收

(C) 甲状旁腺激素相关肽分泌

(D) 甲状旁腺激素分泌

(E) 促甲状腺激素分泌

题目和答案中出现的词根

con-：一起

stip-：挤压

-ation：表示动作的状态（一起挤压的动作，指代腹部肌肉一起收缩以提高腹内压挤压肠道来排便，表便秘）

urin-：尿

re-：重新；反复

spir-：呼吸

bi-：双

lateral：侧面

para-：旁边

thyr-：盾

-oid：类似的（甲状腺的形状为类盾牌状）

lymph-：淋巴的

adeno-：腺体

-pathy：病（淋巴腺体病，指代淋巴结肿大）

inter-：在……之间

stit-：站立（站立在……之间，指代器官间的间质）

hyper-：高

calc-：钙

-emia：血症

tri-：三个

-ol：醇（钙三醇指的是活化形式的维生素 D_3）

macro-：大的

phage：吞噬（大的吞噬指代巨噬细胞）

sorpt：吸

meta-：超过；在……后

-stasis：静止站立

-coccidio（球状）

coccidiosis 球虫病

词根 coccidio-（球状）+ -osis（病态）

例句 Coccidiosis is a common disease in poultry caused by protozoan parasites. 球虫病是由原生动物寄生虫引起的家禽常见疾病。

coccidial 球虫的

词根 coccidio-（球状）+ -al（形容词后缀）

例句 The coccidial infection caused severe diarrhea in the livestock. 球虫感染导致家畜严重腹泻。

coccidiostat 球虫抑制剂

词根 coccidio-（球状）+ -stat（抑制剂）

例句 A coccidiostat is used to control coccidiosis in poultry farming. 球虫抑制剂用于控制家禽养殖中的球虫病。

coccidioidomycosis 球孢子菌病

词根 coccidio-（球状）+ -oid（像……的）+ mycosis（真菌病）

例句 Coccidioidomycosis is a fungal infection that can affect the lungs and skin. 球孢子菌病是一种可以影响肺部和皮肤的

真菌感染。

coccidiocidal 杀灭球虫的

词根 coccidio-（球状）+ -cidal（杀灭的）
例句 Coccidiocidal drugs are effective in treating coccidiosis in livestock. 球虫杀虫药对治疗牲畜的球虫病有效。

coccidectomy 球虫切除术

词根 coccidio-（球状）+ -ectomy（切除术）
例句 In severe cases, coccidectomy might be required to remove infected tissues. 在严重情况下，可能需要进行球虫切除术以去除感染的组织。

col-/ colo-（大肠的）

colon 结肠

词根 col-（大肠）
例句 The colon is the posterior part of the digestive system, responsible for absorbing water and salts. 结肠是消化系统的后部分，负责吸收水分和盐分。

colonoscopy 结肠镜检查

词根 col-（大肠）+ -scopy（检查）
例句 Colonoscopy is a procedure used to examine the inside of the colon for signs of disease. 结肠镜检查是一种用于检查结肠内部是否有疾病迹象的方法。

colitis 结肠炎

词根 col-（大肠）+ -itis（炎症）
例句 Colitis is an inflammation of the colon, often leading to symptoms like diarrhea and abdominal pain. 结肠炎是结肠的炎症，通常导致腹泻和腹痛等症状。

colorectal 结直肠癌

词根 col-（大肠）+ rect-（直肠）+ -al（形容词后缀）

例句 Colorectal cancer is a type of cancer that affects the colon and rectum. 结直肠癌是一种影响结肠和直肠的癌症类型。

colostomy 结肠造口术

词根 col-（大肠）+ -stomy（造口术）

例句 A colostomy is a surgical procedure in which an opening is made in the colon to divert waste. 结肠造口术是一种外科手术，在结肠中开口以引流废物。

colotomy 结肠切开术

词根 col-（大肠）+ -otomy（切开）

例句 Colotomy is a surgical procedure in which a section of the colon is surgically cut open for treatment. 结肠切开术是一种外科手术，即通过切开结肠的某一部分进行治疗。

coloplexy 结肠固定术

词根 col-（大肠）+ -plexy（固定术）

例句 Coloplexy is a procedure used to fix the colon to the abdominal wall. 结肠固定术是一种将结肠固定到腹壁上的手术。

coliform 大肠型杆菌

词根 col-（大肠）+ -form（形状）

例句 Coliform bacteria are bacteria that are commonly found in the intestines and are used as indicators of water contamination. 大肠型细菌是常见于肠道中的细菌，常用作水污染的指示物。

colic 腹绞痛

词根 col-（大肠）+ -ic（形容词后缀的状态）

例句 Colic refers to severe, cramp-like abdominal pain that is often associated with digestive issues. 腹绞痛指的是常与消化问题相关的严重腹部痉挛性疼痛。

colonoscopy biopsy 结肠镜活检

词根 col-（大肠）+ -scopy（检查）+ biopsy（活检）

例句 A colonoscopy biopsy is performed to collect tissue samples from the colon for testing. 结肠镜活检是通过结肠镜检查收集结肠组织样本进行检测。

condyl-（髁）

condyle 髁

词根 condyl-（髁）+ -e（名词后缀）

例句 A condyle is a rounded prominence at the end of a bone, often involved in forming a joint. 髁是骨头末端的一个圆形突出部分，通常参与关节的形成。

condyloma 髁状瘤

词根 condyl-（髁）+ -oma（肿瘤）

例句 Condyloma refers to a benign growth or tumor, often seen in the genital area, caused by the human papillomavirus（HPV）. 髁状瘤是指一种良性肿瘤，常见于生殖器区域，由人乳头状瘤病毒（HPV）引起。

condylomata acuminata 尖锐湿疣

词根 condylom-（髁状瘤）+ -ata（复数后缀）

例句 Condylomata acuminata are a type of genital wart caused by HPV infection, characterized by small, flesh-colored bumps. 尖锐湿疣是一种由HPV感染引起的生殖器疣，表现为小的肉色突起。

condylitis 髁炎

词根 condyl-（髁）+ -itis（炎症）

例句 Condylitis refers to inflammation of the condyle, commonly seen in joints like the knee or elbow. 髁炎是指髁部的炎症，常见于膝关节或肘关节等部位。

subcondylar 髁下的

词根 sub-（下）+ condyl-（髁）+ -ar（形容词后缀）

例句 A subcondylar fracture is a break occurring just below the condyle, often in the jawbone. 髁下骨折是指发生在髁下方的骨折，通常发生在下颌骨。

condyloplasty 髁成形术

词根 condyl-（髁）+ -plasty（修复术）

例句 Condyloplasty is a surgical procedure to reshape or repair a damaged condyle, often in the jaw or knee. 髁成形术是一种对受损髁（常见于颌骨或膝关节）进行重塑或修复的外科手术。

condylomata lata 扁平湿疣

词根 condylom-（髁状瘤）+ -ata（复数后缀）+ lata（广泛的）

例句 Condylomata lata are larger, flat warts that appear in syphilis, typically found in the genital area. 扁平湿疣是梅毒中出现的较大、扁平的疣，通常出现在生殖器区域。

supracondylar 髁上部的

词根 supra-（上）+ condyl-（髁）+ -ar（形容词后缀）

例句 A supracondylar fracture occurs just above the condyle, often seen in the humerus. 髁上骨折是指发生在髁上方的骨折，常见于肱骨。

conio-（灰尘）

coniosis 粉尘病

词根 conio-（灰尘）+ -osis（病态）

例句 Coniosis refers to lung diseases caused by the inhalation of dust, such as pneumoconiosis. 粉尘病是指由吸入灰尘引起的肺部疾病，如尘肺病。

pneumoconiosis 尘肺病

词根 pneumo-（肺）+ conio-（灰尘）+ -osis（病态）

例句 Pneumoconiosis is a condition caused by the accumulation of dust particles in the lungs. 尘肺病是由灰尘颗粒在肺部积聚引起的疾病。

coniometer 尘量计

词根 conio-（灰尘）+ -meter（仪器）

例句 A coniometer is an instrument used to measure the concentration of dust particles in the air. 尘量计是一种用于测量空气中灰尘颗粒浓度的仪器。

coniofibrosis 纤维性肺尘病

词根 conio-（灰尘）+ fibro-（纤维）+ -osis（病态）

例句 Coniofibrosis refers to lung fibrosis caused by inhaling dust particles over time. 纤维性肺尘病是指长期吸入灰尘颗粒而引起的肺纤维化。

coniopathology 尘肺病理学

词根 conio-（灰尘）+ -pathology（病理）

例句 Coniopathology studies the harmful effects of dust on the respiratory system. 尘肺病理学研究灰尘对呼吸系统的有害影响。

coniohazard 尘肺危害

词根 conio-（灰尘）+ hazard（危险）

例句 The coniohazard in coal mines is the inhalation of coal dust, leading to respiratory issues. 煤矿中的尘肺危害是指吸入煤尘，导致呼吸问题。

##织conioviral 尘病毒性的

词根 conio-（灰尘）+ viral（病毒的）

例句 910Conioviral infections are respiratory diseases caused by both dust and viral exposure. 尘病毒性感染是由灰尘和病毒共同引起

的呼吸道疾病。

coniotoxin 尘毒素

词根 conio-（灰尘）+ -toxin（毒素）

例句 Coniotoxin is a harmful substance found in dust that can damage lung tissue. 尘毒素是灰尘中一种有害物质，能够损害肺部组织。

USMLE Step 1 样题

A 45-year-old man is brought to the emergency department 30 minutes after the sudden onset of crushing chest pain. His father, maternal aunt, and paternal uncle all died of myocardial (myo-; cardi-) infarctions under the age of 50 years. Physical examination shows tendinous (tendin-) xanthomas (xanth-; -oma) on the hands and thickened Achilles tendons. Serum lipid studies show a total cholesterol (chole-; stere-; -ol) concentration of 410 mg/dL, HDL-cholesterol (chole-; stere-; -ol) concentration of 30 mg/dL, and triglyceride (tri-; glycer) concentration of 140 mg/dL. The diagnosis of myocardial (myo-; cardi-) infarction is made. This patient most likely has a deficiency of which of the following?

(A) Apo B48

(B) Apo C

(C) HMG-CoA reductase (-ase) activity

(D) LDL receptor

(E) Lipoprotein (lip-) lipase (lip-; -ase) activity

中文翻译

一名 45 岁男性突发剧烈胸痛，30 分钟后被送往急诊科。其父亲、姨母和叔父均在 50 岁前死于心肌梗死。体格检查显示手部肌腱性黄瘤和跟腱增厚。血脂检查显示总胆固醇浓度为 410 mg/dL，HDL 胆固醇浓度为 30 mg/dL，甘油三酯浓度为 140 mg/dL。患者确诊为心肌梗死。该患者最有可能缺乏以下哪项物质？

(A) 载脂蛋白 B48

(B) 载脂蛋白 C

(C) HMG-CoA 还原酶活性

(D) 低密度脂蛋白受体

(E) 脂蛋白脂酶活性

题目和答案中出现的词根

myo-：肌肉

cardi-：心脏

tendin-：肌腱的

xanth-：黄色的（这里指脂肪）

-oma：瘤

chole-：胆

stere：固体的

-ol：醇

tri-：三个

glycer：甘油

-ase：酶

lip-：脂肪

copro-（粪的）

coprology 粪便学

词根 copro-（粪便）+ -logy（学科）

例句 Coprology is the study of feces, including its composition, diseases, and diagnostic value in clinical medicine. 粪便学是研究粪便的学科，包括其成分、疾病以及在临床医学中的诊断价值。

coprolith 粪石

词根 copro-（粪便）+ lith（石）

例句 A coprolith is a hard mass of fecal matter, which can form in the intestines or colon and may lead to obstruction. 粪石是硬化的粪便块，可能在肠道或结肠中形成，并可能导致梗阻。

coproporphyria 粪卟啉症

词根 copro-（粪便）+ porphyria（卟啉症）

例句 Coproporphyria is a type of porphyria, a metabolic disorder that affects the production of heme, leading to symptoms like abdominal pain and neurological issues. 粪卟啉症是一种卟啉症，属于代谢障碍，影响血红素的生产，导致腹痛和神经问题等症状。

coprolithiasis 粪石症

词根 copro-（粪便）+ lithiasis（结石）

例句 Coprolithiasis is the condition where fecal stones form in the intestines or colon, often causing discomfort and sometimes obstruction. 粪石症是指在肠道或结肠中形成粪便结石，通常会引起不适，有时会导致梗阻。

coprophagia 食粪症

词根 copro-（粪便）+ phagia（吞咽）

例句 Coprophagia is the act of consuming feces, which may be observed in certain animals, but can be abnormal and pathological in humans. 食粪症是指吞食粪便的行为，某些动物可能会出现这种情况，但在人类中则为异常和病理性行为。

coprolite 化石粪便

词根 copro-（粪便）+ -lite（石）

例句 Coprolites are fossilized remains of feces that can provide valuable information about ancient diets and ecosystems. 化石粪便是化石化的粪便遗迹，可以为研究古代饮食和生态系统提供有价值的信息。

coprobacillus 粪杆菌

词根 copro-（粪便）+ bacillus（杆菌）

例句 Coprobacillus is a type of bacterium found in feces that plays a role in digestion and fermentation. 粪杆菌是一种在粪便中发现的细菌，在消化和发酵过程中起着作用。

corpus-（体）

corpus 体

词根 corpus-（体）

例句 The corpus is the main part of an organ or structure, such as the corpus of the brain. 体指的是器官或结构的主要部分，如大脑的体部。

corpuscle 小体

词根 corpus-（体）+ -cle（小）

例句 A corpuscle is a small particle or cell, such as a red blood cell. 小体是指像红细胞这样的微小粒子或细胞。

corpuscular 微粒子的

词根 corpus-（体）+ -cular（形容词后缀）

例句 The corpuscular theory suggests that light is made up of small particles. 粒子理论认为光是由小颗粒组成的。

corpus callosum 胼胝体

词根 corpus-（体）+ callosum（硬的）

例句 The corpus callosum is a bundle of nerve fibers connecting the two hemispheres of the brain. 胼胝体是连接大脑两个半球的一束神经纤维。

corpus luteum 黄体

词根 corpus-（体）+ luteum（黄色）

例句 The corpus luteum is a temporary endocrine structure in the ovaries. 黄体是卵巢中的一个暂时性的内分泌结构。

corporal 身体的

词根 corpor-（身体）+ -al（形容词后缀）

例句 Corporal punishment involves physical force to correct behavior. 体罚是通过使用身体力量来纠正行为。

corposome 体小体

词根 corpo-（体）+ -some（体）

例句 A corposome is a tiny particle that is found in the cytoplasm of cells. 体小体是存在于细胞质中的微小颗粒。

corposclerosis 体硬化

词根 corpo-（体）+ -sclerosis（硬化）

例句 Corposclerosis refers to the hardening of the corpus tissue. 体硬化是指体组织的硬化。

corporality 体质

词根 corpor-（身体）+ -ality（性质）

例句 Corporality is the quality or state of having a physical body. 体质是身体的特征或状态。

cortico-（皮质的）

cortex 皮质

词根 cortico-（皮质）

例句 The cortex is the outer layer of an organ, such as the brain or kidney. 皮质是器官（如大脑或肾脏）的外层结构。

corticosteroid 皮质类固醇

词根 cortico-（皮质）+ steroid（类固醇）

例句 Corticosteroids are synthetic drugs that mimic the effects of hormones produced by the adrenal cortex. 皮质类固醇是合成药物，模拟肾上腺皮质产生的激素效应。

cortical 皮质的

词根 cortico-（皮质）+ -al（形容词后缀）

例句 The cortical neurons are responsible for processing sensory information in the brain. 皮层神经元负责处理大脑中的感觉信息。

corticospinal 皮质脊髓的

词根 cortico-（皮质）+ spinal（脊髓的）

例句 The corticospinal tract is a major pathway that carries motor signals from the brain to the spinal cord. 皮质脊髓束是从大脑到脊髓传递运动信号的主要通道。

corticoid 皮质激素

词根 cortico-（皮质）+ -oid（类的）

例句 Corticoids are hormones secreted by the adrenal glands that help regulate various body functions. 皮质激素是肾上腺分泌的激素，有助于调节身体的各种功能。

cortical atrophy 皮质萎缩

词根 cortico-（皮质）+ atrophy（萎缩）

例句 Cortical atrophy refers to the shrinkage or loss of neurons in the brain's cortex. 皮质萎缩指的是大脑皮质中神经元的缩小或丧失。

cortisol 皮质醇

词根 cortico-（皮质）+ -sol（溶解）

例句 Cortisol is a hormone produced by the adrenal cortex in response to stress. 皮质醇是一种由肾上腺皮质在应对压力时产生的激素。

corticosteroid therapy 皮质类固醇治疗

词根 cortico-（皮质）+ steroid（类固醇）+ therapy（治疗）

例句 Corticosteroid therapy is commonly used to reduce inflammation and treat autoimmune diseases. 皮质类固醇治疗常用于减少炎症和治疗自身免疫性疾病。

corticomotor 皮质运动的

词根 cortico-（皮质）+ motor（运动的）

例句 Corticomotor pathways control voluntary movement in the body. 皮质运动通路控制身体的自主运动。

corticotropin 促皮质激素

词根 cortico-（皮质）+ tropin（激素）

例句 Corticotropin is a hormone that stimulates the production of cortisol in the adrenal glands. 促皮质激素是一种刺激肾上腺皮质产生皮质醇的激素。

cranio-（颅的）

cranium 颅的

词根 cranio-（颅的）
例句 The cranium is the part of the skull that encloses the brain. 颅骨是包围大脑的部分。

craniectomy 颅骨切除术

词根 cranio-（颅的）+ -ectomy（切除术）
例句 Craniectomy is a surgical procedure where part of the cranium is removed to relieve pressure on the brain. 颅骨切除术是一种外科手术，切除部分颅骨以减轻大脑的压力。

craniosynostosis 颅缝早闭症

词根 cranio-（颅的）+ syn-（共同）+ -ostosis（骨化）
例句 Craniosynostosis is a condition where the bones in a baby's skull fuse too early, affecting brain growth. 颅缝早闭症是一种婴儿颅骨的骨缝过早融合，影响大脑发育的病症。

cranial 头颅的

词根 cranio-（颅的）+ -al（形容词后缀）
例句 Cranial nerves control motor and sensory functions of the head and neck. 颅神经控制头部和颈部的运动和感觉功能。

craniofacial 颅面的

词根 cranio-（颅的）+ facial（面部的）
例句 Craniofacial surgery involves procedures to treat deformities of the skull and face. 颅面手术包括治疗颅骨和面部畸形的手术。

craniovertebral 颅脊的

词根 cranio-（颅的）+ vertebral（脊椎的）

例句 Craniovertebral junction refers to the area where the skull and spine are connected. 颅脊交界是指颅骨和脊柱连接的区域。

cranioscopy 颅骨检查

词根 cranio-（颅的）+ -scopy（检查）
例句 Cranioscopy is a procedure used to examine the bones of the skull for abnormalities. 颅骨检查是用于检查颅骨骨骼是否有异常的方法。

craniofacial anomalies 颅面异常

词根 cranio-（颅的）+ facial（面部的）+ anomalies（异常）
例句 Craniofacial anomalies are birth defects that affect the structure of the skull and face. 颅面异常是影响颅骨和面部结构的出生缺陷。

craniorachischisis 颅脊裂

词根 cranio-（颅的）+ rachischisis（脊柱裂）
例句 Craniorachischisis is a severe birth defect that results in the open skull and spine, causing neurological issues. 颅脊裂是一种严重的出生缺陷，导致颅骨和脊柱开放，引发神经问题。

cranial nerve 颅神经

词根 cranio-（颅的）+ nerve（神经）
例句 Cranial nerves are responsible for the movement and sensation in the head and neck area. 颅神经负责头部和颈部区域的运动和感觉。

-crasia（异常的混合状态）

dyscrasia 血液病

词根 dys-（异常）+ -crasia（异常的混合状态）
例句 Dyscrasia refers to a disturbance in the body's normal balance of blood components. 血液病指的是身体血液成分正常平衡的

紊乱。

siderocrasia 铁血症

词根 sidero-（铁）+ -crasia（异常的混合状态）

例句 Siderocrasia is a condition characterized by an excess of iron in the body. 铁血症是一种以体内铁元素过多为特征的病症。

hypercrasia 血液过多症

词根 hyper-（过度）+ -crasia（异常的混合状态）

例句 Hypercrasia is the abnormal overproduction of certain blood cells. 血液过多症是某些血细胞的异常增生。

normocrasia 正常血液成分

词根 normo-（正常）+ -crasia（异常的混合状态）

例句 Normocrasia is the normal composition of blood cells in the body. 正常血液成分是指体内血细胞的组成处于正常状态。

myelocrasia 骨髓不和谐

词根 myelo-（骨髓）+ -crasia（异常的混合状态）

例句 Myelocrasia is a disorder of the bone marrow, resulting in an imbalance of blood cell production. 骨髓不和谐是一种骨髓紊乱，导致血细胞生成失衡。

crico-（环状的）

cricoid 环状的

词根 crico-（环状的）+ -id（形容词后缀）

例句 The cricoid cartilage forms a ring around the trachea. 环状软骨围绕气管形成一个环。

cricoarytenoid 环杓的

词根 crico-（环状的）+ arytenoid（杓状）

例句 The cricoarytenoid muscles control the movement of the vocal cords. 环杓肌控制声带的运动。

cricoidectomy 环状软骨切除术

词根 crico-（环状的）+ -ectomy（切除术）

例句 Cricoidectomy is the surgical removal of the cricoid cartilage. 环状软骨切除术是切除环状软骨的手术。

cricoarytenoidotomy 环杓关节切开术

词根 crico-（环状的）+ arytenoid（杓状）+ -otomy（切开）

例句 Cricoarytenoidotomy is the surgical incision of the cricoarytenoid joint. 环杓关节切开术是切开环杓关节的手术。

cricopexy 环状软骨固定术

词根 crico-（环状的）+ -pexy（固定术）

例句 Cricopexy is a surgical procedure to stabilize the cricoid cartilage. 环状软骨固定术是稳定环状软骨的手术。

cricoid cartilage 环状软骨

词根 crico-（环状的）+ cartilage（软骨）

例句 The cricoid cartilage is the only complete ring of cartilage around the trachea. 环状软骨是围绕气管的唯一完整的软骨环。

cricoarytenoid muscles 杓状肌

词根 crico-（环状的）+ arytenoid（杓状）+ muscles（肌肉）

例句 The cricoarytenoid muscles play a key role in controlling speech production. 环杓肌在控制言语发音中起着关键作用。

cricoid pressure 环状软骨压迫

词根 crico-（环状的）+ pressure（压力）

例句 Cricoid pressure is applied during intubation to prevent regurgitation. 在插管过程中施加环状软骨压迫以防止胃内容物反流。

cricoid ring 环状环

词根 crico-（环状的）+ ring（环）

例句 The cricoid ring is essential in maintaining the structure of the trachea. 环状环在维持气管结构方面至关重要。

cricoid ligament 环状韧带

词根 crico-（环状的）+ ligament（韧带）

例句 The cricoid ligament connects the cricoid cartilage to the thyroid cartilage. 环状韧带连接环状软骨和甲状软骨。

USMLE Step 1　样题

A 50-year-old man comes to the office for a follow-up examination. He has a 2-month history of headache (-ache) and shortness of breath with exertion. He also has hypertension (hyper-; -tension) treated with hydrochlorothiazide (hydro-; chloro-) for the past 2 years. His blood pressure is 180/105 mmHg. Ophthalmoscopic (ophthalm-; scop-); examination is most likely to show which of the following in this patient?

(A) Arteriovenous (arterio-; veno-) nicking

(B) Melanocytes (melano-; -cyte) in the uvea

(C) Optic neuritis (neur-; -itis)

(D) Posterior subcapsular (sub-; capsul-) cataracts

(E) Tractional retinal detachment

中文翻译

一位 50 岁的男性前来进行随访检查。他有 2 个月的头痛和劳力性呼吸困难病史。他还患有高血压，过去 2 年一直服用氢氯噻嗪进行治疗。他的血压为 180/105 mmHg。眼底镜检查最可能显示以下哪种情况？

(A) 动静脉狭窄

(B) 葡萄膜中的黑色素细胞

(C) 视神经炎

(D) 后囊下白内障

(E) 牵拉性视网膜脱落

题目和答案中出现的词根

-ache：疼痛

hyper-：高

-tension：张力；压力

hydro-：氢

chloro-：氯

ophthalm-：眼睛的

scop-：镜

arterio-：动脉

veno-：静脉

melano-：黑色的

-cyte：细胞

neur-：神经的

-itis：炎症

sub-：在……下

capsul-：包囊的

-crine（分泌）

endocrine 内分泌

词根 endo-（内部）+ -crine（分泌）

例句 The endocrine system is responsible for secreting hormones that regulate metabolism. 内分泌系统负责分泌调节代谢的激素。

exocrine 外分泌

词根 exo-（外部）+ -crine（分泌）

例句 Exocrine glands secrete their products through ducts to the surface of the body or into cavities. 外分泌腺通过导管将分泌物分泌到身体表面或腔道中。

paracrine 旁分泌

词根 para-（旁边）+ -crine（分泌）

例句 Paracrine signaling involves the secretion of signaling molecules that affect nearby cells. 旁分泌信号传导是指分泌信号分子影响附近细胞的过程。

autocrine 自分泌

词根 auto-（自我）+ -crine（分泌）

例句 Autocrine signaling refers to the secretion of molecules that act on the same cells that produce them. 自分泌信号传导指的是分泌分子作用于其自身分泌的细胞。

neurocrine 神经分泌

词根 neuro-（神经）+ -crine（分泌）

例句 Neurocrine signaling involves the release of neurotransmitters from nerve cells. 神经分泌信号传导是指神经细胞释放神经递质的过程。

apocrine 顶浆分泌

词根 apo-（分离）+ -crine（分泌）

例句 Apocrine glands are a type of exocrine gland that secretes substances through cell membrane shedding. 顶浆分泌腺是外分泌腺的一种，通过细胞膜脱落分泌物质。

endocrinology 内分泌学

词根 endo-（内部）+ -crine（分泌）+ -logy（学科）

例句 Endocrinology is the branch of medicine that deals with disorders of the endocrine glands. 内分泌学是研究内分泌腺疾病的医学分支。

-crit（分离法）

hematocrit 红细胞比容

词根 hemato-（血液）+ -crit（分离法）

例句 The hematocrit test measures the proportion of red blood cells in the blood. 红细胞比容测试测量血液中红细胞的比例。

plasmacrit 血浆分离

词根 plasma-（血浆）+ -crit（分离法）

例句 Plasmacrit refers to the separation of plasma from whole blood. 血浆分离指的是将血浆与全血分离。

spermatocrit 精子比容

词根 sperma-（精子）+ -crit（分离法）

例句 Spermatocrit is a test used to assess the sperm concentration in semen. 精子比容用于评估精液中精子的浓度。

leukocrit 白细胞比容

词根 leuko-（白色）+ -crit（分离法）

例句 Leukocrit is a laboratory measure of the volume percentage of white blood cells in blood. 白细胞比容是实验室中测量血液中白细胞体积百分比的指标。

reticulocrit 网织红细胞比容

词根 reticulo-（网状）+ -crit（分离法）

例句 Reticulocrit measures the proportion of reticulocytes in the blood. 网织红细胞比容测量血液中网织红细胞的比例。

lymphocrit 淋巴细胞比容

词根 lympho-（淋巴）+ -crit（分离法）

例句 Lymphocrit is used to measure the percentage of lymphocytes in blood. 淋巴细胞比容用于测量血液中淋巴细胞的百分比。

cryocrit 冷冻血比容

词根 cryo-（冷）+ -crit（分离法）

例句 Cryocrit is used to measure the volume of red blood cells after freezing. 冷冻血比容用于测量冷冻后红细胞的体积。

critometer 血比容仪

词根 crit-（分离法）+ -ometer（仪器）

例句 A critometer is an instrument used to measure the hematocrit level in blood. 血比容仪是一种用于测量血液中血比容水平的仪器。

USMLE Step 1　样题

A 5-year-old girl is brought to the emergency department because of a 2-day history of fever, urinary (urin-) urgency, and burning pain with urination (urin-; -ation). She has had four similar episodes during the past year. A diagnosis of urinary tract infection is made. Subsequent renal ultrasonography (ultra-; sono-; -graphy) shows one large U-shaped kidney. Which of the following is the most likely embryologic origin of this patient's condition?

(A) Failure of the kidneys to rotate 90 degrees medially

(B) Failure of normal kidney ascent

(C) Failure of one ureteric bud to develop normally

(D) Fusion of the inferior poles of the metanephros (meta-; nephro) during ascent

中文翻译

一名5岁女孩因发热、尿急和排尿灼痛的症状持续2天，被送至急诊科。过去一年中她曾有4次类似的发作。诊断为尿路感染。随后的肾脏超声检查显示一侧肾脏呈巨大U形。以下哪项是该患者病情最可能的胚胎学起源？

(A) 肾脏未能向内旋转90°

(B) 肾脏未能正常上升

(C) 一侧输尿管芽未能正常发育

(D) 后肾上升过程中下极融合

题目和答案中出现的词根

urin-：尿

-ation：表示动作的状态

ultra-：超

sono-：声音的（表示可听见的声音波段）

-graphy：图像

meta：超过；在……后

nephor：肾脏

crypt-（隐）

cryptic 神秘的

词根 crypt-（隐）+ -ic（形容词后缀）

例句 The cryptic message left by the patient confused the medical team. 病人留下的神秘信息让医疗团队感到困惑。

cryptococcus 隐球菌

词根 crypt-（隐）+ -coccus（球菌）

例句 Cryptococcus is a genus of fungi that can cause serious infections in immunocompromised individuals. 隐球菌是一种可以在免疫系统受损的个体中引起严重感染的真菌属。

cryptogenic 隐源性的

词根 crypt-（隐）+ -genic（产生的）

例句 Cryptogenic causes are those whose origin cannot be determined. 隐源性病因是指那些无法确定起源的病因。

cryptorchidism 隐睾症

词根 crypt-（隐）+ orch-（睾丸）+ -idism（疾病）

例句 Cryptorchidism is a condition where one or both testes fail to descend into the scrotum. 隐睾症是一种病症，指一侧或双侧睾丸未能下降到阴囊内。

cryptosporidium 隐孢子虫

词根 crypt-（隐）+ -sporidium（孢子）

例句 Cryptosporidium is a parasite that can cause gastrointestinal illness in humans. 隐孢子虫是一种寄生虫，可以在人类中引起胃肠道疾病。

cryptanalysis 密码分析

词根 crypt-（隐）+ -analysis（分析）

例句 Cryptanalysis is the study of breaking encryption algorithms. 密码分析是研究破解加密算法的学科。

cryptic pregnancy 隐匿性怀孕

词根 crypt-（隐）+ pregnancy（怀孕）

例句 Cryptic pregnancy is a rare condition where a woman is unaware she is pregnant until delivery. 隐匿性怀孕是一种罕见的情况，女性直到分娩时才意识到自己怀孕。

culus-（小）

articulus 小关节

词根 articul-（关节）+ -ulus（小）

例句 The articulus is a small joint or connecting structure in the body. 小关节是指体内的小型关节或连接结构。

ventriculus 小室

词根 ventricul-（心室；胃室）+ -ulus（小）

例句 Ventriculus refers to a small chamber or cavity in the body, such as in the heart or stomach. 小室是指体内的小腔室或空腔，如心脏或胃部中的腔室。

calculus 结石

词根 cal-（石；计算）+ culus（小）

例句 Calculus is a small stone or deposit that forms in various body organs, such as the kidneys. 结石是指在体内不同器官（如肾脏）中形成的小石头或沉积物。

speculum 窥器

词根 spec-（看；观察）+ culum（小）

例句 A speculum is a small instrument used to examine body cavities, such as the vagina. 窥器是一种用于检查体腔（如阴道）的仪器。

nucleus 细胞核

词根 nucl-（核心）+ -us（小）
例句 The nucleus is the small, central part of a cell that contains genetic material. 细胞核是细胞的一个小型核心，包含遗传物质。

corpusculum 小体

词根 corpus-（体）+ culum（小）
例句 A corpusculum is a small body or particle, such as a red blood cell. 小体是指小型的物体或颗粒，如红细胞。

reticulum 网状体

词根 retic-（网）+ ulum（小）
例句 The reticulum is a small network of fibers found in various tissues of the body. 网状体是体内各种组织中发现的小型纤维网络。

cutane/o-（皮肤）

cutaneous 皮肤的

词根 cutane/o-（皮肤）+ -ous（形容词后缀）
例句 Cutaneous melanoma is a type of skin cancer that arises from pigment-producing cells. 皮肤黑色素瘤是一种源自色素产生细胞的皮肤癌。

subcutaneous 皮下的

词根 sub-（下）+ cutane/o-（皮肤）+ -ous（形容词后缀）
例句 Subcutaneous fat is the layer of fat located directly under the skin. 皮下脂肪是位于皮肤下方的脂肪层。

cutaneous t-cell lymphoma 皮肤 T 细胞淋巴瘤

词根 cutane/o-（皮肤）+ T-cell（T 细胞）+ lymphoma（淋巴瘤）
例句 Cutaneous T-cell lymphoma is a cancer of the skin's T-cells. 皮肤 T 细胞淋巴瘤是皮肤 T 细胞的癌症。

cyan-（青紫色）

cyanosis 发绀

词根 cyan-（青紫）+ -osis（病态）
例句 Cyanosis is a condition where there is a bluish tint to the skin, indicating a lack of oxygen in the blood. 发绀是一种皮肤呈现青紫色的病症，表明血液中缺氧。

cyanotic 发绀型心脏病

词根 cyan-（青紫）+ -tic（形容词后缀）
例句 Cyanotic heart disease is a condition that causes low oxygen levels, leading to a bluish hue in the skin. 发绀型心脏病是一种导致血氧水平降低、使皮肤呈现青紫色的病症。

cyanide 氰化物

词根 cyan-（青紫）+ -ide（化合物）
例句 Cyanide is a highly toxic compound that can cause rapid asphyxiation. 氰化物是一种剧毒化合物，可快速导致窒息。

cyanate 氰酸盐

词根 cyan-（青紫）+ -ate（盐或化合物）
例句 Cyanate is a chemical compound that contains the cyanide group. 氰酸盐是一种含有氰化基团的化学化合物。

cyanogen 氰基

词根 cyan-（青紫）+ -gen（产生）
例句 Cyanogen is a chemical compound that produces cyanide ions

when it is decomposed. 氰基是一种化学化合物，在分解时会产生氰离子。

cyanotype 蓝晒

词根 cyan-（青紫）+ -type（类型）
例句 A cyanotype is a photographic printing process that produces blue images. 蓝晒是一种照相印刷过程，能够产生蓝色图像。

cyanothermometer 青紫温度计

词根 cyan-（青紫）+ thermo-（热）+ -meter（计量器）
例句 A cyanothermometer is an instrument used to measure low temperatures in a system that is prone to cold damage. 青紫温度计是一种用于测量易受冷损害系统的低温的仪器。

cyanate ester 氰酸酯

词根 cyan-（青紫）+ -ate（盐）+ ester（酯）
例句 Cyanate esters are used in the production of high-performance composites due to their thermal stability. 氰酸酯由于其热稳定性，常用于生产高性能复合材料。

cyanogen chloride 氰氯

词根 cyan-（青紫）+ -gen（产生）+ chloride（氯化物）
例句 Cyanogen chloride is a highly toxic compound used as a chemical weapon. 氰氯是一种剧毒化合物，曾被用作化学武器。

cyanocobalamin 氰钴胺

词根 cyan-（青紫）+ cobalamin（维生素 B_{12}）
例句 Cyanocobalamin is a synthetic form of vitamin B_{12} used to treat vitamin B_{12} deficiencies. 氰钴胺是合成型的维生素 B_{12}，用于治疗维生素 B_{12} 缺乏症。

USMLE Step 1　样题

A 56-year-old man comes to the office because of a 1-month

history of pain and tingling of his hands and a 6-month history of paresthesia (par-; -esthes) of his feet. As part of the workup, a nerve biopsy (bio-; -psy) specimen is obtained and analyzed at the electron microscopic (micro-; scop-) level. The biopsy (bio-; -psy) specimen shows marked loss of structures labeled by the X's in the photomicrograph (photo-; micro-; -graph) of a normal biopsy (bio-; -psy) specimen shown. The loss of these structures is most likely to cause which of the following neurologic (neuro-) findings in this patient?

(A) Decreased sensitivity of the deep tendon reflex

(B) Impaired stereognosis (stere-; -gnosis)

(C) Loss of pain and temperature sensation

(D) Muscle atrophy (a-; -trophy)

(E) Vasoconstriction (vaso-)

中文翻译

一名 56 岁男性因双手疼痛伴麻木 1 个月、双足感觉异常 6 个月前来就诊。作为诊断的一部分，医生对其进行了神经活检并在电子显微镜下进行分析。活检标本显示，与正常活检标本显微照片中标记为“X”的结构相比，存在显著缺失。这些结构的缺失最可能导致该患者出现以下哪种神经学表现？

(A) 深部腱反射敏感性降低

(B) 立体辨别能力受损

(C) 痛觉和温度觉丧失

(D) 肌肉萎缩

(E) 血管收缩

题目和答案中出现的词根

par-：超过；异常的

-esthes：感觉

bio-：生物

-psy：观察

photo-：像；光

micro：微小的

-graph：图像

neuro-：神经的

stere-：固体的

-gnosis：辨别力

a-：表否定

-trophy：营养

vaso-：血管

cyclo-（环）

cycle 循环

词根 cyclo-（环）

例句 A cycle is a series of events that repeat in a specific order, such as the water cycle. 循环是以特定顺序重复的一系列事件，如水循环。

cyclone 气旋

词根 cyclo-（环）+ -one（形成）

例句 A cyclone is a powerful, rotating storm system that forms over warm ocean waters. 气旋是一种强大的旋转风暴系统，通常形成于温暖的洋面上。

cyclotron 回旋加速器

词根 cyclo-（环）+ -tron（仪器）

例句 A cyclotron is a type of particle accelerator that uses a magnetic field to accelerate charged particles in a circular motion. 回旋加速器是一种利用磁场加速带电粒子沿圆形轨道运动的粒子加速器。

cyclohexane 环己烷

词根 cyclo-（环）+ hexane（六烷）

例句 Cyclohexane is a colorless liquid often used as a solvent in industrial processes. 环己烷是一种无色液体，常用于工业过程中的溶剂。

cyclooxygenase 环氧合酶

词根 cyclo-（环）+ oxygenase（氧化酶）

例句 Cyclooxygenase is an enzyme responsible for the formation of prostaglandins, which mediate inflammation. 环氧合酶是一种负责前列腺素形成的酶，而前列腺素可介导炎症。

cyclin 细胞周期蛋白

词根 cyclo-（环）+ -in（蛋白质）

例句 Cyclins are proteins that regulate the cell cycle by controlling the progression of cells through different stages. 细胞周期蛋白是一类通过控制细胞在不同阶段的进程来调节细胞周期的蛋白质。

cyst-（囊）

cyst 囊

词根 cyst-（囊）

例句 A cyst is a closed sac-like structure that can form in various parts of the body, often filled with fluid or semi-solid material. 囊肿是一种封闭的囊状结构，可以在身体的不同部位形成，通常充

满液体或半固体物质。

cystic 囊性的

词根 cyst-（囊）+ -ic（形容词后缀）
例句 Cystic fibrosis is a genetic disorder that causes severe damage to the lungs and digestive system. 囊性纤维化是一种遗传性疾病，会对肺部和消化系统造成严重损害。

cystectomy 囊肿切除术

词根 cyst-（囊）+ -ectomy（切除术）
例句 Cystectomy is the surgical removal of a cyst from the body. 囊肿切除术是切除体内囊肿的外科手术。

ovarian cyst 卵巢囊肿

词根 ovarian（卵巢的）+ cyst-（囊）
例句 An ovarian cyst is a fluid-filled sac that forms on or inside an ovary. 卵巢囊肿是一个充满液体的囊，形成在卵巢上或卵巢内部。

renal cyst 肾囊肿

词根 renal（肾脏的）+ cyst-（囊）
例句 A renal cyst is a fluid-filled sac that forms on the kidneys. 肾囊肿是一个充满液体的囊，形成在肾脏上。

pilonidal cyst 藏毛囊肿

词根 pilonidal（毛发囊）+ cyst-（囊）
例句 A pilonidal cyst is a pocket of skin filled with hair and debris that forms at the base of the spine. 藏毛囊肿是一种在脊柱底部形成的皮肤囊腔，内含毛发和碎屑。

cystoid 囊状的

词根 cyst-（囊）+ -oid（类似的）
例句 Cystoid lesions are abnormalities that appear as cyst-like structures within tissues. 囊状病变是指在组织中出现类似囊肿的异常

结构。

cystadenoma

词根 cysto-（膀胱）+ aden-（腺体）+ -oma（肿瘤）

例句 Cystadenoma is a type of tumor that arises from glandular tissue and often involves cyst formation. 囊腺瘤是一种来源于腺体组织的肿瘤，通常伴随囊肿形成。

cystic fibrosis

词根 cysto-（膀胱）+ fibros-（纤维化）

例句 Cystic fibrosis is a genetic disorder that affects the lungs, pancreas, and other organs, causing thick mucus to block ducts. 囊性纤维化是一种遗传性疾病，影响肺部、胰腺和其他器官，导致黏稠的黏液堵塞导管。

cysto-（膀胱）

cystitis 膀胱炎

词根 cysto-（膀胱）+ -itis（炎症）

例句 Cystitis is the inflammation of the bladder, commonly caused by urinary tract infections. 膀胱炎是膀胱的炎症，通常由尿路感染引起。

cystoscopy 膀胱镜检查

词根 cysto-（膀胱）+ -scopy（检查仪器）

例句 Cystoscopy is a procedure where a doctor uses a thin tube to look inside the bladder. 膀胱镜检查是指医生使用细管查看膀胱内部。

cystectomy 膀胱切除术

词根 cysto-（膀胱）+ -ectomy（切除术）

例句 Cystectomy is a surgical procedure to remove the bladder, typically done in cases of bladder cancer. 膀胱切除术是一种手术，

通常在膀胱癌的情况下进行。

cystogram 膀胱造影

词根 cysto-（膀胱）+ -gram（图像）

例句 A cystogram is an imaging technique used to examine the bladder using contrast dye. 膀胱造影是一种使用对比剂检查膀胱的成像技术。

cystocele 膀胱膨出

词根 cysto-（膀胱）+ -cele（肿胀；膨出）

例句 Cystocele occurs when the bladder bulges into the vaginal wall, often due to weakened pelvic muscles. 膀胱膨出是指膀胱向阴道壁膨出，通常由骨盆肌肉弱化导致。

cystourethroscopy 膀胱尿道镜检查

词根 cysto-（膀胱）+ urethro-（尿道）+ -scopy（检查）

例句 Cystourethroscopy is a diagnostic procedure used to examine the bladder and urethra. 膀胱尿道镜检查是一种诊断程序，用于检查膀胱和尿道。

cystorrhaphy 膀胱缝合术

词根 cysto-（膀胱）+ -rrhaphy（缝合）

例句 Cystorrhaphy is a surgical procedure that involves suturing the bladder wall. 膀胱缝合术是一种缝合膀胱壁的外科手术。

cyto-（细胞的）

cytology 细胞学

词根 cyto-（细胞）+ -logy（学科）

例句 Cytology is the study of cells, their structure, function, and behavior. 细胞学是研究细胞及其结构、功能和行为的学科。

cytoplasm 细胞质

词根 cyto-（细胞）+ -plasm（质）

例句 Cytoplasm is the gel-like substance inside a cell where most cellular processes occur. 细胞质是细胞内部的凝胶状物质，绝大多数细胞活动在此进行。

cytoskeleton 细胞骨架

词根 cyto-（细胞）+ -skeleton（骨架）

例句 The cytoskeleton provides structural support and shape to a cell. 细胞骨架为细胞提供结构和形状支持。

cytokine 细胞因子

词根 cyto-（细胞）+ -kine（因子）

例句 Cytokines are signaling proteins that help cells communicate with each other. 细胞因子是帮助细胞相互沟通的信号蛋白。

cytotoxic 细胞毒性的

词根 cyto-（细胞）+ toxic（有毒的）

例句 Cytotoxic drugs are used to kill cancer cells by damaging their DNA. 细胞毒性药物通过破坏癌细胞的 DNA 来杀死癌细胞。

cytogenetics 细胞遗传学

词根 cyto-（细胞）+ -genetics（遗传学）

例句 Cytogenetics is the branch of genetics that studies the structure and function of chromosomes. 细胞遗传学是遗传学的一个分支，研究染色体的结构和功能。

cytometer 细胞计数器

词根 cyto-（细胞）+ -meter（测量仪器）

例句 A cytometer is used to measure the physical and chemical properties of cells. 细胞计数器用于测量细胞的物理和化学特性。

cytotoxicity 细胞毒性

词根 cyto-（细胞）+ toxic（有毒的）+ -ity（名词后缀）
例句 Cytotoxicity refers to the ability of a substance to kill or damage cells. 细胞毒性指的是物质杀死或损害细胞的能力。

cytosine 胞嘧啶

词根 cyto-（细胞）+ -sine（含氮碱基）
例句 Cytosine is a nucleotide base that pairs with guanine in DNA and RNA. 胞嘧啶是一种核苷酸碱基，在 DNA 和 RNA 中与鸟嘌呤配对。

cytokinesis 细胞质分裂

词根 cyto-（细胞）+ -kinesis（运动）
例句 Cytokinesis is the process during cell division in which the cytoplasm divides, resulting in two daughter cells. 细胞质分裂是细胞分裂过程中细胞质发生分裂，最终形成两个子细胞的过程。

USMLE Step 1　样题

A 3-week-old girl delivered at term with no complications is brought to the physician by her mother because of a 1-week history of yellow eyes and skin, tan-colored stools, and dark brown urine. The newborn has been breast-feeding without difficulty. She is alert and appears to be in no distress (dis-; -tress). She is at the 50th percentile for length and weight. Physical examination shows scleral icterus and jaundice. There is mild hepatomegaly; the spleen is not palpable. Laboratory studies show:

Hemoglobin (hemo-; -globin) 14.4 g/dL

Hematocrit (hemato-; -crit) 43%

Leukocyte (leuko-; -cyte) count 8,000/mm^3

Serum Albumin 3.5 g/dL

Bilirubin (bili-; -rubin), total 14 mg/dL

Direct 12.5 mg/dL

AST 50 U/L

ALT 45 U/L

Which of the following is the most likely diagnosis?

(A) Biliary atresia (a-; -tresia)

(B) Crigler-Najjar syndrome, type I

(C) Gilbert syndrome

(D) Hemolytic (hemo-; lyt) disease of the newborn

(E) Physiologic jaundice (jaun-)

中文翻译

一名足月顺产、无并发症的 3 周龄女婴，因出现黄疸（眼睛和皮肤发黄）、陶土色粪便及深褐色尿液症状达 1 周，被其母亲带至医生处就诊。该新生儿母乳喂养情况良好，无喂养困难。她意识清醒，无明显不适表现。其身长和体重均处于正常范围内。体格检查显示存在巩膜黄染和黄疸，肝脏轻度肿大，脾脏大小正常。实验室检查结果如下：

血红蛋白 14.4 g/dL

红细胞压积 43%

白细胞计数 8,000/ mm^3

血清白蛋白 3.5 g/dL

总胆红素 14 mg/dL

直接胆红素 12.5 mg/dL

AST 50 单位 / L

ALT 45 单位 / L

以下哪项是最可能的诊断？

(A) 胆道闭锁

(B) Crigler-Najjar 综合征 I 型

(C) Gilbert 综合征

(D) 新生儿溶血病

(E) 生理性黄疸

题目和答案中出现的词根

dis-：分开

-tress：用力

hepato-：肝脏的

mega-：大

hemo-：血

-globin：球蛋白

hemato-：血

-crit：分离法

leuko-：白色的

-cyte：细胞

bili-：胆的

-rubin：红色

a-：表示否定

-tresia：孔（否定加孔表示闭锁）

-lyt：溶解

jaun：黄色的

dacryo-（眼泪的）

dacryoma 泪腺肿瘤

词根 dacryo-（眼泪）+ -oma（肿瘤）

例句 Dacryoma is a type of benign tumor that occurs in the tear glands. 泪腺肿瘤是一种发生在泪腺的良性肿瘤。

dacryocystitis 泪囊炎

词根 dacryo-（眼泪）+ cyst-（囊）+ -itis（炎症）

例句 Dacryocystitis is the infection and inflammation of the tear sac, usually caused by a blocked tear duct. 泪囊炎是泪囊的感染和炎症，通常由泪管堵塞引起。

dacryocystorhinostomy 泪囊鼻吻合术

词根 dacryo-（眼泪）+ cysto-（囊）+ rhin-（鼻）+ -ostomy（造口术）

例句 Dacryocystorhinostomy is a surgical procedure to create a new drainage pathway for tears from the eye to the nose. 泪囊鼻腔吻合术是一种通过手术创建新的引流通道，使泪液从眼部引流至鼻部的外科手术。

dacryoadenitis 泪腺炎

词根 dacryo-（眼泪）+ aden-（腺体）+ -itis（炎症）

例句 Dacryoadenitis is the inflammation of the tear-producing glands, which can cause swelling and discomfort. 泪腺炎是泪腺的炎症，可能引起肿胀和不适。

dacryorrhea 溢泪症

词根 dacryo-（眼泪）+ -rrhea（流出）

例句 Dacryorrhea is the excessive flow of tears from the eyes, often due to irritation or infection. 溢泪症是眼泪过度流出，通常是由刺激或感染引起的。

USMLE Step 1 样题

A 46-year-old woman comes to the physician because of a 3-day history of intermittent (inter-; mitt-) pain with urination (urin-) and increased urinary (urin-) frequency. She says that she had one similar episode (epi-; -sode) during the past 6 months. She also has had irregular (ir-) menses, and her last menstrual (menstru-) period occurred 2 months ago. She has not had fever, nausea, vomiting, or blood in her urine. She is sexually active with one male partner. Physical examination shows no abnormalities. Urinalysis shows:

RBC 3–5/hpf

WBC 10–20/hpf

Nitrites positive

Leukocyte (leuk-; -cyte) esterase (-ase) positive

Bacteria positive

Which of the following is the strongest predisposing risk factor for the development of this patient's condition?

(A) Leiomyomata (leio-; myo-) uterus

(B) Perimenopause (peri-; meno-; pause)

(C) Pregnancy

(D) Sexual intercourse

中文翻译

一名46岁女性因过去3天出现间歇性排尿疼痛和排尿次数增加而就医。她表示在过去6个月内有过一次类似发作。她还有月经不规律的病史，末次月经发生在2个月前。她没有发热、恶心、呕吐或血尿症状。她与一名男性伴侣有性生活。体格检查未见异常。尿液分析结果如下：

红细胞 3 ～ 5 个 / 高倍视野

白细胞 10 ～ 20 个 / 高倍视野

亚硝酸盐 阳性

白细胞酯酶 阳性

细菌 阳性

以下哪项是该患者病情发展的最强风险因素？

(A) 子宫肌瘤

(B) 围绝经期

(C) 妊娠

(D) 性生活

题目和答案中出现的词根

inter-：在……之间

mitt-：时间区间

urin-：尿

epi-：在……上（或旁）

-sode：道路（在旅途旁边，指的是发作，通常是间歇性的发作期，旅途指的是正常的人生旅途，而正常人生旅途旁就是间歇发病期）

ir-：表否定

menstru-：每个月的

leuk-：白色的

-cyte：细胞

-ase：酶

leio-：平滑的

myo-：肌肉

peri-：外周

meno-：每个月

-pause：停止

-dactyly（指头的）

polydactyly 多指症

词根 poly-（多）+ dactyly（指头的）

例句 Polydactyly is a condition where a person has more than five fingers or toes. 多指症是一种人拥有超过五根手指或脚趾的病症。

syndactyly 并指症

词根 syn-（联合）+ dactyly（指头的）

例句 Syndactyly is a congenital condition where two or more fingers are fused together. 并指症是一种先天性病症，指两根或多根手指融合在一起。

brachydactyly 短指症

词根 brachy-（短）+ dactyly（指头的）

例句 Brachydactyly refers to abnormally short fingers or toes. 短指症指的是手指或脚趾异常短小的情况。

macrodactyly 大指症

词根 macro-（大）+ dactyly（指头的）

例句 Macrodactyly is a condition characterized by unusually large fingers or toes. 大指症是指手指或脚趾异常大的情况。

de-（去除）

defibrillator 除颤器

词根 de-（去除）+ fibrill-（纤颤）+ -ator（器具）

例句 A defibrillator is a device used to restore a normal heart rhythm by delivering a shock to the heart. 除颤器是一种通过向心脏传送电击来恢复正常心律的设备。

decontamination 去污

词根 de-（去除）+ contamination（污染）

例句 Decontamination is the process of removing harmful substances or pathogens from surfaces or objects. 去污是去除物体表面有害物质或病原体的过程。

decalcification 去钙化

词根 de-（去除）+ calc-（钙）+ -fication（化）

例句 Decalcification refers to the process of removing calcium from bones or teeth. 去钙化指的是去除骨骼或牙齿中的钙的过程。

dehydration 脱水

词根 de-（去除）+ hydr-（水）+ -ation（过程）

例句 Dehydration is the loss of body fluids, which can lead to serious health issues if not treated. 脱水是体液的流失，如果不治疗，可能会导致严重的健康问题。

denervation 去神经化

词根 de-（去除）+ nerv-（神经）+ -ation（过程）

例句 Denervation involves the removal of nerve supply to a part of the body. 去神经化指去除身体某部分的神经供应。

dem-/demo-（人口）

demography 人口统计学

词根 demo-（人口）+ -graphy（记录）

例句 Demography is the statistical study of populations, including the structure and dynamics of a society. 人口统计学是对人口的统计研究，包括社会结构和社会动态的研究。

demographic 人口的；人口统计的

词根 demo-（人口）+ -ic（形容词后缀）

例句 Demographic changes, such as population growth and aging, can have significant effects on society. 人口变化，如人口增长和老龄化，可能对社会产生重大影响。

demography-based research 基于人口统计学的研究

词根 demo-（人口）+ graph-（记录）+ -based（基于）

例句 Demography-based research helps in understanding trends in population growth, migration, and aging. 基于人口统计学的研究有助于理解人口增长、迁移和老龄化的趋势。

dent-/（o）dont-（牙齿的）

dentist 牙医

词根 dent-（牙齿）+ -ist（从事某种职业的人）

例句 A dentist is a healthcare professional who specializes in the diagnosis, treatment, and prevention of oral diseases. 牙医是专门从事口腔疾病诊断、治疗和预防的医疗专业人员。

dentistry 牙科

词根 dent-（牙齿）+ -istry（学科）

例句 Dentistry is the branch of medicine focused on the study, diagnosis, prevention, and treatment of dental and oral health issues. 牙科是医学的一个分支，专注于口腔健康问题的研究、诊断、预防和治疗。

dental 牙齿的

词根 dent-（牙齿）+ -al（形容词后缀）

例句 Dental health is essential for overall well-being, and regular checkups are necessary for maintaining good oral hygiene. 牙齿健康对整体健康至关重要，定期检查牙齿对于保持良好的口腔卫生是必要的。

dentition 牙列

词根 dent-（牙齿）+ -ition（状态）

例句 Dentition refers to the development, arrangement, and condition of a person's teeth. 牙列指的是一个人牙齿的发育、排列和状态。

denture 假牙

词根 dent-（牙齿）+ -ure（名词后缀）

例句 A denture is a removable replacement for missing teeth, designed to restore function and appearance. 假牙是一种可拆卸的牙齿替代物，用于恢复牙齿功能和外观。

endodontics 牙髓学

词根 endo-（内部）+ dont-（牙齿）+ -ics（学科）

例句 Endodontics is a branch of dentistry focused on the diagnosis and treatment of diseases and injuries of the dental pulp. 牙髓学是牙科的一个分支，专注于牙髓疾病和损伤的诊断与治疗。

periodontics 牙周学

词根 periodont-（牙周）+ -ics（学科）

例句 Periodontics is a branch of dentistry that deals with the prevention, diagnosis, and treatment of periodontal disease. 牙周学是牙科的一个分支，专注于牙周病的预防、诊断和治疗。

dentalgia 牙痛

词根 dent-（牙齿）+ -algia（痛）

例句 Dentalgia is the pain or discomfort that occurs in the teeth or surrounding tissues, often due to cavities or infections. 牙痛是发生在牙齿或周围组织的疼痛或不适，通常是由蛀牙或感染引起的。

dentifrice 牙洁剂

词根 dent-（牙齿）+ -frice（摩擦）

例句 Dentifrice is a substance used to clean and polish teeth, commonly known as toothpaste. 牙洁剂是用于清洁和抛光牙齿的物质，通常被称为牙膏。

orthodontics 正畸学

词根 ortho-（正直）+ dont-（牙齿）+ -ics（学科）

例句 Orthodontics is the dental specialty that focuses on the correction of misaligned teeth and jaws. 正畸学是牙科专业之一，专注于矫正错位的牙齿和颌骨。

dentate 有齿的

词根 dent-（牙齿）+ -ate（形容词后缀）

例句 Dentate refers to having a toothed or serrated edge, often used to describe certain types of leaves or structures in the mouth. 有齿的指的是具有齿状或锯齿状边缘，通常用于描述某些类型的叶子或口腔结构。

hypodontia 少牙症

词根 hypo-（缺乏）+ odont-（牙齿）+ -ia（病症）

例句 Hypodontia is a condition where a person is born with fewer teeth than normal, often due to genetic factors. 少牙症是指一个人生来缺少牙齿，通常与遗传因素有关。

macrodontia 巨牙症

词根 macro-（大）+ odont-（牙齿）+ -ia（病症）

例句 Macrodontia is a condition characterized by abnormally large teeth, which can lead to dental problems. 巨牙症是一种特征为牙齿异常增大的疾病，可能导致牙齿问题。

odontogenic 牙源性的

词根 odont-（牙齿）+ -genic（产生的）

例句 Odontogenic tumors are tumors that originate from tooth-forming tissues. 牙源性肿瘤是指起源于牙齿形成组织的肿瘤。

deoxy-（脱氧）

deoxyribonucleic acid（DNA）脱氧核糖核酸

词根 deoxy-（脱氧）+ ribonucleic acid（核糖核酸）

例句 Deoxyribonucleic acid（DNA）carries genetic information in cells. 脱氧核糖核酸（DNA）在细胞中携带遗传信息。

deoxyadenosine 脱氧腺苷

词根 deoxy-（脱氧）+ adenosine（腺苷）

例句 Deoxyadenosine is a molecule that is a building block of DNA. 脱氧腺苷是一种构成 DNA 的基本分子单元。

deoxythymidine 脱氧胸苷

词根 deoxy-（脱氧）+ thymidine（胸苷）

例句 Deoxythymidine is a nucleoside involved in the synthesis of

DNA. 脱氧胸苷是参与 DNA 合成的核苷。

deoxyribose 脱氧核糖

词根 deoxy-（脱氧）+ ribose（核糖）
例句 Deoxyribose is a sugar found in DNA that lacks one oxygen atom compared to ribose in RNA. 脱氧核糖是 DNA 中的一种糖，与 RNA 中的核糖相比，缺少一个氧原子。

deoxyguanosine 脱氧鸟苷

词根 deoxy-（脱氧）+ guanosine（鸟苷）
例句 Deoxyguanosine is a purine nucleoside that is part of the structure of DNA. 脱氧鸟苷是嘌呤核苷，是 DNA 结构的一部分。

USMLE Step 1 样题

A 46-year-old woman comes to the physician because of a 1-month history of fatigue, weakness, and palpitations. She has advanced kidney disease as a result of continued use of combination analgesics (an-; alges-) for low back pain. She has hypertension (hyper-; -tension) well controlled with a loop diuretic, a β-adrenergic (adren-) blocker, and a dihydropyridine (di-; hydro-) calcium (calc-) channel blocker. She has a history of gastritis (gastr-; -itis) and hemorrhoids (hemo-; rrho-; -oid) associated with occult blood in the stools. She is in no acute distress (dis-; -tress). Her temperature is 36.8°C (98.2°F), pulse is 74/min, respirations (re-; spir-; -ation) are 14/min, and blood pressure is 150/86 mmHg. Physical examination shows mild midepigastric (mid-; epi-; gastr-) tenderness to palpation and 2+ edema of the lower extremities. Cardiac examination shows an S4 gallop. Test of the stool for occult blood is positive. Laboratory studies show:

Hemoglobin (hemo-; -globin) 8.8 g/dL

Hematocrit (hemato-; -crit) 26.8%

Mean corpuscular (corpuscu-) volume 82 μm³

Serum Ferritin 262 ng/mL

Folate 284 ng/mL (N=150–450)

Total iron 60 μg/dL

Transferrin (trans-; ferr-) saturation 22% (N=20%–50%)

Lactate dehydrogenase (de-; hydr-; gen-; -ase) 62 U/L

Which of the following is the most likely cause of this patient's anemia?

(A) Bone marrow suppression

(B) Decreased erythropoietin (erythr-; -poietin) production

(C) Intravascular (intra-) hemolysis (hemo-; -lysis)

(D) Iron deficiency anemia (an-; -emia)

(E) Splenic sequestration

中文翻译

一名 46 岁女性因过去 1 个月出现疲劳、虚弱和心悸而就医。她因长期使用复方止痛药治疗腰痛，导致晚期肾病。她有高血压，服用袢利尿剂、β-肾上腺素受体阻滞剂和二氢吡啶类钙通道阻滞剂，血压控制效果良好。她有胃炎和痔疮病史，伴有粪便隐血。她无急性不适症状。体温 36.8℃（98.2℉），脉搏 74 次 / 分钟，呼吸 14 次 / 分钟，血压 150/86 mmHg。体格检查显示轻度上腹中部压痛，双下肢 2+ 级水肿。心脏检查发现 S4 奔马律。粪便隐血试验阳性。实验室检查结果如下：

血红蛋白 8.8 g/dL

血细胞比容 26.8%

平均红细胞体积 82 μm³

血清铁蛋白 262 ng/mL

叶酸 284 ng/mL（正常范围：150 ～ 450）

总铁 60 μg/dL

转铁蛋白饱和度 22%（正常范围：20% ～ 50%）

乳酸脱氢酶 62 U/L

以下哪项是该患者贫血最可能的原因？

(A) 骨髓抑制

(B) 促红细胞生成素生成减少

(C) 血管内溶血

(D) 缺铁性贫血

(E) 脾脏隔离

题目和答案中出现的词根

an-：表示否定

alges-：疼痛

hyper-：高

-tension：张力；压力

adren-：肾上腺

di-：双

hydro-：氢

calc-：钙

gastr-：胃的

-itis：炎症

hemo-：血

rrho-：流动

-oid：类似的（类似血液流动的感觉，指代痔疮）

dis-：分开

-tress：用力

re-：重新；反复

spir-：呼吸

-ation：表示动作的状态

mid-：在……中间

epi-：在……上

hemo-：血

-globin：球蛋白

hemato-：血

-crit：分离法

corpuscu-：肉体的，这里指红细胞本体

trans-：转；跨

ferr-：铁

de-：去掉

gen-：产生

-ase：酶（去掉氢产生的酶，即脱氢酶）

erythr-：红色的

-poietin：发生；生成（生成红色的，即促红素）

intra-：在……内

-lysis：分解

an-：表示否定

-emia：血症

derm-（皮肤）

dermatology 皮肤学

词根 derm-（皮肤）+ -ology（学科）

例句 Dermatology is the branch of medicine that focuses on the diagnosis and treatment of skin diseases. 皮肤学是专注于皮肤疾病诊断和治疗的医学分支。

dermatitis 皮肤炎

词根 derm-（皮肤）+ -itis（炎症）

例句 Dermatitis is the inflammation of the skin, often resulting in redness, itching, and swelling. 皮肤炎是皮肤的炎症，常表现为红肿、瘙痒和肿胀。

dermabrasion 皮肤磨削术

词根 derm-（皮肤）+ abras-（磨损）

例句 Dermabrasion is a procedure used to remove the outer layers of the skin to treat scars or wrinkles. 皮肤磨削术是一种用来去除皮肤外层，以治疗疤痕或皱纹的手术。

dermatoplasty 皮肤成形术

词根 derm-（皮肤）+ -plasty（修复手术）

例句 Dermatoplasty is the surgical repair or reconstruction of the skin. 皮肤成形术是对皮肤进行修复或重建的外科手术。

dermis 真皮

词根 derm-（皮肤）

例句 The dermis is the thick layer of living tissue beneath the epidermis, containing blood vessels and nerves. 真皮是位于表皮下的厚层活组织，包含血管和神经。

-desis（融合固定）

arthrodesis 关节融合术

词根 arthr-（关节）+ -desis（融合固定）

例句 Arthrodesis is a surgical procedure to fuse two bones in a joint to eliminate movement. 关节融合术是一种外科手术，用于将关节中的两块骨头融合在一起，以消除关节活动。

spondylodesis 脊柱融合术

词根 spondyl-（脊椎）+ -desis（融合固定）

例句 Spondylodesis is a procedure to fuse two or more vertebrae in the spine. 脊椎融合术是将脊柱中的两块或更多椎骨融合的手术。

tenodesis 肌腱固定术

词根 teno-（肌腱）+ -desis（融合固定）

例句 Tenodesis is the surgical procedure used to attach a tendon to a bone. 肌腱固定术是将肌腱固定到骨头上的外科手术。

tarsodesis 踝骨融合术

词根 tars-（踝）+ -desis（融合固定）

例句 Tarsodesis is a procedure to fuse the bones in the ankle joint. 踝骨融合术是将踝关节中的骨骼融合的手术。

chondrodesis 软骨融合术

词根 chondro-（软骨）+ -desis（融合固定）

例句 Chondrodesis is a surgical technique used to fuse cartilage and bone in certain joints. 软骨融合术是一种用于融合软骨与骨骼的手术。

didym-（睾丸，强调成对）

didymus 双胞胎；睾丸

词根 didym-（睾丸）

例句 Didymus refers to a paired organ, such as the testicles in males. 该词指成对的器官，例如男性的睾丸。

didymitis 睾丸炎

词根 didym-（睾丸）+ -itis（炎症）

例句 Didymitis is the inflammation of the testicles, often caused by infections. 睾丸炎是睾丸的炎症，通常由感染引起。

didymectomy 睾丸切除术

词根 didym-（睾丸）+ -ectomy（切除术）

例句 Didymectomy is the surgical removal of one or both testicles. 睾丸切除术是切除一个或两个睾丸的外科手术。

didymoepididymitis 睾丸附睾炎

词根 didym-（睾丸）+ epi-（表面）+ didym-（睾丸）+ -itis（炎症）

例句 Didymoepididymitis is the inflammation of both testicles and the epididymis, often caused by bacterial infections. 睾丸附睾炎是睾丸和附睾的炎症，通常由细菌感染引起。

didymus cryptorchidism 隐睾症

词根 didym-（睾丸）+ crypt-（隐藏）+ orchid-（睾丸）+ -ism（病态）

例句 Didymus cryptorchidism is a condition in which the testicles fail to descend into the scrotum. 隐睾症是一种病症，指睾丸未能降入阴囊。

D

USMLE Step 1 样题

A 72-year-old man comes to the physician for a health maintenance examination. He has no personal or family history of major medical illnesses. He has never smoked cigarettes (cigar-; -ette). Pulse oximetry (oxi-; -metry) on room air shows an oxygen saturation of 98%. Physical examination shows plethoric (plethor-) skin and splenomegaly (splen-; mega-). Laboratory studies show:

Hemoglobin (hemo-; -globin) 21.1 g/dL

Hematocrit (hemato-; -crit) 61%

Leukocyte (leuk-; -cyte) count 15,000/mm^3

Segmented neutrophils (neutro-; -phil) 68%

Basophils (baso-; -phil) 4%

Lymphocytes (lymph-; -cyte) 28%

Platelet (plate-; -let) count 501,000/mm^3

Leukocyte (leuk-; -cyte) alkaline (alkali-) phosphatase (phosph-; -ase) increased

A peripheral (peri-; pher-) blood smear shows occasional giant platelets (plate-; -let). The primary hematologic (hemato-) defect in this patient most likely occurred in which of the following cells?

(A) Erythroid (erthr-; -oid) progenitor (pro-; genit-)

(B) Hematopoietic stem (hemato-; poiet)

(C) Lymphatic (lymph-) progenitor (pro-; genit-)

(D) Megakaryocyte (mega-; karyo-; -cyte) progenitor (pro-; genit-)

(E) Pluripotent (pluri-; potent) stem

中文翻译

一名 72 岁男性前来就诊，进行健康检查。他无个人或家族重大疾病史，从不吸烟。室温空气下脉搏血氧饱和度为 98%。体格检查显示皮肤多血质和脾肿大。实验室检查结果如下：

血红蛋白 21.1 g/dL

血细胞比容 61%

白细胞计数 15,000/mm³

中性分叶核粒细胞 68%

嗜碱性粒细胞 4%

淋巴细胞 28%

血小板计数 501,000/mm³

白细胞碱性磷酸酶升高

外周血涂片显示偶见巨大血小板

该患者的主要血液学缺陷最有可能发生在以下哪种细胞中？

(A) 红系祖细胞

(B) 造血干细胞

(C) 淋巴祖细胞

(D) 巨核细胞祖细胞

(E) 多能干细胞

题目和答案中出现的词根

cigar-：雪茄

-ette：小的（小雪茄指普通香烟）

oxi-：氧气的

-metry：测量仪

splen-：脾脏

mega-：大

hemo-：血

-globin：球蛋白

hemato-：血

-crit：分离法

leuk-：白色的

-cyte：细胞

neutro-：中性的

-phil：嗜

baso-：碱性的

lymph-：淋巴的

plate-：板状的

-lets：小

alkali-：溶液碱性的

phosph-：磷

-ase：酶

erthr-：红色的

-oid：类似的

pro-：在……之前

genit-：产生

-poiet：产生

mega-：大

karyo-：细胞核

pluri-：多个

potent：能力

dips-（渴）

polydipsia 多饮症

词根 poly-（多）+ dips-（渴）

例句 Polydipsia is a condition characterized by excessive thirst and fluid consumption. 多饮症是一种以过度口渴和过量饮水为特征的病症。

dipsomania 饮酒狂

词根 dips-（渴）+ -mania（狂躁）

例句 Dipsomania refers to an intense craving or obsession with drinking alcohol. 饮酒狂是指对饮酒的强烈渴望或痴迷。

dipsesis 渴症

词根 dips-（渴）+ -esis（病态）

例句 Dipsesis is the medical term for abnormal thirst, often a symptom of diabetes. 渴症是异常口渴的医学术语，通常是糖尿病的症状。

dipsic 渴的

词根 dips-（渴）+ -ic（形容词后缀）

例句 The dipsic patient constantly seeks water due to an overwhelming thirst. 患有渴症的病人因极度口渴而不断寻找水。

dipsotoxicosis 渴毒症

词根 dips-（渴）+ tox-（毒）+ -icosis（病态）

例句 Dipsotoxicosis refers to a condition in which excessive thirst leads to the consumption of harmful substances. 渴毒症指的是过度口渴导致摄入有害物质的病症。

diverticulo-（袋状的）

diverticulitis 憩室炎

词根 diverticulo-（袋状的）+ -itis（炎症）

例句 Diverticulitis is the infection and inflammation of the diverticula in the colon, often leading to abdominal pain and fever. 憩室炎是结肠中憩室的感染和炎症，常导致腹痛和发热。

diverticulosis 憩室症

词根 diverticulo-（袋状的）+ -osis（病态）

例句 Diverticulosis refers to the presence of diverticula in the colon without inflammation. 憩室症是指结肠内存在憩室，但没有炎症。

diverticulectomy 憩室切除术

词根 diverticulo-（袋状的）+ -ectomy（切除术）

例句 Diverticulectomy is the surgical removal of diverticula from the digestive tract. 憩室切除术是从消化道中切除憩室的外科手术。

diverticulography 憩室造影

词根 diverticulo-（袋状的）+ -graphy（成像）

例句 Diverticulography is a diagnostic imaging technique used to visualize diverticula in the colon. 憩室造影是一种用于观察结肠中憩室的成像技术。

diverticular disease 憩室病

词根 diverticulo-（袋状的）+ disease（疾病）

例句 Diverticular disease involves the formation of pouches in the colon, which can become inflamed or infected. 憩室病是指结肠内形成囊状突起，这些突起可能会发生炎症或感染。

doch-（导管的）

choledochal 胆总管的

词根 choledoch-（胆总管）+ -al（与……有关的）

例句 The choledochal duct carries bile from the liver to the duodenum. 胆总管将胆汁从肝脏输送到十二指肠。

choledochitis 胆总管炎

词根 choledoch-（胆总管）+ -itis（炎症）

例句 Choledochitis is the inflammation of the common bile duct, often caused by a bacterial infection. 胆总管炎是胆总管的炎症，通常由细菌感染引起。

choledochectomy 胆总管切除术

词根 choledoch-（胆总管）+ -ectomy（切除术）

例句 Choledochectomy is the surgical removal of the common bile duct, typically performed in severe cases of bile duct disease. 胆总管切除术是指手术切除胆总管，通常用于治疗严重的胆管疾病。

choledochostomy 胆总管造口术

词根 choledoch-（胆总管）+ -ostomy（造口术）

例句 A choledochostomy is performed to create an opening in the bile duct to relieve a blockage. 胆总管造口术是通过在胆管中创建一个开口以缓解堵塞。

choledocholithiasis 胆总管结石

词根 choledoch-（胆总管）+ -lithiasis（结石形成）

例句 Choledocholithiasis occurs when gallstones are present in the common bile duct, causing pain and potential blockage. 胆总管结石是指胆石产生于胆总管内，可能导致疼痛和堵塞。

choledochorrhaphy 胆总管缝合术

词根 choledoch-（胆总管）+ -rrhaphy（缝合术）

例句 Choledochorrhaphy is a surgical procedure used to repair a tear or rupture in the common bile duct. 胆总管缝合术是用于修复胆总管撕裂或破裂的外科手术。

choledochal cyst 胆总管囊肿

词根 choledoch-（胆总管）+ -al（形容词后缀）

例句 A choledochal cyst is a rare congenital condition where a cyst forms in the common bile duct. 胆总管囊肿是一种罕见的先天性疾病，指胆总管中形成囊肿。

choledochoduodenostomy 胆总管十二指肠造口术

词根 choledoch-（胆总管）+ duoden-（十二指肠）+ -ostomy（造口术）

例句 Choledochoduodenostomy is a surgical procedure where the common bile duct is connected to the duodenum to relieve bile duct obstructions. 胆总管十二指肠造口术是一种手术，通过将胆总管与十二指肠连接来缓解胆管堵塞。

-dynia（疼痛）

gastrodynia 胃痛

词根 gastro-（胃）+ -dynia（疼痛）

例句 Gastrodynia refers to pain in the stomach area, often related to digestive issues. 胃痛指的是胃部区域的疼痛，通常与消化问题有关。

neuralgia 神经痛

词根 neur-（神经）+ -algia（疼痛）

例句 Neuralgia is a type of pain that occurs along the path of a nerve. 神经痛是一种沿神经路径发生的疼痛类型。

myalgia 肌肉痛

词根 myo-（肌肉）+ -algia（疼痛）

例句 Myalgia refers to muscle pain, which can be caused by overuse or injury. 肌肉痛是指肌肉的疼痛，可能由过度使用或受伤引起。

arthralgia 关节痛

词根 arthr-（关节）+ -algia（疼痛）

例句 Arthralgia is pain in the joints, often a symptom of arthritis. 关节痛是关节的疼痛，通常是关节炎的症状。

cephalodynia 头痛

词根 cephalo-（头）+ -dynia（疼痛）

例句 Cephalodynia is the term used for headaches. 头痛是指头部的疼痛。

dys-（困难的）

dysfunction 功能障碍

词根 dys-（困难）+ function（功能）

例句 Dysfunction refers to abnormal or impaired functioning of an organ or system. 功能障碍指的是器官或系统的异常或功能受损。

dysphagia 吞咽困难症

词根 dys-（困难）+ phag-（吃）+ -ia（病态）

例句 Dysphagia is a condition characterized by difficulty swallowing. 吞咽困难症是一种以吞咽困难为特征的病症。

dyslexia 阅读障碍

词根 dys-（困难）+ lex-（词语）+ -ia（病态）

例句 Dyslexia is a learning disorder that makes it difficult to read, write, and spell correctly. 阅读障碍是一种学习障碍，导致阅读、

写作困难。

dyspnea 呼吸困难

词根 dys-（困难）+ pnea（呼吸）

例句 Dyspnea is the medical term for difficulty breathing, often associated with respiratory disorders. 呼吸困难是医学上用于描述呼吸费力的术语，通常与呼吸系统疾病有关。

E

E

echino-（棘状的）

echinococcosis 棘球蚴病

词根 echino-（棘状的）+ coccus（球形）+ -osis（病理状态）

例句 Echinococcosis is a parasitic infection caused by the Echinococcus species, leading to cyst formation in various organs. 棘球蚴病是由棘球绦虫引起的寄生虫感染，导致在多个器官中形成囊肿。

echinococcus 棘球绦虫

词根 echino-（棘状的）+ coccus（球形）

例句 Echinococcus is a genus of parasitic tapeworms that can cause cysts in organs such as the liver and lungs. 棘球绦虫是一种寄生性绦虫，可能在肝脏和肺等器官中引起囊肿。

echinoderm 棘皮动物

词根 echino-（棘状的）+ derm-（皮肤）

例句 Echinoderms are marine animals like starfish and sea urchins that have spiny skin. 棘皮动物是像海星和海胆这样的海洋动物，具有刺状皮肤。

echinocandin 棘皮霉素

词根 echino-（棘状的）+ candin（霉素）

例句 Echinocandin is an antifungal drug used to treat infections caused by Candida and other fungi. 棘皮霉素是一种抗真菌药物，用于治疗由念珠菌和其他真菌引起的感染。

echinopathy 棘皮病

词根 echino-（棘状的）+ -pathy（疾病）

例句 Echinopathy refers to diseases related to or caused by echinococci, such as echinococcosis. 棘皮病指的是与棘球绦虫相关或由其引起的疾病，如棘球蚴病。

echinocytosis 刺球状细胞症

词根 echino-（棘状的）+ cytosis（细胞增多）

例句 Echinocytosis refers to a condition where red blood cells appear spiny or jagged under a microscope, often seen in conditions like uremia or after certain toxin exposures. 刺球状细胞症是指在显微镜下红细胞呈现出刺状或不规则形状，通常见于尿毒症或接触某些毒素后。

echinocyte 刺球状细胞

词根 echino-（棘状的）+ cyte（细胞）

例句 Echinocytes are red blood cells that have a spiny appearance due to changes in their membrane, which can be associated with various disorders. 刺球状细胞是指因细胞膜变化而呈现刺状外观的红细胞，可能与多种疾病相关。

echinoid 刺状的

词根 echino-（棘状的）+ -oid（类似）

例句 Echinoid cells resemble the shape of spiny structures, often seen in conditions where red blood cells undergo deformities. 刺状的细胞具有刺状结构的形态，通常见于红细胞发生变形的病症。

-ectasis（扩张）

bronchiectasis 支气管扩张

词根 bronchi-（支气管）+ -ectasis（扩张）

例句 Bronchiectasis is a condition where the airways in the lungs become widened, leading to mucus buildup and infection. 支气管扩张是一种肺部气道变宽的病症，导致黏液积聚和感染。

cardiectasis 心脏扩张

词根 cardi-（心脏）+ -ectasis（扩张）

例句 Cardiectasis refers to the abnormal dilation of the heart chambers, often due to heart disease. 心脏扩张是指心脏腔室的异常扩张，通常由心脏病引起。

pulmonary ectasis 肺扩张

词根 pulmon-（肺）+ -ectasis（扩张）

例句 Pulmonary ectasis is the expansion of the lungs' air sacs, which can lead to difficulty breathing. 肺扩张是肺部气囊的扩张，可能导致呼吸困难。

vasectasis 血管扩张

词根 vas-（血管）+ -ectasis（扩张）

例句 Vasectasis is the dilation or expansion of blood vessels, which can cause swelling. 血管扩张是血管的扩张，可能导致肿胀。

cholangiectasis 胆管扩张

词根 cholangi-（胆管）+ -ectasis（扩张）

例句 Cholangiectasis refers to the dilation of the bile ducts, often seen in liver disease. 胆管扩张是胆管的扩张，通常出现在肝病中。

USMLE Step 1 样题

A 45-year-old woman comes to the office for a follow-up examination 2 weeks after she sustained a vertebral fracture at L1. The fracture occurred spontaneously and there is no history of trauma to the area or other fractures. She gained 27 kg during the 6 months before the fracture occurred. Her only medication is hydromorphone (hydro-) as needed for pain. She is 163 cm tall and now weighs 100 kg; BMI is 38 kg/m^2. Temperature is 37.0°C

(98.6°F), pulse is 86/min, respirations (re-; spir-; -ation) are 12/min, and blood pressure is 145/98 mmHg. Physical examination shows central obesity and purple striae over the abdomen bilaterally (bi-; -lateral). The lower extremities appear thin. Results of laboratory studies are shown:

Plasma Renin activity 5.0 ng/mL/h (N=0.6–4.0)

Metanephrine (meta-; nephr-) 0.3 nmol/L (N<0.4)

Serum Cortisol (corti-; -ol), random 43 μg/dL

Adrenocorticotropic (adren-; corti-; -tropic) hormone 120 pg/mL (N<120)

Aldosterone (aldo-; ster-; -one) 8 ng/dL (N=2–9)

Urine 24-hour free cortisol (corti-; -ol) excretion (ex-; cret-; -ion) 340 μg/24 h (N=3.5–45)

The most likely cause of the fracture in this patient is an increase in which of the following processes?

(A) Calcium absorption (ab-; sorpt-; -ion)

(B) Calcium excretion (ex-; cret-; -ion)

(C) Osteoblast (osteo-; -blast) proliferation (pro-; life-; -ation)

(D) Osteoclast (osteo-; -clast) proliferation

(E) Phosphorus absorption (ab-; sorpt-; -ion)

(F) Phosphorus excretion (ex-; cret-; -ion)

中文翻译

一名 45 岁女性在 L1 椎体骨折后 2 周来复诊。骨折为自发性发生，无该部位外伤或其他骨折史。在骨折发生前的 6 个月内，她体重增加了 27 kg。她唯一服用的药物是按需服用的氢吗啡酮，用以止痛。她身高 163 cm，现体重 100 kg；BMI 为 38 kg/m²。体温 37.0℃（98.6℉），脉搏 86 次 / 分钟，呼吸 12 次 / 分钟，血压 145/98 mmHg。体格检查显示中心性肥胖，腹部双侧紫纹，下肢外观纤细。实验室检查结果如下：

血浆肾素活性 5.0 ng/mL/h（正常值：0.6 ～ 4.0）

甲氧基肾上腺素 0.3 nmol/L（正常值：<0.4）

随机血清皮质醇 43 μg/dL

促肾上腺皮质激素 120 pg/mL（正常值：<120）

醛固酮 8 ng/dL（正常值：2 ～ 9）

24 小时尿游离皮质醇排泄量 340 μg/24 h（正常值：3.5～45）

该患者骨折最可能的病因是以下哪种生理过程增强？

(A) 钙吸收

(B) 钙排泄

(C) 成骨细胞增殖

(D) 破骨细胞增殖

(E) 磷吸收

(F) 磷排泄

题目和答案中出现的词根

hydro-：氢

re-：重新；反复

spir：呼吸

-ation：表示动作的状态

bi-：双

lateral：侧面

meta-：超过；在……后

nephr-：肾（改变后的肾，指代肾上腺激素代谢物）

corti-：皮质

-ol：醇

adren-：肾上腺

corti-：皮质

-tropic：营养的（肾上腺皮质营养，指促肾上腺皮质激素的）

ex-：向外

cret-：分离

-ion：表示动作（向外分离的动作，指的是外分泌）

ab-：表否定

sorpt：吸（指吸收，即离开原来的位置如肠腔）

osteo-：骨

-blast：前体

-clast：破坏

-ectomy（切除）

appendectomy 阑尾切除术

词根 append-（阑尾）+ -ectomy（切除术）

例句 Appendectomy is a surgical procedure to remove the appendix, typically due to appendicitis. 阑尾切除术是去除阑尾的外科手术，通常是因为阑尾炎。

mastectomy 乳房切除术

词根 mast-（乳房）+ -ectomy（切除术）

例句 Mastectomy is the surgical removal of one or both breasts, often performed for breast cancer. 乳房切除术是去除单侧或双侧乳房的外科手术，通常用于治疗乳腺癌。

hysterectomy 子宫切除术

词根 hyster-（子宫）+ -ectomy（切除术）

例句 Hysterectomy is the removal of the uterus, commonly performed due to conditions like uterine fibroids or cancer. 子宫切除术是去除子宫的手术，常见于子宫肌瘤或癌症等情况。

gastrectomy 胃切除术

词根 gastr-（胃）+ -ectomy（切除术）

例句 Gastrectomy is the surgical removal of part or all of the stomach, often performed for gastric cancer. 胃切除术是部分或全部去除胃的手术，通常用于治疗胃癌。

thyroidectomy 甲状腺切除术

词根 thyroid-（甲状腺）+ -ectomy（切除术）

例句 Thyroidectomy is the surgical removal of all or part of the thyroid gland, often due to thyroid cancer or hyperthyroidism. 甲状腺切除术是去除部分或全部甲状腺的外科手术，通常是因甲状腺癌或甲亢。

-emesis（吐）

emesis 呕吐

词根 emesis（呕吐）

例句 Emesis is the medical term for vomiting, which is the forceful expulsion of stomach contents through the mouth. 呕吐是医学术语，指通过口腔强力排出胃内容物。

hyperemesis 剧烈呕吐

词根 hyper-（过度）+ emesis（呕吐）

例句 Hyperemesis is a condition characterized by severe and persistent vomiting, often seen in pregnancy. 剧烈呕吐是一种以严重且持续的呕吐为特征的病症，常见于妊娠期。

hyperemesis gravidarum 妊娠剧吐

词根 hyper-（过度）+ emesis（呕吐）+ gravidarum（怀孕）

例句 Hyperemesis gravidarum is an extreme form of morning sickness that can lead to dehydration. 妊娠剧吐是一种严重的孕吐，可能导致脱水。

projectile emesis 喷射性呕吐

词根 projectile（喷射的）+ emesis（呕吐）

例句 Projectile emesis is a type of vomiting where the expelled contents travel a considerable distance. 喷射性呕吐是一种呕吐类型，胃内容物可以喷射到较远的距离。

-emia（血症）

anemia 贫血

词根 an-（缺乏）+ -emia（血症）

例句 Anemia is a condition where there is a lack of red blood cells or hemoglobin, leading to fatigue and weakness. 贫血是指红细胞或血红蛋白缺乏的病症，导致疲劳和虚弱。

leukemia 白血病

词根 leuk-（白）+ -emia（血症）

例句 Leukemia is a cancer of the blood or bone marrow that results in the overproduction of white blood cells. 白血病是一种血液或骨髓的癌症，导致白细胞过度产生。

hypoglycemia 低血糖症

词根 hypo-（低）+ glyc-（糖）+ -emia（血症）

例句 Hypoglycemia occurs when the blood sugar levels drop too low, leading to symptoms like shaking and dizziness. 低血糖症是血糖水平过低时发生的病症，导致颤抖和头晕等症状。

hyperkalemia 高钾血症

词根 hyper-（高）+ kal-（钾）+ -emia（血症）

例句 Hyperkalemia is a condition where there is too much potassium in the blood, which can affect heart function. 高钾血症是指血液中钾离子过多，可能影响心脏功能。

uremia 尿毒症

词根 ur-（尿）+ -emia（血症）

例句 Uremia is the buildup of waste products in the blood due to kidney failure. 尿毒症是肾功能衰竭导致废物在血液中积累。

septicemia 败血症

词根 septic-（感染）+ -emia（血症）

例句 Septicemia is a serious bloodstream infection that can lead to sepsis. 败血症是一种严重的血液感染，可能导致脓毒症。

polycythemia 红细胞增多症

词根 poly-（多）+ cyt-（细胞）+ -emia（血症）

例句 Polycythemia is a condition where there are too many red blood cells in the blood, leading to thickened blood. 红细胞增多症是指血液中红细胞过多，导致血液变稠的病症。

hypoxemia 低氧血症

词根 hypo-（低）+ ox-（氧）+ -emia（血症）

例句 Hypoxemia is a condition where there is an abnormally low level of oxygen in the blood. 低氧血症是指血液中的氧气含量异常低。

USMLE Step 1 样题

A 2-week-old male newborn is brought to the office for a well-child examination. He was delivered following an uncomplicated (un-), spontaneous vaginal delivery at 41 weeks' gestation. The mother has no history of serious illness and did not receive prenatal (pre-; natal) care. Her only medication is a prenatal (pre-; natal) vitamin. She has consumed large amounts of vodka nightly for 10 years. Which of the following examination findings is most likely to be present in this patient?

(A) Hypospadias (hypo-; spad-)

(B) Limb hypoplasia (hypo-; -plasia)

(C) Neck webbing

(D) Short palpebral (palpebr-) fissures

(E) Spasticity

中文翻译

一名 2 周龄男婴被带到诊室进行健康检查。该患儿为妊娠 41 周时经无并发症的自然阴道分娩出生。母亲无严重疾病史，未接受产前检查。她唯一服用的药物是产前维生素。她在过去 10 年中每晚大量饮用伏特加酒。该患儿最可能出现以下哪项体检结果？

(A) 尿道下裂

(B) 肢体发育不全

(C) 颈部蹼状皮肤

(D) 睑裂短小

(E) 痉挛状态

题目和答案中出现的词根

un-：表否定

pre-：在……之前

-natal：出生

hypo-：低

spad-：开口

-plasia：生长（在生长之下，指代发育不良，即处在生长之下的水平）

palpebr-：眼睑的

-ence（状态）

prevalence 患病率；流行程度

词根 preval-（普遍）+ -ence（状态）

例句 The prevalence of diabetes has significantly increased in recent years, especially in urban populations. 近年来，糖尿病的患病率显著增加，尤其是在城市居民中。

recurrence 复发

词根 re-（再）+ curr-（发生）+ -ence（状态）

例句 Recurrence of cancer after treatment remains a significant challenge for oncologists. 癌症复发仍然是肿瘤学家面临的重要挑战。

emergence 出现

词根 emerg-（出现）+ -ence（状态）

例句 The emergence of antibiotic-resistant bacteria poses a significant threat to public health worldwide. 抗生素耐药细菌的出现对全球公共健康构成了重大威胁。

incontinence 失禁

词根 in-（否定）+ contin-（控制）+ -ence（状态）

例句 Urinary incontinence is a common condition in elderly patients, affecting their quality of life. 尿失禁是老年患者中常见的病症，影响生活质量。

convalescence 恢复期

词根 convalesc-（恢复）+ -ence（状态）

例句 The patient is in the convalescence stage and is gradually regaining strength after surgery. 患者正处于手术后恢复期，体力逐渐恢复。

coherence 连贯性

词根 co-（共同）+ her-（黏合）+ -ence（状态）

例句 Cognitive coherence is an important factor in assessing mental health conditions such as schizophrenia. 认知连贯性是评估精神分裂症等精神健康状况的重要因素。

defervescence 退热

词根 de-（降低）+ ferv-（热）+ -ence（状态）

例句 The patient' s defervescence indicates that the infection is under control and the fever is subsiding. 患者的退热表明感染得到控制，发热正在消退。

dependence 依赖

词根 depend-（依靠）+ -ence（状态）

例句 Opioid dependence is a serious medical condition requiring comprehensive treatment and support. 阿片类药物依赖是一种需要综合治疗的严重医学状况。

persistence 持续性

词根 persist-（坚持）+ -ence（状态）

例句 The persistence of symptoms such as chronic pain often complicates the management of certain conditions. 慢性疼痛等症状的持续存在常常使某些病情的管理更加复杂。

obsolescence 退化；衰退

词根 obsoles-（衰退）+ -ence（状态）

例句 Obsolescence of certain brain functions is often observed in neurodegenerative diseases such as Alzheimer's. 在阿尔茨海默病等神经退行性疾病中，某些大脑功能的退化很常见。

effervescence 冒泡；兴奋状态

词根 ef-（向外）+ ferv-（沸腾）+ -ence（状态）

例句 Effervescence can be observed in some chemical reactions, such as those in carbonated drinks or biological processes. 在某些化学反应中，如碳酸饮料反应或生物过程，可以观察到冒泡现象。

preeminence 显著作用

词根 pre-（在前）+ emin-（突出）+ -ence（状态）

例句 The preeminence of certain genetic factors can influence a patient's susceptibility to diseases. 某些遗传因素的显著作用可能会影响患者对疾病的易感性。

resilience 恢复力

词根 resil-（弹回）+ -ence（状态）

例句 Psychological resilience is an important factor in helping patients recover from traumatic events or chronic illnesses. 心理恢复力是帮助患者从创伤事件或慢性疾病中恢复的重要因素。

eminence 突出

词根 emin-（突出）+ -ence（状态）

例句 The eminence of a particular symptom in a clinical setting often guides the course of diagnosis and treatment. 在临床环境中，某一特定症状的显著性通常会指导诊断和治疗过程。

flatulence 胃肠胀气

词根 flatul-（气体）+ -ence（状态）

例句 Flatulence can be a symptom of various gastrointestinal disorders, such as irritable bowel syndrome. 胃肠胀气可能是多种胃肠道疾病的症状，例如肠易激综合征。

diffidence 自信缺乏

词根 dif-（远离）+ fid-（信任）+ -ence（状态）

例句 In medical consultations, diffidence in expressing symptoms can lead to delayed or missed diagnoses. 在医疗咨询中，患者对症状表达缺乏自信可能导致诊断延迟或遗漏。

encephalo-（脑）

encephalitis 脑炎

词根 encephalo-（脑）+ -itis（炎症）

例句 Encephalitis is the inflammation of the brain, often caused by viral infections. 脑炎是脑部的炎症，通常由病毒感染引起。

encephalopathy 脑病

词根 encephalo-（脑）+ -pathy（疾病）

例句 Encephalopathy refers to any disease that affects the structure or function of the brain. 脑病指的是影响大脑结构或功能的疾病。

encephalogram 脑电图

词根 encephalo-（脑）+ -gram（图像）

例句 An encephalogram is a diagnostic test used to measure brain activity and function. 脑电图是用于测量大脑活动和功能的诊断测试。

encephalomyelitis 脑脊髓炎

词根 encephalo-（脑）+ myel-（脊髓）+ -itis（炎症）

例句 Encephalomyelitis is the inflammation of both the brain and the spinal cord. 脑脊髓炎是指大脑和脊髓的炎症。

encephalograph 脑图仪

词根 encephalo-（脑）+ -graph（记录仪器）

例句 An encephalograph is a medical device used to record electrical activity in the brain. 脑图仪是一种用于记录大脑电活动的医学设备。

endo-（内侧的）

endoscope 内窥镜

词根 endo-（内）+ scope（镜子）

例句 An endoscope is a medical instrument used to view the inside of a body cavity or organ. 内窥镜是一种用于观察体腔或器官内部的医学仪器。

endometriosis 子宫内膜异位症

词根 endo-（内）+ metri-（子宫）+ -osis（病态）

例句 Endometriosis is a painful condition where tissue similar to the lining of the uterus grows outside the uterus. 子宫内膜异位症是一种疼痛性病症，特征为类似子宫内膜的组织在子宫外生长。

endocrine 内分泌的

词根 endo-（内）+ crine（分泌）

例句 Endocrine glands are responsible for producing hormones that regulate various bodily functions. 内分泌腺负责产生调节身体各种功能的激素。

endocarditis 心内膜炎

词根 endo-（内）+ card-（心脏）+ -itis（炎症）

例句 Endocarditis is the inflammation of the inner lining of the heart chambers, often caused by bacterial infections. 心内膜炎是心脏腔室内膜的炎症，通常由细菌感染引起。

endothermic 吸热的

词根 endo-（内）+ therm-（热）+ -ic（形容词后缀）

例句 Endothermic reactions are chemical reactions that absorb heat from their surroundings. 吸热反应是指从周围环境吸收热量的化学反应。

entero-（肠道）

enteritis 肠炎

词根 entero-（肠道）+ -itis（炎症）

例句 Enteritis is the inflammation of the intestines, which can lead to symptoms like diarrhea and abdominal pain. 肠炎是肠道的炎症，可能导致腹泻和腹痛等症状。

enteropathy 肠病

词根 entero-（肠道）+ -pathy（疾病）

例句 Enteropathy refers to any disease affecting the intestines, including conditions like Crohn' s disease. 肠病指的是影响肠道的疾病，包括克罗恩病等病症。

enterocolitis 小肠结肠炎

词根 entero-（肠道）+ col-（结肠）+ -itis（炎症）

例句 Enterocolitis is the inflammation of both the small intestine and the colon, often caused by infections. 小肠结肠炎是小肠和结肠的炎症，通常由感染引起。

enterostomy 肠造口术

词根 entero-（肠道）+ -stomy（造口术）

例句 Enterostomy is a surgical procedure in which a part of the intestine is brought to the surface of the abdomen. 肠造口术是一种将部分肠管引至腹壁表面的外科手术。

enteric nervous system 肠神经系统

词根 entero-（肠道）+ -ic（形容词后缀）

例句 The enteric nervous system is a complex network of neurons that controls gastrointestinal function. 肠神经系统是控制胃肠功能的复杂神经网络。

USMLE Step 1 官网样题

A 5-year-old girl is brought to the office by her mother because of a 6-hour history of bloody diarrhea (dia-; -rrhea). She is interactive (inter-; -act) and in no acute distress (dis-; -tress). Her blood pressure is 90/55 mmHg. Abdominal examination shows normoactive (norm-) bowel sounds. Stool cultures are obtained, and the patient's mother is advised to give the girl plenty of fluids. Five days later, the patient develops decreased urine output and is brought back to the office. Her blood pressure is now 135/88 mmHg. Physical examination shows pallor. Laboratory studies show:

Hemoglobin (hemo-; -globin) 8.5 g/dL (N=11–15)

Hematocrit (hemato-; -crit) 26% (N=28%–45%)

Platelet (plate-; -let) count 45,000/mm^3 (N=150,000–400,000)

Serum creatinine 3.3 mg/dL (N=0.3–0.7)

Which of the following infectious agents is the most likely cause of these findings?

(A) Campylobacter (campylo-; -bacter) jejuni

(B) Escherichia coli

(C) Rotavirus (rota-)

(D) Salmonella enterica (enter-) serovar enteritidis (enter-; -itis)

(E) Yersinia pestis

中文翻译

一名5岁女童被母亲带至诊室就诊，主诉持续6小时的血性腹泻。患儿神志清醒，无急性痛苦表现。血压90/55 mmHg。腹部查体显示肠鸣音正常。已留取粪便培养标本，并嘱患儿母亲给患儿多补充水分。5天后，患儿出现尿量减少，再次被带至诊室。此时血压升至135/88 mmHg。体格检查发现患儿面色苍白。实验室检查结果如下：

血红蛋白8.5 g/dL（正常值：11～15）

血细胞比容26%（正常值：28%～45%）

血小板计数45,000/mm³（正常值：150,000～400,000）

血清肌酐3.3 mg/dL（正常值：0.3～0.7）

以下哪种病原体最可能是这些表现的病因？

(A) 空肠弯曲菌

(B) 大肠埃希菌

(C) 轮状病毒

(D) 肠沙门氏菌

(E) 鼠疫耶尔森菌

题目和答案中出现的词根

dia-：通过（这里指通过肠道）

-rrhea：流出（通过肠道流出，指腹泻）

inter-：在……之间

-act：作用

dis-：分开

-tress：用力

norm：正常的

hemo-：血

-globin：球蛋白

hemato-：血

-crit：分离法

plate-：板状的

-lets：小

campylo-：弯曲的

-bacter：杆菌

rota-：轮状的

enter-：肠道的

-itis：炎症

episi-（外阴）

episiotomy 会阴切开术

词根 episi-（外阴）+ -otomy（切开术）

例句 Episiotomy is performed during childbirth to prevent severe perineal tears. 会阴切开术是在分娩过程中进行的，以防止严重的会阴撕裂。

episioplasty 会阴成形术

词根 episi-（外阴）+ -plasty（修复术）

例句 Episioplasty is used to reconstruct the perineum after injury. 会阴成形术用于受伤后的会阴重建。

episioperineoplasty 会阴整形术

词根 episi-（外阴）+ perineo-（会阴）+ -plasty（整形术）

例句 Episioperineoplasty helps restore function and appearance to the perineal area. 会阴整形术有助于恢复会阴区域的功能和外观。

episiorrhaphy 会阴缝合术

词根 episi-（外阴）+ -rrhaphy（缝合术）

例句 Episiorrhaphy is required when perineal tears occur during childbirth. 当分娩中发生会阴撕裂时，需要进行会阴缝合术。

episiostenosis 外阴狭窄

词根 episi-（外阴）+ -stenosis（狭窄）

例句 Episiostenosis can develop due to scar tissue formation after surgery. 外阴狭窄可能由于手术后瘢痕组织形成而发展。

episioclysis 会阴灌洗术

词根 episi-（外阴）+ -clysis（灌洗术）

例句 Episioclysis is used to cleanse the perineal area in cases of infection. 会阴灌洗术用于清洁感染的会阴区域。

episiotomy repair 会阴切开术修复

词根 episi-（外阴）+ -tomy（切开术）+ repair（修复）

例句 Episiotomy repair is necessary to close the incision made during delivery. 会阴切开术修复用于闭合分娩过程中切开的切口。

episiodynia 会阴痛

词根 episi-（外阴）+ -dynia（疼痛）

例句 Episiodynia can be a symptom of perineal trauma after childbirth. 会阴痛可能是分娩后会阴损伤的症状。

episiosclerosis 外阴硬化

词根 episi-（外阴）+ -sclerosis（硬化）

例句 Episiosclerosis is associated with chronic inflammatory conditions of the perineum. 外阴硬化与会阴慢性炎症有关。

episiotracheloplasty 外阴子宫颈成形术

词根 episi-（外阴）+ trachelo-（子宫颈）+ -plasty（修复术）

例句 Episiotracheloplasty is a reconstructive surgery involving both the vulva and cervix. 外阴子宫颈成形术是外阴和子宫颈的重建手术。

eryth-（红色）

erythrocyte 红细胞

词根 eryth-（红色）+ -cyte（细胞）

例句 Erythrocytes transport oxygen throughout the body. 红细胞负责将氧气输送到全身。

erythropoiesis 红细胞生成

词根 eryth-（红色）+ -poiesis（生成）

例句 Erythropoiesis occurs in the bone marrow. 红细胞生成发生在骨髓中。

erythropoietin 促红细胞生成素

词根 eryth-（红色）+ -poietin（生成素）

例句 Erythropoietin stimulates red blood cell production. 促红细胞生成素促进红细胞的生成。

erythroblast 红细胞母细胞

词根 eryth-（红色）+ -blast（幼细胞）

例句 Erythroblasts are immature red blood cells in the bone marrow. 红细胞母细胞是骨髓中的未成熟红细胞。

erythremia 红血病

词根 eryth-（红色）+ -emia（血症）

例句 Erythremia is characterized by an excess of red blood cells. 红血病的特征是红细胞过量。

erythroderma 红皮病

词根 eryth-（红色）+ -derma（皮肤）

例句 Erythroderma causes widespread skin redness and scaling. 红

皮病导致皮肤大面积发红和脱屑。

erythrocytosis 红细胞增多症

词根 eryth-（红色）+ -cytosis（细胞增多）
例句 Erythrocytosis results in increased red blood cell count. 红细胞增多症导致红细胞数量增加。

erythroclasis 红细胞破裂

词根 eryth-（红色）+ -clasis（破裂）
例句 Erythroclasis refers to the destruction of red blood cells. 红细胞破裂指的是红细胞的破坏。

erythroenzymopathy 红细胞酶病

词根 eryth-（红色）+ enzyme（酶）+ -pathy（病症）
例句 Erythroenzymopathy affects red blood cell enzyme function. 红细胞酶病影响红细胞的酶功能。

erythrophobia 红色恐惧症

词根 eryth-（红色）+ -phobia（恐惧）
例句 Erythrophobia is the fear of redness or blushing. 红色恐惧症是对红色或脸红的恐惧。

eu-（正常的；良好的）

euphoria 愉悦感

词根 eu-（良好）+ phor-（携带）+ -ia（状态）
例句 Euphoria is a state of extreme happiness. 愉悦感是一种极度幸福的状态。

euthanasia 安乐死

词根 eu-（良好）+ thanatos（死亡）
例句 Euthanasia is used to relieve unbearable suffering. 安乐死用于缓解无法忍受的痛苦。

eugenics 优生学

词根 eu-（良好）+ gen-（基因）+ -ics（学科）

例句 Eugenics studies methods to improve genetic traits. 优生学研究改善遗传特征的方法。

eubiotics 良性生物学

词根 eu-（良好）+ bio-（生命）+ -tics（学科）

例句 Eubiotics focuses on maintaining a balanced microbiome. 良性生物学关注维持微生物群的平衡。

euthyroid 甲状腺功能正常

词根 eu-（正常）+ thyroid（甲状腺）

例句 Euthyroid patients have normal thyroid hormone levels. 甲状腺功能正常的患者甲状腺激素水平正常。

extra-（外）

extracellular 细胞外的

词根 extra-（外）+ cellular（细胞的）

例句 Extracellular fluid surrounds and supports the cells. 细胞外液环绕并支撑着细胞。

extrathoracic 胸腔外的

词根 extra-（外）+ thoracic（胸腔的）

例句 Extrathoracic airway obstruction affects breathing. 胸腔外气道阻塞会影响呼吸。

extracorporeal 体外的

词根 extra-（外）+ corporeal（身体的）

例句 Extracorporeal circulation is used in heart-lung machines. 体外循环用于心肺机。

extraperitoneal 腹膜外的

词根 extra-（外）+ peritoneal（腹膜的）

例句 Extraperitoneal injuries require specific surgical approaches. 腹膜外损伤需要特定的外科处理。

extracranial 颅外的

词根 extra-（外）+ cranial（颅骨的）

例句 Extracranial blood flow is important in stroke evaluation. 颅外血流在中风评估中很重要。

extravascular 血管外的

词根 extra-（外）+ vascular（血管的）

例句 Extravascular hemolysis occurs outside the blood vessels. 血管外溶血发生在血管外。

extrauterine 子宫外的

词根 extra-（外）+ uterine（子宫的）

例句 Extrauterine pregnancy is also called ectopic pregnancy. 宫外孕也称为异位妊娠。

USMLE Step 1 样题

A 72-year-old man is brought to the office because of a 6-month history of increasing fatigue and a 1-month history of numbness of his feet. Physical examination shows marked pallor. Proprioception (proprio-; cept-; -ion) and sensation to vibration are decreased in the lower extremities. Laboratory studies show:

Hemoglobin 7.6 g/dL

Mean corpuscular volume 117 μm^3

Reticulocyte count 0%

Serum vitamin B_{12} 23.6 pg/mL (N=200–900)

Histopathology of a gastric mucosal biopsy specimen shows atrophic gastritis (gastr-; -itis) with extensive lymphocyte (lymph-; -cyte) infiltration. Serologic studies will most likely show autoantibodies (auto-; anti-; body) to which of the following labeled cell types in the photomicrograph (photo-; micro-; -graphy) of normal mucosa or to one of its secretory products? (Image is ignored)

中文翻译

一名 72 岁男性因 6 个月来日益加重的疲乏感及 1 个月来足部麻木感被送至诊室。体格检查显示患者明显苍白，下肢本体感觉及振动觉减退。实验室检查结果如下：

血红蛋白 7.6 g/dL

平均红细胞体积 117 μm^3

网织红细胞计数 0%

血清维生素 B_{12} 23.6 pg/mL（正常值：200 ~ 900）

胃黏膜活检标本的组织病理学检查显示萎缩性胃炎伴广泛淋巴细胞浸润。血清学检查最可能检测到针对正常黏膜显微照片中哪种标记细胞类型或其分泌产物的自身抗体？（图片省略）

题目和答案中出现的词根

proprio-：自己

cept-：感觉

-ion：动作（感觉自己的动作，即为本体感知）

hemo-：血

-globin：球蛋白

corpuscu-：肉体的，这里指红细胞本体

reticul-：网状的

-cyte：细胞

gastr-：胃的

-itis：炎症

lymph-：淋巴

auto-：自我

anti-：抗

-body：体（自我抗体，即自身免疫性抗体）

photo-：像；光

micro-：微小的

-graphy：图像（微小图像照片，即显微镜照片）

fibro-（纤维）

fibroblast 成纤维细胞

词根 fibro-（纤维）+ -blast（幼细胞）
例句 Fibroblasts produce collagen and extracellular matrix. 成纤维细胞合成胶原蛋白和细胞外基质。

fibrosis 纤维化

词根 fibro-（纤维）+ -osis（病变）
例句 Lung fibrosis can lead to severe respiratory issues. 肺纤维化可能导致严重的呼吸问题。

fibrocartilage 纤维软骨

词根 fibro-（纤维）+ cartilage（软骨）
例句 Fibrocartilage provides support and shock absorption in joints. 纤维软骨在关节中起支撑和减震作用。

fibromyalgia 纤维肌痛

词根 fibro-（纤维）+ myo-（肌肉）+ -algia（疼痛）
例句 Fibromyalgia is a chronic condition causing widespread pain. 纤维肌痛是一种导致全身疼痛的慢性疾病。

fibroadenoma 纤维腺瘤

词根 fibro-（纤维）+ aden-（腺）+ -oma（瘤）
例句 Fibroadenomas are common benign breast tumors. 纤维腺瘤是常见的乳腺良性肿瘤。

fibroelastosis 纤维弹性组织增生

词根 fibro-（纤维）+ elast-（弹性）+ -osis（病变）
例句 Fibroelastosis affects the heart's endocardium. 纤维弹性组织

增生影响心脏的心内膜。

fibrochondrogenesis 纤维软骨形成异常

词根 fibro-（纤维）+ chondro-（软骨）+ -genesis（生成）
例句 Fibrochondrogenesis is a rare genetic disorder affecting cartilage development. 纤维软骨形成异常是一种影响软骨发育的罕见遗传病。

fibroplasia 纤维增生

词根 fibro-（纤维）+ -plasia（增生）
例句 Fibroplasia is a key process in wound healing. 纤维增生是伤口愈合的关键过程。

fibrosarcoma 纤维肉瘤

词根 fibro-（纤维）+ -sarcoma（肉瘤）
例句 Fibrosarcoma is a malignant tumor derived from fibrous tissue. 纤维肉瘤是一种源自纤维组织的恶性肿瘤。

fibroepithelial tumor 纤维上皮肿瘤

词根 fibro-（纤维）+ epithelial（上皮的）+ tumor（肿瘤）
例句 Fibroepithelial tumors are often benign growths in the skin. 纤维上皮肿瘤通常是皮肤的良性增生。

flatul-（气）

flatulence 腹胀

词根 flatul-（气）+ -ence（状态）
例句 Flatulence is caused by excessive gas production in the intestines. 腹胀是由肠道内产生过量气体引起的。

flatulogenic 引起胀气的

词根 flatul-（气）+ -genic（生成的）
例句 Certain foods are flatulogenic and may cause bloating. 某些

食物容易引起胀气。

flatulopathy 肠胀气病

词根 flatul-（气）+ -pathy（病变）

例句 Flatulopathy is a disorder characterized by excessive gas accumulation. 肠胀气病是一种以过量气体积聚为特征的疾病。

flatulosity 胀气

词根 flatul-（气）+ -osity（状态）

例句 Flatulosity often results from poor digestion or food intolerance. 胀气通常是消化不良或食物不耐受的结果。

flatulent colic 腹胀绞痛

词根 flatul-（气）+ -ent（形容词后缀）+ colic（绞痛）

例句 Flatulent colic can cause severe discomfort in infants. 腹胀绞痛可能会导致婴儿严重不适。

flatuliform 类似胀气的

词根 flatul-（气）+ -iform（形状）

例句 Flatuliform distension can be mistaken for other gastrointestinal issues. 类似胀气的腹胀可能会被误认为是其他胃肠问题。

flatulency 肠道胀气

词根 flatul-（气）+ -ency（状态）

例句 Flatulency is a common symptom in digestive disorders. 肠道胀气是消化系统疾病的常见症状。

flatulodynia 胀气性疼痛

词根 flatul-（气）+ -dynia（疼痛）

例句 Flatulodynia can be relieved by dietary modifications. 胀气性疼痛可以通过饮食调整来缓解。

flatuloviscous 气体黏性的

词根 flatul-（气）+ viscous（黏性）

例句 Flatuloviscous secretions can affect bowel movement. 气体黏性分泌物可能影响排便。

USMLE Step 2 CK 样题

An 18-month-old boy is brought to the emergency department by his mother 30 minutes after he fell from his bed onto the floor. Two months ago, he sustained a fracture of the right humerus when he fell while playing in the park. The fracture healed quickly with immobilization (im-; mobil-) and casting. His mother sustained several bone fractures in early childhood, but she currently does not have any medical concerns. On arrival, the boy is crying. Pulse is 162/min, respirations (re-; spir-; -ation) are 48/min, and blood pressure is 122/80 mmHg. Examination discloses bluish sclera and ecchymoses (ec-; chym-; -osis) and tenderness over the right tibia. X-ray of the right lower extremity confirms a fracture of the tibia. The right lower extremity is immobilized (im-; mobil-) with a cast. Limitation of physical activity is recommended to prevent future fractures. Given this patient's condition, it is most appropriate for which of the following types of screening to be done regularly?

(A) Audiography (audio-; -graphy)

(B) DEXA scan

(C) Echocardiography (echo-; cardio-; -graphy)

(D) Retinal examination

(E) Serum calcium and vitamin D concentrations

F

中文翻译

一名18个月大的男婴从床上跌落至地面，30分钟后被其母亲送至急诊科。两个月前，他在公园玩耍时摔倒，导致右肱骨骨折，通过固定和石膏治疗后骨折迅速愈合。其母亲在幼儿时期曾多次骨折，但目前无任何健康问题。入院时，男童正在哭泣。脉搏162次/分钟，呼吸48次/分钟，血压122/80 mmHg。检查发现巩膜呈蓝色，右胫骨处有瘀斑和压痛。右下肢X线检查显示胫骨骨折。右下肢已用石膏固定。建议限制其活动以防止未来再次骨折。鉴于该患者的病情，以下哪种类型的定期筛查最为合适？

(A) 听力检查

(B) DEXA扫描

(C) 心脏超声检查

(D) 视网膜检查

(E) 血清钙和维生素D浓度检测

题目和答案中出现的词根

im-：表否定

mobil：移动

re-：重新；反复

spir：呼吸

-ation：表示动作的状态

ec-：向外

chym-：液体

-osis：病理状态（液体向外流动的病理状态，指的是淤斑，即皮下有血液从血管向外流动）

audio-：听力的

-graphy：图像

echo-：回声

cardio-：心脏的

flav-（黄色）

flavoprotein 黄素蛋白

词根 flav-（黄色）+ protein（蛋白）

例句 Flavoproteins are involved in cellular respiration and metabolism. 黄素蛋白参与细胞呼吸和代谢。

flavin adenine dinucleotide（FAD）黄素腺嘌呤二核苷酸

词根 flav-（黄色）+ adenine（腺嘌呤）+ dinucleotide（二核苷酸）

例句 FAD acts as a coenzyme in redox reactions. FAD 作为氧化还原反应的辅酶。

flavin mononucleotide（FMN）黄素单核苷酸

词根 flav-（黄色）+ mono-（单个）+ nucleotide（核苷酸）

例句 FMN is essential for electron transport in mitochondria. FMN 在线粒体电子传递过程中起重要作用。

flavivirus 黄病毒

词根 flav-（黄色）+ virus（病毒）

例句 Flavivirus includes pathogens like dengue and Zika viruses. 黄病毒包括登革热病毒和寨卡病毒等病原体。

flavine 黄素

词根 flav-（黄色）

例句 Flavine compounds are essential in many enzymatic processes. 黄素化合物在许多酶促反应中至关重要。

flavonoid 类黄酮

词根 flav-（黄色）+ -oid（类似）

例句 Flavonoids have antioxidant properties and benefit cardiovascular health. 类黄酮具有抗氧化特性，有益于心血管健康。

flavobacterium 黄杆菌

词根 flav-（黄色）+ bacterium（细菌）

例句 Flavobacterium species are common in aquatic environments. 黄杆菌属细菌常见于水生环境中。

flavomycin 黄霉素

词根 flav-（黄色）+ -mycin（抗生素）

例句 Flavomycin is used as a growth promoter in livestock. 黄霉素用于促进牲畜生长。

flavoenzyme 黄素酶

词根 flav-（黄色）+ enzyme（酶）

例句 Flavoenzymes are involved in oxidation-reduction reactions. 黄素酶参与氧化还原反应。

follic-（滤泡）

follicle 滤泡

词根 follic-（滤泡）

例句 The hair follicle is the part of the skin that produces hair. 毛囊是皮肤产生头发的部分。

folliculitis 滤泡炎

词根 follic-（滤泡）+ -itis（炎症）

例句 Folliculitis is an inflammation of the hair follicles, often caused by infection. 滤泡炎是毛囊的炎症，通常由感染引起。

follicular phase 滤泡期

词根 follic-（滤泡）+ -ular（形容词后缀）+ phase（阶段）

例句 The follicular phase is the part of the menstrual cycle that begins on the first day of menstruation. 滤泡期是月经周期的一个阶段，从月经第一天开始。

follicular cyst 滤泡囊肿

词根 follic-（滤泡）+ -ar（形容词后缀）+ cyst（囊肿）

例句 A follicular cyst forms when the follicle fails to release an egg. 滤泡囊肿形成是因为滤泡未能释放卵子。

folliculogenesis 滤泡生成

词根 follic-（滤泡）+ -genesis（生成）

例句 Folliculogenesis is the process by which ovarian follicles develop. 滤泡生成是卵巢滤泡发育的过程。

folliculopathy 滤泡病

词根 follic-（滤泡）+ -pathy（病变）

例句 Folliculopathy refers to any disorder affecting the hair follicles. 滤泡病指影响毛囊的疾病。

follicular lymphoma 滤泡淋巴瘤

词根 follic-（滤泡）+ -ar（形容词后缀）+ lymphoma（淋巴瘤）

例句 Follicular lymphoma is a type of cancer that affects the lymph nodes. 滤泡淋巴瘤是一种影响淋巴结的癌症。

follicular hyperplasia 滤泡增生

词根 follic-（滤泡）+ hyper-（过度）+ -plasia（增生）

例句 Follicular hyperplasia is a common response to infection or inflammation. 滤泡增生是对感染或炎症的常见反应。

follicular thyroid cancer 滤泡型甲状腺癌

词根 follic-（滤泡）+ thyroid（甲状腺）+ cancer（癌）

例句 Follicular thyroid cancer is a malignant tumor that develops in the thyroid gland. 滤泡型甲状腺癌是甲状腺腺体中发展起来的恶性肿瘤。

follicular dendritic cell 滤泡树突状细胞

词根 follic-（滤泡）+ dendritic（树突状）+ cell（细胞）
例句 Follicular dendritic cells play a key role in immune response. 滤泡树突状细胞在免疫反应中起着关键作用。

fuso-（梭状）

fusospirochetal necrosis 梭杆菌 - 螺旋体性坏死

词根 fuso-（梭状）+ spirochet-（螺旋体）+ -al（形容词后缀）+ necrosis（坏死）
例句 Fusospirochetal necrosis is associated with severe tissue destruction, especially in the oral cavity. 梭杆菌 - 螺旋体性坏死与严重的组织破坏有关，尤其是口腔组织。

fusiform widening 梭形扩宽

词根 fuso-（梭状）+ form（形态）+ widening（扩宽）
例句 Fusiform widening of the arteries is often seen in vascular diseases. 梭形扩宽常见于血管疾病中，尤其是在动脉中。

fusospirochetal pharyngitis 梭杆菌 - 螺旋体性咽炎

词根 fuso-（梭状）+ spirochet-（螺旋体）+ -al（形容词后缀）+ pharyngitis（咽炎）
例句 Fusospirochetal pharyngitis is a throat infection caused by a combination of fusobacteria and spirochetes. 梭杆菌 - 螺旋体性咽炎是由梭杆菌和螺旋体结合引起的咽部感染。

fusospirochetal stomatitis 梭杆菌 - 螺旋体性口腔炎

词根 fuso-（梭状）+ spirochet-（螺旋体）+ -al（形容词后缀）+ stomatitis（口炎）

例句 Fusospirochetal stomatitis results in painful swelling and ulceration of the gums and mouth. 梭杆菌 - 螺旋体性口腔炎导致牙龈和口腔的疼痛、肿胀和溃疡。

fusiform aneurysmal dilatation 梭形动脉瘤扩张

词根 fuso-（梭状）+ form（形状）+ aneurysm（动脉瘤）+ dilatation（扩张）

例句 Fusiform aneurysmal dilatation is an abnormal widening of a blood vessel in a spindle shape. 梭形动脉瘤扩张是血管异常扩张为梭形。

fusospirochetal gingival infection 梭杆菌 - 螺旋体性牙龈感染

词根 fuso-（梭状）+ spirochet-（螺旋体）+ gingiv-（牙龈）+ infection（感染）

例句 Fusospirochetal gingival infection is linked to severe gum diseases and bad breath. 梭杆菌 - 螺旋体性牙龈感染与严重的牙龈疾病和口臭有关。

fusiform lesion 梭形病变

词根 fuso-（梭状）+ form（形状）+ lesion（病变）

例句 A fusiform lesion on the brain can lead to neurological symptoms. 大脑上的梭形病变可能会导致神经症状。

fusiform body 梭形体

词根 fuso-（梭状）+ form（形状）+ body（体）

例句 The fusiform body in the body refers to a shape that tapers at both ends. 体内的梭形体指的是两端逐渐变细的形状。

fusospirochetal tonsillitis 梭杆菌 - 螺旋体性扁桃体炎

词根 fuso-（梭状）+ spirochet-（螺旋体）+ -al（形容词后缀）+ tonsillitis（扁桃体炎）

例句 Fusospirochetal tonsillitis leads to inflamed tonsils and severe throat pain. 梭杆菌 - 螺旋体性扁桃体炎导致扁桃体肿胀和严重的喉咙痛。

G

galacto-（乳相关的）

galactorrhea 乳溢

词根 galacto-（乳汁）+ -rrhea（流出）

例句 Galactorrhea can occur due to hormonal imbalances or pituitary tumors. 乳溢可能是激素失调或垂体肿瘤引起的。

galactosemia 半乳糖血症

词根 galacto-（乳糖）+ -emia（血症）

例句 Galactosemia is a genetic disorder affecting the metabolism of galactose. 半乳糖血症是一种影响半乳糖代谢的遗传疾病。

galactagogue 催乳剂

词根 galacto-（乳汁）+ -agogue（促进分泌的药物）

例句 Fenugreek is often used as a galactagogue to boost milk production. 胡芦巴常用作催乳剂来促进乳汁分泌。

galactopoiesis 乳汁生成

词根 galacto-（乳汁）+ -poiesis（生成）

例句 Prolactin is a hormone involved in galactopoiesis. 催乳素是参与乳汁生成的激素。

galactose 半乳糖

词根 galacto-（乳糖）+ -ose（糖）

例句 Galactose is a simple sugar found in milk. 半乳糖是牛奶含有的一种单糖。

galactosidase 半乳糖苷酶

词根 galacto-（乳糖）+ -sidase（酶）

例句 Galactosidase enzymes are responsible for breaking down lactose. 半乳糖苷酶负责分解乳糖。

galactocele 乳腺囊肿

词根 galacto-（乳汁）+ -cele（囊肿）
例句 A galactocele forms when milk is trapped within a duct. 乳腺囊肿是由于乳汁滞留在乳腺管中形成的。

galactolipid 乳脂类

词根 galacto-（乳）+ lipid（脂质）
例句 Galactolipids are important in cellular membranes and milk fat. 乳脂类在细胞膜和乳脂中具有重要作用。

galactose kinase deficiency 半乳糖激酶缺乏症

词根 galacto-（乳糖）+ kinase（激酶）+ deficiency（缺乏）
例句 Galactose kinase deficiency can lead to galactosemia. 半乳糖激酶缺乏症可导致半乳糖血症。

galactolysis 乳糖分解

词根 galacto-（乳糖）+ -lysis（分解）
例句 Galactolysis refers to the breakdown of galactose into simpler molecules. 乳糖分解是指将半乳糖分解为更简单的分子。

USMLE Step 2 CK 样题

Two weeks after undergoing open cholecystectomy (chole-; cyst-; -ectomy) for gangrenous (gangren-) cholecystitis (chole; cyst-; -itis), a 47-year-old woman comes to the clinic for removal of surgical staples. She was treated with oral vancomycin (-mycin) for Clostridioides (clostri-; -oides) difficile colitis (col-; -itis) during hospitalization. She has type 2 diabetes mellitus. Current medications are metformin (met-; form-) and pantoprazole (panto-; -prazole). She reports loose stools four times daily during the past

2 weeks. In addition to wearing a clean isolation gown, which of the following is the most appropriate precaution (pre-; caut) for the physician to take?

(A) Washing hands thoroughly with alcohol gel

(B) Washing hands thoroughly with soap and water

(C) Wearing a surgical mask

(D) Wearing sterile gloves and preparing the staple skin line with chlorhexidine (chlor-; hex-, -idine)

(E) No additional precautions are necessary

中文翻译

一名 47 岁女性在因坏疽性胆囊炎接受开放性胆囊切除术后两周，来到门诊拆除手术缝合钉。她在住院期间因艰难梭菌结肠炎接受了口服万古霉素治疗。她患有 2 型糖尿病。目前使用的药物为二甲双胍和泮托拉唑。过去两周，她每天有 4 次稀便。除穿戴隔离衣外，医生应采取以下哪项最适当的预防措施？

(A) 用酒精凝胶彻底洗手

(B) 用肥皂和水彻底洗手

(C) 佩戴外科口罩

(D) 佩戴无菌手套并用氯己定对缝合钉所在皮肤区域进行消毒

(E) 无须额外预防措施

题目和答案中出现的词根

chole-：胆

cyst-：囊

-ectomy：切除术

gangren-：坏死

-itis：炎症

-mycin：抗生素

col-：大肠

met-：甲基

form-：甲酸

panto-：全面的

-prazole：离子泵抑制剂药物

pre-：在……之前

caut-：警惕

chlor-：氯

hex-：六

-dine：含氨化合物

gastro-（胃）

gastritis 胃炎

词根 gastro-（胃）+ -itis（炎症）

例句 Gastritis can result from excessive alcohol consumption or infection. 胃炎可能由过度饮酒或感染引起。

gastroenterology 胃肠病学

词根 gastro-（胃）+ entero-（肠）+ -logy（学科）

例句 Gastroenterology focuses on the digestive system and its disorders. 胃肠病学专注于消化系统及其相关疾病。

gastrectomy 胃切除术

词根 gastro-（胃）+ -ectomy（切除）

例句 A gastrectomy may be performed to treat stomach cancer. 胃切除术可用于治疗胃癌。

gastroesophageal reflux disease 胃食管反流病

词根 gastro-（胃）+ esophago-（食管）

例句 Gastroesophageal reflux disease causes acid from the stomach to flow backward. 胃食管反流病导致胃酸反流至食管。

gastroparesis 胃轻瘫

词根 gastro-（胃）+ -paresis（瘫痪）

例句 Gastroparesis leads to delayed stomach emptying, causing discomfort. 胃轻瘫会导致胃排空延迟，造成不适。

gastrostomy 胃造口术

词根 gastro-（胃）+ -stomy（造口术）

例句 A gastrostomy is performed to create an opening into the stomach for feeding. 胃造口术是为了在胃中创建一个供食物输入的开口。

gastroenteritis 胃肠炎

词根 gastro-（胃）+ entero-（肠）+ -itis（炎症）

例句 Gastroenteritis is commonly caused by viral or bacterial infections. 胃肠炎通常由病毒或细菌感染引起。

gastroplasty 胃成形术

词根 gastro-（胃）+ -plasty（成形术）

例句 Gastroplasty is a surgical procedure to reduce stomach size. 胃成形术是一种缩小胃部大小的手术。

gastrocolic reflex 胃结肠反射

词根 gastro-（胃）+ colic（结肠）

例句 The gastrocolic reflex is triggered after eating, promoting bowel movements. 胃结肠反射在进食后被触发，促进排便。

gastrointestinal bleeding 胃肠道出血

词根 gastro-（胃）+ intestino-（肠）+ -al（形容词后缀）

例句 Gastrointestinal bleeding may be caused by ulcers or tumors. 胃肠道出血可能由溃疡或肿瘤引起。

-genesis（生长；发育）

embryogenesis 胚胎发生

词根 embryo-（胚胎）+ -genesis（发育）

例句 Embryogenesis is a critical period during development when organs begin to form. 胚胎发生是器官开始形成的关键发育阶段。

osteogenesis 成骨

词根 osteo-（骨）+ -genesis（生长）

例句 Osteogenesis involves the process of bone formation. 成骨指骨骼的形成过程。

carcinogenesis 致癌过程

词根 carcino-（癌）+ -genesis（生长）

例句 Carcinogenesis is a multi-step process that can lead to tumor formation. 致癌过程是一个多步骤过程，可能导致肿瘤形成。

neurogenesis 神经发生

词根 neuro-（神经）+ -genesis（生长）

例句 Neurogenesis is the process by which new neurons are formed in the brain. 神经发生是大脑中生成新神经元的过程。

spermatogenesis 精子生成

词根 spermato-（精子）+ -genesis（生长）

例句 Spermatogenesis occurs in the testes and is vital for reproduction. 精子生成发生在睾丸中，对繁殖至关重要。

pathogenesis 病理发生

词根 patho-（疾病）+ -genesis（生长）

例句 Pathogenesis refers to the development of a disease. 病理发生是指疾病的发展过程。

angiogenesis 血管生成

词根 angio-（血管）+ -genesis（生长）

例句 Angiogenesis is essential for wound healing. 血管生成对伤口愈合至关重要。

tumorigenesis 肿瘤发生

词根 tumori-（肿瘤）+ -genesis（发生）

例句 Tumorigenesis is linked to genetic mutations and abnormal cell growth. 肿瘤发生与基因突变和细胞异常生长有关。

histogenesis 组织生成

词根 histo-（组织）+ -genesis（生长）

例句 Histogenesis describes the formation of tissues from undifferentiated cells. 组织生成描述的是未分化细胞形成组织的过程。

biogenesis 生物发生论

词根 bio-（生命）+ -genesis（生长）

例句 Biogenesis is the concept that life arises from pre-existing life. 生物发生论是生命起源于已存在生命的概念。

gingivo-（牙龈的）

gingivitis 牙龈炎

词根 gingivo-（牙龈）+ -itis（炎症）

例句 Gingivitis is a common gum disease caused by plaque build-up. 牙龈炎是一种常见的由牙菌斑堆积引起的牙龈疾病。

gingivectomy 牙龈切除术

词根 gingivo-（牙龈）+ -ectomy（切除）

例句 Gingivectomy is performed to remove diseased gum tissue. 牙龈切除术用于切除患病的牙龈组织。

gingivoplasty 牙龈成形术

词根 gingivo-（牙龈）+ -plasty（成形术）

例句 Gingivoplasty is done to reshape and contour the gums. 牙龈成形术用于重塑和调整牙龈形状。

gingival hyperplasia 牙龈增生

词根 gingivo-（牙龈）+ hyper-（过度）+ -plasia（增生）

例句 Gingival hyperplasia can be caused by certain medications. 牙龈增生可能由某些药物引起。

gingival recession 牙龈萎缩

词根 gingivo-（牙龈）+ recession（后退）

例句 Gingival recession is a common problem that exposes the tooth roots. 牙龈萎缩是一个常见问题，会导致牙根暴露。

gingivostomatitis 牙龈口腔炎

词根 gingivo-（牙龈）+ stomato-（口腔）+ -itis（炎症）

例句 Gingivostomatitis is often seen in children with viral infections. 牙龈口腔炎常见于患病毒感染的儿童。

gingival sulcus 牙龈沟

词根 gingivo-（牙龈）+ sulcus（沟）

例句 The gingival sulcus is the space between the tooth and gum. 牙龈沟是牙齿和牙龈之间的空间。

gingival epithelium 牙龈上皮

词根 gingivo-（牙龈）+ epithelium（上皮）

例句 The gingival epithelium acts as a barrier against bacteria. 牙

龈上皮是抵抗细菌的屏障。

gingivobuccal sulcus 牙龈颊沟

词根 gingivo-（牙龈）+ buccal（颊部）+ sulcus（沟）

例句 Inflammation in the gingivobuccal sulcus can lead to discomfort while eating. 牙龈颊沟的炎症可能导致进食时不适。

gingivobuccal carcinoma 牙龈颊癌

词根 gingivo-（牙龈）+ buccal（颊）+ carcinoma（癌）

例句 Gingivobuccal carcinoma is a type of oral cancer affecting the gums and cheek. 牙龈颊癌是一种影响牙龈和颊部的口腔癌。

glio-（胶质）

glioblastoma 胶质母细胞瘤

词根 glio-（胶质）+ -blastoma（母细胞瘤）

例句 Glioblastoma is an aggressive brain tumor with a poor prognosis. 胶质母细胞瘤是一种具有较差预后的侵袭性脑瘤。

glioma 胶质瘤

词根 glio-（胶质）+ -oma（肿瘤）

例句 Gliomas are the most common type of primary brain tumor. 胶质瘤是最常见的原发性脑肿瘤类型。

glial cells 神经胶质细胞

词根 glio-（胶质）+ cells（细胞）

例句 Glial cells provide support and protection to neurons. 神经胶质细胞为神经元提供支持和保护。

gliopathy 胶质病

词根 glio-（胶质）+ -pathy（病）

例句 Gliopathy refers to diseases affecting glial cells. 胶质病是指影响胶质细胞的疾病。

gliogenesis 胶质细胞生成

词根 glio-（胶质）+ -genesis（生成）

例句 Gliogenesis is crucial for maintaining central nervous system integrity. 胶质细胞生成对维持中枢神经系统的完整性至关重要。

neuroglia 神经胶质

词根 neuro-（神经）+ glio-（胶质）

例句 Neuroglia play an important role in the immune response of the brain. 神经胶质在大脑的免疫反应中起重要作用。

gliotoxicity 胶质毒性

词根 glio-（胶质）+ -toxicity（毒性）

例句 Gliotoxicity can result from neuroinflammation or exposure to toxins. 胶质毒性可能由神经炎症或毒素暴露引起。

glial scar 胶质瘢痕

词根 glio-（胶质）+ scar（瘢痕）

例句 Glial scars form after brain injuries and may inhibit neural repair. 脑损伤后会形成胶质瘢痕，可能抑制神经修复。

microgliosis 小胶质细胞增生

词根 micro-（小）+ glio-（胶质）+ -osis（病症）

例句 Microgliosis is often seen in neurodegenerative diseases. 小胶质细胞增生常见于神经退行性疾病。

astrogliosis 星形胶质细胞增生

词根 astro-（星形）+ glio-（胶质）+ -osis（增生）

例句 Astrogliosis is a reactive process in response to brain injury. 星形胶质细胞增生是对脑损伤的一种反应性过程。

globul-（球）

globulin 球蛋白

词根 globul-（球）+ -in（蛋白质）

例句 Globulin levels in the blood can indicate immune system activity. 血液中的球蛋白水平可以反映免疫系统的活性。

immunoglobulin 免疫球蛋白

词根 immuno-（免疫）+ globul-（球）+ -in（蛋白质）

例句 Immunoglobulin plays a vital role in defending the body against infections. 免疫球蛋白在抵御感染中起重要作用。

cryoglobulin 冷球蛋白

词根 cryo-（冷）+ globul-（球）+ -in（蛋白质）

例句 Cryoglobulins can precipitate at low temperatures, leading to vascular complications. 冷球蛋白在低温下可能沉淀，导致血管并发症。

globulite 小球晶

词根 globul-（球）+ -ite（小物体）

例句 Globulites are small spherical inclusions found in volcanic rocks. 小球晶是火山岩中发现的小球状夹杂物。

lipoglobulin 脂球蛋白

词根 lipo-（脂肪）+ globul-（球）+ -in（蛋白质）

例句 Lipoglobulins transport lipids through the bloodstream. 脂球蛋白通过血流运输脂质。

macroglobulin 大球蛋白

词根 macro-（大）+ globul-（球）+ -in（蛋白质）

例句 Elevated macroglobulin levels can indicate an underlying blood disorder. 大球蛋白升高可能表明潜在的血液疾病。

paraglobulin 副球蛋白

词根 para-（旁）+ globul-（球）+ -in（蛋白质）
例句 Paraglobulin is associated with plasma proteins. 副球蛋白与血浆蛋白有关。

globulomerule 小球器

词根 globul-（球）+ -merule（小体）
例句 Globulomerule plays a role in cellular energy production. 小球器在细胞能量产生中起作用。

globuliform 球形的

词根 globul-（球）+ form（形态）
例句 Certain bacteria are globuliform in shape. 某些细菌呈球形。

microglobulin 微球蛋白

词根 micro-（小）+ globul-（球）+ -in（蛋白质）
例句 Beta-2 microglobulin levels are used to monitor kidney function. β2- 微球蛋白水平用于监测肾功能。

glomerulo-（肾小球的）

glomerulonephritis 肾小球肾炎

词根 glomerulo-（肾小球）+ nephr-（肾）+ -itis（炎症）
例句 Glomerulonephritis often results from infections or autoimmune conditions. 肾小球肾炎通常由感染或自身免疫疾病引起。

glomerulosclerosis 肾小球硬化

词根 glomerulo-（肾小球）+ sclerosis（硬化）
例句 Glomerulosclerosis can lead to kidney failure if not treated promptly. 如果未及时治疗，肾小球硬化可能导致肾衰竭。

glomerulopathy 肾小球病

词根 glomerulo-（肾小球）+ -pathy（病）

例句 Various types of glomerulopathy affect kidney function in different ways. 不同类型的肾小球病以不同方式影响肾功能。

glomerular filtration rate 肾小球滤过率

词根 glomerulo-（肾小球）+ filtration（过滤）

例句 The glomerular filtration rate is a key indicator of kidney function. 肾小球滤过率是衡量肾功能的重要指标。

glomerulocystic kidney disease 肾小球囊性病

词根 glomerulo-（肾小球）+ cystic（囊性的）

例句 Glomerulocystic kidney disease involves cyst formation within the glomeruli. 肾小球囊性病指肾小球中的囊肿形成。

glomerulonephrosis 肾小球变性

词根 glomerulo-（肾小球）+ nephro-（肾）+ -osis（状态）

例句 Glomerulonephrosis is often associated with proteinuria. 肾小球变性通常伴有蛋白尿。

mesangial glomerulopathy 系膜性肾小球病

词根 mesangial（系膜的）+ glomerulo-（肾小球）+ -pathy（病）

例句 Mesangial glomerulopathy affects the cells that support the glomerular capillaries. 系膜性肾小球病影响支持肾小球毛细血管的细胞。

immune glomerulonephritis 免疫性肾小球肾炎

词根 immune（免疫）+ glomerulo-（肾小球）+ -nephritis（肾炎）

例句 Immune glomerulonephritis is triggered by an abnormal immune response. 免疫性肾小球肾炎由异常的免疫反应引发。

focal segmental glomerulosclerosis 局灶性节段性肾小球硬化

词根 glomerulo-（肾小球）+ sclerosis（硬化）

例句 Focal segmental glomerulosclerosis is a major cause of nephrotic syndrome. 局灶性节段性肾小球硬化是肾病综合征的主要原因之一。

glomerular capillaries 肾小球毛细血管

词根 glomerulo-（肾小球）+ capillaries（毛细血管）
例句 Glomerular capillaries are vital for filtering blood in the kidneys. 肾小球毛细血管对血液过滤至关重要。

glosso-/glott-（舌头）

glossitis 舌炎

词根 glosso-（舌头）+ -itis（炎症）
例句 Glossitis is characterized by swelling and inflammation of the tongue. 舌炎的特征是舌头肿胀和发炎。

glossalgia 舌痛

词根 glosso-（舌头）+ -algia（疼痛）
例句 Glossalgia can be caused by nerve damage or oral infections. 舌痛可能由神经损伤或口腔感染引起。

glossectomy 舌切除术

词根 glosso-（舌头）+ -ectomy（切除）
例句 Glossectomy is performed to remove part or all of the tongue in cancer cases. 舌切除术用于癌症患者部分或全部舌头的切除。

glossolalia 舌语症

词根 glosso-（舌头）+ -lalia（说话）
例句 Glossolalia is commonly associated with religious or ecstatic states. 舌语症通常与宗教或狂喜状态有关。

glottis 声门

词根 glott-（舌头或声门）

例句 The glottis plays a crucial role in phonation and breathing. 声门在发声和呼吸中起重要作用。

subglottic stenosis 舌下狭窄

词根 sub-（下）+ glott-（舌头）+ stenosis（狭窄）
例句 Subglottic stenosis can cause breathing difficulties. 声门下狭窄可能导致呼吸困难。

epiglottitis 会厌炎

词根 epi-（上）+ glott-（舌头）+ -itis（炎症）
例句 Epiglottitis is a medical emergency due to its risk of airway obstruction. 会厌炎是一种急症，因为它可能导致气道阻塞。

hypoglossal nerve 舌下神经

词根 hypo-（下）+ glosso-（舌头）
例句 The hypoglossal nerve controls the movement of the tongue. 舌下神经控制舌头的运动。

glossophobia 演讲恐惧症

词根 glosso-（舌头）+ -phobia（恐惧）
例句 Glossophobia, or the fear of public speaking, affects many people. 演讲恐惧症，即对公开演讲的恐惧，影响了许多人。

glossoplegia 舌瘫

词根 glosso-（舌头）+ -plegia（瘫痪）
例句 Glossoplegia can result from neurological damage or stroke. 舌瘫可能由神经损伤或中风引起。

USMLE Step 2 CK　样题

A 72-year-old man comes to the clinic because of a 3-week history of visual changes in his right eye. During this period, he has noticed that the lines of his daily crossword puzzle look curved, and the blinds in his apartment appear wavy. He wears magnifying lenses for reading. He has not had pain in his eye or photophobia (photo-; -phobia). He has no history of trauma to the area. On examination, visual acuity is 20/200 in the right eye and 20/100 in the left eye. Both pupils are round and reactive (re-; -act) to light. Palpation of both globes through closed eyelids shows no abnormalities. There is normal red reflex (re-; -flex) bilaterally (bi-; -lateral). The lenses appear clear. Which of the following is the most likely diagnosis?

(A) Cataracts

(B) Central retinal artery occlusion

(C) Closed-angle glaucoma (glau-; -oma)

(D) Macular degeneration (de-; gener-; -ation)

(E) Temporal arteritis (arter-; -itis)

中文翻译

一名72岁男性因过去3周右眼视力变化来就诊。在此期间，他注意到每天填写的填字游戏的线条变得弯曲，公寓的百叶窗呈波浪状。他使用放大镜阅读。他没有眼痛或畏光症状，也无该部位外伤史。检查显示右眼视力为20/200，左眼为20/100。双侧瞳孔呈圆形，对光反应正常。闭眼触诊双侧眼球未见异常。双侧红光反射正常。晶状体看起来透明。以下哪项是最可能的诊断？

(A) 白内障

(B) 视网膜中央动脉闭塞

(C) 闭角型青光眼

(D) 黄斑变性

(E) 颞动脉炎

题目和答案中出现的词根

photo-：像；光

-phobia：害怕

re-：重新；反复

-act：作用

-flex：弯曲（指的是电信号在反射弧神经的传导，从中央神经系统传出到外周肌肉，再弯曲返回中央神经系统）

bi-：双

lateral：侧

glau-：蓝灰色

-oma：瘤（蓝灰色肿瘤，指的是青光眼。眼内压增高导致角膜水肿，看起来像角膜的肿瘤，并导致其看起来为蓝灰色）

de-：去掉

gener-：生长

-ation：表示动作的状态

arter-：动脉的

-itis：炎症

glyco-（葡萄糖）

glycemia 血糖

词根 glyco-（葡萄糖）+ -emia（血液中的状态）

例句 Abnormal glycemia levels can indicate diabetes. 血糖水平异常可能是糖尿病的迹象。

glycogen 糖原

词根 glyco-（葡萄糖）+ -gen（生成）

例句 The liver stores excess glucose in the form of glycogen. 肝脏以糖原的形式储存多余的葡萄糖。

hypoglycemia 低血糖

词根 hypo-（低）+ glyco-（葡萄糖）+ -emia（血症）

例句 Hypoglycemia can cause dizziness, confusion, and fainting. 低血糖可能引起头晕、意识混乱和昏厥。

hyperglycemia 高血糖

词根 hyper-（高）+ glyco-（葡萄糖）+ -emia（血症）

例句 Hyperglycemia is a common symptom of uncontrolled diabetes. 高血糖是血糖控制不佳的糖尿病患者的常见症状。

glycolysis 糖酵解

词根 glyco-（葡萄糖）+ -lysis（分解）

例句 Glycolysis is the process of breaking down glucose to produce energy. 糖酵解是分解葡萄糖以产生能量的过程。

glycosuria 糖尿

词根 glyco-（葡萄糖）+ -uria（尿液）

例句 Glycosuria occurs when excess glucose is excreted in the urine. 糖尿是在尿液中排出过量葡萄糖的现象。

glycosylation 糖基化

词根 glyco-（糖）+ -sylation（结合）

例句 Protein glycosylation plays a key role in cell communication and immune responses. 蛋白质糖基化在细胞通信和免疫反应中起关键作用。

glycosaminoglycan 糖胺聚糖

词根 glyco-（糖）+ amino-（胺）+ -glycan（多糖）

例句 Glycosaminoglycans are important components of connective tissue. 糖胺聚糖是结缔组织的重要成分。

glycoside 苷

词根 glyco-（糖）+ -side（化合物）
例句 Glycosides are natural compounds found in many plants. 苷类是在许多植物中发现的天然化合物。

glycogenesis 糖原生成

词根 glyco-（葡萄糖）+ -genesis（生成）
例句 Glycogenesis occurs when excess glucose is converted to glycogen for storage. 当多余的葡萄糖转化为糖原以便储存时，就会发生糖原生成。

-gnath-（下巴）

prognathism 下颌前突

词根 pro-（向前）+ -gnath-（下巴）+ -ism（状态或特征）
例句 Prognathism can lead to functional and aesthetic concerns in patients. 下颌前突可能会导致患者的功能和美学问题。

micrognathia 小颌畸形

词根 micro-（小）+ -gnath-（下巴）+ -ia（病症）
例句 Micrognathia is often seen in congenital syndromes like Pierre Robin sequence. 小颌畸形常见于先天性综合征，如皮埃尔 - 罗宾综合征。

brachygnathia 短下颌

词根 brachy-（短）+ -gnath-（下巴）+ -ia（病症）
例句 Brachygnathia can affect chewing and speaking ability. 短下颌可能影响咀嚼和说话能力。

macrognathia 巨颌畸形

词根 macro-（大）+ -gnath-（下巴）+ -ia（病症）

例句 Macrognathia is characterized by an unusually large jaw. 巨颌畸形的特征是下颌异常增大。

orthognathic surgery 正颌手术

词根 ortho-（正）+ -gnath-（下巴）+ -ic（形容词后缀）+ surgery（手术）

例句 Orthognathic surgery corrects jaw misalignment to improve function and appearance. 正颌手术可以纠正下颌错位，改善功能和外观。

gnathalgia 下巴疼痛

词根 -gnath-（下巴）+ algia（疼痛）

例句 Gnathalgia may be associated with temporomandibular joint disorders. 下巴疼痛可能与颞下颌关节疾病有关。

gnathoplasty 下巴成形术

词根 -gnath-（下巴）+ -plasty（成形术）

例句 Gnathoplasty is performed to reshape the jaw for both functional and aesthetic reasons. 下巴成形术是为了改善颌部功能及美观而进行的颌骨重塑手术。

gnathostome 有颌脊椎动物

词根 -gnath-（下巴）+ stome（开口）

例句 Gnathostomes represent the majority of vertebrates with jaws. 有颌脊椎动物代表了大多数具有下颌的脊椎动物。

gnathic nerve 下巴神经

词根 -gnath-（下巴）+ -ic（形容词后缀）+ nerve（神经）

例句 The gnathic nerve controls sensation and movement in the jaw region. 下巴神经控制下颌区域的感觉和运动。

gnathodynamometer 下颌动力计

词根 -gnath-（下巴）+ dynamo-（力量）+ meter（测量仪器）

例句 The gnathodynamometer measures the strength of the jaw muscles. 下颌动力计用于测量下颌肌肉的力量。

USMLE Step 2 CK 样题

A 4-month-old female infant is recovering (re-; -cover) in the hospital 5 days after uncomplicated (un-) surgical repair of a ventricular septal defect via median sternotomy (stern-; -otomy) utilizing cardiopulmonary (cardio-; pulmon-) bypass. She was extubated (ex-; tub-) on postoperative (post-) day 1 and by postoperative (post-) day 4. she was no longer receiving any inotropic (ino-; -trop) infusions (in-; -fus) or intravenous (intra-; veno-) drugs. She is breast-feeding well; plans are made for discharge (dis-; -charge) from the hospital the next morning. However, on the next morning she develops a temperature of 38.8°C (101.8°F), cool and clammy skin, cold distal extremities, delayed capillary (capill-) refill, and minimal urine output. Cardiac rhythm strip and tracing of arterial (arter-) blood pressure are shown. Which of the following is the most appropriate next step in evaluation?

(A) Cardiac catheterization

(B) CT angiography (angio-; -graphy)

(C) Echocardiography (echo-; cardio-; -graphy)

(D) Electrophysiology (electro-; physi-; -ology) study

(E) MRI of the heart

中文翻译

一名4月龄女婴因室间隔缺损接受了无并发症的手术修补治疗（经胸骨正中切口，采用体外循环），术后第5天仍在医院康复。患儿于术后第1天拔除气管插管，至术后第4天，不再接受强心剂或静脉给药治疗。患儿母乳喂养良好；计划次日早晨出院。然而，次日早晨，患儿出现体温38.8℃（101.8℉）、皮肤湿冷、四肢末端发凉、毛细血管再充盈延迟以及尿量极少等症状。心电图和动脉血压描记图如下所示（图片省略）。以下哪项是下一步评估的最合适措施？

(A) 心导管检查

(B) CT 血管造影

(C) 心脏超声检查

(D) 电生理学检查

(E) 心脏 MRI

题目和答案中出现的词根

re-：重新；反复

-cover：获得

un-：表示否定

stern-：胸骨

-otomy：切开术

cardio-：心脏的

pulmon-：肺的

ex-：向外

tub-：管

post-：在……之后

ino-：肌纤维的

-trop：改变

in-：向内

fus-：倾泻

intra：在……内

veno-：静脉

dis-：离开

-charge：负担

capill-：毛发

arter-：动脉

angio-：血管

-graphy：图像

echo-：回声

cardio-：心脏

electro-：电的

physi- ：生理

-ology：学科

gonado/gono-（生殖的）

gonadotropin 促性腺激素

词根 gonado-（性腺）+ -tropin（刺激素）

例句 Gonadotropins are hormones that regulate reproductive function. 促性腺激素是调节生殖功能的激素。

gonorrhea 淋病

词根 gono-（生殖）+ -rrhea（流出）

例句 Gonorrhea is a sexually transmitted infection caused by Neisseria gonorrhoeae. 淋病是一种由淋病奈瑟球菌引起的性传播感染。

gonadal dysgenesis 性腺发育不良

词根 gonado-（性腺）+ dys-（不良）+ genesis（生成）

例句 Gonadal dysgenesis can result in infertility. 性腺发育不良可能导致不孕。

gonocyte 生殖细胞

词根 gono-（生殖）+ -cyte（细胞）

例句 Gonocytes develop into mature sperm or egg cells. 生殖细胞发育成成熟的精子或卵细胞。

gonadoblastoma 性腺母细胞瘤

词根 gonado-（性腺）+ -blastoma（母细胞瘤）

例句 Gonadoblastoma is a rare tumor seen in patients with gonadal dysgenesis. 性腺母细胞瘤是性腺发育不良患者中罕见的肿瘤。

gonadectomy 性腺切除术

词根 gonado-（性腺）+ -ectomy（切除）

例句 Gonadectomy is performed in cases of gonadal tumors. 因性腺肿瘤进行性腺切除术。

gonadogenesis 性腺发育

词根 gonado-（性腺）+ -genesis（生长）

例句 Gonadogenesis is a critical stage in sexual development. 性腺发育是性发育中的关键阶段。

gonococcal infection 淋病奈瑟球菌感染

词根 gono-（生殖）+ cocci（球菌）

例句 A gonococcal infection may cause urethritis or pelvic inflammatory disease. 淋病奈瑟球菌感染可能导致尿道炎或盆腔炎。

gonadotropin-releasing hormone 促性腺激素释放激素

词根 gonado-（性腺）+ tropin（刺激素）

例句 The gonadotropin-releasing hormone regulates the production of gonadotropins. 促性腺激素释放激素调节促性腺激素的生成。

gonoblast 生殖母细胞

词根 gono-（生殖）+ -blast（未成熟细胞）

例句 Gonoblasts give rise to mature gametes in reproductive organs. 生殖母细胞在生殖器官中生成成熟配子。

–gram / –graph / –graphy（图；影像）

electrocardiogram 心电图

词根 electro-（电）+ cardio-（心脏）+ -gram（图）

例句 The electrocardiogram is used to monitor heart activity. 心电图用于监测心脏活动。

sonogram 超声成像

词根 sono-（声音）+ -gram（图）

例句 A sonogram helps visualize internal organs using sound waves. 超声成像利用声波帮助观察内脏器官。

mammography 乳房 X 线片

词根 mammo-（乳房）+ -graphy（影像）

例句 Mammography is used to detect breast cancer in its early stages. 乳房 X 线片用于检测早期乳腺癌。

radiograph X 线片

词根 radio-（辐射）+ -graph（影像）

例句 The radiograph revealed a fracture in the patient's femur. X 线片显示患者的股骨骨折。

angiography 血管造影

词根 angio-（血管）+ -graphy（影像）

例句 Angiography is performed to examine blockages in blood vessels. 血管造影用于检查血管中的阻塞情况。

echocardiography 超声心动图

词根 echo-（回声）+ cardio-（心脏）+ -graphy（影像）

例句 Echocardiography uses sound waves to create images of the heart. 超声心动图利用声波生成心脏图像。

tomography 断层摄影术

词根 tomo-（切片）+ -graphy（影像）

例句 Tomography provides cross-sectional images of the body. 断层摄影术生成身体的横截面图像。

sialography 唾腺造影术

词根 sialo-（唾液）+ -graphy（影像）

例句 Sialography is used to visualize the salivary glands. 唾腺造影术用于观察唾腺。

kymograph 波动记录仪

词根 kymo-（波动）+ -graph（图）

例句 The kymograph is used to record pressure changes in fluids. 波动记录仪用于记录液体中的压力变化。

arteriography 动脉造影

词根 arterio-（动脉）+ -graphy（影像）

例句 Arteriography is essential for detecting arterial blockages. 动脉造影对检测动脉阻塞至关重要。

cholangiogram 胆管造影

词根 cholangio-（胆管）+ -gram（影像）

例句 The cholangiogram highlights bile duct blockages. 胆管造影显示胆管阻塞情况。

spirogram 肺活量曲线图

词根 spiro-（呼吸）+ -gram（图）

例句 The spirogram measures a patient's lung function. 肺活量曲线图测量患者的肺功能。

myelogram 脊髓造影

词根 myelo-（脊髓）+ -gram（影像）

例句 A myelogram can diagnose spinal cord compression. 脊髓造影可以诊断脊髓压迫。

gravi-（重；严重）

myasthenia gravis 重症肌无力

词根 myo-（肌肉）+ asthenia（无力）+ gravis（严重）

例句 Myasthenia gravis is an autoimmune disorder that affects muscle strength. 重症肌无力是一种影响肌肉力量的自身免疫疾病。

gravimetric analysis 重量分析

词根 gravi-（重）+ metric（测量）

例句 Gravimetric analysis is a laboratory technique used to measure substances by weight. 重量分析是一种通过称量物质来测定含量的实验室技术。

gravid uterus 妊娠子宫

词根 gravi-（重）+ uterus（子宫）

例句 The gravid uterus increases in size as pregnancy progresses. 随着妊娠进展，子宫逐渐增大。

gravitational pull 重力吸引

词根 gravi-（重）+ -tion（动作或状态）

例句 Gravitational pull keeps planets in orbit around the sun. 重力吸引使行星围绕太阳运行。

gravidity 孕次

词根 gravi-（重）+ -ity（状态）

例句 Gravidity refers to the number of times a woman has been pregnant. 孕次指一个女性怀孕的次数。

gravitation 引力

词根 gravi-（重）+ -ation（过程）

例句 Gravitation is the force that pulls objects toward each other. 引力是使物体相互吸引的力。

gravimeter 重力计

词根 gravi-（重）+ -meter（测量仪器）

例句 A gravimeter measures variations in the Earth' s gravitational field. 重力计用于测量地球引力场的变化。

gravitational collapse 引力塌缩

词根 gravi-（重）+ collapse（塌缩）

例句 Gravitational collapse occurs when a massive star' s core collapses under its own weight. 引力塌缩是指大质量恒星的核心在自身重量作用下塌缩。

gravistimulation 重力刺激

词根 gravi-（重）+ stimulation（刺激）

例句 Gravistimulation influences the growth direction of plant roots. 重力刺激影响植物根部的生长方向。

gravitropism 向重性

词根 gravi-（重）+ tropism（趋向）

例句 Gravitropism is the growth response of plants to gravity. 向重性是植物对重力的生长反应。

gyneco-（女性）

G

gynecology 妇科学

词根 gyneco-（女性）+ -logy（学科）

例句 Gynecology focuses on the health of the female reproductive system. 妇科学专注于女性生殖系统的健康。

gynecologist 妇科医生

词根 gyneco-（女性）+ -logist（专家）

例句 A gynecologist diagnoses and treats conditions affecting the female reproductive system. 妇科医生诊断并治疗影响女性生殖系统的疾病。

gynecomastia 男性乳房发育

词根 gyneco-（女性）+ -mastia（乳房）

例句 Gynecomastia can result from hormonal imbalances or certain medications. 男性乳房发育可能是激素失调或某些药物引起的。

gynecoid pelvis 女性型骨盆

词根 gyneco-（女性）+ -oid（形状）

例句 A gynecoid pelvis is ideal for childbirth due to its rounded shape. 女性型骨盆因其圆形结构适合分娩。

gynecopathology 女性病理学

词根 gyneco-（女性）+ pathology（病理学）

例句 Gynecopathology studies diseases specific to the female body. 女性病理学研究特定于女性的疾病。

gynecoid obesity 女性型肥胖

词根 gyneco-（女性）+ -oid（形状）+ obesity（肥胖）

例句 Gynecoid obesity is characterized by fat distribution around the hips and thighs. 女性型肥胖的特征是脂肪主要分布在臀部和大腿周围。

gynecotokology 妇产学

词根 gyneco-（女性）+ tokology（分娩学）
例句 Gynecotokology deals with the study of labor and delivery in women. 妇产学涉及女性分娩过程的研究。

gynecocracy 女性统治

词根 gyneco-（女性）+ -cracy（统治）
例句 In a gynecocracy, women hold the primary power in governance. 在女性统治的制度下，女性掌握主要的治理权。

gynephobia 对女性的恐惧

词根 gyneco-（女性）+ -phobia（恐惧）
例句 Gynephobia can stem from traumatic experiences or cultural influences. 对女性的恐惧可能源于创伤经历或文化影响。

gyneco-oncology 妇科肿瘤学

词根 gyneco-（女性）+ oncology（肿瘤学）
例句 Gyneco-oncology focuses on cancers affecting the female reproductive system. 妇科肿瘤学研究影响女性生殖系统的癌症。

H

haplo-（单）

haploid 单倍体

H

词根 haplo-（单）+ -oid（形状）

例句 Haploid cells have half the number of chromosomes compared to diploid cells. 单倍体细胞的染色体数量是二倍体细胞的一半。

haplosufficient 单倍体充足的

词根 haplo-（单）+ sufficient（足够的）

例句 A haplosufficient gene is one that is capable of performing its function with just one allele. 单倍体充足基因是指仅凭一个等位基因就能发挥作用的基因。

haplotype 单倍型

词根 haplo-（单）+ type（类型）

例句 A haplotype is a group of genes inherited together from a single parent. 单倍型是一组来自单一亲本的基因共同遗传。

haploidization 单倍体化

词根 haplo-（单）+ -ization（转化过程）

例句 Haploidization is the process where a cell or organism reduces its chromosome number to half. 单倍体化是一个细胞或生物将其染色体数目减半的过程。

haplotyping 单倍型分型

词根 haplo-（单）+ typing（分型）

例句 Haplotyping is used in genetic research to identify specific gene variations. 单倍型分型在遗传研究中用于识别特定的基因变异。

haplodiploid 单倍二倍体

词根 haplo-（单）+ diploid（双倍体）

例句 Haplodiploid species have a reproductive system where males are haploid and females are diploid. 单倍二倍体物种的生殖系统特点是雄性为单倍体，雌性为双倍体。

haplotaxonomy 单倍型分类学

词根 haplo-（单）+ taxonomy（分类学）

例句 Haplotaxonomy is the classification of organisms based on their haplotypes. 单倍型分类学是基于单倍型对生物进行分类的学科。

haploidentical 单倍体同源

词根 haplo-（单）+ identical（相同的）

例句 Haploidentical stem cell transplantation involves using stem cells from a partially matched donor. 单倍体同源干细胞移植指使用来自部分匹配供体的干细胞。

hema-/hemo-（血的）

hemoglobin 血红蛋白

词根 hemo-（血）+ globin（蛋白质）

例句 Hemoglobin carries oxygen from the lungs to the rest of the body. 血红蛋白将氧气从肺部运输到身体其他部位。

hemophilia 血友病

词根 hemo-（血）+ -philia（倾向）

例句 Hemophilia is a genetic disorder where blood doesn't clot properly. 血友病是一种遗传性疾病，导致血液无法正常凝固。

hematology 血液学

词根 hema-（血）+ -logy（学科）

例句 Hematology is the branch of medicine that focuses on blood and blood disorders. 血液学是医学的一个分支，专注于血液及其相关疾病的研究。

hemorrhage 出血

词根 hemo-（血）+ -rrhage（流出）
例句 The patient suffered from a hemorrhage after the surgery. 患者在手术后出现了出血。

hematoma 血肿

词根 hema-（血）+ -toma（肿瘤）
例句 A hematoma forms when blood collects outside of blood vessels. 血肿是血液积聚在血管外形成的。

hemocytometer 血细胞计数器

词根 hemo-（血）+ cyto-（细胞）+ -meter（计量器）
例句 A hemocytometer is used to count the number of blood cells in a sample. 血细胞计数器用于计算样本中的血细胞数量。

hemostasis 止血

词根 hemo-（血）+ -stasis（停止）
例句 Hemostasis is the process of stopping bleeding, either through clotting or surgical methods. 止血是通过凝血或手术方法停止出血的过程。

hemoptysis 咯血

词根 hemo-（血）+ ptysis（咳嗽）
例句 Hemoptysis can be a symptom of lung diseases such as tuberculosis. 咯血可能是肺部疾病如肺结核的症状。

hemochromatosis 血色病

词根 hemo-（血）+ chromato-（颜色）+ -osis（病症）
例句 Hemochromatosis is a genetic disorder causing excessive iron

absorption into the bloodstream. 血色病是一种遗传性疾病，导致过量的铁被吸收到血液中。

hematuria 血尿

词根 hemo-（血）+ -uria（尿液）

例句 Hematuria is the presence of blood in the urine, often caused by urinary tract infections. 血尿是尿液中出现血液，通常由尿路感染引起。

hemoglobinopathy 血红蛋白病

词根 hemo-（血）+ globin（蛋白质）+ -pathy（病）

例句 Sickle cell disease is a type of hemoglobinopathy that affects red blood cells. 镰状细胞病是一种影响红细胞的血红蛋白病。

hemangioma 血管瘤

词根 hemo-（血）+ angi-（血管）+ -oma（肿瘤）

例句 Hemangiomas are benign tumors formed by abnormal blood vessels. 血管瘤是由异常血管形成的良性肿瘤。

USMLE Step 2 CK 样题

A 17-year-old girl comes to the office because of a 3-month history of daily moderate epigastric (epi-; gastri-) pain that is more severe after meals. Three weeks ago, she had watery diarrhea (dia-; -rrhea) for 2 days, which resolved spontaneously. She has not had vomiting. She has no history of serious illness and takes no medications. Vital signs are within normal limits. Examination, including abdominal examination, shows no abnormalities. Which of the following is most likely to confirm the diagnosis?

(A) CT scan of the abdomen

(B) Endoscopy (endo-; -scop)

(C) Examination of the stool for ova and parasites

(D) Stool culture

(E) Upper gastrointestinal (gastro-; instestin-) series

中文翻译

一名 17 岁女孩因过去 3 个月每天出现中度上腹痛而就诊，饭后疼痛加重。3 周前，她曾有为期 2 天的水样腹泻，之后自行缓解，无呕吐症状。既往无严重疾病史，未服用任何药物。生命体征正常。腹部检查等未发现异常。以下哪项检查最有可能确诊？

(A) 腹部 CT 检查

(B) 内镜检查

(C) 粪便虫卵和寄生虫检查

(D) 粪便培养

(E) 上消化道造影

题目和答案中出现的词根

epi：在……之上

gastri：胃的

dia-：通过（这里指通过肠道）

-rrhea：流出（通过肠道流出，指腹泻）

endo-：内

-scop：镜子检查

gastro-：胃

instestin-：肠道

hemi-（半）

hemisphere 半球；大脑半球

词根 hemi-（半）+ sphere（球）

例句 The earth is divided into two hemispheres, the northern and southern hemispheres. 地球被分为两个半球，北半球和南半球。

hemiplegia 偏瘫

词根 hemi-（半）+ plegia（瘫痪）

例句 Hemiplegia is a condition where one side of the body is paralyzed. 偏瘫是指身体的一侧瘫痪。

hemianopia 偏盲

词根 hemi-（半）+ anopia（盲）

例句 Hemianopia is a loss of vision in half of the visual field, often due to brain injury. 偏盲是指一半视觉丧失，通常由脑损伤导致。

hemiparasite 半寄生植物

词根 hemi-（半）+ parasite（寄生虫）

例句 A hemiparasite is a plant that partially depends on another for nutrients. 半寄生植物是部分依赖其他植物提供养分的植物。

hemiparalysis 半身麻痹

词根 hemi-（半）+ paralysis（麻痹）

例句 Hemiparalysis affects only one side of the body, often caused by stroke. 半身麻痹只影响身体的一侧，通常由中风引起。

hemicrania 偏头痛

词根 hemi-（半）+ crania（头颅）

例句 Hemicrania refers to pain occurring on one side of the head, typically due to migraines. 偏头痛是指头部一侧的疼痛。

heminectomy 半侧肢体切除术

词根 hemi-（半）+ -ectomy（切除）

例句 Heminectomy is a surgical procedure to remove part of a limb. 半侧肢体切除术是一种切除肢体部分组织的外科手术。

hemispherectomy 半球切除术

词根 hemi-（半）+ sphere（球）+ -ectomy（切除）

例句 Hemispherectomy is a surgical procedure to remove part of the brain in extreme cases of epilepsy. 半球切除术是一种在极端癫痫病例中切除部分大脑的手术。

hemianalgesia 半侧无痛觉

词根 hemi-（半）+ analgesia（无痛觉）

例句 Hemianalgesia is a condition where there is a loss of pain sensation on one side of the body. 半侧无痛觉是指身体一侧失去痛觉的情况。

hepat-/hepato-（肝脏的）

hepatitis 肝炎

词根 hepat-（肝脏）+ -itis（炎症）

例句 Hepatitis is an inflammation of the liver, often caused by viruses or alcohol. 肝炎是肝脏的炎症，通常由病毒或酒精引起。

hepatomegaly 肝脏肿大

词根 hepato-（肝脏）+ -megaly（肿大）

例句 Hepatomegaly is often a sign of liver disease, such as cirrhosis or hepatitis. 肝脏肿大通常是肝脏疾病的标志,如肝硬化或肝炎。

hepatocellular carcinoma 肝细胞癌

词根 hepato-（肝脏）+ cellular（细胞的）+ carcinoma（癌症）

例句 Hepatocellular carcinoma is the most common type of liver cancer. 肝细胞癌是最常见的肝癌类型。

hepatopathy 肝病

词根 hepato-（肝脏）+ -pathy（病）
例句 Hepatopathy includes any disease or dysfunction of the liver. 肝病包括任何肝脏的疾病或功能障碍。

hepatobiliary 肝胆的

词根 hepato-（肝脏）+ biliary（胆道的）
例句 Hepatobiliary disorders affect both the liver and the bile ducts. 肝胆疾病影响肝脏和胆道。

hepatomegaly 肝脏肿大

词根 hepato-（肝脏）+ megaly（肿大）
例句 Hepatomegaly is a condition where the liver becomes enlarged, often due to infection or inflammation. 肝脏肿大是指肝脏变大，通常是由感染或炎症引起的。

hepatotoxicity 肝毒性

词根 hepato-（肝脏）+ toxic（毒性）
例句 Hepatotoxicity is the occurrence of liver damage due to exposure to toxins or medications. 肝毒性是指暴露于毒素或药物而导致的肝脏损害。

hepatocyst 肝囊肿

词根 hepato-（肝脏）+ cyst（囊肿）
例句 Hepatocysts are fluid-filled sacs that develop in the liver. 肝囊肿是发生在肝脏中的充满液体的囊泡。

hepatoplasty 肝脏整形术

词根 hepato-（肝脏）+ -plasty（整形术）
例句 Hepatoplasty is a type of surgery used to treat liver damage. 肝脏整形术是一种治疗肝脏损伤的手术。

hepatocellular 肝细胞的

词根 hepato-（肝脏）+ cellular（细胞的）

例句 Hepatocellular damage is often seen in viral infections like hepatitis. 肝细胞损伤通常见于如肝炎等病毒感染。

hepatic 肝脏的

词根 hepat-（肝脏）+ -ic（形容词后缀）

例句 Hepatic diseases can severely affect a person's ability to process toxins. 肝脏疾病会严重影响人体代谢毒素的能力。

hetero-（异）

heterosexual 异性恋的

词根 hetero-（异）+ sexual（性别）

例句 Heterosexual individuals are attracted to people of the opposite sex. 异性恋者被异性吸引。

heterogeneity 异质性

词根 hetero-（异）+ -geniety（性质）

例句 Heterogeneity in a population refers to the presence of diverse characteristics. 人群中的异质性指的是多样化特征的存在。

heterochromia 异色症

词根 hetero-（异）+ chromia（颜色）

例句 Heterochromia is a condition where a person has two different colored eyes. 异色症是指一个人拥有两只颜色不同的眼睛。

heterozygous 杂合子

词根 hetero-（异）+ -zygous（配子）

例句 A heterozygous individual has two different alleles for a specific gene. 杂合子个体在特定基因上携带两个不同的等位基因。

heteromorphic 异形的

词根 hetero-（异）+ morph-（形状）

例句 Heteromorphic organisms exhibit a variety of shapes or forms. 异形生物表现出各种形态或外形。

heteropolymer 异种聚合物

词根 hetero-（异）+ polymer（聚合物）

例句 Heteropolymers are made from different types of monomers. 异种聚合物是由不同类型的单体组成的。

heterolysis 异解

词根 hetero-（异）+ -lysis（分解）

例句 Heterolysis is the process of splitting a compound into different components. 异解是指将化合物分解成不同成分的过程。

hidr-（汗）

hyperhidrosis 多汗症

词根 hyper-（高）+ hidr-（汗）+ -osis（状态）

例句 Hyperhidrosis is a condition characterized by excessive sweating. 多汗症是一种以过度出汗为特征的疾病。

anhidrosis 无汗症

词根 an-（无）+ hidr-（汗）+ -osis（状态）

例句 Anhidrosis is a condition where a person is unable to sweat. 无汗症是指一个人无法出汗的状况。

hidrosis 汗腺分泌

词根 hidr-（汗）+ -osis（状态）

例句 Hidrosis is the process of sweating or perspiring. 汗腺分泌是排汗的过程。

hidrocystoma 汗腺囊肿

词根 hidr-（汗）+ cyst-（囊肿）+ -oma（肿瘤）

例句 Hidrocystoma is a benign tumor of the sweat glands. 汗腺囊肿是一种良性的汗腺肿瘤。

hidrotherapy 水疗法

词根 hidr-（汗）+ therapy（疗法）

例句 Hidrotherapy uses the therapeutic benefits of water to treat various conditions. 水疗法利用水的治疗效果来治疗各种疾病。

hidrosadenitis 汗腺炎

词根 hidr-（汗）+ aden-（腺体）+ -itis（炎症）

例句 Hidrosadenitis is an inflammation of the sweat glands, often resulting in painful lumps. 汗腺炎是汗腺的炎症，通常会出现疼痛的肿块。

hidrotic 出汗的

词根 hidr-（汗）+ -otic（形容词后缀）

例句 Hidrotic medications can help manage excessive sweating. 多汗症治疗药物有助于控制过度出汗。

hidrotic dermatitis 汗疹

词根 hidr-（汗）+ derm-（皮肤）+ -itis（炎症）

例句 Hidrotic dermatitis is a rash caused by excessive sweating. 汗疹是由过度出汗引起的皮疹。

hidrosurgery 汗腺手术

词根 hidr-（汗）+ surgery（手术）

例句 Hidrosurgery is performed to treat conditions like hyperhidrosis. 汗腺手术用于治疗像多汗症这样的病症。

hidrosalpingectomy 汗腺输卵管切除术

词根 hidr-（汗）+ salping-（输卵管）+ -ectomy（切除）

例句 Hidrosalpingectomy is a surgery to remove affected sweat glands or tissue. 汗腺输卵管切除术是切除受影响的汗腺或组织的手术。

histo-（组织）

histology 组织学

词根 histo-（组织）+ -logy（学科）
例句 Histology is the study of the microscopic structure of tissues. 组织学是研究组织微观结构的学科。

histopathology 组织病理学

词根 histo-（组织）+ patho-（病）+ -logy（学科）
例句 Histopathology involves the examination of tissues to diagnose diseases. 组织病理学指通过检查组织来诊断疾病。

histogenesis 组织发生

词根 histo-（组织）+ -genesis（生成）
例句 Histogenesis refers to the process of tissue formation from embryonic cells. 组织发生是指胚胎细胞形成组织的过程。

histone 组蛋白

词根 histo-（组织）+ -one（化学物质）
例句 Histones are proteins that help package DNA into the nucleus of cells. 组蛋白是协助将 DNA 包裹进细胞核内的蛋白质。

histochemistry 组织化学

词根 histo-（组织）+ chemistry（化学）
例句 Histochemistry involves the chemical analysis of tissue samples to understand their composition. 组织化学涉及对组织样本的化学分析，以了解其组成。

histocompatibility 组织相容性

词根 histo-（组织）+ compatibility（相容性）

例句 Histocompatibility is crucial in organ transplantation to prevent rejection. 组织相容性在器官移植中对于防止排斥反应至关重要。

histopathologic 组织病理的

词根 histo-（组织）+ patho-（病）+ -logic（形容词后缀）

例句 Histopathologic analysis is essential for diagnosing various types of cancer. 组织病理分析对于诊断各种类型的癌症至关重要。

histotrophic 组织营养的

词根 histo-（组织）+ -trophic（营养的）

例句 The histotrophic method is used to study the nutritional support provided to embryos during early development. 组织营养法被用来研究胚胎在早期发育过程中所获得的营养支持。

histodifferentiation 组织分化

词根 histo-（组织）+ -differentiation（分化）

例句 Histodifferentiation describes how cells develop into specialized tissue types. 组织分化描述了细胞如何发育成特定的组织类型。

USMLE Step 2 CK 样题

A 23-year-old man comes to the emergency department because of a 1-hour history of intermittent (inter-; mitt-) coughing spasms that began suddenly while he was attempting to clean mold from his garage with a mixture of acetic acid and cleaning agents. The cough is not productive. He reports shortness of breath only during the coughing spasms. Medical history is unremarkable (un-) and he takes no medications. He does not smoke cigarettes (cigar-; -ette), drink alcoholic beverages, or use other substances. He is 180 cm tall and weighs 75 kg; BMI is 23 kg/m^2 . Vital signs are within normal limits. Pulse oximetry (oxi-; -metry) on room air shows an oxygen saturation of 94%. The patient has periodic paroxysmal (par-; oxysm-) coughing during the examination. Oropharynx (oro-; -pharynx) is clear. Auscultation of the lungs discloses bilateral (bi-; lateral) wheezes throughout all lung fields. There is no use of accessory muscles of respiration (re-; spir-; -ation). The remainder of the physical examination discloses no abnormalities. Chest X-ray shows mild hyperexpansion (hyper-) of the lungs bilaterally (bi-; -lateral). Results of arterial blood gas analysis on room air are shown:

PO_2 72 mmHg

PCO_2 38 mmHg

pH 7.41

HCO_3^- 23 mEq/L

Which of the following is the most appropriate initial step in management?

(A) Albuterol therapy

(B) Bronchoscopy (bronch-; -scopy)

(C) CT scan of the chest

(D) Intubation (in-; -tube)

(E) Methylprednisolone (methy-) therapy

中文翻译

一名 23 岁男性因突发间歇性咳嗽痉挛 1 小时前往急诊科就诊。症状于其试图使用醋酸与清洁剂混合物清理车库霉菌时突然发作。咳嗽无痰，仅在咳嗽痉挛期间出现呼吸困难。既往病史无特殊，未服用任何药物。他不吸烟、不饮酒，亦不使用其他药物。患者身高 180 cm，体重 75 kg，BMI 为 23 kg/m^2。生命体征均正常。室内空气下脉搏血氧饱和度为 94%。查体期间患者有周期性阵发性咳嗽。口咽部清晰。肺部听诊显示双肺全野可闻及干啰音。未使用呼吸辅助肌。其余体格检查未见异常。胸部 X 线片显示双肺轻度过度充气。室内空气下动脉血气分析结果如下：

动脉血氧分压 72 mmHg

动脉血二氧化碳分压 38 mmHg

pH 值 7.41

碳酸氢根 23 mEq/L

以下哪项是治疗中最合适的初始措施？

(A) 沙丁胺醇治疗

(B) 支气管镜检查

(C) 胸部 CT 扫描

(D) 气管插管

(E) 甲泼尼龙治疗

题目和答案中出现的词根

inter-：在……之间

mitt-：时间区间

un-：表否定

cigar-：雪茄

-ette：小

oxi-：氧气的

-metry：测量仪

par-：超越；异常

oxysm-：尖锐

oro-：口

-pharynx：咽喉

bi-：双

lateral：侧

re-：重新；反复

spir：呼吸

-ation：表示动作的状态

hyper：高

bronch-：支气管

-scopy：镜

in-：向内

-tube：管

methy-：甲基

-holic（热爱）

alcoholic 酗酒者

词根 alco-（酒）+ -holic（热爱）

例句 An alcoholic person often struggles with dependency and health problems. 酗酒者常常面临酒精依赖和健康问题。

workaholic 工作狂

词根 work（工作）+ -holic（热爱）

例句 A workaholic is someone who spends excessive time working, often at the cost of personal life. 工作狂是指一个人花费过多时间工作，通常以个人生活为代价。

shopaholic 购物狂

词根 shop（购物）+ -holic（热爱）

例句 A shopaholic often feels compelled to buy items, even when unnecessary. 购物狂通常会感到强烈的购买冲动，即使不需要也会购物。

gamblingaholic 赌博成瘾者

词根 gambling-（赌博）+ -holic（热爱）

例句 A gamblingaholic may engage in excessive gambling, resulting in financial and emotional distress. 赌博成瘾者可能会沉迷于赌博，导致财务和情感困扰。

foodaholic 美食家

词根 food（食物）+ -holic（热爱）

例句 A foodaholic is always trying new dishes and exploring different cuisines. 美食家总是尝试新的菜肴，探索不同的美食。

USMLE Step 2 CK　样题

A 43-year-old man comes to the office because of a 2-week history of fatigue and mild pain in his right armpit. He has not had fever or weight loss. Medical history is remarkable for type 2 diabetes mellitus and hypercholesterolemia (hyper-; chole-; ster-; -ol; -emia). Medications are metformin (met-; form-), simvastatin (-statin), and aspirin. He is a social worker and frequently visits clients in homeless shelters. He lives alone with two dogs and a cat and has one male sexual partner. Vital signs are within normal limits. He appears well. Examination of the right upper extremity shows an erythematous (erythema-) axilla with a 4-cm, mobile, tender, nonfluctuant axillary lymph node and a tender, 1-cm epitrochlear (epi-; trochle-) lymph node. Abdominal examination shows no hepatosplenomegaly (hepato-; splen-; mega-). Which of the following is the most likely diagnosis?

(A) Castleman disease

(B) Cat-scratch disease

(C) Hidradenitis (hidr-; aden-; -itis) suppurativa

(D) T-cell lymphoma (lymph-; -oma)

(E) Tuberculosis (tuber-; -osis)

中文翻译

一名 43 岁男性因持续 2 周的疲劳感及右侧腋窝轻度疼痛前来就诊。患者无发热或体重减轻症状。患者有 2 型糖尿病及高胆固醇血症，长期服用二甲双胍、辛伐他汀及阿司匹林。患者职业为社工，常前往流浪者收容所探访服务对象。他独居，与两只狗和一只猫共同生活，有一名男性性伴侣。生命体征正常，一般状况良好。右侧上肢检查显示腋窝皮肤发红，触及一枚 4 cm 大小、可移动、压痛明显且无波动感的腋窝淋巴结，另见一枚 1 cm 大小、有压痛的上内上髁淋巴结。腹部查体未发现肝脾肿大。以下哪项是最可能的诊断？

(A) 卡斯尔曼病

(B) 猫抓病

(C) 化脓性汗腺炎

(D) T 细胞淋巴瘤

(E) 结核病

题目和答案中出现的词根

hyper-：高

chole-：胆

ster-：固体的

-ol：醇

-emia：血症

met-：甲基

form-：甲酸

-statin：静止

erythema-：红色的

epi-：在……上（或旁）

trochle-：滑车

hepato-：肝脏的

splen-：脾脏的

mega-：大

hidr-：汗

aden-：腺体

-itis：炎症

lymph-：淋巴

-oma：瘤

tuber-：结节

-osis：病理状态（结节病态，指代结核病，因为它的I期表现为肺部的多发结节）

homeo-（稳定）

homeostasis 内稳态

词根 homeo-（稳定）+ -stasis（状态）

例句 Homeostasis refers to the maintenance of stable internal conditions in an organism. 内稳态指的是有机体维持稳定的内环境。

homeothermic 恒温的

词根 homeo-（稳定）+ thermic（温度）

例句 Homeothermic animals can regulate their body temperature within a narrow range. 恒温动物能够将体温维持在一个狭窄的波动范围内。

homeobox 同源盒

词根 homeo-（稳定）+ -box（盒）

例句 Homeobox genes control the body plan development in animals and plants. 同源盒基因在动物和植物的身体构型发育中起控制作用。

homeopathy 同种疗法

词根 homeo-（稳定）+ patho-（病）+ -pathy（疗法）

例句 Homeopathy is a form of alternative medicine that uses highly diluted substances. 同种疗法是一种使用高度稀释物质的替代医学形式。

homeodomain 同源结构域

词根 homeo-（稳定）+ domain（区域）

例句 The homeodomain is a part of a protein that binds to DNA to regulate gene expression. 同源结构域是蛋白质的一部分，它与 DNA 结合以调节基因表达。

homeorhesis 同向流

词根 homeo-（稳定）+ -rhesis（流动）

例句 Homeorhesis refers to the tendency of an organism to return to a stable state after a disturbance. 同向流指的是有机体在受到干扰后趋向于恢复稳定状态。

homeodimerization 同源二聚化

词根 homeo-（稳定）+ dimerization（二聚化）

例句 Homeodimerization occurs when two homeodomain-containing proteins form a complex. 同源二聚化发生在两个含有同源结构域的蛋白质形成复合物时。

homeostatic 稳态的

词根 homeo-（稳定）+ -static（稳定的）

例句 The homeostatic mechanisms in the body ensure internal conditions remain constant despite external changes. 体内的稳态机制确保外部变化时内环境保持不变。

homeometric 同种尺度的

词根 homeo-（稳定）+ metric（测量）

例句 Homeometric regulation ensures that organisms remain stable in their physical dimensions. 同量调节确保生物体在物理尺寸上保持稳定。

homo-（同）

homogeneous 同质的

词根 homo-（同）+ -geneous（性质）

例句 A homogeneous mixture has components that are uniformly distributed throughout. 同质混合物是指其成分均匀分布的混合物。

homogenize 使均匀

词根 homo-（同）+ -genize（使……化）

例句 The milk is homogenized to ensure the fat particles are evenly distributed. 牛奶被均质化，以确保脂肪颗粒均匀分布。

homosexual 同性恋的

词根 homo-（同）+ sexual（性别）

例句 A homosexual person is attracted to individuals of the same sex. 同性恋者会被同性别的人吸引。

homogenization 均质化

词根 homo-（同）+ -ization（过程）

例句 Homogenization is the process of making something uniform in composition or texture. 均质化是使某物在组成或质地上变得均匀的过程。

homocysteine 同型半胱氨酸

词根 homo-（同）+ cysteine（半胱氨酸）

例句 High levels of homocysteine in the blood can increase the risk of cardiovascular disease. 血液中高水平的同型半胱氨酸可能会增加患心血管疾病的风险。

homologous 同源的

词根 homo-（同）+ logous（相似的）

例句 Homologous chromosomes carry the same genes but may have different alleles. 同源染色体携带相同的基因，但可能具有不同的等位基因。

homologation 同源化

词根 homo-（同）+ -logation（使成为）

例句 Homologation is the process of making something standard or legally acceptable. 同源化是使某物变得标准化或合理化的过程。

H

homocentral 同心的

词根 homo-（同）+ central（中心的）
例句 Homocentral structures are those that have the same center point. 同心结构是指具有相同中心点的结构。

homogeneity 同质性

词根 homo-（同）+ -geneity（性质）
例句 The homogeneity of the group allowed for smooth decision-making. 群体的同质性使得决策过程顺利进行。

homotropic 同向的

词根 homo-（同）+ -tropic（趋向的）
例句 Homotropic interactions refer to molecules or factors that interact in a similar manner. 同向相互作用指的是以相似方式相互作用的分子或因素。

hydro-（氢；水）

hydrogen 氢气

词根 hydro-（氢）+ -gen（生成）
例句 Hydrogen is the lightest element in the periodic table. 氢是元素周期表中最轻的元素。

hydrotherapy 水疗

词根 hydro-（水）+ therapy（疗法）
例句 Hydrotherapy is used to treat various injuries by utilizing water's therapeutic effects. 水疗通过利用水的治疗效果来治疗各种损伤。

hydrocarbon 碳氢化合物

词根 hydro-（氢）+ carbon（碳）
例句 Hydrocarbons are organic compounds made entirely of hydro-

gen and carbon. 碳氢化合物是完全由氢和碳组成的有机化合物。

hydrophobia 水恐惧症

词根 hydro-（水）+ phobia（恐惧）
例句 Hydrophobia is the irrational fear of water, often linked to rabies infection. 水恐惧症是对水的非理性恐惧，常与狂犬病感染有关。

hydration 水合作用

词根 hydro-（水）+ -ation（作用）
例句 Proper hydration is essential for maintaining optimal health. 适当的水合作用对维持健康至关重要。

hyper-（高）

hypertension 高血压

词根 hyper-（高）+ tension（压力）
例句 Hypertension is a condition where the blood pressure in the arteries is consistently too high. 高血压是一种动脉血压持续过高的疾病。

hyperactive 过度活跃的

词根 hyper-（高）+ active（活跃的）
例句 Children with ADHD are often hyperactive and have difficulty focusing. 患有注意力缺陷多动障碍的孩子通常过度活跃，难以集中注意力。

hyperglycemia 高血糖

词根 hyper-（高）+ glycemia（血糖）
例句 Hyperglycemia is a condition where the blood glucose levels are higher than normal. 高血糖是一种血糖水平高于正常范围的状态。

hyperthyroidism 甲亢

词根 hyper-（高）+ thyroid（甲状腺）+ -ism（病症）

例句 Hyperthyroidism occurs when the thyroid gland overproduces hormones. 甲亢是指甲状腺过度分泌激素。

hyperventilation 过度通气

词根 hyper-（高）+ ventilation（通气）

例句 Hyperventilation can lead to dizziness and fainting due to low carbon dioxide levels. 过度通气可能是二氧化碳水平过低，导致头晕和昏厥。

hyperopia 远视

词根 hyper-（高）+ -opia（视力）

例句 Hyperopia is a condition where distant objects are seen more clearly than nearby ones. 远视是一种看远处物体比近处物体更清晰的情况。

hyperpigmentation 皮肤色素沉着过度

词根 hyper-（高）+ pigmentation（色素沉着）

例句 Hyperpigmentation occurs when there is an excess production of melanin in the skin. 皮肤色素沉着过度是指皮肤中黑色素的过量生成。

hypercalcemia 高钙血症

词根 hyper-（高）+ calcemia（钙）

例句 Hypercalcemia is a condition characterized by elevated calcium levels in the blood. 高钙血症是一种以血液中钙水平升高为特征的疾病。

hyperplasia 增生

词根 hyper-（高）+ -plasia（增生）

例句 Hyperplasia is the abnormal increase in the number of cells in a tissue or organ. 增生是指组织或器官中细胞数目异常增多的情况。

hypno-（睡眠的）

hypnosis 催眠

词根 hypno-（睡眠）+ -sis（名词后缀）

例句 Hypnosis is a state of focused attention and heightened suggestibility, often used for therapeutic purposes. 催眠是一种高度集中注意力和增强暗示性的状态，通常用于治疗目的。

hypnotherapy 催眠疗法

词根 hypno-（睡眠）+ therapy（治疗）

例句 Hypnotherapy uses hypnosis to help treat conditions like stress, pain, and anxiety. 催眠疗法利用催眠帮助治疗诸如压力大、疼痛和焦虑等病症。

hypnotic 催眠药；催眠的

词根 hypno-（睡眠）+ -tic（形容词后缀）

例句 Hypnotic drugs are substances used to induce sleep or calmness in patients with sleep disorders. 催眠药是用于诱导睡眠或安抚患有睡眠障碍患者的物质。

hypnotherapy session 催眠治疗会话

词根 hypno-（睡眠）+ therapy（治疗）+ session（会话）

例句 A hypnotherapy session may involve guiding the patient into a relaxed state to address their emotional issues. 催眠治疗会话能引导患者进入放松状态，以解决他们的情绪问题。

hypnogram 睡眠图

词根 hypno-（睡眠）+ -gram（图表）

例句 A hypnogram is a graphical representation of a person' s sleep stages throughout the night. 睡眠图是显示一个人整个晚上睡眠阶段的图形。

hypnologist 催眠学专家

词根 hypno-（睡眠）+ -logist（学者）

例句 A hypnologist is a professional who specializes in the study and practice of hypnosis. 催眠学专家是专门从事催眠研究和实践的专业人员。

hypnogenic 催眠诱导的

词根 hypno-（睡眠）+ -genic（生成的）

例句 Hypnogenic suggestions are those that promote a state of hypnosis in a person. 催眠诱导性建议是指那些促使人进入催眠状态的建议。

hypnagogic 入睡时的；睡前的

词根 hypno-（睡眠）+ -agogic（引导的）

例句 Hypnagogic hallucinations are vivid dreams or sensations that occur as a person is falling asleep. 入睡时的幻觉是指人在即将入睡时发生的生动梦境或感觉。

hypnopompic 从睡梦中醒来的

词根 hypno-（睡眠）+ -pompic（引导的）

例句 Hypnopompic experiences occur during the transition from sleep to wakefulness, sometimes involving vivid dreams. 从睡梦中醒来的经历发生在从睡眠到觉醒的过渡过程中，有时伴随着生动的梦境。

hypnotherapy treatment 催眠治疗

词根 hypno-（睡眠）+ therapy（治疗）+ treatment（治疗）

例句 Hypnotherapy treatment can help patients manage chronic pain, stress, and certain phobias. 催眠治疗有助于患者缓解慢性疼痛、压力和某些恐惧症。

hypnopedia 催眠学习法

词根 hypno-（睡眠）+ -pedia（教育）

例句 Hypnopedia is the practice of attempting to learn new information during sleep, though it is not scientifically proven to be effective. 催眠学习法是指尝试在睡眠中学习新信息的做法，尽管科学上并未证明其有效性。

hypnotherapists 催眠治疗师

词根 hypno-（睡眠）+ therapist（治疗师）
例句 Hypnotherapists are trained professionals who use hypnosis as a therapeutic tool to help patients overcome various conditions. 催眠治疗师是经过训练的专业人员，使用催眠作为治疗工具帮助患者克服各种病症。

hypnotization 催眠化

词根 hypno-（睡眠）+ -ization（过程）
例句 Hypnotization is the process of inducing hypnosis, typically for therapeutic purposes. 催眠化是指引发催眠的过程，通常用于治疗目的。

hypnoreflex 催眠反射

词根 hypno-（睡眠）+ reflex（反射）
例句 Hypnoreflex is a reflex action that occurs when an individual is in a hypnotic state, often involving physical or emotional responses. 催眠反射是在催眠状态下发生的反射动作，通常包括身体或情感反应。

hypo-（低）

hypotension 低血压

词根 hypo-（低）+ tension（压力）
例句 Hypotension can cause dizziness and fainting due to insufficient blood flow. 低血压指血流不足导致头晕和昏厥。

hypoglycemia 低血糖

词根 hypo-（低）+ glycemia（血糖）

例句 Hypoglycemia occurs when blood sugar levels drop too low. 低血糖是指血糖水平降得过低的情况。

hypothermia 低体温

词根 hypo-（低）+ thermia（温度）

例句 Hypothermia occurs when the body temperature drops below the normal range. 低体温发生在体温降至正常范围以下时。

hypoxia 缺氧

词根 hypo-（低）+ -oxia（氧气）

例句 Hypoxia is a condition in which there is a deficiency of oxygen in the tissues. 缺氧是指组织中氧气不足的状态。

hypoallergenic 低过敏性

词根 hypo-（低）+ allergenic（过敏的）

例句 Hypoallergenic products are designed to minimize the risk of allergic reactions. 低过敏性产品旨在降低过敏反应的风险。

hypodermic 皮下注射的

词根 hypo-（低）+ dermic（皮肤的）

例句 Hypodermic needles are used for injecting medications under the skin. 皮下注射针用于将药物注射到皮肤下。

hypothyroidism 甲状腺功能减退

词根 hypo-（低）+ thyroid（甲状腺）+ -ism（病症）

例句 Hypothyroidism occurs when the thyroid gland produces insufficient hormones. 甲状腺功能减退是指甲状腺分泌激素不足。

hypostasis 坠积性淤血

词根 hypo-（低）+ -stasis（停滞）

例句 Hypostasis refers to the pooling of blood in the lowest parts of the body. 坠积性淤血指的是血液积聚在身体最低部位的现象。

USMLE Step 2 CK 样题

An 87-year-old man is admitted to the hospital because of a 4-day history of moderate abdominal cramps, nausea, and vomiting. He has not had a bowel movement or passed gas in the past 24 hours. He has colon cancer metastatic (meta-; stat-) to the lungs, liver, and peritoneum (peri-; -tone). Eighteen months ago, he underwent a low anterior resection (re-; sect-) for T3N2 rectal cancer. Six months ago, exploratory laparotomy (lapar-; -otomy) showed diffuse carcinomatosis (carcin-; -oma; -osis) and bowel obstruction, and an ileotransverse (ileo-; trans-) bypass was performed. The patient and his family were informed of the findings and advised that he would not be a candidate for a laparotomy (lapar-; -otomy) in the future because there would be no surgical options to treat another obstruction. The patient has no other history of serious illness. Medications are 5-fluorouracil and bevacizumab (-mab). Temperature is 37.2°C (99.0°F), pulse is 100/min, respirations (re-; spir-; -ation) are 20/min, and blood pressure is 130/80 mmHg. The abdomen is distended and mildly tender to palpation. There are no peritoneal signs. CT scan of the abdomen shows a mid-jejunal small-bowel obstruction, multiple intraperitoneal (intra-) tumor deposits, and ascites. The physician recommends insertion of nasogastric (naso-; gastri-) and percutaneous (per-; cutan-) endoscopic (endo-; scop-) gastrostomy (gastr-; -stomy) tubes. The patient and his family request that the patient undergo a laparotomy (lapar-; -otomy) and intestinal bypass. Which of the following is the most appropriate next step in management?

(A) Abide by the wishes of the patient and his family

(B) Alter the chemotherapy (chemo-) regimen

(C) Explain the futility of the operation to the patient and his family

(D) Offer to transfer the patient to another facility

(E) Suggest external beam radiation therapy

中文翻译

一名 87 岁男性因 4 天来中度腹部绞痛、恶心和呕吐被送往医院。在过去 24 小时内，他没有排便或排气。他患有结肠癌，已转移至肺、肝和腹膜。18 个月前，他因 T3N2 直肠癌接受了低位前切除术。6 个月前，探查性开腹手术显示广泛癌扩散和肠梗阻，他因此接受了回肠横结肠旁路手术。当时已告知患者及其家属手术结果，并建议未来不再进行开腹手术，因为没有手术方法可治疗再次发生的梗阻。患者无其他严重疾病史。目前使用的药物为 5- 氟尿嘧啶和贝伐珠单抗。体温 37.2℃（99.0℉），脉搏 100 次 / 分钟，呼吸 20 次 / 分钟，血压 130/80 mmHg。腹部膨隆，触诊时有轻度压痛，无腹膜刺激征。腹部 CT 扫描显示空肠中段小肠梗阻、腹腔内多发肿瘤转移灶和腹水。医生建议插入鼻胃管和经皮内镜胃造瘘管。患者及其家属要求进行开腹手术和肠道旁路手术。以下哪项是最适合的下一步治疗措施？

(A) 遵循患者及其家属的意愿

(B) 更改化疗方案

(C) 向患者及其家属解释手术的无益性

(D) 提议将患者转院至其他医疗机构

(E) 进行体外放疗

题目和答案中出现的词根

meta-：超过，在……后

-stat：静止站立

peri-：外周

-tone：延伸（延伸到周围，指代腹膜，即从腹腔向周围延伸的膜）

re：再；回；离开

sect-：切

lapar-：腹部

-otomy：切开

carcin-：上皮细胞恶变

-oma：瘤

-osis：病理状态

ileo-：回肠

trans-：跨；转

-mab：是 monoclone antibody 的缩写，指代单克隆抗体

re-：重新；反复

spir：呼吸

-ation：表示动作的状态

intra-：在……内

naso-：鼻

gastri-：胃

-stomy：切开术，属于 -otomy 的同义变异

per-：经过

cutan-：皮肤

endo-：内

scop-：视野

chemo-：化学的

H

hystero-（子宫）

hysterectomy 子宫切除术

词根 hystero-（子宫）+ -ectomy（切除）

例句 A hysterectomy is a surgical procedure to remove the uterus. 子宫切除术是去除子宫的外科手术。

hysteroscopy 子宫镜检查

词根 hystero-（子宫）+ -scopy（镜检查）

例句 Hysteroscopy is a procedure used to examine the inside of the uterus. 子宫镜检查是一种用来检查子宫内部的方法。

hysteropexy 子宫固定术

词根 hystero-（子宫）+ -pexy（固定术）

例句 Hysteropexy is a procedure where the uterus is surgically fixed in place to treat prolapse. 子宫固定术是一种手术，通过将子宫固定在原位来治疗子宫脱垂。

hysterosalpingography 子宫输卵管造影

词根 hystero-（子宫）+ salpingo-（输卵管）+ -graphy（造影）

例句 Hysterosalpingography is an imaging test used to examine the uterus and fallopian tubes. 子宫输卵管造影是一种成像检查，用于检查子宫和输卵管。

hysteroptosis 子宫脱垂

词根 hystero-（子宫）+ -ptosis（脱垂）

例句 Hysteroptosis is a condition where the uterus falls into the vaginal canal due to weakened pelvic muscles. 子宫脱垂是一种由于盆腔肌肉变弱，子宫下垂进入阴道的情况。

hysterosalpingectomy 子宫输卵管切除术

词根 hystero-（子宫）+ salping-（输卵管）+ -ectomy（切除）
例句 Hysterosalpingectomy is a surgery that removes both the uterus and fallopian tubes. 子宫输卵管切除术是一种同时切除子宫和输卵管的手术。

hysterotomy 子宫剖开术

词根 hystero-（子宫）+ -tomy（切开）
例句 A hysterotomy is sometimes performed during cesarean deliveries. 子宫剖开术有时在剖宫产中进行。

I

–ia（情况）

anemia 贫血

词根 an-（无）+ -emia（血液中的状态）

例句 Anemia is a condition characterized by a deficiency of red blood cells. 贫血是由红细胞不足引起的情况。

dysphoria 不悦感

词根 dys-（不良）+ -phoria（情感状态）

例句 Dysphoria is a state of unease or dissatisfaction. 不悦感是一种不安或不满的情绪状态。

insomnia 失眠症

词根 in-（不）+ somno-（睡眠）+ -ia（情况）

例句 Insomnia refers to the condition of being unable to fall or stay asleep. 失眠症是指无法入睡或保持睡眠的状态。

pneumonia 肺炎

词根 pneumon-（肺）+ -ia（情况）

例句 Pneumonia is an infection that causes inflammation in the lungs. 肺炎是导致肺部炎症的感染。

hypothermia 低体温症

词根 hypo-（低）+ therm-（温度）+ -ia（情况）

例句 Hypothermia occurs when the body temperature drops below normal levels. 低体温症发生在体温降至正常水平以下时。

-icidal（杀）

bactericidal 杀菌的

词根 bacteri-（细菌）+ -cidal（杀）

例句 Bactericidal agents are used to kill bacteria and prevent infections. 杀菌剂用于杀死细菌并防止感染。

virucidal 杀病毒的

词根 viru-（病毒）+ -cidal（杀）

例句 Virucidal disinfectants are effective in killing viruses on surfaces. 杀病毒的消毒剂可有效杀灭物体表面的病毒。

fungicidal 杀真菌的

词根 fungi-（真菌）+ -cidal（杀）

例句 Fungicidal treatments are used to eliminate fungal infections in plants and animals. 杀真菌的治疗用于消除植物和动物中的真菌感染。

insecticidal 杀虫的

词根 insecti-（昆虫）+ -cidal（杀）

例句 Insecticidal sprays are commonly used to control pest infestations. 杀虫喷雾常用于控制害虫的侵扰。

algicidal 杀藻的

词根 algi-（藻）+ -cidal（杀）

例句 Algicidal products are used to remove harmful algae from water sources. 杀藻产品用于清除水源中的有害藻类。

larvicidal 杀幼虫的

词根 larvi-（幼虫）+ -cidal（杀）

例句 Larvicidal treatments help reduce the number of insect larvae in stagnant water. 杀幼虫的处理帮助减少静水中的昆虫幼虫数量。

molluscicidal 杀软体动物的

词根 mollusci-（软体动物）+ -cidal（杀）

例句 Molluscicidal compounds are used to control mollusk populations, particularly in aquatic environments. 杀软体动物的化合物用于控制软体动物种群，尤其是在水生环境中。

herbicidal 除草的

词根 herbi-（草）+ -cidal（杀）

例句 Herbicidal chemicals are widely used in agriculture to control unwanted weeds. 除草化学品在农业中广泛用于控制杂草。

spermicidal 杀精的

词根 spermi-（精子）+ -cidal（杀）

例句 Spermicidal creams or gels are used as contraceptives to kill sperm. 杀精霜或凝胶作为避孕药物杀死精子。

USMLE Step 2 CK 样题

A 19-year-old man is brought to the emergency department (ED) by ambulance 15 minutes after he was stabbed in the chest during a fight. The stab wound is located medially to the left nipple. At the scene, pulse was 105/min, respirations (re-; spir-; -ation) were 18/min, and blood pressure was 120/80 mmHg. Pulse oximetry (oxi-; -metry) on room air showed an oxygen saturation of 96%. Two large-bore intravenous (intra-; veno-) catheters were placed en route to the ED, and lactated Ringer solution was initiated. On arrival in the trauma bay, the patient develops a pulse of 130/min and blood pressure of 80/40 mmHg. There is jugular venous distention. Results of focused assessment with sonography (sono-; -graphy) for trauma (FAST) are most likely to lead to which of the following next steps for this patient?

(A) CT scan of the chest and abdomen with contrast

(B) Exploratory laparotomy (lapar-; -otomy)

(C) Needle decompression and chest tube placement

(D) Pericardiocentesis (peri-; cardio-; -centesis)

(E) Peritoneal (peri-; ton-) lavage

中文翻译

一名 19 岁男性在斗殴中被刺伤胸部，15 分钟后由救护车送往急诊科。刺伤位于左乳头内侧。在现场，患者脉搏为 105 次 / 分钟，呼吸为 18 次 / 分钟，血压为 120/80 mmHg。在室温空气下的脉搏血氧饱和度为 96%。在前往急诊科的途中，患者已被置入两根大口径静脉导管，并开始输注乳酸林格液。到达创伤急救室时，患者脉搏增至 130 次 / 分钟，血压降至 80/40 mmHg，出现颈静脉怒张。创伤超声快速评估的结果最可能提示以下哪项作为患者的下一步治疗？

(A) 胸部和腹部增强 CT 扫描

(B) 探查性开腹手术

(C) 针刺减压和胸管置入

(D) 心包穿刺术

(E) 腹腔灌洗

题目和答案中出现的词根

re-：重新；反复

spir：呼吸

-ation：表示动作的状态

oxi-：氧气的

-metry：测量仪

intra-：在……内

veno-：静脉

sono-：声音的

-graphy：图像

lapar-：腹部

-otomy：切开

peri-：外周

cardio-：心脏

centesis：穿刺术

peri-：外周

tone：延伸

-icity（状态）

multiplicity 多样性

词根 multi-（多）+ -icity（状态）

例句 The multiplicity of factors involved in climate change makes it a complex issue. 气候变化所涉及的多种因素使其成为一个复杂的问题。

plasticity 可塑性

词根 plastic-（塑料）+ -icity（状态）

例句 Plasticity refers to the ability of a material to undergo permanent deformation without breaking. 可塑性是指一种材料在不破裂的情况下发生永久变形的能力。

elasticity 弹性

词根 elastic-（弹性）+ -icity（状态）

例句 Elasticity is the ability of a material to return to its original shape after being stretched or compressed. 弹性是指材料在拉伸或压缩后恢复原状的能力。

idio-（特发的；自发的；个体的）

idiopathic 特发性的

词根 idio-（特发的）+ pathic（疾病的）

例句 The doctor diagnosed the patient with idiopathic pulmonary fibrosis. 医生诊断患者患有特发性肺纤维化。

idiopathy 特发病

词根 idio-（特发的）+ pathy（疾病）

例句 Idiopathy refers to a disease with no known cause. 特发病指的是没有已知病因的疾病。

idioglossia 自语症

词根 idio-（自发的）+ glossia（舌；语言）

例句 Idioglossia is a speech disorder where a child speaks in a unique, unintelligible language. 自语症是一种儿童说出独特但无法理解的语言的言语障碍。

idiotropic 自向性的

词根 idio-（自发的）+ tropic（方向的）

例句 The patient's behavior was described as idiotropic, focusing inward rather than engaging with others. 患者的行为被描述为自

向性的，专注于自身而不是与他人互动。

idioblast 特异细胞

词根 idio-（自发的）+ blast（幼细胞）

例句 Idioblasts are specialized plant cells, but similar unique cells are found in human tissue. 特异细胞是植物中的特殊细胞，但在人类组织中也发现了类似的独特细胞。

idioplasm 原质基因

词根 idio-（个体的）+ plasm（质；细胞质）

例句 Idioplasm contains hereditary material that determines individual traits. 原质基因含有决定个体特征的遗传物质。

idiocy 白痴症（旧称，现在多用 intellectual disability）

词根 idio-（个体的）+ -cy（状态）

例句 In historical medical literature, idiocy was used to describe severe intellectual disability. 在医学文献中，白痴症曾用于描述严重的智力障碍。

idiotype 个体型

词根 idio-（个体的）+ type（类型）

例句 An idiotype is a unique set of antigenic determinants in an antibody molecule. 个体型是抗体分子中特有的一组抗原决定簇。

idiopsychology 个体心理学

词根 idio-（个体的）+ psychology（心理学）

例句 Idiopsychology focuses on studying individual mental processes rather than group dynamics. 个体心理学专注于研究个体的心理过程，而不是群体动力学。

USMLE Step 2 CK　样题

A 22-year-old man is brought to the emergency department

by his girlfriend 30 minutes after she found him unconscious (un-) in his home. She last saw him yesterday and he appeared well. He has a history of cocaine and heroin use, and also use of prescription narcotic analgesics (an-; alges-) that he obtains from friends. On arrival, he is lethargic. Temperature is 35.0°C (95.0°F), pulse is 68/min, respirations (re-; spir-; -ation) are 8/min, and blood pressure is 96/50 mmHg. Pulse oximetry (oxi-; -metry) on room air shows an oxygen saturation of 96%. The left lower extremity is cyanotic (cyan-) and cold to the touch. The remainder of the examination shows no abnormalities. Results of serum studies are shown:

K^+ 5.5 mEq/L

HCO_3^- 18 mEq/L

Creatinine 1 mg/dL

Creatine kinase (-ase) 50,000 U/L

This patient is at greatest risk for which of the following conditions?

(A) Acute kidney injury

(B) Acute liver failure

(C) Cardiac arrhythmia (a-; rhyth-)

(D) Hypocalcemia (hypo-; cal-; -emia)

(E) Hypophosphatemia (hypo-; phosph-; -emia)

中文翻译

一名 22 岁男性由其女友带至急诊科，此前 30 分钟她发现他在家中不省人事。她最后一次见他是在昨天，当时他看起来正常。

他有可卡因和海洛因使用史，并且长期使用从朋友处获得的处方阿片类镇痛药。到达时，他呈嗜睡状态。体温 35.0℃（95.0℉），脉搏 68 次 / 分钟，呼吸 8 次 / 分钟，血压 96/50 mmHg。在室温空气下的脉搏血氧饱和度为 96%。左下肢发绀，触之冰冷。其余体检无异常。血清检查结果如下：

钾 5.5 mEq/L

碳酸氢根 18 mEq/L

肌酐 1 mg/dL

肌酸激酶 50,000 U/L

该患者最可能面临以下哪种疾病的风险？

(A) 急性肾损伤

(B) 急性肝衰竭

(C) 心律失常

(D) 低钙血症

(E) 低磷酸血症

题目和答案中出现的词根

un-：表示否定

an-：表示否定

algesi-：疼痛

re-：重新；反复

spir：呼吸

-ation：表示动作的状态

oxi-：氧气的

-metry：测量仪

cyan-：蓝色

-ase：酶

a-：表示否定

rhyth-：节律

hypo-：低

cal-：钙

-emia：血症

phosph-：磷

-idium（小体）

clostridium 梭状芽孢杆菌

词根 clostr-（梭状芽孢）+ -idium（指小型或某种属）

例句 Clostridium is a genus of bacteria, including species that cause diseases like botulism, tetanus, and gas gangrene. 梭状芽孢杆菌是一个细菌属，包含引起肉毒中毒、破伤风和气性坏疽的种类。

coccidium 球虫

词根 cocc-（球形）+ -idium（指小型或某种属）

例句 Coccidium is a genus of protozoan parasites that cause coccidiosis in animals, leading to digestive issues. 球虫是一个原生动物寄生虫属，导致动物发生球虫病，引起消化问题。

cystidium 囊状体

词根 cyst-（囊）+ -idium（小型结构）

例句 Cystidium is a structure found in certain fungi and plants, often serving as a reproductive or storage body. 囊状体是某些真菌和植物中发现的结构，通常作为繁殖或储存器官。

bacillidium 芽孢杆菌属

词根 bacill-（芽孢）+ -idium（表示属或类型）

例句 Bacillidium is used to refer to a genus of bacteria, including species involved in various infections. 芽孢杆菌属是一种细菌属，包括导致各种感染的细菌种类。

sarcomidium 肉瘤小体

词根 sarcom-（肉瘤）+ -idium（小型体）

例句 Sarcomidium refers to small, tumor-like growths found in certain sarcomas. 肉瘤小体是指在某些肉瘤中发现的小型肿瘤状生长物。

helminthidium 蠕虫小体

词根 helminth-（蠕虫）+ -idium（小型体）

例句 Helminthidium refers to small, worm-like forms in parasitic infections that may affect the digestive system. 蠕虫小体是指寄生感染中类似蠕虫的小型生物体，可能影响消化系统。

phyllidium 叶状体

词根 phyll-（叶）+ -idium（小体）

例句 Phyllidium refers to a leaf-like structure found in certain plants or parasites. 叶状体是某些植物或寄生虫中存在的叶片状结构。

endocystidium 内囊小体

词根 endo-（内）+ cyst-（囊）+ -idium（小体）

例句 Endocystidium refers to a small cyst-like structure inside certain cells or organisms. 内囊小体是指在某些细胞或生物体内发现的小型囊泡状结构。

mycelidium 菌丝小体

词根 mycel-（菌丝）+ -idium（小体）

例句 Mycelidium refers to a small mycelium-like structure found in certain fungi. 菌丝小体是某些真菌中存在的小型菌丝状结构。

gonidium 配子小体

词根 gon-（配子）+ -idium（小体）

例句 Gonidium refers to a reproductive cell or structure in certain algae and protozoans. 配子小体是某些藻类和原生动物中的生殖细胞或结构。

-imum（的）

maximum 最大值

词根 max-（最大）+ -imum（的）
例句 The maximum allowable dosage of the medication should not exceed the prescribed limit. 药物的最大允许剂量不应超过规定的限度。

minimum 最小值

词根 min-（最小）+ -imum（的）
例句 The minimum requirement for the study is a sample size of at least 100 participants. 研究的最小样本量为 100 名参与者。

optimum 最佳

词根 opt-（最佳）+ -imum（的）
例句 The optimum temperature for enzyme activity is usually specified in laboratory protocols. 酶活性的最佳温度通常在实验室协议中规定。

maximum tolerated dose 最大耐受剂量

词根 max-（最大）+ -imum（的）+ dose（剂量）
例句 The maximum tolerated dose is the highest dose of a drug that can be given without causing unacceptable side effects. 最大耐受剂量是可以服用，而不会引起不可接受的副作用的最高剂量。

momentum 瞬间的

词根 moment-（瞬间）+ -um（名词后缀）
例句 The momentum of the patient's recovery was monitored closely to adjust treatment plans. 密切监测患者的康复进展，以便调整治疗方案。

-in（物质）

melanin 黑色素

词根 melan-（黑色的）+ in（物质）

例句 Melanin is responsible for the pigmentation of skin, hair, and eyes. 黑色素负责皮肤、头发和眼睛的着色。

keratin 角蛋白

词根 kerat-（角化的）+ in（物质）

例句 Keratin is a protein found in hair, nails, and skin that provides strength and structure. 角蛋白是存在于头发、指甲和皮肤中的蛋白质，为这些组织提供强度和结构。

vitamin 维生素

词根 vita-（生命必需的）+ in（物质）

例句 Vitamins are essential nutrients that the body needs to funct-ion properly. 维生素是身体正常运作所必需的营养物质。

adrenalin 肾上腺素

词根 adren-（肾上腺的）+ in（物质）

例句 Adrenalin is a hormone that increases the body' s alertness and physical performance during stress. 肾上腺素是一种激素，在压力下增加身体的警觉性并增强身体表现。

caffeine 咖啡因

词根 caff-（咖啡的）+ in（物质）

例句 Caffeine is a stimulant found in coffee, tea, and some sodas. 咖啡因是一种刺激物，存在于咖啡、茶和一些汽水中。

serotonin 血清素

词根 sero-（血清的）+ in（物质）

例句 Serotonin is a neurotransmitter that affects mood, sleep, and appetite. 血清素是影响情绪、睡眠和食欲的神经递质。

histamine 组胺

词根 histo-（组织的）+ in（物质）
例句 Histamine is a compound involved in immune responses and allergic reactions. 组胺是一种参与免疫反应和过敏反应的化合物。

ino-（纤维）

inosine 肌苷

词根 ino-（纤维）+ -sine（类）
例句 Inosine is involved in the metabolism of purine nucleotides. 肌苷参与嘌呤核苷酸的代谢。

inositol 肌醇

词根 ino-（纤维）+ -sitol（醇）
例句 Inositol plays a role in cell signaling and is important for the nervous system. 肌醇在细胞信号传导中起着作用，对神经系统也很重要。

inotropism 变力作用

词根 ino-（纤维）+ tropism（趋向；作用）
例句 Inotropism refers to the effect of increasing or decreasing the force of contraction of muscle fibers, especially heart muscle. 变力作用是指增加或减少肌纤维收缩力量的作用，尤其是心肌。

inotropy 肌力变化性

词根 ino-（纤维）+ -tropy（变化性）
例句 Inotropy refers to the force of contraction of the heart muscle fibers. 肌力变化性指的是心肌纤维的收缩力量。

inoskeleton 纤维骨架

词根 ino-（纤维）+ skeleton（骨架）

例句 The inoskeleton provides structural integrity to the cell by forming a fibrous framework. 纤维骨架通过形成纤维框架为细胞提供完整结构。

inofibril 纤维小管

词根 ino-（纤维）+ fibril（小纤维）

例句 Inofibrils are very fine fiber-like structures that are part of the cellular matrix. 纤维小管是细胞基质的一部分，类似纤维的细小结构。

inotissue 纤维组织

词根 ino-（纤维）+ tissue（组织）

例句 Inotissue refers to fibrous tissues found in various organs that provide structure and support. 纤维组织是存在于各种器官中的纤维，为器官提供结构和支撑。

inter-（间）

intercellular 细胞间的

词根 inter-（间）+ cellular（细胞的）

例句 The intercellular space is the area between the cells in tissues. 细胞间隙是组织中细胞之间的区域。

intermittent 间歇性的

词根 inter-（间）+ mitt-（送）+ -ent（形容词后缀）

例句 Intermittent pain is pain that comes and goes. 间歇性疼痛是时有时无的疼痛。

intercostal 肋间的

词根 inter-（间）+ costal（肋骨的）

例句 The intercostal muscles are located between the ribs. 肋间肌位于肋骨之间。

interleukin 白介素

词根 inter-（间）+ leuk-（白细胞）+ -in（物质）
例句 Interleukins are cytokines that play a role in immune responses. 白介素是参与免疫反应的细胞因子。

interdisciplinary 跨学科的

词根 inter-（间）+ disciplin-（学科）+ -ary（形容词后缀）
例句 Interdisciplinary care involves professionals from multiple fields working together. 跨学科护理涉及来自多个领域的专业人员协同工作。

intervertebral 椎间的

词根 inter-（间）+ vertebr-（脊椎）+ -al（形容词后缀）
例句 Intervertebral discs are the shock absorbers between the vertebrae. 椎间盘是脊椎之间的减震结构。

interosseous 骨间的

词根 inter-（间）+ osse-（骨）+ -ous（形容词后缀）
例句 The interosseous membrane connects the bones of the forearm. 骨间膜连接前臂的骨骼。

interruption 中断

词根 inter-（间）+ rupt-（断裂）+ -ion（名词后缀）
例句 The interruption of blood flow can lead to tissue damage. 血流中断可能导致组织损伤。

interferon 干扰素

词根 inter-（间）+ feron（带来；产生）
例句 Interferons are proteins that help protect cells from viral infections. 干扰素是帮助保护细胞免受病毒感染的蛋白质。

intercalated 插入的

词根 inter-（间）+ calat-（插入）+ -ed（形容词后缀）

例句 Intercalated discs are specialized connections between heart muscle cells. 插入盘是心脏肌肉细胞之间的特化连接。

interdigital 指间的

词根 inter-（间）+ digit-（手指）+ -al（形容词后缀）

例句 Interdigital spaces are the areas between the fingers or toes. 指间隙是手指或脚趾之间的区域。

intervention 干预

词根 inter-（间）+ ven-（来）+ -tion（名词后缀）

例句 Early medical intervention can prevent complications in certain diseases. 早期的医疗干预可以预防某些疾病的并发症。

interspinal 脊椎间的

词根 inter-（间）+ spinal（脊椎的）

例句 The interspinal muscles are located between the spinal vertebrae. 脊椎间肌位于脊椎椎骨之间。

intermittent claudication 间歇性跛行

词根 inter-（间）+ mitt-（送）+ -ent（形容词后缀）

例句 Intermittent claudication occurs when there is insufficient blood flow to the muscles, causing pain while walking. 间歇性跛行发生在肌肉血流不足时，使人走路时会感到疼痛。

intercalary 插入的；间歇的

词根 inter-（间）+ calary（插入的）

例句 Intercalary bones are bones that are inserted into the normal bone structure, like the patella. 插入骨是插入到正常骨结构中的骨骼，例如髌骨。

interosseous membrane 骨间膜

词根 inter-（间）+ osseous（骨的）+ membrane（膜）

例句 The interosseous membrane connects the radius and ulna in the forearm. 骨间膜连接前臂的桡骨和尺骨。

interphase 间期

词根 inter-（间）+ phase（阶段）
例句 Interphase is the phase of the cell cycle in which the cell grows and DNA is replicated. 间期是细胞周期的某一阶段，细胞在此阶段生长并复制 DNA。

intra-（内）

intravenous 静脉内的

词根 intra-（内）+ venous（静脉的）
例句 Intravenous therapy involves administering fluids directly into the bloodstream through the veins. 静脉内治疗是通过静脉直接将药液输送到血液中。

intramuscular 肌肉内的

词根 intra-（内）+ muscular（肌肉的）
例句 Intramuscular injections are often used to administer vaccines and other medications. 肌肉注射常用于接种疫苗和其他药物的给药。

intraocular 眼内的

词根 intra-（内）+ ocular（眼睛的）
例句 Intraocular pressure is the fluid pressure within the eye. 眼内压是眼睛内部的液体压力。

intrauterine 子宫内的

词根 intra-（内）+ uterine（子宫的）
例句 Intrauterine devices are commonly used as a form of contraception. 子宫内装置常用作避孕方法。

intra-abdominal 腹腔内的

词根 intra-（内）+ abdominal（腹部的）

例句 Intra-abdominal infections can occur when bacteria invade the abdominal cavity. 腹腔内感染可能发生在细菌侵入腹腔时。

intraspinal 脊髓内的

词根 intra-（内）+ spinal（脊柱的）

例句 Intraspinal injections are used to deliver medication directly to the spinal cord. 脊髓内注射用于将药物直接输送到脊髓。

intrahepatic 肝内的

词根 intra-（内）+ hepatic（肝脏的）

例句 Intrahepatic bile duct obstruction can lead to jaundice and liver damage. 肝内胆管梗阻可导致黄疸和肝脏损伤。

intra-articular 关节内的

词根 intra-（内）+ articular（关节的）

例句 Intra-articular injections can help reduce inflammation in the joints. 关节内注射可以帮助减轻关节的炎症。

intracellular 细胞内的

词根 intra-（内）+ cellular（细胞的）

例句 Intracellular processes involve the reactions that occur inside a cell. 细胞内过程涉及发生在细胞内部的反应。

ir-（不）

irreversible 不可逆的

词根 ir-（不）+ reversible（可逆的）

例句 The damage caused to the liver was irreversible, leading to liver failure. 肝脏的损伤是不可逆的，并会导致肝衰竭。

irregular 不规则的

词根 ir-（不）+ regular（规则的）

例句 Irregular heartbeats can indicate a potential arrhythmia. 不规则的心跳可能表示潜在的心律失常。

irreconcilable 不可调和的

词根 ir-（不）+ reconcilable（可调和的）

例句 The two diagnoses were irreconcilable, requiring further investigation. 两种诊断相互矛盾，不可调和，需要进一步调查。

irrelevant 不相关的

词根 ir-（不）+ relevant（相关的）

例句 The study found that certain factors were irrelevant to the patient's condition. 研究发现某些因素与患者的病情无关。

irrefutable 不可辩驳的

词根 ir-（不）+ refutable（可反驳的）

例句 The medical evidence presented was irrefutable and led to the correct diagnosis. 提供的医学证据是不可辩驳的，并促成了正确的诊断。

irreflexive 不反射的

词根 ir-（不）+ reflexive（反射的）

例句 Irreflexive movements may indicate damage to the nervous system. 非反射性运动可能表明神经系统受损。

irresponsible 不负责任的

词根 ir-（不）+ responsible（负责任的）

例句 The doctor's irresponsible actions led to complications in the patient's recovery. 医生的不负责任行为导致患者康复过程中的并发症。

irreparable 不可修复的

词根 ir-（不）+ reparable（可修复的）

例句 The heart valve damage was deemed irreparable, requiring a transplant. 心脏瓣膜的损伤被认为是不可修复的，需要进行移植。

irresistible 不可抗拒的

词根 ir-（不）+ resistible（可抗拒的）

例句 The patient experienced an irresistible urge to consume certain foods, a symptom of a disorder. 患者出现了难以抗拒的食欲，这是某种疾病的症状。

USMLE Step 2 CK 官网样题

A 32-year-old nulligravid (null-; -gravid) woman comes to the office because she has been unable to conceive during the past 12 months. She and her husband have unprotected (un-) sexual intercourse three times weekly. Two years ago, she was involved in a motor vehicle collision; CT scan at that time showed absence (ab-; -sen) of the left kidney. She has no other history of serious illness, and her only medication is a prenatal (pre-; -natal) vitamin. She has no known allergies. Vital signs are within normal limits. Pelvic examination shows no abnormalities. Hysterosalpingography (hyster-; salpin-; -graphy) is shown. When this patient conceives, she is at greatest risk for which of the following pregnancy complications?

(A) Fetal macrosomia (macro-; som-)

(B) Multiple gestation

(C) Oligohydramnios (oligo-; hydr-; amnio-)

(D) Preeclampsia (pre-; -eclampsia)

(E) Preterm (pre-; -term) labor

中文翻译

一名 32 岁未孕女性来就医，因为她在过去 12 个月内未能怀孕。她和丈夫每周进行 3 次无保护性交。两年前，她遭遇了一场车祸，当时的CT扫描显示左肾缺失。她无其他严重疾病史，唯一服用的药物是孕前维生素。她没有已知的过敏史。生命体征正常。盆腔检查未发现异常。子宫输卵管造影结果已显示。当该患者怀孕时，她最可能出现以下哪种妊娠并发症？

(A) 胎儿巨大儿症

(B) 多胎妊娠

(C) 羊水过少

(D) 子痫前期

(E) 早产

题目和答案中出现的词根

null-：没有

gravid：怀孕

un-：表示否定

ab-：表否定

-sen：感觉

pre-：在……之前

-natal：出生

hyster-：子宫

salpin-：输卵管

-graphy：图像

macro-：大的

som-：身体

oligo-：少的

hydr-：氢，这里指水

amnio-：羊膜的

-eclampsia：癫痫

-term：这里指的是预产期

isch（io）-（坐骨的）

ischiocavernosus 坐骨海绵体肌

词根 ischio-（坐骨）+ cavernosus（海绵体的）

例句 The ischiocavernosus muscle plays a role in erectile function by regulating blood flow to the genital region. 坐骨海绵体肌通过调节生殖器区域的血液流动，在勃起功能中起着作用。

ischial 坐骨的

词根 isch-（坐骨）+ -al（形容词后缀）

例句 Ischial bursitis refers to the inflammation of the bursa near the ischium, often due to prolonged sitting. 坐骨滑囊炎是指坐骨附近滑囊的炎症，通常是由长期久坐引起的。

ischorectal 坐骨直肠的

词根 ischio-（坐骨）+ rectal（直肠的）

例句 Ischorectal abscesses are infections that occur in the space between the ischium and rectum. 坐骨直肠脓肿是发生在坐骨和直肠之间的感染。

ischiorrhagia 坐骨出血

词根 ischio-（坐骨）+ -rrhagia（出血）

例句 Ischiorrhagia is a rare condition that causes bleeding in the ischial region. 坐骨出血是一种罕见的疾病，指坐骨区域的出血。

ischialgia 坐骨神经痛

词根 isch-（坐骨）+ -algia（疼痛）

例句 Ischialgia refers to pain that originates from the ischium or sciatic nerve. 坐骨神经痛指的是源自坐骨或坐骨神经的疼痛。

ischiorrhaphy 坐骨缝合术

词根 ischio-（坐骨）+ -rrhaphy（缝合术）

例句 Ischiorrhaphy is a surgical procedure to repair damaged tissue in the ischium area. 坐骨缝合术是一种修复坐骨区域受损组织的外科手术。

ischial tuberosity 坐骨结节

词根 isch-（坐骨）+ tuberosity（结节）

例句 The ischial tuberosity is the part of the pelvis that supports the weight when sitting. 坐骨结节是骨盆的一部分，支撑坐姿时体重。

isch-（压制）

ischemia 缺血

词根 isch-（压制）+ -emia（血液中的状态）

例句 Ischemia occurs when there is a restriction in blood supply to tissues, leading to oxygen deficiency. 缺血发生在血液供应受限时，导致组织缺氧。

ischemic 缺血的

词根 isch-（压制）+ -emic（血液的）

例句 Ischemic heart disease results from the reduced blood flow to the heart muscle. 缺血性心脏病是由心肌血流减少所致。

ischemia reperfusion injury 缺血再灌注损伤

词根 isch-（压制）+ -emia（血液中的状态）+ reperfusion（再灌注）+ injury（损伤）

例句 Ischemia reperfusion injury occurs when blood flow returns to tissue after a period of ischemia, causing damage. 缺血再灌注损伤是指组织在缺血一段时间后，血液重新灌注所引发的损伤。

-ism（情况）

autism 自闭症

词根 auto-（自己）+ -ism（情况）

例句 Autism is a developmental disorder characterized by difficulties in social interaction and communication. 自闭症是一种发育障碍，特征为社交互动和沟通的困难。

hyperthyroidism 甲状腺功能亢进症

词根 hyper-（过度）+ thyroid-（甲状腺）+ -ism（情况）

例句 Hyperthyroidism is a condition where the thyroid gland produces too much thyroid hormone. 甲状腺功能亢进症是一种甲状腺分泌过多甲状腺激素的病症。

hypothyroidism 甲状腺功能减退症

词根 hypo-（不足）+ thyroid-（甲状腺）+ -ism（情况）

例句 Hypothyroidism occurs when the thyroid gland does not produce enough thyroid hormones. 甲状腺功能减退症发生在甲状腺未能产生足够的甲状腺激素时。

alcoholism 酗酒症

词根 alcohol-（酒精）+ -ism（情况）

例句 Alcoholism is a medical condition characterized by an inability to control alcohol consumption. 酗酒症是一种病症，特征是无法控制的饮酒行为。

astigmatism 散光

词根 astigmat-（散光）+ -ism（情况）

例句 Astigmatism is a refractive error in the eye, leading to blurred or distorted vision. 散光是眼睛的屈光误差，导致视力模糊或扭曲。

USMLE Step 2 CK 样题

A 40-year-old man comes to the office during the summer because of a 3-day history of fever, diffuse muscle aches, fatigue, and sore throat. He has had no sick contacts. Medical history is unremarkable (un-) and he takes no medications. He received the influenza virus vaccine this year. Ten days ago, he returned from a trip to Malaysia, where he says he enjoyed the local food and nightlife. Temperature is 38.8°C (101.8°F), pulse is 90/min, respirations (re-; spir-; -ation) are 16/min, and blood pressure is 126/70 mmHg. The remainder of the examination shows no abnormalities. Results of laboratory studies are shown:

Blood hemoglobin (hemo-; -globin) 10 g/dL

MCV 90 μm^3

WBC 2400/mm^3

Neutrophils (neutro-; -phil), segmented 60%

Neutrophils (neutro-; -phil), bands 5%

Lymphocytes (lymph-; -cyte) 5%

Monocytes (mono-; -cyte) 20%

Eosinophils (eosino-; -phil) 4%

Basophils (baso-; -phil) 6%

Platelet (plate-; -let) count 350,000/mm^3

Red cell distribution width 14%

Monospot test result is negative. Which of the following is the most appropriate next step in diagnosis?

(A) Cytomegalovirus (cyto-; mega-) serologic (sero-) testing

(B) Epstein-Barr virus serologic (sero-) testing

(C) Hemagglutination (hem-; agglut-) inhibition assay

(D) HIV RNA polymerase (poly-; mer-; -ase) chain reaction testing

(E) Serum hepatitis (hepa-;-itis) B surface antigen testing

中文翻译

一名40岁男性在夏季因3天来的发热、全身肌肉酸痛、疲劳和咽喉痛来就诊。他没有接触过任何病人。既往病史无特殊，无用药史。他今年接种了流感疫苗。10天前，他从马来西亚旅行返回，他表示在那里享受了当地美食和夜生活。体温38.8℃（101.8℉），脉搏90次/分钟，呼吸16次/分钟，血压126/70 mmHg。其余体检结果无异常。实验室检查结果如下：

血红蛋白 10 g/dL

平均红细胞体积 90 μm³

白细胞计数 2,400/mm³

分叶核中性粒细胞 60%

带状核中性粒细胞 5%

淋巴细胞 5%

单核细胞 20%

嗜酸性粒细胞 4%

嗜碱性粒细胞 6%

血小板计数 350,000/mm^3

红细胞分布宽度 14%

单核细胞增多症斑点试验阴性

以下哪项是诊断中最适当的下一步？

(A) 巨细胞病毒血清学检测

(B) 爱泼斯坦 - 巴尔病毒血清学检测

(C) 血凝抑制试验

(D) HIV RNA 聚合酶链反应检测

(E) 血清乙型肝炎表面抗原检测

题目和答案中出现的词根

un-：表示否定

re-：重新；反复

spir-：呼吸

-ation：表示动作的状态

hemo-：血

-globin-：球蛋白

neutro-：中性的

-phil：嗜

lymph-：淋巴的

-cyte：细胞

mono-：单个的（这里指单核的）

eosino-：酸性的

baso-：碱性的

plate-：板状的

-lets：小

cyto-: 细胞

mega-: 大

sero-: 血清

hem-: 血的，属于 hemo- 的同义变异

agglut-: 凝聚

poly-: 多

mer-: 部分

-ase: 酶

hepa-: 肝脏的

-itis: 炎症

iso-（等同的）

isotope 同位素

词根 iso-（相同）+ -tope（位置）

例句 An isotope is a form of an element with the same number of protons but different numbers of neutrons. 同位素是元素的一种形式，指具有相同数量的质子，但中子数量不同。

isomer 同分异构体

词根 iso-（相同）+ -mer（部分）

例句 Isomers are molecules that have the same chemical composition but differ in structure. 同分异构体是具有相同化学成分但结构不同的分子。

isometric 等度的

词根 iso-（相同）+ metric（测量的）

例句 Isometric exercises involve the contraction of muscles without changing their length. 等长运动是指肌肉在收缩时长度保持不变的运动。

isothermal 等温的

词根 iso-（相同）+ thermal（热的）

例句 An isothermal process is one that occurs at a constant temperature. 等温过程是指在恒定温度下发生的过程。

isomerism 同分异构现象

词根 iso-（相同）+ -merism（状态）

例句 Isomerism is the phenomenon where molecules with the same molecular formula have different structural arrangements. 同分异构现象是指分子式相同但排列结构不同的现象。

isomerization 异构化

词根 iso-（相同）+ -merization（聚合）

例句 Isomerization is the process of changing a molecule into one of its isomers. 异构化是将分子转变为其同分异构体的过程。

isoenzymes 同工酶

词根 iso-（相同）+ enzyme（酶）

例句 Isoenzymes are enzymes that catalyze the same reaction but differ in their molecular structure. 同工酶是催化相同反应但在分子结构上不同的酶。

-itis（炎症）

arthritis 关节炎

词根 arthr-（关节）+ -itis（炎症）

例句 Arthritis is an inflammation of the joints that causes pain and stiffness. 关节炎是关节的炎症，导致关节疼痛和僵硬。

gastritis 胃炎

词根 gastr-（胃）+ -itis（炎症）

例句 Gastritis is an inflammation of the stomach lining, often caused by infection or stress. 胃炎是胃黏膜的炎症，通常由感染或压力引起。

tonsillitis 扁桃体炎

词根 tonsill-（扁桃体）+ -itis（炎症）

例句 Tonsillitis causes swelling and pain in the tonsils, often due to an infection. 扁桃体炎导致扁桃体肿胀和疼痛，通常是由感染引起的。

bronchitis 支气管炎

词根 bronch-（支气管）+ -itis（炎症）

例句 Bronchitis is the inflammation of the bronchi in the lungs, often caused by a viral infection. 支气管炎是肺部支气管的炎症，通常由病毒感染引起。

dermatitis 皮炎

词根 derm-（皮肤）+ -itis（炎症）

例句 Dermatitis is a condition that causes inflammation, redness, and itching of the skin. 皮炎是一种导致皮肤发炎、红肿和瘙痒的疾病。

sinusitis 鼻窦炎

词根 sinus-（鼻窦）+ -itis（炎症）

例句 Sinusitis is an inflammation of the sinuses, often caused by a bacterial or viral infection. 鼻窦炎是鼻窦的炎症，通常由细菌或病毒感染引起。

meningitis 脑膜炎

词根 mening-（脑膜）+ -itis（炎症）

例句 Meningitis is an infection of the protective membranes surrounding the brain and spinal cord. 脑膜炎是包绕大脑和脊髓的保护膜的感染。

pneumonitis 肺炎

词根 pneumon-（肺）+ -itis（炎症）

例句 Pneumonitis is inflammation of the lung tissue, often caused by inhaling irritants. 肺炎是肺组织的炎症，通常由吸入刺激物引起。

cystitis 膀胱炎

词根 cyst-（膀胱）+ -itis（炎症）

例句 Cystitis is inflammation of the bladder, often caused by a urinary tract infection. 膀胱炎是膀胱的炎症，通常由尿路感染引起。

endometritis 子宫内膜炎

词根 endomet-（子宫内膜）+ -itis（炎症）

例句 Endometritis is an infection of the lining of the uterus, often associated with childbirth or surgery. 子宫内膜炎是子宫内膜的感染，通常与分娩或手术相关。

-ity（状态）

purity 纯净

词根 pur-（纯洁）+ -ity（状态）

例句 Purity of water is essential for safe drinking and health. 水的纯净度对安全饮用和健康至关重要。

sensitivity 敏感性

词根 sens-（感觉）+ -ity（状态）

例句 Sensitivity to light can be a symptom of an underlying eye condition. 对光的敏感性强可能是潜在眼病的症状。

flexibility 灵活性

词根 flex-（弯曲）+ -ity（状态）

例句 Flexibility is a key skill in adapting to new work environments. 保持灵活性是适应新工作环境的关键技能。

creativity 创造力

词根 creat-（创造）+ -ity（状态）

例句 Creativity is the ability to think of new and original ideas. 创造力是指产生新颖和独特想法的能力。

diversity 多样性

词根 diver-（不同）+ -ity（状态）

例句 Diversity in the workplace fosters innovation and creativity. 工作场所的多样性促进了创新创造。

juxta-（旁；静态）

juxtapose 并列；放置在一起

词根 juxta-（旁）+ pose（放置）
例句 The artist chose to juxtapose bright colors with dark tones to create contrast. 艺术家选择将明亮的颜色与暗色调并列，以创造对比效果。

juxtaposition 并列；放置

词根 juxta-（旁）+ position（位置）
例句 The juxtaposition of old and new architecture in the city makes it unique. 城市中新旧建筑的并列使得它独具特色。

juxtamedullary 髓旁的

词根 juxta-（旁）+ medullary（髓的）
例句 Juxtamedullary nephrons are located near the inner part of the kidney, close to the medulla. 髓旁肾单位位于靠近肾脏内部的髓部区域。

juxtacortical 皮层旁的

词根 juxta-（旁）+ cortical（皮层的）
例句 Juxtacortical areas of the brain are located next to the cortical regions. 皮层旁区域位于大脑的皮层区域旁边。

juxtaglomerular 肾小球旁的

词根 juxta-（旁）+ glomerular（肾小球的）
例句 The juxtaglomerular apparatus plays a crucial role in regulating blood pressure and kidney function. 肾小球旁装置在调节血压和肾脏功能中起着至关重要的作用。

juxtacellular 细胞旁的

词根 juxta-（旁）+ cellular（细胞的）

例句 Juxtacellular signaling is essential for the communication between neighboring cells. 细胞旁信号传递对于邻近细胞之间的交流至关重要。

juxtasternal 胸骨旁的

词根 juxta-（旁）+ sternal（胸骨的）

例句 The juxtasternal region is located next to the sternum in the chest. 胸骨旁区域位于胸部的胸骨旁。

juxtafacial 面部旁的

词根 juxta-（旁）+ facial（面部的）

例句 The juxtafacial structures refer to those anatomical features located adjacent to the face. 面部旁结构指的是位于面部旁边的解剖特征。

USMLE Step 2 CK　样题

A 57-year-old woman comes to the emergency department because of a 2-day history of fever, chills, and sore throat. She is on day 6 of a 7-day course of trimethoprim (tri-; meth-) sulfamethoxazole (sulfa-; meth-; -oxazole) for treatment of cystitis. She has been taking lisinopril (lisi-; -pril) nightly for 2 years for treatment of hypertension (hyper-; -tension). She has no other history of serious illness and takes no other medications. Temperature is 38.6°C (101.4°F), pulse is 84/min, respirations (re-; spir-; -ation) are 16/min, and blood pressure is 118/76 mmHg. Examination shows erythema (eryth-; -ema) of the pharynx but no exudates. No other abnormalities are noted. Results of laboratory studies are shown:

Blood hematocrit (hemato-; -crit) 38%

WBC 2,200/mm^3

Neutrophils (neutro-; -phil), segmented 16%

Neutrophils, bands 4%

Lymphocytes (lymph-; -cyte) 64%

Monocytes (mono-; -cyte) 16%

Platelet (plate-; -let) count 225,000/mm^3

Which of the following is the most likely explanation for these findings?

(A) Acute mononucleosis (mono-; nucle-; -osis)

(B) Acute myelogenous (myelo-; gen-) leukemia (leuk-; -emia)

(C) Adverse effect of trimethoprim (tri-; meth-) -sulfamethoxazole (sulfa-; meth-; -oxazole)

(D) Allergic reaction to lisinopril (lisi-; -pril)

(E) Myelofibrosis (myelo-; fibro-; -osis)

(F) Sepsis syndrome

中文翻译

一名 57 岁女性因 2 天来的发热、寒战和咽喉痛来到急诊科。她目前正在接受为期 7 天的甲氧苄啶 - 磺胺甲恶唑治疗膀胱炎，今日是第 6 天。她因高血压已服用 2 年赖诺普利，每晚一次。她无其他严重疾病史，也未服用其他药物。体温 38.6℃（101.4℉），脉搏 84 次 / 分钟，呼吸 16 次 / 分钟，血压 118/76 mmHg。检查显示咽部红斑，但无渗出物。未发现其他异常。实验室检查结果如下：

血细胞比容 38%

白细胞计数 2,200/mm³

分叶核中性粒细胞 16%

带状核中性粒细胞 4%

淋巴细胞 64%

单核细胞 16%

血小板计数 225,000/mm³

以下哪项是最可能解释这些检查结果的原因？

(A) 急性单核细胞增多症

(B) 急性髓系白血病

(C) 甲氧苄啶 - 磺胺甲恶唑的不良反应

(D) 对赖诺普利的过敏反应

(E) 骨髓纤维化

(F) 脓毒症综合征

题目和答案中出现的词根

tri-：三个

meth-：甲基（methy 的同义变异）

sulfa：硫基

oxazole：含有氧和氮的五元环（咪唑）

lisi-：赖氨酸残基

-pril：普利（血管紧张素转换酶抑制剂的通用后缀）

hyper-：高

-tension：张力；压力

re-：重新；反复

spir：呼吸

-ation：表示动作的状态

eryth-：红色

-ema：病理状态（红色的病理状态指代红斑）

hemato-：血

-crit：分离法

neutro-：中性的

-phil：嗜

lymph-：淋巴

-cyte：细胞

mono-：单个的

plate-：板状的

-lets：小

nucle-：核

-osis：病理状态

myelo-：骨髓的

gen-：产生

leuk-：白色的

-emia：血症（白色血症指代白血病）

fibro-：纤维的

K

kal-（钾）

kalium 钾

词根 kal-（钾）

例句 Kalium is the Latin name for potassium, an essential element in the human body. 词为钾的拉丁名称，钾是人体必需的元素。

kaliphilia 喜钾症

词根 kal-（钾）+ -philia（倾向）

例句 Kaliphilia is an uncommon condition where a person has an excessive need for potassium. 喜钾症是一种罕见的情况，指一个人对钾有过度需求。

hypokalemia 低钾血症

词根 hypo-（低）+ kal-（钾）+ -emia（血液状态）

例句 Hypokalemia occurs when potassium levels in the blood drop too low, leading to muscle weakness. 低钾血症发生在血液中的钾水平过低时，导致肌肉无力。

hyperkalemia 高钾血症

词根 hyper-（高）+ kal-（钾）+ -emia（血液状态）

例句 Hyperkalemia is a condition where the potassium levels in the blood are too high. 高钾血症是血液中的钾水平过高的情况。

karyo-（核的）

karyotype 核型

词根 karyo-（核）+ -type（类型）

例句 A karyotype analysis is used to examine an individual's chromosome composition for genetic disorders. 核型分析用于检查个体染色体组成，以发现遗传疾病。

karyokinesis 核分裂

词根 karyo-（核）+ -kinesis（分裂）
例句 Karyokinesis is a critical step in cell division where the nucleus divides into two. 核分裂是细胞分裂中核分裂成两个的重要步骤。

karyogamy 核融合

词根 karyo-（核）+ -gamy（融合）
例句 Karyogamy occurs during sexual reproduction when the nuclei of two cells fuse. 核融合发生在有性生殖过程中，当两个细胞的细胞核融合时。

karyoplasm 核质

词根 karyo-（核）+ -plasm（物质）
例句 Karyoplasm is the substance found within the nuclear envelope, surrounding the genetic material. 核质是存在于核膜内，包围遗传物质的物质。

karyosome 核小体

词根 karyo-（核）+ -some（体）
例句 Karyosomes are visible structures within the nucleus during certain stages of cell division. 核小体是细胞分裂的某些阶段中可以在细胞核中观察到的结构。

karyorrhexis 核破裂

词根 karyo-（核）+ -rrhexis（破裂）
例句 Karyorrhexis is the fragmentation of the cell nucleus, often occurring during cell death. 核破裂是细胞核的碎片化，通常发生在细胞死亡时。

karyogenesis 核形成

词根 karyo-（核）+ -genesis（生成）

例句 Karyogenesis refers to the process of nucleus formation during the early stages of cell development. 核形成是指细胞发育早期的细胞核形成过程。

karyolysis 核溶解

词根 karyo-（核）+ -lysis（溶解）

例句 Karyolysis involves the dissolution of the nucleus, typically as a result of cell death. 核溶解是指细胞核的溶解，通常是细胞死亡的结果。

karyoclastic 核破裂的

词根 karyo-（核）+ -clastic（破裂的）

例句 Karyoclastic changes occur in cells undergoing apoptosis, leading to the breakdown of the nucleus. 核碎裂变化发生在经历凋亡的细胞中，导致细胞核解体。

karyotaxis 核排列

词根 karyo-（核）+ -taxis（排列；运动）

例句 Karyotaxis refers to the arrangement and positioning of the nucleus within the cell. 核排列是指细胞内细胞核的排列和定位。

karyochromatism 核染色质现象

词根 karyo-（核）+ chromat-（色）+ -ism（现象）

例句 Karyochromatism describes the staining properties of nuclear chromatin observed under a microscope. 核染色质现象描述了在显微镜下观察到的核染色质的染色特性。

karyopherin 核转运蛋白

词根 karyo-（核）+ -pherin（运送）

例句 Karyopherins are proteins that transport molecules into and out of the cell nucleus. 核转运蛋白是将分子运入和运出细胞核的

蛋白质。

karyoschisis 核裂解

词根 karyo-（核）+ -schisis（裂开）

例句 Karyoschisis is the splitting of the nucleus during pathological conditions. 核裂解是在病理条件下发生的细胞核分裂现象。

karyocyte 核细胞

词根 karyo-（核）+ -cyte（细胞）

例句 A karyocyte is any cell that contains a distinct nucleus, such as a eukaryotic cell. 核细胞是指任何含有明确细胞核的细胞，例如真核细胞。

kerato-（角质）

keratosis 角化症

词根 kerato-（角质）+ -osis（病症）

例句 Keratosis is a skin condition characterized by the overproduction of keratin, leading to thickened skin. 角化症是一种以角蛋白过度生成和皮肤增厚为特征的皮肤病。

keratitis 角膜炎

词根 kerato-（角质）+ -itis（炎症）

例句 Keratitis is an inflammation of the cornea, often caused by infection or trauma. 角膜炎是角膜的炎症，通常由感染或创伤引起。

keratocyte 角质细胞

词根 kerato-（角质）+ -cyte（细胞）

例句 Keratocytes are responsible for producing and maintaining the structural integrity of keratinized tissues. 角质细胞负责生成和维持角质化组织的结构完整性。

keratoderma 角化皮肤病

词根 kerato-（角质）+ -derma（皮肤）

例句 Keratoderma is characterized by thickened skin, typically on the palms and soles. 角化皮肤病的特征是皮肤增厚，通常出现在手掌和脚底。

keratoplasty 角膜移植术

词根 kerato-（角质）+ -plasty（成形术）

例句 Keratoplasty is a surgical procedure to replace damaged or diseased corneal tissue with healthy tissue. 角膜移植术是一种用健康组织替换受损或患病角膜组织的手术。

keratoconus 圆锥角膜

词根 kerato-（角质）+ -conus（圆锥）

例句 Keratoconus is a progressive condition where the cornea thins and bulges into a cone shape. 圆锥角膜是一种进行性疾病，角膜变薄并向外凸成圆锥形。

keratogenous 角质生成的

词根 kerato-（角质）+ -genous（生成）

例句 Keratogenous tissues are those that contribute to the formation of keratin. 角质生成组织是指那些参与角蛋白生成的组织。

keratophyte 角质寄生菌

词根 kerato-（角质）+ -phyte（植物）

例句 Keratophytes are types of fungi that grow on keratinized tissues, such as nails and skin. 角质寄生菌是一类生长在角质组织上的真菌，如指甲和皮肤。

keratolysis 角质溶解

词根 kerato-（角质）+ -lysis（溶解）

例句 Keratolysis is a condition where the outer layer of skin breaks down due to bacterial activity or moisture. 角质溶解是指皮肤外层

由于细菌活动或水分而分解的情况。

keratometer 角膜曲率计

词根 kerato-（角质）+ -meter（测量仪）

例句 A keratometer is used to measure the curvature of the cornea, often for fitting contact lenses. 角膜曲率计用于测量角膜的曲率，通常用于配制隐形眼镜。

USMLE Step 2 CK 样题

A 20-year-old woman comes to the office because of a 1-year history of a lump on her left ear that appeared 2 months after she had the ear pierced. Physical examination shows the findings in the photograph. Which of the following is the most appropriate initial treatment for this patient?

(A) Corticosteroid (cortico-; ster-; -oid) injection

(B) Cryotherapy (cryo-)

(C) Laser ablation (ab-; lat-; -ion)

(D) Needle aspiration (a-; spir-; -ation)

(E) Wide excision

中文翻译

一名 20 岁女性来就诊，因左耳出现肿块已持续 1 年，该肿块在她耳部穿孔 2 个月后出现。以下哪项是该患者最适当的初始治疗方法？

(A) 皮质类固醇注射

(B) 冷冻疗法

(C) 激光消融

(D) 针吸

(E) 广泛切除

题目和答案中出现的词根

cortico-：肾上腺皮质的

ster-：固体的

-oid：类似的

cryo-：冷的

ab-：表否定

lat-：带着

-ion：表示动作

a-：这里是朝向的意思

spir-：呼吸

-ation：表示动作的状态

-kine（动）

kinetics 动力学

词根 kine-（动）+ -ics（学科）

例句 Kinetics is the branch of physics that studies the motion of objects and the forces that cause them to move. 动力学是物理学的一个分支，研究物体的运动及导致其运动的力。

kinesiology 运动学

词根 kine-（动）+ -ology（学科）

例句 Kinesiology is the scientific study of human movement. 运动学是对人类运动的科学研究。

kinetochore 动粒

词根 kine-（动）+ -tophore（携带）

例句 The kinetochore is a protein structure on the centromere that attaches to spindle fibers during cell division. 动粒是位于着丝粒上的一种蛋白质结构，在细胞分裂时与纺锤体纤维连接。

kinesiotherapy 运动疗法

词根 kine-（动）+ -therapy（治疗）

例句 Kinesiotherapy is the therapeutic use of physical movement to treat injuries or diseases. 运动疗法是通过物理运动治疗损伤或疾病的一种方法。

hyperkinesis 过动症

词根 hyper-（过度）+ kine-（动）+ -sis（状态）

例句 Hyperkinesis is a condition characterized by excessive movement or hyperactivity. 过动症是一种表现为过度运动或过度活跃的状态。

kinemometer 运动计量仪

词根 kine-（动）+ -mometer（计量器）

例句 A kinemometer is a device used to measure the speed and motion of moving objects. 运动计量仪是一种用于测量运动物体速度的设备。

kinesiology tape 运动学胶带

词根 kine-（动）+ -ology（学科）+ tape（胶带）

例句 Kinesiology tape is used to support muscles and joints without restricting movement. 运动学胶带用于支持肌肉和关节，而不限制运动。

kinetoplasm 运动质

词根 kine-（动）+ -plasm（质）

例句 Kinetoplasm is the part of the cytoplasm involved in cell movement and transport. 运动质是细胞质的一部分，涉及细胞运动和运输。

koil-（凹的）

koilonychia 匙状甲

词根 koil-（凹形）+ onychia（甲状）

例句 Koilonychia refers to the condition where the nails become concave or spoon-shaped, often seen in iron deficiency anemia. 匙状甲指的是指甲呈凹形或匙状，通常见于缺铁性贫血。

koilocytosis 凹细胞症

词根 koil-（凹形）+ cytosis（细胞）

例句 Koilocytosis is the presence of abnormally shaped cells with a hollow or irregular appearance, often found in HPV-infected cells. 凹细胞症是指细胞出现形态异常、具有空洞或不规则外观，通常见于 HPV 感染的细胞中。

koilocyte 凹细胞

词根 koil-（凹形）+ cyte（细胞）

例句 A koilocyte is an abnormal cell with a perinuclear clear zone, often associated with human papillomavirus（HPV）infection. 凹细胞是具有细胞核周围清晰区域的异常细胞，通常与人类乳头状瘤病毒（HPV）感染相关。

koilocytopathic 凹细胞病理的

词根 koil-（凹形）+ cytopath-（细胞病理）+ -ic（形容词后缀）

例句 Koilocytopathic changes are pathological changes in cells, especially due to viral infections like HPV, that affect the cellular structure. 凹细胞病理变化是指细胞中的病理变化，特别是由 HPV 等病毒感染引起的，其影响细胞结构。

koilodysplasia 凹细胞发育不良

词根 koil-（凹形）+ dys-（不正常）+ -plasia（增生）

例句 Koilodysplasia refers to abnormal development or growth of koilocytes, which is often associated with HPV infection and cervical dysplasia. 凹细胞发育不良是指凹细胞的异常发育或生长，通常与 HPV 感染和宫颈发育不良相关。

kyph（o）-（脊柱前后弯曲）

kyphosis 脊柱后凸

词根 kyph-（脊柱后弯曲）+ -osis（病症）

例句 Kyphosis is an excessive outward curvature of the spine, leading to a hunched posture. 脊柱后凸是脊柱向外过度弯曲，导致驼背姿势。

kyphoscoliosis 脊柱后侧凸

词根 kypho-（脊柱后弯曲）+ scolio-（弯曲）+ -osis（病症）

例句 Kyphoscoliosis is a spinal deformity that involves both lateral and posterior curvatures. 脊柱后侧凸是一种既有侧弯又有后凸的脊柱畸形。

kyphotic 后凸的

词根 kyph-（脊柱后弯曲）+ -otic（形容词后缀）

例句 A kyphotic posture can develop due to poor posture or underlying spinal conditions. 后凸姿势可能是由不良姿势或潜在的脊柱疾病引起的。

kyphoplasty 脊柱成形术

词根 kypho-（脊柱后弯曲）+ -plasty（成形术）

例句 Kyphoplasty is a surgical procedure used to treat vertebral compression fractures. 脊柱成形术是一种用于治疗椎体压缩性骨折的手术。

K

kyphotomy 后凸切开术

词根 kypho-（脊柱后弯曲）+ -tomy（切开术）

例句 Kyphotomy involves surgically correcting severe kyphosis to alleviate pain and restore mobility. 后凸切开术通过手术矫正严重的脊柱后凸，以缓解疼痛并恢复活动能力。

kyphocervical 颈部后凸的

词根 kypho-（脊柱后弯曲）+ cervical（颈部的）

例句 Kyphocervical deformities can result from trauma or degenerative conditions. 颈部后凸畸形可能由创伤或退行性疾病引起。

kyphoplasty balloon 脊柱成形球囊

词根 kypho-（脊柱后弯曲）+ plasty（成形术）+ balloon（球囊）

例句 During kyphoplasty, a balloon is inserted to restore vertebral height before injecting bone cement. 在脊柱成形术中，会插入一个球囊以恢复椎体高度，然后注入骨水泥。

kyphostatic 静态后凸的

词根 kypho-（脊柱后弯曲）+ -static（静止的）

例句 Kyphostatic conditions refer to long-term spinal curvatures without progressive worsening. 静态后凸是指长期的脊柱后弯曲而无进行性恶化。

kyphostenosis 脊柱后凸狭窄

词根 kypho-（脊柱后弯曲）+ -stenosis（狭窄）

例句 Kyphostenosis involves the narrowing of the spinal canal due to excessive kyphotic curvature. 脊柱后凸狭窄是过度后凸导致脊柱管变窄。

lact-（乳）

lactation 泌乳

词根 lact-（乳）+ -ation（过程）

例句 Lactation is the process by which mammals produce and secrete milk to feed their young. 泌乳是哺乳动物产生并分泌乳汁喂养幼崽的过程。

lactose 乳糖

词根 lact-（乳）+ -ose（糖）

例句 Lactose is a sugar found in milk that provides energy to newborns. 乳糖是牛奶中的一种糖，为新生儿提供能量。

lactase 乳糖酶

词根 lact-（乳）+ -ase（酶）

例句 Lactase is the enzyme responsible for breaking down lactose into glucose and galactose. 乳糖酶是一种将乳糖分解为葡萄糖和半乳糖的酶。

lactic acid 乳酸

词根 lact-（乳）+ -ic acid（酸）

例句 Lactic acid builds up in muscles during intense exercise, causing temporary fatigue. 剧烈运动时，乳酸在肌肉中堆积，导致暂时性疲劳。

lactobacillus 乳酸杆菌

词根 lact-（乳）+ -bacillus（杆菌）

例句 Lactobacillus is a type of beneficial bacteria found in fermented foods and the gut. 乳酸杆菌是一种存在于发酵食品和肠道中的有益细菌。

lactiferous 产乳的

词根 lact-（乳）+ -ferous（携带的）

例句 Lactiferous ducts transport milk from the mammary glands to the nipple. 乳腺管将乳汁从乳腺输送到乳头。

lactalbumin 乳清蛋白

词根 lact-（乳）+ albumin（蛋白）

例句 Lactalbumin is a protein found in milk that aids in infant nutrition. 乳清蛋白是牛奶中的一种蛋白质，有助于婴儿的营养吸收。

lactoglobulin 乳球蛋白

词根 lact-（乳）+ globulin（球蛋白）

例句 Lactoglobulin is one of the main proteins found in whey and contributes to its nutritional value. 乳球蛋白是乳清中的主要蛋白质之一，为乳清提供营养价值。

lactogenesis 乳生成

词根 lact-（乳）+ -genesis（生成）

例句 Lactogenesis refers to the onset of milk production after childbirth. 乳生成是指分娩后乳汁的生成。

lactonase 乳酮酶

词根 lact-（乳）+ -ase（酶）

例句 Lactonase is an enzyme involved in the hydrolysis of lactones. 乳酮酶是一种参与乳酮水解的酶。

laryng-（喉）

laryngitis 喉炎

词根 laryng-（喉）+ -itis（炎症）

例句 Laryngitis is an inflammation of the voice box, often resulting in hoarseness or loss of voice. 喉炎是声带的炎症，通常导致声音嘶哑或失声。

laryngoscopy 喉镜检查

词根 laryng-（喉）+ -scopy（镜检查）

例句 A laryngoscopy is performed to examine the larynx for abnormalities or lesions. 喉镜检查用于观察喉部的异常或病变。

laryngeal 喉部的

词根 laryng-（喉）+ -eal（形容词后缀）

例句 Laryngeal cancer can affect a person's ability to speak and swallow. 喉癌可能影响一个人的说话和吞咽能力。

laryngospasm 喉痉挛

词根 laryng-（喉）+ -spasm（痉挛）

例句 Laryngospasm is a sudden closure of the vocal cords, often causing difficulty breathing. 喉痉挛是声带突然关闭，常导致呼吸困难。

laryngectomy 喉切除术

词根 laryng-（喉）+ -ectomy（切除术）

例句 A laryngectomy is a surgical procedure to remove the larynx, often due to cancer. 喉切除术是一种外科手术，通常因喉癌而进行。

laryngopharynx 咽喉

词根 laryng-（喉）+ pharynx（咽）

例句 The laryngopharynx is the part of the throat that connects the larynx to the esophagus. 咽喉是连接喉部和食管的咽喉部分。

laryngotracheitis 喉气管炎

词根 laryng-（喉）+ trache-（气管）+ -itis（炎症）

例句 Laryngotracheitis is an infection that causes inflammation of the larynx and trachea. 喉气管炎是一种导致喉和气管发炎的感染。

laryngostenosis 喉狭窄

词根 laryng-（喉）+ -stenosis（狭窄）

例句 Laryngostenosis is a narrowing of the larynx, often leading to breathing difficulties. 喉狭窄是喉部变窄，通常会导致呼吸困难。

laryngotomy 喉切开术

词根 laryng-（喉）+ -tomy（切开术）

例句 Laryngotomy is a surgical incision into the larynx to restore breathing. 喉切开术是一种切开喉部以恢复呼吸的外科手术。

laryngomalacia 喉软化症

词根 laryng-（喉）+ -malacia（软化）

例句 Laryngomalacia is a condition seen in infants, where the larynx is soft and collapses during breathing. 喉软化症是一种婴儿常见的疾病，表现为喉部软组织在呼吸时容易塌陷。

lateral-（侧；边）

bilateral 双侧的

词根 bi-（双）+ lateral（侧）

例句 Bilateral symmetry is common in animals, with body structures mirrored on both sides. 双侧对称在动物中很常见，指身体结构在两侧对称。

unilateral 单侧的

词根 uni-（单）+ lateral（侧）

例句 The patient was diagnosed with unilateral hearing loss in the right ear. 患者被诊断出右耳单侧听力丧失。

ipsilateral 同侧的

词根 ipsi-（相同）+ lateral（侧）

例句 Ipsilateral paralysis affects the same side of the body as the brain lesion. 同侧瘫痪影响与脑损伤同侧的身体部分瘫痪。

contralateral 对侧的

词根 contra-（相对）+ lateral（侧）

例句 A stroke in the left hemisphere can cause contralateral weakness on the right side of the body. 左脑半球的中风可能导致身体右侧的对侧无力。

lateralization 侧化

词根 lateral（侧）+ -ization（过程）

例句 Lateralization of brain function means that certain cognitive functions are specialized in one hemisphere. 大脑功能侧化意味着某些认知功能在一个半球中更为突出。

lateral epicondylitis 肱骨外上髁炎

词根 lateral（侧）+ epicondyle（上髁）+ -itis（炎症）

例句 Lateral epicondylitis, commonly known as tennis elbow, is caused by overuse of the forearm muscles. 肱骨外上髁炎，又称网球肘，是由前臂肌肉过度使用引起的。

lateral recumbent 侧卧位

词根 lateral（侧）+ recumbent（卧位）

例句 The lateral recumbent position is often used in first aid to maintain an open airway. 侧卧位常用于急救中保持呼吸道通畅。

lateral line 侧线

词根 lateral（侧）+ line（线）

例句 Fish use their lateral line to detect movements and vibrations in the water. 鱼利用侧线感知水中的运动和振动。

lateral displacement 侧向位移

词根 lateral（侧）+ displacement（位移）

例句 Lateral displacement of the patella can result from ligament injuries. 髌骨的侧向位移可能由韧带损伤引起。

lateral sclerosis 侧索硬化症

词根 lateral（侧）+ sclerosis（硬化）

例句 Amyotrophic lateral sclerosis（ALS）is a progressive neurodegenerative disease affecting motor neurons. 肌萎缩侧索硬化症（ALS）是一种影响运动神经元的进行性神经退行性疾病。

USMLE Step 2 CK　样题

A 50-year-old man comes to the office because of a 3-day history of mild headache and intermittent (inter-; mitt-) confusion. He has a 30-year history of schizophrenia (schiz-; pren-) and a 5-year history of emphysema (em-; phys-; -ema). Medications are clozapine (-apine), sertraline, and inhaled beclomethasone (meth-; -asone) and salmeterol. He also receives home oxygen therapy. He smoked two packs of cigarettes (cigar-; -ette) daily for 33 years but quit 5 years ago. Temperature is 36.8°C (98.2°F), respirations (re-; spir-; -ation) are 20/min, pulse is 90/min, and blood pressure is 115/70 mmHg. Examination shows moist mucous membranes. Lungs are clear to auscultation (auscult-; -ation). There is no peripheral edema. Neurologic (neuro-) examination shows no focal findings. Results of a complete blood count are within the reference ranges. Results of other laboratory studies are shown:

Serum Na^+ 116 mEq/L

K^+ 4 mEq/L

Cl^- 90 mEq/L

Urea nitrogen 10 mg/dL

Creatinine 1 mg/dL

Glucose 100 mg/dL

Which of the following is the most appropriate next step in management?

(A) CT scan of the chest

(B) Measurement of serum cortisol and TSH concentrations

(C) Measurement of serum uric acid concentration

(D) Measurement of urine and plasma osmolarity

(E) MRI of the brain

中文翻译

一名 50 岁男性来就诊，因 3 天来轻度头痛和间歇性意识模糊。他有 30 年精神分裂症病史和 5 年肺气肿病史。目前服用的药物包括氯氮平、舍曲林，以及吸入式倍氯米松和沙美特罗。他还接受家庭氧疗。他有 33 年每天吸两包烟的吸烟史，但 5 年前已戒烟。体温 36.8℃（98.2℉），呼吸 20 次 / 分钟，脉搏 90 次 / 分钟，血压 115/70 mmHg。检查显示黏膜湿润。肺部听诊清晰，无周围水肿。神经系统检查未发现局灶性异常。全血细胞计数结果在参考范围内。其他实验室检查结果如下：

血清钠 116 mEq/L

钾 4 mEq/L

氯 90 mEq/L

尿素氮 10 mg/dL

肌酐 1 mg/dL

葡萄糖 100 mg/dL

以下哪项是最适当的下一步检查？

(A) 胸部 CT 扫描

(B) 测量血清皮质醇和 TSH 浓度

(C) 测量血清尿酸浓度

(D) 测量尿液和血浆渗透压

(E) 脑部 MRI

题目和答案中出现的词根

inter-：在……之间

mitt-：时间区间

schiz-：分裂

pren-：意识

em-：在内的

phys-：气体

-ema：病态

-apine：三环抗抑郁药

meth-：甲基

-asone：糖皮质激素相关

cigar-：雪茄

-ette：小的

re-：重新；反复

spir：呼吸

-ation：表示动作的状态

auscult-：听

neuro-：神经的

leio-（平滑肌的）

leiomyoma 平滑肌瘤

词根 leio-（平滑肌）+ -myoma（肌瘤）

例句 Leiomyoma is a benign tumor that arises from smooth muscle tissue, commonly found in the uterus. 平滑肌瘤是一种良性肿瘤，

通常在子宫的平滑肌组织中形成。

leiomyosarcoma 平滑肌肉瘤

词根 leio-（平滑肌）+ -myo（肌肉）+ -sarcoma（肉瘤）

例句 Leiomyosarcoma is a rare malignant tumor that originates in smooth muscle cells. 平滑肌肉瘤是一种罕见的恶性肿瘤，起源于平滑肌细胞。

leiomyositis 平滑肌炎

词根 leio-（平滑肌）+ -myo（肌肉）+ -itis（炎症）

例句 Leiomyositis refers to the inflammation of smooth muscle, often due to infections or autoimmune disorders. 平滑肌炎是平滑肌的炎症，通常由感染或自身免疫疾病引起。

leiomyofibroma 平滑肌纤维瘤

词根 leio-（平滑肌）+ -fibro（纤维）+ -oma（肿瘤）

例句 Leiomyofibroma is a rare tumor consisting of both smooth muscle and fibrous tissue. 平滑肌纤维瘤是一种由平滑肌和纤维组织构成的罕见肿瘤。

leiomyoblastoma 平滑肌母细胞瘤

词根 leio-（平滑肌）+ -blast（母细胞）+ -oma（肿瘤）

例句 Leiomyoblastoma arises from immature smooth muscle cells and can be either benign or malignant. 平滑肌母细胞瘤起源于未成熟的平滑肌细胞，可能是良性或恶性。

leiomyopathy 平滑肌病

词根 leio-（平滑肌）+ -myopathy（肌病）

例句 Leiomyopathy is a disease affecting the smooth muscles, leading to weakness and dysfunction. 平滑肌病是一种影响平滑肌的疾病，导致肌肉无力和功能障碍。

leiomyonecrosis 平滑肌坏死

词根 leio-（平滑肌）+ -necrosis（坏死）

例句 Leiomyonecrosis refers to the death of smooth muscle tissue due to insufficient blood supply. 平滑肌坏死是血液供应不足导致的平滑肌组织死亡。

leiomyocarcinoma 平滑肌癌

词根 leio-（平滑肌）+ -carcinoma（癌）
例句 Leiomyocarcinoma is a rare cancerous growth in smooth muscle, commonly occurring in the uterus or digestive tract. 平滑肌癌是一种罕见的癌性增生，常见于子宫或消化道。

leiomyomatosis 多发性平滑肌瘤

词根 leio-（平滑肌）+ -myomatosis（多发性肌瘤）
例句 Leiomyomatosis involves the development of multiple leiomyomas in an organ or tissue. 多发性平滑肌瘤是指在器官或组织中出现多个平滑肌瘤。

leiomyodystrophy 平滑肌营养不良

词根 leio-（平滑肌）+ -dystrophy（营养障碍）
例句 Leiomyodystrophy is a condition characterized by progressive degeneration of smooth muscle fibers. 平滑肌营养不良是一种以平滑肌纤维逐渐退化为特征的疾病。

lepto-（细）

leptomeninges 软脑膜

词根 lepto-（细）+ meninges（脑膜）
例句 The leptomeninges consist of the two delicate layers of the meninges, the pia mater and arachnoid mater. 软脑膜由脑膜的两层薄层组成，即软膜和蛛网膜。

leptospirosis 钩端螺旋体病

词根 lepto-（细）+ spiro（螺旋）+ -osis（病症）

例句 Leptospirosis is a bacterial infection caused by spiral-shaped bacteria, often transmitted through contaminated water. 钩端螺旋体病是一种由螺旋形细菌引起的细菌感染，通常通过受污染的水传播。

leptodermic 薄皮的

词根 lepto-（细）+ dermic（皮肤的）
例句 Leptodermic refers to individuals with very thin and delicate skin. 此词用于形容皮肤非常薄和细腻。

leptocephalus 细头幼体

词根 lepto-（细）+ cephalus（头部）
例句 Leptocephalus is the larval stage of certain fish, characterized by a thin, transparent body. 细头幼体是某些鱼类的幼虫阶段，具有细长而透明的身体。

leptorrhine 细鼻的

词根 lepto-（细）+ rhine（鼻子）
例句 Leptorrhine describes individuals with a long and narrow nose structure. 此词指拥有细长的鼻结构。

leptotrichia 细发杆菌属

词根 lepto-（细）+ trichia（毛发）
例句 Leptotrichia are bacteria that typically inhabit the human mouth and gastrointestinal tract. 细发杆菌是通常寄生于人体口腔和胃肠道中的细菌。

leptophonia 声音微弱

词根 lepto-（细；弱）+ phonia（声音）
例句 Leptophonia is a condition characterized by abnormally weak or soft voice. 声音微弱是一种声音异常低弱或柔和的病症。

leptomeningitis 软脑膜炎

词根 lepto-（细）+ meningitis（脑膜炎）

例句 Leptomeningitis is the inflammation of the thin meninges covering the brain and spinal cord. 软脑膜炎是覆盖大脑和脊髓的薄脑膜的炎症。

leptosomatic 细体型的

词根 lepto-（细）+ somatic（身体的）

例句 Leptosomatic individuals have a slender body type with long limbs and little fat. 细体型的人体型瘦长，四肢修长，脂肪较少。

leptocardia 细心脏症

词根 lepto-（细）+ cardia（心脏）

例句 Leptocardia is a rare congenital condition involving an abnormally thin or underdeveloped heart. 细心脏症是一种罕见的先天性疾病，表现为心脏异常薄或发育不良。

L

leuko-（白色的）

leukocyte 白细胞

词根 leuko-（白色的）+ -cyte（细胞）

例句 Leukocytes are a crucial part of the immune system, helping to fight infections and diseases. 白细胞是免疫系统的重要组成部分，有助于抵抗感染和疾病。

leukemia 白血病

词根 leuko-（白色的）+ -emia（血液中的病症）

例句 Leukemia is a cancer of the blood-forming tissues, leading to an overproduction of abnormal white blood cells. 白血病是一种血液生成组织的癌症，导致异常白细胞过度增生。

leukopenia 白细胞减少

词根 leuko-（白色的）+ -penia（减少）
例句 Leukopenia occurs when the white blood cell count is lower than normal, increasing the risk of infections. 白细胞减少是指白细胞计数低于正常水平，患感染的风险增加。

leukocytosis 白细胞增多症

词根 leuko-（白色的）+ -cytosis（细胞增多）
例句 Leukocytosis is often a sign of infection or inflammation in the body. 白细胞增多症通常是体内感染或炎症的标志。

leukoderma 白斑病

词根 leuko-（白色的）+ -derma（皮肤）
例句 Leukoderma refers to localized loss of pigmentation in the skin, resulting in white patches. 白斑病是指皮肤局部色素消失，形成白色斑块。

leukopathy 白病症

词根 leuko-（白色的）+ -pathy（病）
例句 Leukopathy refers to any disease associated with abnormal white matter in the body, particularly in the brain. 白病症是指与体内，尤其是大脑白质异常有关的疾病。

leukoencephalopathy 白质脑病

词根 leuko-（白色的）+ encephalo-（脑）+ -pathy（病）
例句 Leukoencephalopathy is a condition affecting the white matter of the brain, often leading to neurological symptoms. 白质脑病是一种影响大脑白质的疾病，通常引发神经症状。

leukocytoclastic 白细胞破裂的

词根 leuko-（白色的）+ cyto-（细胞）+ -clastic（破裂）
例句 Leukocytoclastic vasculitis is an inflammation of small blood

vessels caused by the breakdown of white blood cells. 白细胞破裂性血管炎是白细胞破裂引起的小血管炎症。

leukoblast 白细胞母细胞

词根 leuko-（白色的）+ -blast（未成熟细胞）
例句 Leukoblasts are immature white blood cells typically found in bone marrow during cell development. 白细胞母细胞是细胞发育过程中骨髓中常见的未成熟白细胞。

leukorrhea 白带增多

词根 leuko-（白色的）+ -rrhea（流出）
例句 Leukorrhea is a condition characterized by a thick white or yellowish vaginal discharge, often due to infection. 白带增多是以白色或黄白色阴道分泌物增多为特征的病症，通常由感染引起。

lipo-（脂肪的）

lipolysis 脂肪分解

词根 lipo-（脂肪）+ -lysis（分解）
例句 Lipolysis is the breakdown of fats and lipids to release energy. 脂肪分解是脂肪和类脂被分解以释放能量的过程。

lipoma 脂肪瘤

词根 lipo-（脂肪）+ -oma（肿瘤）
例句 A lipoma is a benign tumor composed of fatty tissue, often found under the skin. 脂肪瘤是一种由脂肪组织组成的良性肿瘤，通常在皮肤下发现。

lipid 脂质

词根 lipo-（脂肪）+ -id（物质）
例句 Lipids include fats, oils, and cholesterol, which play key roles

in energy storage and cell structure. 脂质包括脂肪、油和胆固醇，在能量储存和细胞结构中起着重要作用。

lipoprotein 脂蛋白

词根 lipo-（脂肪）+ protein（蛋白）

例句 Lipoproteins are molecules that transport fats and cholesterol in the bloodstream. 脂蛋白是运输脂肪和胆固醇的分子。

lipogenesis 脂肪生成

词根 lipo-（脂肪）+ -genesis（生成）

例句 Lipogenesis is the process by which the body converts excess carbohydrates into fat. 脂肪生成是指身体将多余的碳水化合物转化为脂肪的过程。

lipodystrophy 脂肪代谢障碍

词根 lipo-（脂肪）+ -dystrophy（营养障碍）

例句 Lipodystrophy is a condition characterized by abnormal distribution or loss of fat in the body. 脂肪代谢障碍是以身体脂肪分布异常或丧失为特征的病症。

lipofuscin 脂褐素

词根 lipo-（脂肪）+ fuscin（褐色物质）

例句 Lipofuscin is an age-related pigment that accumulates in cells, particularly in the heart and brain. 脂褐素是一种与年龄相关的色素，积累在细胞中，特别是心脏和大脑中。

lipemia 血脂过多

词根 lipo-（脂肪）+ -emia（血液中的状态）

例句 Lipemia is a condition in which there is an excess of lipids in the blood. 血脂过多是指血液中脂质过多的状态。

liposuction 吸脂术

词根 lipo-（脂肪）+ -suction（吸取）

例句 Liposuction is a cosmetic procedure that removes excess fat from specific areas of the body. 吸脂术是一种去除身体特定部位多余脂肪的美容手术。

lipoatrophy 脂肪萎缩

词根 lipo-（脂肪）+ -atrophy（萎缩）

例句 Lipoatrophy is the localized loss of fat tissue, often seen as a side effect of certain medications. 脂肪萎缩是局部脂肪组织丧失，通常是某些药物的副作用。

USMLE Step 2 CK 样题

An 18-year-old patient comes to the emergency department because of a 2-day history of severe abdominal pain. The pain began in the middle of the abdomen after a large meal but now is localized to the right lower quadrant (quad-). The patient also has a 2-month history of intermittent (inter-; mitt-) diarrhea (dia-; -rrhea). Three weeks ago, the patient had an upper respiratory (re-; spir-) tract infection that resolved spontaneously. The patient currently takes no medications. The patient identifies as nonbinary (non-) and uses they/they pronouns; their assigned sex at birth was male. They do not smoke cigarettes (cigar-; ette) or use other substances. Temperature is 37.8℃ (100.0°F), pulse is 80/min, respirations (re-; spir-; -ation) are 20/min, and blood pressure is 110/70 mmHg. Abdominal examination shows fullness and tenderness to palpation of the right lower quadrant (quad-). Leukocyte (leuk-; -cyte) count is 11,000/mm^3. Which of the following is the most appropriate next step in diagnosis?

(A) Abdominal ultrasonography (ultra-; sono-; -graphy) of the right lower quadrant (quad-)

(B) Air-contrast barium enema

(C) CT scan of the abdomen

(D) Technetium 99m scan of the bowel

(E) Upper gastrointestinal (gastro-; intestin-) series with small bowel follow-through

中文翻译

一名 18 岁患者因 2 天来严重腹痛来到急诊科。疼痛在饱餐后始于腹部中央，但现在局限于右下腹。患者还有 2 个月的间歇性腹泻史。3 周前，患者曾患上呼吸道感染，已自行痊愈。患者目前未服用任何药物。患者自认为其无性别；出生时被认定为男性。其不吸烟也不使用其他药物。体温 37.8°C（100.0°F），脉搏 80 次 / 分钟，呼吸 20 次 / 分钟，血压 110/70 mmHg。腹部检查显示右下腹饱满并有触痛。白细胞计数为 11,000/mm^3。以下哪项是诊断中最适当的下一步？

(A) 右下腹部超声检查

(B) 空气对比钡剂灌肠

(C) 腹部 CT 扫描

(D) 肠道锝 -99m 扫描

(E) 上消化道钡剂造影联合小肠透视

题目和答案中出现的词根

quad-：四个

inter-：在……之间

mitt-：时间区间

dia-：通过

-rrhea：流出

re-：重新；反复

spir：呼吸

non-：表示否定

cigar-：雪茄

-ette：小的

leuk-：白色的

-cyte：细胞

ultra-：超

sono-：声音的

-graphy：图像

gastro-：胃

intestin-：肠

-listhesis（滑动）

spondylolisthesis 脊椎滑脱

词根 spondylo-（脊椎）+ -listhesis（滑动）

例句 Spondylolisthesis occurs when a vertebra slips out of place relative to the one below it. 脊椎滑脱是指一个椎骨相对于下方椎骨滑出原位。

retrolisthesis 后滑脱

词根 retro-（后）+ -listhesis（滑动）

例句 Retrolisthesis is a condition where a vertebra moves backward relative to the vertebra below. 后滑脱是指一个椎骨相对于下方椎

骨向后移位。

anterolisthesis 前滑脱

词根 antero-（前）+ -listhesis（滑动）
例句 Anterolisthesis involves the forward displacement of a vertebra over the one beneath it. 前滑脱是指椎骨相对于下方椎骨向前移位。

lateral listhesis 侧滑脱

词根 lateral（侧）+ -listhesis（滑动）
例句 Lateral listhesis is a sideways slippage of the vertebra, often caused by spinal deformities. 侧滑脱是椎骨向侧面移位，通常由脊柱畸形引起。

cervical listhesis 颈椎滑脱

词根 cervical（颈部的）+ -listhesis（滑动）
例句 Cervical listhesis occurs when a vertebra in the neck region moves out of alignment. 颈椎滑脱是指颈部椎骨偏离正常位置。

lumbosacral listhesis 腰骶滑脱

词根 lumbo-（腰部）+ sacral（骶部）+ -listhesis（滑动）
例句 Lumbosacral listhesis is common in the lower spine and can cause nerve compression. 腰骶滑脱常见于下腰部脊柱，可导致神经受压。

posterolisthesis 后位滑脱

词根 postero-（后）+ -listhesis（滑动）
例句 Posterolisthesis describes a vertebra sliding backward, leading to instability. 后位滑脱是指椎骨向后移位，导致脊柱不稳。

degenerative listhesis 退行性滑脱

词根 degenerative（退化的）+ -listhesis（滑动）
例句 Degenerative listhesis is commonly seen in older adults due

to disc degeneration. 退行性滑脱在老年人中较为常见，通常由椎间盘退化引起。

multilevel listhesis 多层滑脱

词根 multi-（多）+ -listhesis（滑动）

例句 Multilevel listhesis involves slippage at multiple spinal levels, leading to severe symptoms. 多层滑脱指多个脊柱层面的移位，可能导致严重症状。

-lith（石）

nephrolithiasis 肾结石病

词根 nephro-（肾）+ -lith（石）+ -iasis（病症）

例句 Nephrolithiasis refers to the presence of kidney stones that can cause severe pain. 肾结石病指肾脏中存在结石，可能引起剧烈疼痛。

cholelithiasis 胆结石病

词根 chole-（胆）+ -lith（石）+ -iasis（病症）

例句 Cholelithiasis is a condition characterized by the formation of stones in the gallbladder. 胆结石病是胆囊内形成结石的一种疾病。

lithotripsy 碎石术

词根 lith-（石）+ -tripsy（碎裂）

例句 Lithotripsy is a procedure that uses shock waves to break up stones in the kidney or gallbladder. 碎石术是一种利用冲击波碎裂肾结石或胆结石的手术。

urolithiasis 尿路结石

词根 uro-（尿）+ -lith（石）+ -iasis（病症）

例句 Urolithiasis occurs when stones form in any part of the urinary tract. 尿路结石是指结石形成在尿路的任何部位。

sialolithiasis 涎石病

词根 sialo-（唾液）+ -lith（石）+ -iasis（病症）

例句 Sialolithiasis is caused by the formation of stones in the salivary glands. 涎石病是唾液腺内形成结石所引起的疾病。

lithiasis 结石症

词根 lith-（石）+ -iasis（病症）

例句 Lithiasis is a general term for any condition involving stone formation in the body. 结石症是指身体内任何涉及结石形成的病症。

enterolithiasis 肠石症

词根 entero-（肠）+ -lith（石）+ -iasis（病症）

例句 Enterolithiasis refers to the presence of stones within the intestines. 肠石症是指肠内出现结石。

pancreatolithiasis 胰腺结石病

词根 pancreato-（胰腺）+ -lith（石）+ -iasis（病症）

例句 Pancreatolithiasis occurs when stones form in the ducts of the pancreas. 胰腺结石病是胰腺导管中形成结石的一种疾病。

otolith 耳石

词根 oto-（耳）+ -lith（石）

例句 Otoliths are small stones in the inner ear that help with balance and spatial orientation. 耳石是内耳中的小石头，有助于保持平衡和空间感知。

hepatolithiasis 肝内结石

词根 hepato-（肝）+ -lith（石）+ -iasis（病症）

例句 Hepatolithiasis is a rare condition involving the formation of stones within the liver bile ducts. 肝内结石是一种罕见疾病，指肝胆管内形成结石。

USMLE Step 2 CK 样题

A 68-year-old man comes to the office because of a 3-month history of moderate low back pain that extends into both legs. He first noticed the pain while standing in the ticket line at a theater. At that time, the pain was accompanied by tingling in both legs. The symptoms recurred (re-; -cur) a few days later as he was standing in the grocery checkout line. The pain has not responded to ibuprofen or naproxen but improves with sitting or lying down. Prior to onset of the pain, the patient typically walked for 30 minutes four times weekly. He discontinued (dis-) his walking regimen 2 months ago because it seemed to trigger his back pain. He has hypertension (hyper-; tension) and hyperlipidemia (hyper-; lipid-; -emia). Medications are hydrochlorothiazide (hydro-; chloro-; -thiazide) -triamterene, simvastatin (-statin), and aspirin. The patient has smoked one pack of cigarettes (cigar-; -ette) daily for 40 years. Pulse is 74/min and blood pressure is 140/90 mmHg. Lungs are clear to auscultation (auscult-; -ation); expiration (ex-; spir-; -ation) phase is delayed. On cardiac examination, a grade 2/6 systolic crescendo (cresc-; -endo)-decrescendo (decresc-; -endo) murmur is heard at the upper right sternal border. There is trace ankle edema bilaterally (bi-; -lateral); ankle brachial index is 1.0. Musculoskeletal (musculo-; skele-) and neurologic (neuro-) examinations show no abnormalities. Which of the following is the most likely diagnosis?

(A) Abdominal aortic aneurysm

(B) Osteoporosis (osteo-; por-; -osis)

(C) Peripheral neuropathy (neuro-; -pathy)

(D) Spinal stenosis (sten-; -osis)

(E) Vascular claudication (claudi-; -ation)

中文翻译

一名 68 岁男性来就诊，因 3 个月来中度腰痛且疼痛延伸至双腿。他首次注意到疼痛是在剧院售票处排队站立时。当时，疼痛伴有麻木感。几天后，他在杂货店排队结账站立时症状再次出现。疼痛对抗炎药如布洛芬或萘普生无反应，但坐下或躺下时有所缓解。在疼痛出现之前，患者通常每周 4 次步行 30 分钟。两个月前，他因步行似乎会引发腰痛而停止了步行锻炼。他有高血压和高脂血症病史。目前服用的药物包括氢氯噻嗪 - 氨苯蝶啶、辛伐他汀和阿司匹林。患者有 40 年每天吸 1 包烟的吸烟史。脉搏 74 次 / 分钟，血压 140/90 mmHg。肺部听诊清晰，呼气相延长。心脏检查在右上胸骨旁听到 2/6 级收缩期渐强 - 渐弱杂音。双侧踝部有轻微水肿；踝臂指数为 1.0。肌肉骨骼和神经系统检查无异常。以下哪项是最可能的诊断？

(A) 腹主动脉瘤

(B) 骨质疏松症

(C) 周围神经病变

(D) 脊柱狭窄

(E) 血管性跛行

题目和答案中出现的词根

re-：重新；反复

-cur：跑（再次跑过来指的是复发）

dis-：离开

hyper-：高

-tension：张力；压力

lipid-：脂肪

-emia：血症

hydro-：氢

chloro-：氯

-thiazide：噻嗪

-statin：静止（这里指把合成胆固醇的关键酶 HMG-CoA 还原酶静止，通常代指降脂药物）

cigar-：雪茄

-ette：小的

auscult-：听

-ation：表示动作的状态

ex-：向外

spir-：呼吸

cresc-：变大

-endo：和音乐相关的声音（变大的声音指的是音量渐强）

decresc-：变小

bi-：双

-lateral：侧

musculo-：肌肉的

skele-：骨骼的

neuro-：神经的

osteo-：骨

por：孔

-osis：病理状态

-pathy：病

sten-：窄的

claudi-：跛的

lord-（弯曲）

lordosis 脊柱前凸

词根 lord-（弯曲）+ -osis（病症）

例句 Lordosis is an exaggerated inward curvature of the lower spine, commonly referred to as swayback. 脊柱前凸是下脊柱过度向内弯曲的现象，通常称为马鞍背。

cervical lordosis 颈椎前凸

词根 cervical（颈部的）+ lord-（弯曲）+ -osis（病症）

例句 Cervical lordosis refers to the normal or abnormal inward curve of the neck region of the spine. 颈椎前凸是指颈部脊柱的正常或异常内弯。

lumbar lordosis 腰椎前凸

词根 lumbar（腰部的）+ lord-（弯曲）+ -osis（病症）

例句 Lumbar lordosis is common in pregnant women due to the added weight and pressure on the lower back. 腰椎前凸在孕妇中很常见，是额外的体重和对腰部的压力导致的。

hyperlordosis 过度前凸

词根 hyper-（过度）+ lord-（弯曲）+ -osis（病症）

例句 Hyperlordosis can lead to lower back pain and difficulty standing for long periods. 过度前凸可能导致腰部疼痛和长时间站立的困难。

hypolordosis 前凸不足

词根 hypo-（不足）+ lord-（弯曲）+ -osis（病症）

例句 Hypolordosis, or a flattened spinal curve, can result in reduced flexibility and back pain. 前凸不足或脊柱弯曲变平，可能导致灵活性降低和背部疼痛。

lordotic posture 前凸姿势

词根 lord-（弯曲）+ -otic（形容词后缀）

例句 A lordotic posture is characterized by an exaggerated inward curve of the lower back. 前凸姿势的特征是腰部有明显的内弯。

lordotome 脊柱矫正器

词根 lord-（弯曲）+ -tome（切开工具）

例句 A lordotome may be used during surgery to correct spinal deformities. 脊柱矫正器可能在手术中用于矫正脊柱畸形。

lordoscoliosis 脊柱前侧凸

词根 lord-（弯曲）+ scolio-（弯曲）+ -osis（病症）

例句 Lordoscoliosis is a complex spinal deformity involving both lateral and anterior curvatures. 脊柱前侧凸是一种复杂的脊柱畸形，包括侧弯和前凸。

lordoplastic surgery 脊柱矫正术

词根 lord-（弯曲）+ -plasty（成形术）

例句 Lordoplastic surgery aims to correct excessive spinal curvatures to restore proper posture. 脊柱矫正术旨在矫正过度弯曲的脊柱，恢复正常姿势。

lordoarthrosis 脊柱前凸关节病

词根 lord-（弯曲）+ arthro-（关节）+ -osis（病症）

例句 Lordoarthrosis refers to joint degeneration associated with abnormal spinal curvature. 脊柱前凸关节病是与异常脊柱弯曲有关的关节退化。

lux-（脱位）

luxation 脱位

词根 lux-（脱位）+ -ation（过程）
例句 Luxation occurs when a bone is displaced from its joint, often causing severe pain and immobility. 脱位是指骨头从关节中脱出，通常引起剧烈疼痛和活动受限。

subluxation 半脱位

词根 sub-（下）+ lux-（脱位）+ -ation（过程）
例句 Subluxation is a partial dislocation where the joint surfaces remain partially in contact. 半脱位是指关节表面部分接触但未完全脱出的情况。

reluxation 复发性脱位

词根 re-（再）+ lux-（脱位）+ -ation（过程）
例句 Reluxation is common in shoulder joints and may require surgical correction. 复发性脱位在肩关节中较为常见，可能需要手术矫正。

hip luxation 髋关节脱位

词根 hip（髋）+ lux-（脱位）+ -ation（过程）
例句 Hip luxation can occur due to trauma or congenital conditions and often leads to difficulty walking. 髋关节脱位可能由外伤或先天性疾病引起，通常导致行走困难。

temporomandibular luxation 颞下颌关节脱位

词根 temporomandibular（颞下颌）+ lux-（脱位）+ -ation（过程）
例句 Temporomandibular luxation occurs when the lower jaw dislocates from its normal position. 颞下颌关节脱位是下颌骨脱离正常位置的一种现象。

lymph-（淋巴）

lymphocyte 淋巴细胞

词根 lymph-（淋巴）+ -cyte（细胞）

例句 Lymphocytes are white blood cells that play a critical role in immune responses. 淋巴细胞是白细胞的重要组成部分，在免疫反应中起关键作用。

lymphoma 淋巴瘤

词根 lymph-（淋巴）+ -oma（肿瘤）

例句 Lymphoma is a type of cancer that affects the lymphatic system. 淋巴瘤是一种影响淋巴系统的癌症。

lymphadenopathy 淋巴结病

词根 lymph-（淋巴）+ adeno-（腺）+ -pathy（病症）

例句 Lymphadenopathy is characterized by swollen or enlarged lymph nodes, often due to infection. 淋巴结病的特征是淋巴结肿大，通常由感染引起。

lymphatic system 淋巴系统

词根 lymph-（淋巴）+ -atic（形容词后缀）

例句 The lymphatic system is responsible for transporting lymph and maintaining fluid balance. 淋巴系统负责运输淋巴液并维持体液平衡。

-lysis（分解）

hemolysis 溶血

词根 hemo-（血）+ -lysis（分解）

例句 Hemolysis is the destruction of red blood cells, releasing hemoglobin into the bloodstream. 溶血是红细胞破裂并将血红蛋白释放到血液中的过程。

hydrolysis 水解

词根 hydro-（水）+ -lysis（分解）

例句 Hydrolysis is a chemical reaction in which water breaks down a compound into smaller molecules. 水解是一种化学反应，水将化合物分解成较小的分子。

glycolysis 糖酵解

词根 glyco-（糖）+ -lysis（分解）

例句 Glycolysis is the metabolic pathway that breaks down glucose to produce energy. 糖酵解是分解葡萄糖以产生能量的代谢途径。

proteolysis 蛋白质分解

词根 proteo-（蛋白质）+ -lysis（分解）

例句 Proteolysis involves the breakdown of proteins into smaller peptides or amino acids. 蛋白质分解是指蛋白质分解成较小的肽或氨基酸的过程。

lipolysis 脂肪分解

词根 lipo-（脂肪）+ -lysis（分解）

例句 Lipolysis is the process by which fats are broken down into glycerol and fatty acids. 脂肪分解是将脂肪分解成甘油和脂肪酸的过程。

autolysis 自溶

词根 auto-（自身）+ -lysis（分解）

例句 Autolysis occurs when a cell self-destructs by digesting its own components. 自溶是指细胞通过消化自身成分而自我破坏。

electrolysis 电解

词根 electro-（电）+ -lysis（分解）

例句 Electrolysis is the process of using electrical energy to drive a non-spontaneous chemical reaction. 电解是利用电能驱动非自发化学反应的过程。

paralysis 瘫痪

词根 para-（旁）+ -lysis（松弛；分解）
例句 Paralysis occurs when muscles lose their ability to function due to nerve damage. 瘫痪是指神经损伤导致肌肉失去功能。

fibrinolysis 纤维蛋白溶解

词根 fibrino-（纤维蛋白）+ -lysis（分解）
例句 Fibrinolysis is a process that prevents blood clots from growing and becoming problematic. 纤维蛋白溶解是一种防止血栓增大并引发问题的过程。

lysis 溶解

词根 -lysis（分解；溶解）
例句 Bacterial lysis occurs when the cell walls are broken down, resulting in cell death. 细菌溶解是指细胞壁破裂，导致细菌死亡的过程。

-lyte（溶质）

electrolyte 电解质

词根 electro-（电）+ -lyte（溶质）
例句 Electrolytes are minerals that help maintain fluid balance and proper muscle and nerve function. 电解质是帮助维持体液平衡和肌肉、神经正常功能的矿物质。

hemolyte 血液溶质

词根 hemo-（血）+ -lyte（溶质）
例句 Hemolytes are substances released when red blood cells rupture during hemolysis. 血液溶质是红细胞在溶血过程中破裂时释放出的物质。

hydrolyte 水溶质

词根 hydro-（水）+ -lyte（溶质）

例句 A hydrolyte is a compound that dissolves in water and contributes to the formation of ions. 水溶质是溶解在水中并产生离子的化合物。

cryolyte 低温电解质

词根 cryo-（低温）+ -lyte（溶质）

例句 Cryolytes are used in low-temperature electrochemical reactions, such as in cryogenic environments. 低温电解质用于低温电化学反应中，例如在低温环境下。

metalyte 金属溶质

词根 meta-（变化）+ -lyte（溶质）

例句 Metalytes refer to metal-based substances that dissolve in specific solvents to produce ions. 金属溶质是指溶解在特定溶剂中产生离子的金属基物质。

oxylyte 氧溶质

词根 oxy-（氧）+ -lyte（溶质）

例句 Oxylytes are oxygen-carrying solutions used in oxygen therapy or medical treatments. 氧溶质是用于氧疗或其他治疗的携氧溶液。

isolyte 等电解质溶液

词根 iso-（相等）+ -lyte（溶质）

例句 Isolyte solutions are used in medical treatments to restore the body's electrolyte balance. 等电解质溶液用于治疗中，以恢复身体的电解质平衡。

thermolyte 热溶质

词根 thermo-（热）+ -lyte（溶质）

例句 Thermolytic reactions occur when thermolytes are subjected to high temperatures, causing them to decompose. 热溶质在高温下分解时会引发热分解反应。

alkalolyte 碱性溶质

词根 alkalo-（碱）+ -lyte（溶质）

例句 Alkalolytes are basic compounds that dissolve in water to form alkaline solutions. 碱性溶质是溶解在水中形成碱性溶液的化合物。

solvolyte 溶剂溶质

词根 solvo-（溶解）+ -lyte（溶质）

例句 Solvolytes are substances that can be dissolved or broken down by specific solvents. 溶剂溶质是指能够被特定溶剂溶解或分解的物质。

USMLE Step 2 CK 样题

A 32-year-old man comes to the office because of a 3-month history of a painless (-less) rash over his arms. During the past month, he also has had a 3.2-kg weight loss despite no change in appetite. He has no history of serious illness and takes no medications. He is 175 cm tall and weighs 72 kg; BMI is 23 kg/m^2. Pulse is 98/min; other vital signs are within normal limits. Lungs are clear to auscultation (auscult-; -ation). Cardiac examination shows no abnormalities. A photograph of the left upper extremity is shown. Similar findings are noted over the right upper extremity. Which of the following is the most likely cause of this patient's dermatologic (dermat-) findings?

(A) Actinic (actin-) keratosis (kerat-; -osis)

(B) Dermatitis (dermat-; -itis) herpetiformis (herpet-; -iformis)

(C) Kaposi sarcoma (sarc-; -oma)

(D) Lichen planus

(E) Seborrheic (sebo-; rrhe-) dermatitis (dermat-; -itis)

中文翻译

一名 32 岁男性前来就诊，因 3 个月来手臂出现无痛性皮疹。近 1 个月来，他体重减轻了 3.2 kg，尽管食欲未变。他无严重疾病史，也未服用任何药物。他身高 175 cm，体重 72 kg；BMI 为 23 kg/m²。脉搏 98 次 / 分钟；其他生命体征正常。肺部听诊清晰。心脏检查无异常。左上肢的照片显示皮疹情况，右上肢也有类似表现。以下哪项是该患者皮肤表现的最可能原因？

(A) 光化性角化病

(B) 疱疹样皮炎

(C) 卡波西肉瘤

(D) 扁平苔藓

(E) 脂溢性皮炎

题目和答案中出现的词根

-less：表否定

auscult-：听

-ation：表示动作的状态

dermat-：皮肤的

actin-：光线的

kerat-：角化的

-osis：病理状态

-itis：炎症

herpet-：匍匐的（疱疹的生长方式）

-iformis：像……的形状

sarc-：肉体的

-oma：瘤

sebo-：脂肪的

rrhe-：流出的，是 rrhea 的同义变异

macro-（大）

macrophage 巨噬细胞

词根 macro-（大）+ -phage（吞噬）

例句 Macrophages play a key role in the immune system by engulfing and destroying pathogens. 巨噬细胞通过吞噬和摧毁病原体，在免疫系统中发挥重要作用。

macrocephaly 巨头症

词根 macro-（大）+ -cephaly（头）

例句 Macrocephaly is a condition where the head is abnormally large, often due to excess brain fluid. 巨头症是指头部异常增大，通常是由脑内液体过多引起的。

macroglossia 巨舌症

词根 macro-（大）+ glossia（舌）

例句 Macroglossia is characterized by an enlarged tongue, which may cause difficulty breathing and speaking. 巨舌症的特征是舌头增大，可能导致呼吸和说话困难。

macrocytosis 大细胞增多症

词根 macro-（大）+ -cytosis（细胞增多）

例句 Macrocytosis is a blood condition involving an increased number of abnormally large red blood cells. 大细胞增多症是一种血液疾病，指异常大的红细胞数量增加。

macronucleus 大核

词根 macro-（大）+ nucleus（核）

例句 A macronucleus is a large, prominent nucleus found in some unicellular organisms, such as ciliates. 大核是某些单细胞生物（如

纤毛虫）中的大型细胞核。

macropodia 巨足症

词根 macro-（大）+ pod（足）+ -ia（病症）

例句 Macropodia refers to abnormally large feet, which can result from genetic or developmental factors. 巨足症是指遗传或发育原因导致的足部异常增大。

macrovascular 大血管的

词根 macro-（大）+ vascular（血管）

例句 Macrovascular complications are common in diabetic patients and affect large blood vessels. 大血管并发症在糖尿病患者中常见，影响大血管的功能。

macroenvironment 宏观环境

词根 macro-（大）+ environment（环境）

例句 The macroenvironment includes external factors such as economic conditions and cultural trends. 宏观环境包括经济状况和文化趋势等外部因素。

macrophthalmia 大眼症

词根 macro-（大）+ ophthalmia（眼睛）

例句 Macrophthalmia is a condition where the eyes are larger than normal, which may affect vision. 大眼症是指眼睛比正常水平大，可能影响视力。

macromolecule 大分子

词根 macro-（大）+ molecule（分子）

例句 Proteins, nucleic acids, and polysaccharides are examples of macromolecules essential for life. 蛋白质、核酸和多糖是生命所必需的大分子。

mal-（错误的）

malnutrition 营养不良

词根 mal-（错误；不足）+ nutrition（营养）

例句 Malnutrition occurs when the body does not receive enough nutrients to maintain proper health. 营养不良是指身体未摄入足够的营养以维持健康。

malfunction 功能失调

词根 mal-（错误）+ function（功能）

例句 A malfunction in the heart valve can lead to improper blood flow and health complications. 心脏瓣膜功能失调可能导致血液流动异常及健康问题。

malformation 畸形

词根 mal-（错误）+ formation（形成）

例句 Malformation of the spine can cause conditions such as scoliosis or kyphosis. 脊柱畸形可能导致脊柱侧弯或后凸等病症。

malaise 不适感

词根 mal-（不好）+ aise（舒适）

例句 Malaise is often one of the first signs of an underlying infection or illness. 不适感通常是潜在感染或疾病的早期信号之一。

malpractice 医疗事故

词根 mal-（错误）+ practice（实践）

例句 The surgeon was sued for malpractice after the patient suffered complications. 患者出现并发症后，外科医生因医疗事故被起诉。

malodorous 恶臭的

词根 mal-（坏的）+ odorous（有气味的）

例句 The stagnant water became malodorous due to bacterial growth. 由于细菌滋生，静止的水散发出恶臭。

malignancy 恶性肿瘤

词根 mal-（坏的）+ ignancy（状态）

例句 Malignancy in the lungs can lead to life-threatening complications if left untreated. 肺部的恶性肿瘤如果不及时治疗可能引发致命并发症。

malcontent 不满者

词根 mal-（不满）+ content（满足）

例句 The malcontent workers went on strike to protest against poor working conditions. 不满的工人为抗议恶劣的工作环境而罢工。

malevolent 恶意的

词根 mal-（坏的）+ volent（意图）

例句 His malevolent actions caused harm to several innocent people. 他的恶意行为伤害了几名无辜者。

malabsorption 吸收不良

词根 mal-（不好）+ absorption（吸收）

例句 Malabsorption can lead to weight loss and nutrient deficiencies. 吸收不良可能导致体重下降和营养缺乏。

-malacia（软）

osteomalacia 骨软化症

词根 osteo-（骨）+ -malacia（软）

例句 Osteomalacia is a condition characterized by softening of the bones due to vitamin D deficiency. 骨软化症是维生素 D 缺乏导致

骨骼软化的一种疾病。

chondromalacia 软骨软化症

词根 chondro-（软骨）+ -malacia（软）

例句 Chondromalacia affects the cartilage under the kneecap, causing pain during movement. 软骨软化症影响膝盖下方的软骨，在运动时会引起疼痛。

tracheomalacia 气管软化症

词根 tracheo-（气管）+ -malacia（软）

例句 Tracheomalacia occurs when the walls of the trachea become weak and collapse during breathing. 气管软化症是指气管壁变薄弱并在呼吸时塌陷。

laryngomalacia 喉软化症

词根 laryngo-（喉）+ -malacia（软）

例句 Laryngomalacia is a common condition in infants, where the soft tissues of the larynx collapse during breathing. 喉软化症是婴儿中常见的一种疾病，喉部软组织在呼吸时会塌陷。

keratomalacia 角膜软化症

词根 kerato-（角膜）+ -malacia（软）

例句 Keratomalacia is caused by a severe deficiency of vitamin A, leading to softening and ulceration of the cornea. 角膜软化症由维生素 A 严重缺乏引起，导致角膜软化和溃疡。

bronchomalacia 支气管软化症

词根 broncho-（支气管）+ -malacia（软）

例句 Bronchomalacia is characterized by weakened bronchial walls, leading to airway obstruction. 支气管软化症的特征是支气管壁变薄弱，导致气道阻塞。

cardiomalacia 心脏软化

词根 cardio-（心脏）+ -malacia（软）

例句 Cardiomalacia can occur after a heart attack, resulting in softening of the heart muscle. 心脏软化可能在心脏病发作后发生，导致心肌软化。

myelomalacia 脊髓软化症

词根 myelo-（脊髓）+ -malacia（软）

例句 Myelomalacia is a serious condition involving softening of the spinal cord due to trauma or lack of blood flow. 脊髓软化症是一种严重疾病，通常由创伤或血液供应不足引起。

encephalomalacia 脑软化症

词根 encephalo-（脑）+ -malacia（软）

例句 Encephalomalacia is the softening of brain tissue often caused by a stroke or severe injury. 脑软化症是由中风或严重损伤引起的脑组织软化。

arteriomalacia 动脉软化症

词根 arterio-（动脉）+ -malacia（软）

例句 Arteriomalacia can weaken blood vessels and increase the risk of aneurysms. 动脉软化症会削弱血管，增加动脉瘤的风险。

mast-（乳房的）

mastitis 乳腺炎

词根 mast-（乳房）+ -itis（炎症）

例句 Mastitis is an inflammation of breast tissue, often associated with breastfeeding. 乳腺炎是乳房组织的炎症，通常与哺乳有关。

mastectomy 乳房切除术

词根 mast-（乳房）+ -ectomy（切除）

例句 A mastectomy is a surgical procedure performed to remove one or both breasts, often due to cancer. 乳房切除术是切除单侧或双侧乳房的手术，通常是由于乳腺癌。

mastalgia 乳房疼痛

词根 mast-（乳房）+ -algia（疼痛）

例句 Mastalgia is a common condition among women, often related to hormonal changes. 乳房疼痛在女性中很常见，通常与激素变化有关。

mastopathy 乳房病

词根 mast-（乳房）+ -pathy（病症）

例句 Mastopathy includes benign conditions of the breast, such as fibrocystic changes. 乳房病包括乳房的良性病变，如纤维囊性改变。

mastodynia 乳房痛

词根 mast-（乳房）+ -dynia（疼痛）

例句 Mastodynia can be cyclic or non-cyclic and is often linked to the menstrual cycle. 乳房痛可以是周期性的或非周期性的，通常与月经周期有关。

mastopexy 乳房提升术

词根 mast-（乳房）+ -pexy（固定术）

例句 Mastopexy is a cosmetic procedure to lift and reshape sagging breasts. 乳房提升术是一种提升和重塑下垂乳房的美容手术。

mastocytosis 肥大细胞增多症

词根 mast-（乳房；肥大细胞）+ -cytosis（细胞增多）

例句 Mastocytosis is a rare condition involving an abnormal accumulation of mast cells in tissues. 肥大细胞增多症是一种罕见疾病，指组织中肥大细胞的异常积聚。

mastocarcinoma 乳腺癌

词根 mast-（乳房）+ carcinoma（癌）

例句 Mastocarcinoma is a malignant tumor originating in the breast tissue. 乳腺癌是起源于乳房组织的恶性肿瘤。

mastorrhagia 乳房出血

词根 mast-（乳房）+ -rrhagia（出血）

例句 Mastorrhagia is a rare condition characterized by bleeding from the breast. 乳房出血是一种以乳房出血为特征的罕见病症。

mastadenitis 乳腺炎

词根 mast-（乳房）+ aden-（腺）+ -itis（炎症）

例句 Mastadenitis refers to inflammation of the mammary glands, often resulting from bacterial infection. 乳腺炎是乳腺腺体的炎症，通常由细菌感染引起。

megalo-/-megaly（大）

hepatomegaly 肝肿大

词根 hepato-（肝）+ -megaly（大）

例句 Hepatomegaly is often a sign of liver disease or infection, such as hepatitis. 肝肿大通常是肝病或感染（如肝炎）的症状。

splenomegaly 脾肿大

词根 spleno-（脾）+ -megaly（大）

例句 Splenomegaly occurs due to infections, liver diseases, or blood disorders. 脾肿大可能由感染、肝病或血液疾病引起。

cardiomegaly 心脏肥大

词根 cardio-（心脏）+ -megaly（大）

例句 Cardiomegaly can result from high blood pressure or heart failure. 心脏肥大可能是由高血压或心力衰竭引起的。

acromegaly 肢端肥大症

词根 acro-（四肢）+ -megaly（大）

例句 Acromegaly is a hormonal disorder that results from excess growth hormone, leading to enlarged extremities. 肢端肥大症是一

种生长激素过量导致的激素紊乱，表现为四肢增大。

gastromegaly 胃肿大

词根 gastro-（胃）+ -megaly（大）
例句 Gastromegaly can be caused by chronic overeating or underlying gastrointestinal issues. 胃肿大可能由长期暴饮暴食或胃肠道疾病引起。

megaloblast 大幼红细胞

词根 megalo-（大）+ -blast（幼细胞）
例句 Megaloblasts are abnormal, large red blood cell precursors found in certain types of anemia. 大幼红细胞是某些类型贫血中发现的异常增大的红细胞前体。

megalomania 夸大妄想症

词根 megalo-（大）+ -mania（狂热）
例句 Megalomania is a mental disorder where a person has delusional fantasies of power and grandeur. 夸大妄想症是一种精神疾病，患者有获得权力、变得伟大的妄想。

osteomegaly 骨增大

词根 osteo-（骨）+ -megaly（大）
例句 Osteomegaly can occur due to metabolic bone diseases, such as Paget's disease. 骨增大可能由代谢性骨病引起，如佩吉特病。

nephromegaly 肾脏肿大

词根 nephro-（肾脏）+ -megaly（大）
例句 Nephromegaly is commonly caused by kidney infections, tumors, or cysts. 肾脏肿大通常由肾脏感染、肿瘤或囊肿引起。

encephalomegaly 脑增大

词根 encephalo-（脑）+ -megaly（大）
例句 Encephalomegaly may result from hydrocephalus or brain inflammation. 脑增大可能是由脑积水或脑部炎症引起的。

USMLE Step 2 CK 样题

A 15-year-old boy is brought to the office 2 hours after he awoke with weakness of the right side of his face. He has a 2-week history of intermittent (inter-; -mitt) headache (-ache), sensitivity to light, and mild to moderate neck pain. He has no history of serious illness. His only medication is acetaminophen (acet-; amin-;-ophen) as needed. He lives in New Jersey and has not traveled outside of the state during the past 6 months. Temperature is 37.4°C (99.3°F), pulse is 78/min and regular, and blood pressure is 108/70 mmHg. Flexion of the neck elicits moderate pain and resistance. The right eyelids do not close completely. Ocular movements are normal. There is no evidence of ptosis. The right side of the forehead (fore-) does not wrinkle when the patient looks up. There is severe weakness of the right corner of the mouth. There are no abnormalities of the left side of the face. Muscle strength in the jaw, tongue, and palate is normal and symmetric. There is no dysarthria (dys-; arthr-). Muscle strength is 5/5 in all extremities. Coordination (co-) and sensation are intact. Gait is normal. A lumbar puncture is performed, and opening pressure is 180 mmH_2O. Cerebrospinal (cerebro-) fluid analysis results are shown:

Glucose 60 mg/dL

Total protein 52 mg/dL

WBC 85/mm^3

Segmented neutrophils (neutro-; -phil) 30%

Lymphocytes (lymph-; -cyte) 70%

RBC 1/mm³

Which of the following is the most appropriate next step in diagnosis?

(A) Measurement of serum angiotensin (angio-; -tens) -converting enzyme activity

(B) Measurement of serum Lyme (Borrelia burgdorferi) antibody (anti-) concentration

(C) Polymerase chain reaction test for cytomegalovirus (cyto-; megalo-)

(D) Serum antinuclear (anti-; nucle-) antibody (anti-) assay

(E) Serum protein electrophoresis (electro-; phor-; -esis)

中文翻译

一名 15 岁男孩在醒来后 2 小时因右侧面部无力被带到门诊。他有 2 周的间歇性头痛、光敏感和轻中度颈部疼痛病史。他无严重疾病史。唯一使用的药物是按需服用的对乙酰氨基酚。他住在新泽西州，过去 6 个月内未离开过该州。体温 37.4℃（99.3℉），脉搏 78 次 / 分钟且规律，血压 108/70 mmHg。颈部屈曲引起中度疼痛和阻力。右侧眼睑无法完全闭合。眼球运动正常。无眼睑下垂证据。患者抬头时，右侧额头无皱纹。右侧嘴角严重无力。面部左侧无异常。颌部、舌头和腭的肌肉力量正常且对称。无构音障碍。四肢肌肉力量均为 5/5 级。协调和感觉功能完整。步态正常。进行了腰椎穿刺，开放压为 180 mmH_2O。脑脊液分析结果如下：

葡萄糖 60 mg/dL

总蛋白 52 mg/dL

白细胞 85/mm³

分叶核中性粒细胞 30%

淋巴细胞 70%

红细胞 1/mm³

以下哪项是诊断中最适当的下一步？

(A) 测量血清血管紧张素转换酶活性

(B) 测量血清莱姆病（伯氏疏螺旋体）抗体浓度

(C) 巨细胞病毒的聚合酶链反应检测

(D) 血清抗核抗体检测

(E) 血清蛋白电泳

题目和答案中出现的词根

inter-：在……之间

mitt-：时间区间

-ache：疼痛

acet-：乙酰基

amin-：胺

-ophen：芳香环

fore-：前

dys-：困难的

arthr-：关节（这里代指发音，即产生发音的关节和肌肉的协同运动）

co-：协同的

cerebro-：脑的

neutro-：中性的

-phil：嗜

lymph-：淋巴

-cyte：细胞

angio-：血管

-tens：张力

anti-：抗

cyto-：细胞

megalo：巨大的

nucle：细胞核

electro-：电的

phor-：携带

-esis：过程（携带电的过程指代电泳）

melano-（黑色）

melanoma 黑色素瘤

词根 melano-（黑色）+ -oma（肿瘤）

例句 Melanoma is a dangerous form of skin cancer that develops from pigment-producing cells. 黑色素瘤是一种危险的皮肤癌，由色素细胞恶变发展而来。

melanin 黑色素

词根 melano-（黑色）+ -in（物质）

例句 Melanin is a pigment that gives color to the skin, hair, and eyes. 黑色素是赋予皮肤、头发和眼睛颜色的色素。

melanocyte 黑色素细胞

词根 melano-（黑色）+ -cyte（细胞）

例句 Melanocytes are cells that produce melanin and protect the skin from UV damage. 黑色素细胞是生成黑色素并保护皮肤免

受紫外线伤害的细胞。

melanodermic 黑皮肤的

词根 melano-（黑色）+ -dermic（皮肤的）

例句 Melanodermic conditions are characterized by excessive pigmentation of the skin. 黑皮肤病的特征是皮肤色素过多。

melanogenesis 黑色素生成

词根 melano-（黑色）+ -genesis（生成）

例句 Melanogenesis occurs in response to sun exposure, increasing melanin production to protect the skin. 黑色素生成是在阳光照射下增加黑色素以保护皮肤的过程。

melanopathy 黑色素病

词根 melano-（黑色）+ -pathy（病）

例句 Melanopathy refers to disorders affecting melanin production or distribution in the body. 黑色素病是影响身体内黑色素生成或分布的疾病。

melanoderma 皮肤黑变病

词根 melano-（黑色）+ -derma（皮肤）

例句 Melanoderma can result from prolonged sun exposure or hormonal imbalances. 皮肤黑变病可能由长期日晒或激素失衡引起。

melanocholia 黑胆质症

词根 melano-（黑）+ cholia（胆汁）

例句 Melanocholia, historically linked to melancholia, was believed to arise from an excess of black bile. 黑胆质症，历史上与忧郁症有关，被认为是由过多黑胆汁引起的。

melanuria 黑尿症

词根 melano-（黑色）+ -uria（尿液）

例句 Melanuria is characterized by dark or black-colored urine, often indicating metabolic disorders. 黑尿症的特征是尿液呈深色或黑色，通常表明代谢异常。

melanosarcoma 黑色素肉瘤

词根 melano-（黑色）+ -sarcoma（肉瘤）

例句 Melanosarcoma is a malignant tumor arising from melanocytes. 黑色素肉瘤是由黑色素细胞引起的恶性肿瘤。

mening-（脑膜）

meningitis 脑膜炎

词根 mening-（脑膜）+ -itis（炎症）

例句 Meningitis is an inflammation of the protective membranes covering the brain and spinal cord. 脑膜炎是覆盖大脑和脊髓的保护膜的炎症。

meningocele 脑膜膨出

词根 mening-（脑膜）+ -cele（膨出）

例句 A meningocele occurs when the meninges protrude through a defect in the skull or spinal column. 脑膜膨出是指脑膜通过颅骨或脊柱的缺陷突出。

meningoencephalitis 脑膜脑炎

词根 mening-（脑膜）+ encephalo-（脑）+ -itis（炎症）

例句 Meningoencephalitis is a severe condition involving inflammation of both the meninges and the brain. 脑膜脑炎是一种严重的病症，指脑膜和大脑的炎症。

meningomyelitis 脑膜脊髓炎

词根 mening-（脑膜）+ myelo-（脊髓）+ -itis（炎症）

例句 Meningomyelitis refers to inflammation of both the spinal cord and its protective meninges. 脑膜脊髓炎是指脊髓及其保护性脑膜的炎症。

meningococcal disease 脑膜炎球菌病

词根 mening-（脑膜）+ coccal（球菌的）

例句 Meningococcal disease is a serious bacterial infection that can lead to meningitis or septicemia. 脑膜炎球菌病是一种严重的细菌感染，可导致脑膜炎或败血症。

meningopathy 脑膜病

词根 mening-（脑膜）+ -pathy（病）

例句 Meningopathy is a general term for any disorder affecting the meninges. 脑膜病是指影响脑膜的任何疾病。

meningoencephalocele 脑膜脑膨出

词根 mening-（脑膜）+ encephalo-（脑）+ -cele（膨出）

例句 Meningoencephalocele occurs when both brain tissue and meninges herniate through a skull defect. 脑膜脑膨出是指脑组织和脑膜通过颅骨缺陷膨出。

meningioma 脑膜瘤

词根 mening-（脑膜）+ -oma（肿瘤）

例句 Meningioma is a type of tumor that originates in the meninges, the protective layers surrounding the brain and spinal cord. 脑膜瘤是一种源自脑膜的肿瘤，脑膜是包围大脑和脊髓的保护层。

meningoblastoma 脑膜母细胞瘤

词根 mening-（脑膜）+ -blastoma（母细胞瘤）

例句 Meningoblastoma is a rare tumor originating from embryonic cells in the meninges. 脑膜母细胞瘤是一种起源于脑膜中胚胎细胞的罕见肿瘤。

meningoradiculitis 脑膜神经根炎

词根 mening-（脑膜）+ radiculo-（神经根）+ -itis（炎症）

例句 Meningoradiculitis is an inflammatory condition affecting both the meninges and the nerve roots. 脑膜神经根炎是一种影响脑膜和神经根的炎症性疾病。

meno-（月经的）

menorrhea 正常月经

词根 meno-（月经）+ -rrhea（流出）

例句 Menorrhea refers to the regular menstrual flow experienced by women of reproductive age. 正常月经是育龄女性定期经历的月经。

amenorrhea 闭经

词根 a-（无）+ meno-（月经）+ -rrhea（流出）

例句 Amenorrhea is the absence of menstruation, which may be caused by hormonal imbalances or other health conditions. 闭经是指月经停止，可能由激素失衡或其他健康问题引起。

dysmenorrhea 痛经

词根 dys-（困难、痛苦）+ meno-（月经）+ -rrhea（流出）

例句 Dysmenorrhea causes severe menstrual cramps and discomfort during menstruation. 痛经在月经期间引起严重的经痛和不适。

menopause 绝经

词根 meno-（月经）+ -pause（停止）

例句 Menopause marks the end of a woman's menstrual cycles, typically occurring in middle age. 绝经标志着女性月经周期的结束，通常发生在中年。

menometrorrhagia 经间期出血

词根 meno-（月经）+ metro-（子宫）+ -rrhagia（出血）

例句 Menometrorrhagia involves heavy or prolonged bleeding between menstrual periods. 经间期出血是指月经间期出现大量或长时间出血。

menorrhagia 月经过多

词根 meno-（月经）+ -rrhagia（过多流出）

例句 Menorrhagia is characterized by heavy or prolonged menstrual bleeding. 月经过多是指月经流量过大或持续时间过长。

oligomenorrhea 月经稀少

词根 oligo-（少）+ meno-（月经）+ -rrhea（流出）

例句 Oligomenorrhea is a condition where menstrual periods are infrequent or irregular. 月经稀少是指月经周期不规律或间隔时间较长。

hypomenorrhea 月经过少

词根 hypo-（不足）+ meno-（月经）+ -rrhea（流出）

例句 Hypomenorrhea is characterized by a reduced menstrual flow, which can indicate hormonal issues. 月经过少的特征是月经流量减少，可能表明激素问题。

polymenorrhea 月经频发

词根 poly-（多）+ meno-（月经）+ -rrhea（流出）

例句 Polymenorrhea occurs when menstrual periods happen more frequently than normal. 月经频发是指月经频繁于正常次数发生。

menostasis 月经停滞

词根 meno-（月经）+ -stasis（停滞）

例句 Menostasis refers to the cessation of menstrual flow due to obstructions or other conditions. 月经停滞是指阻塞或其他原因导致月经停止。

-mere（部分）

centromere 着丝粒

词根 centro-（中心）+ -mere（部分）

例句 The centromere is the part of a chromosome that links sister chromatids during cell division. 着丝粒是染色体中连接姐妹染色单体的部分，在细胞分裂中起重要作用。

sarcomere 肌节

词根 sarco-（肌肉）+ -mere（部分）
例句 A sarcomere is the basic contractile unit of striated muscle fibers. 肌节是横纹肌纤维的基本收缩单位。

telomere 端粒

词根 telo-（末端）+ -mere（部分）
例句 Telomeres protect the ends of chromosomes from deterioration or fusion with neighboring chromosomes. 端粒保护染色体的末端免受损伤或与邻近染色体融合。

blastomere 卵裂球

词根 blasto-（胚胎）+ -mere（部分）
例句 A blastomere is a type of cell produced by division of the fertilized egg during early embryonic development. 卵裂球是受精卵在早期胚胎发育过程中分裂产生的一种细胞。

chromomere 染色小体

词根 chrom-（色）+ -mere（部分）
例句 A chromomere is a bead-like structure on a chromosome that appears during prophase of cell division. 染色小体是在细胞分裂前期染色体上出现的珠状结构。

myomere 肌节

词根 myo-（肌肉）+ -mere（部分）
例句 Myomeres are segmented muscle fibers found in the body of vertebrates. 肌节是脊椎动物体内的分段肌肉纤维。

monomere 单体

词根 mono-（一个）+ -mere（部分）

例句 Monomeres are single molecules that can combine to form polymers. 单体是可以结合形成聚合物的单个分子。

isomere 同分异构体

词根 iso-（相同）+ -mere（部分）

例句 Isomeres have the same molecular formula but different structural arrangements. 同分异构体具有相同的分子式，但结构排列不同。

polymere 聚合物

词根 poly-（多）+ -mere（部分）

例句 Polymers are large molecules made by linking together many smaller units called monomers. 聚合物是由许多称为单体的小单位连接而成的大分子。

meta-（转化）

metabolism 新陈代谢

词根 meta-（转化）+ -bolism（代谢）

例句 Metabolism is the process by which the body converts food into energy and building materials. 新陈代谢是身体将食物转化为能量和结构材料的过程。

metamorphosis 变形

词根 meta-（转化）+ -morphosis（形态变化）

例句 Metamorphosis is the biological process by which a caterpillar turns into a butterfly. 变形是毛毛虫转变为蝴蝶的生物过程。

metastasis 转移

词根 meta-（转化）+ -stasis（停留、扩散）

例句 Metastasis occurs when cancer cells spread from the primary site to other parts of the body. 癌细胞转移是指癌细胞从原发部位扩散到身体的其他部位。

metaplasia 化生

词根 meta-（转化）+ -plasia（形成）

例句 Metaplasia involves the transformation of one type of cell into another, often as an adaptive response. 化生是指一种细胞类型转化为另一种，通常是适应性反应。

metachromasia 变色现象

词根 meta-（转化）+ chrom-（颜色）+ -asia（状态）

例句 Metachromasia refers to the staining of tissues in different colors due to chemical properties. 变色现象是指由于化学性质不同，组织被染成不同颜色。

metabolite 代谢物

词根 meta-（转化）+ -bolite（物质）

例句 Metabolites are the intermediates and products of metabolism, essential for cellular processes. 代谢物是新陈代谢中的中间产物和最终产物，对于细胞过程至关重要。

USMLE Step 2 CK 样题

A 50-year-old woman comes to the office for a health maintenance examination. She feels well. Medical history is unremarkable (un-) and she takes no medications. There is no family history of serious illness. Physical examination, including breast examination, discloses no abnormalities. Mammography (mammo-; -graphy) shows a cluster of 20 pleomorphic (pleo-; morph-) microcalcifications (micro-; calc-) in a 1-cm area at the 2-o'clock position of the right breast. Which of the following is the most likely diagnosis?

(A) Ductal carcinoma (carcin-; -oma) in situ

(B) Fat necrosis

(C) Fibroadenoma (fibro-; aden-; -oma)

(D) Mastitis (mast-; -itis)

(E) Sclerosing (scler-) adenosis (aden-; -osis)

中文翻译

一名 50 岁女性来到门诊进行体检。她感觉良好。既往病史无特殊，未服用任何药物。家族无严重疾病史。乳房检查未发现异常。乳腺 X 线检查显示右乳房 2 点钟位置 1 cm 区域内有 20 个多形性微钙化灶。以下哪项是最可能的诊断？

(A) 原位导管癌

(B) 脂肪坏死

(C) 纤维腺瘤

(D) 乳腺炎

(E) 硬化性腺病

题目和答案中出现的词根

un-：表否定

mammo-：乳房

-graphy：图像

pleo-：多的

morph-：形状

micro-：微小的

calc-：钙

calcin：癌

-oma：瘤

fibro-：纤维的

aden：腺

mast-：乳房

-itis：炎症

scler-：硬的

-osis：病理状态

metri-（子宫）

endometritis 子宫内膜炎

词根 endo-（内部）+ metri-（子宫）+ -itis（炎症）

例句 Endometritis is an inflammation of the inner lining of the uterus, often due to infection. 子宫内膜炎是子宫内膜的炎症，通常由感染引起。

metritis 子宫炎

词根 metri-（子宫）+ -itis（炎症）

例句 Metritis refers to inflammation of the uterus, often occurring after childbirth or abortion. 子宫炎是子宫的炎症，通常发生在分娩或流产后。

perimetritis 子宫周围炎

词根 peri-（周围）+ metri-（子宫）+ -itis（炎症）

例句 Perimetritis is an inflammation of the tissue surrounding the uterus, often due to pelvic infections. 子宫周围炎是子宫周围组织的炎症，通常由盆腔感染引起。

myometrium 子宫肌层

词根 myo-（肌肉）+ metri-（子宫）+ -um（结构）

例句 The myometrium is the thick, muscular layer of the uterus that contracts during childbirth. 子宫肌层是子宫厚实的肌肉层，

在分娩时收缩。

endometrium 子宫内膜

词根 endo-（内部）+ metri-（子宫）+ -um（结构）

例句 The endometrium is the innermost layer of the uterus and is shed during menstruation. 子宫内膜是子宫最内层，会在月经期间脱落。

parametritis 子宫旁炎

词根 para-（旁边）+ metri-（子宫）+ -itis（炎症）

例句 Parametritis involves inflammation of the tissues adjacent to the uterus. 子宫旁炎是指子宫旁边组织的炎症。

metrodynia 子宫痛

词根 metri-（子宫）+ -dynia（疼痛）

例句 Metrodynia is characterized by severe uterine pain, often related to menstrual disorders. 子宫痛的特征是严重的子宫疼痛，通常与月经紊乱有关。

metrostaxis 子宫渗血

词根 metri-（子宫）+ -staxis（滴流、渗血）

例句 Metrostaxis refers to slow and continuous bleeding from the uterus, often due to trauma or infection. 子宫渗血是指子宫持续缓慢出血，通常由创伤或感染引起。

-metry（测量）

geometry 几何学

词根 geo-（地球）+ -metry（测量）

例句 Geometry is the branch of mathematics concerned with the properties and relationships of points, lines, and shapes. 几何学是研究点、线和形状的性质及其关系的数学分支。

optometry 验光

词根 opto-（视力）+ -metry（测量）

例句 Optometry involves the examination of eyes to measure vision and prescribe corrective lenses. 验光是对眼睛进行检查，以测量视力并配制矫正镜片的过程。

biometry 生物测量

词根 bio-（生命）+ -metry（测量）

例句 Biometry is the application of statistical analysis to biological data. 生物测量是将统计分析应用于生物数据的一种方法。

thermometry 温度测量

词根 thermo-（热）+ -metry（测量）

例句 Thermometry is essential in medical diagnostics to monitor body temperature. 温度测量在医学诊断中至关重要，用于监测体温。

audiometry 听力测量

词根 audio-（听觉）+ -metry（测量）

例句 Audiometry tests are used to assess a person's hearing capabilities and detect hearing loss. 听力测量用于评估一个人的听力能力并检测听力损失。

anthropometry 人体测量

词根 anthropo-（人类）+ -metry（测量）

例句 Anthropometry is commonly used in ergonomic design to ensure proper fit and function of equipment. 人体测量常用于人体工程学设计，以确保设备的合适和功能。

spirometry 肺活量测定

词根 spiro-（呼吸）+ -metry（测量）

例句 Spirometry is a pulmonary function test that measures how much air a person can inhale and exhale. 肺活量测定是一种测量

人吸入和呼出空气量的肺功能测试。

barometry 气压测量

词根 baro-（压力）+ -metry（测量）
例句 Barometry is used to monitor atmospheric pressure, which can help predict weather changes. 气压测量用于监测大气压力，有助于预测天气变化。

photometry 光度测量

词根 photo-（光）+ -metry（测量）
例句 Photometry is used to measure the intensity of light in various environments. 光度测量用于测量不同环境中的光强。

craniometry 颅骨测量

词根 cranio-（颅骨）+ -metry（测量）
例句 Craniometry was historically used to study human evolution and skull structure. 颅骨测量曾被用于研究人类进化和头骨结构。

micell-（微胶粒）

micelle 胶束

词根 micell-（微胶粒）
例句 Micelles are aggregates of surfactant molecules dispersed in a liquid, often used in cleaning products. 胶束是分散在液体中的表面活性剂分子聚集体，常用于清洁产品中。

micellization 胶束化

词根 micell-（微胶粒）+ -ization（过程）
例句 Micellization occurs when surfactant molecules form micelles in a solution. 胶束化是指表面活性剂分子在溶液中形成胶束的过程。

polymeric micelle 聚合物胶束

词根 poly-（多）+ micell-（微胶粒）

例句 Polymeric micelles are used in drug delivery to enhance the solubility of poorly water-soluble drugs. 聚合物胶束用于药物递送，增强难溶于水药物的溶解性。

reverse micelle 反胶束

词根 reverse（反转）+ micell-（微胶粒）
例句 Reverse micelles are formed in nonpolar solvents, where the hydrophilic ends of surfactants are in the center. 反胶束是在非极性溶剂中形成的，此时表面活性剂的亲水端在中心。

micellar water 胶束水

词根 micell-（微胶粒）+ water（水）
例句 Micellar water is a popular skincare product that cleanses and removes makeup using micelles. 胶束水是一种受欢迎的护肤产品，通过胶束来清洁和卸妆。

micellar solubilization 胶束增溶

词根 micell-（微胶粒）+ solubilization（溶解）
例句 Micellar solubilization is used to dissolve poorly water-soluble drugs in aqueous solutions. 胶束增溶用于将难溶于水的药物溶解在水溶液中。

micellar phase 胶束相

词根 micell-（微胶粒）+ phase（相）
例句 The micellar phase refers to the formation of micelles in a system, which can alter the system's properties. 胶束相指的是系统中胶束的形成，这可以改变系统的性质。

micellar carrier 胶束载体

词根 micell-（微胶粒）+ carrier（载体）
例句 Micellar carriers are used in drug delivery systems to transport hydrophobic drugs. 胶束载体用于药物递送系统，以运输疏水性药物。

micell-forming agents 胶束形成剂

词根 micell-（微胶粒）+ forming agents（形成剂）

例句 Micell-forming agents are added to solutions to induce the formation of micelles. 胶束形成剂被添加到溶液中以诱导胶束的形成。

micellar aggregates 胶束聚集体

词根 micell-（微胶粒）+ aggregates（聚集体）

例句 Micellar aggregates are clusters of micelles that play a role in the solubilization of nonpolar substances. 胶束聚集体是胶束的聚集体，在增溶非极性物质中起重要作用。

USMLE Step 2 CK　样题

A 42-year-old nulligravid (null-; -gravid) woman comes to the office because of a 6-month history of hot flashes and intermittent (inter-; -mitt) palpitations (palpit-; -ation). Her last menstrual period was 6 months ago. Menses previously occurred at regular 29-day intervals (inter-; -val) but gradually had occurred less frequently during the past 2 years. She underwent ovarian cystectomy (cyst-; -ectomy) 13 years ago for a small benign teratoma (terat-; -oma). She used an oral contraceptive (contra-; -cept) for 12 years until tubal ligation 6 years ago. Her mother and sister had menopause (meno-; -pause) at the ages of 47 and 49 years, respectively. The patient has smoked one pack of cigarettes (cigar-; -ette) daily for 26 years. She is sexually active and monogamous (mono-; gam-) with one male partner. She is 170 cm tall and weighs 86 kg; BMI is 30 kg/m^2 . Pulse is 82/min and blood pressure is 130/85 mmHg. Physical examination, including pelvic examination, discloses no abnormalities. Which of the following is the most appropriate next step in diagnosis?

(A) Measurement of serum follicle-stimulating hormone concentration

(B) Measurement of serum luteinizing hormone concentration

(C) Measurement of serum testosterone (test-;ster-; -one) concentration

(D) ECG

(E) Pelvic ultrasonography (ultra-; sono-; -graphy)

中文翻译

一名 42 岁未孕女性来到诊所，因 6 个月来出现潮热和间歇性心悸。她最后一次月经是在 6 个月前。此前月经周期为规律的 29 天，但在过去 2 年中逐渐变得不规律。她 13 年前因小型良性畸胎瘤接受了卵巢囊肿切除术。她曾使用口服避孕药 12 年，直到 6 年前进行了输卵管结扎术。她的母亲和姐姐分别在 47 岁和 49 岁时进入更年期。患者有 26 年每天吸一包烟的吸烟史。她与一名男性保持单一性关系。她身高 170 cm，体重 86 kg；BMI 为 30 kg/m²。脉搏 82 次 / 分钟，血压 130/85 mmHg。盆腔检查未发现异常。以下哪项是诊断中最适当的下一步？

(A) 测量血清卵泡刺激激素浓度

(B) 测量血清黄体生成素浓度

(C) 测量血清睾酮浓度

(D) 心电图检查

(E) 盆腔超声检查

题目和答案中出现的词根

null-：没有

-gravid：怀孕

inter-：在……之间

mitt-：时间区间

palpit-：快速敲击

-ation：表示动作的状态

inter-：在……之间

-val：空间

cyst-：囊

-ectomy：切除术

terat-：怪物

-oma：瘤

contra-：反

-cept：获得

meno-：每个月

-pause：停止

cigar-：雪茄

-ette：小的

mono-：单个的

gam-：婚姻

test-：睾丸

ster-：固体的

-one：酮

ultra-：超

sono-：声音的

-graphy：图像

micro-（小）

microscope 显微镜

词根 micro-（小）+ -scope（观察）

例句 A microscope is an essential tool in biology for observing small structures, such as cells. 显微镜是生物学中观察小结构（如细胞）的重要工具。

microorganism 微生物

词根 micro-（小）+ organism（生物）

例句 Microorganisms, such as bacteria and fungi, play important roles in ecosystems. 微生物（如细菌和真菌）在生态系统中起着重要作用。

microcephaly 小头症

词根 micro-（小）+ -cephaly（头）

例句 Microcephaly is a condition in which an infant’s head is significantly smaller than expected. 小头症是指婴儿的头部明显小于正常预期。

microbiology 微生物学

词根 micro-（小）+ -biology（生物学）

例句 Microbiology is the study of microscopic organisms, including viruses, bacteria, and fungi. 微生物学是研究微小生物体（包括病毒、细菌和真菌）的学科。

microvascular 微血管的

词根 micro-（小）+ vascular（血管的）

例句 Microvascular complications are common in diabetes, affecting small blood vessels in the eyes and kidneys. 糖尿病常见微血管

并发症，影响眼睛和肾脏中的小血管。

microcosm 微观世界

词根 micro-（小）+ -cosm（宇宙）

例句 A microcosm can represent a small-scale version of a larger system, such as a classroom mirroring society. 微观世界可以代表更大系统的小型缩影，例如教室反映社会。

micrometer 微米测量仪

词根 micro-（小）+ -meter（测量仪）

例句 A micrometer is a device used to measure extremely small distances or thicknesses. 微米测量仪是一种用于测量极小距离或厚度的仪器。

micrograph 显微照片

词根 micro-（小）+ -graph（记录）

例句 A micrograph provides a photographic record of objects observed under a microscope. 显微照片是显微镜下观测对象的摄影记录。

microanatomy 微观解剖学

词根 micro-（小）+ anatomy（解剖学）

例句 Microanatomy focuses on the structures within tissues and cells that are too small to see with the naked eye. 微观解剖学研究肉眼无法观察的组织和细胞内部结构。

microangiopathy 微血管病

词根 micro-（小）+ angio-（血管）+ -pathy（病）

例句 Microangiopathy is a disease affecting the small blood vessels, commonly seen in diabetic patients. 微血管病是影响小血管的疾病，常见于糖尿病患者。

mito-（线；丝）

mitochondria 线粒体

词根 mito-（线）+ chondria（粒）

例句 Mitochondria are known as the powerhouse of the cell, responsible for producing energy. 线粒体被称为细胞的能量工厂，负责生产能量。

mitosis 有丝分裂

词根 mito-（线）+ -sis（过程）

例句 Mitosis is a process of cell division that results in two genetically identical daughter cells. 有丝分裂是细胞分裂的过程，产生两个基因完全相同的子细胞。

mitomycin 丝裂霉素

词根 mito-（丝）+ mycin（抗生素）

例句 Mitomycin is an anticancer drug that inhibits DNA synthesis by blocking cell division. 丝裂霉素是一种抗癌药，通过阻断细胞分裂来抑制 DNA 合成。

mitophagy 线粒体自噬

词根 mito-（线粒体）+ -phagy（吞噬）

例句 Mitophagy is the process by which damaged mitochondria are degraded and recycled by the cell. 线粒体自噬是细胞降解和回收受损线粒体的过程。

mitotic spindle 有丝分裂纺锤体

词根 mito-（丝）+ spindle（纺锤体）

例句 The mitotic spindle plays a crucial role in separating chromosomes during cell division. 有丝分裂纺锤体在细胞分裂过程中

起到分离染色体的关键作用。

mitofusin 线粒体融合蛋白

词根 mito-（线粒体）+ -fusin（融合）

例句 Mitofusin proteins help in the fusion of mitochondria, which is essential for maintaining cellular energy balance. 线粒体融合蛋白有助于线粒体的融合，对于维持细胞能量平衡至关重要。

mitoplasm 线粒体质

词根 mito-（线粒体）+ plasm（质）

例句 The mitoplasm contains enzymes crucial for energy production within the mitochondria. 线粒体质含有在线粒体内能量生产过程中起重要作用的酶。

mitogenesis 线粒体生成

词根 mito-（线粒体）+ genesis（生成）

例句 Mitogenesis involves the biogenesis of new mitochondria within cells, which is critical for energy metabolism. 线粒体生成指细胞内新线粒体的生物合成，是能量代谢的重要组成部分。

mitofibril 线粒纤维

词根 mito-（线）+ fibril（纤维）

例句 Mitofibrils are structures within cells that consist of mitochondria and help maintain cellular function. 线粒纤维是细胞内由线粒体组成的结构，有助于维持细胞功能。

USMLE Step 2 CK　样题

A 68-year-old woman returns to the office for a follow-up examination. One month ago, urinalysis (urin-; -lysis) showed protein during workup of a suspected urinary tract infection. At that time, the patient was prescribed a 3-day course of oral cephalexin (cephal-). Today, she says her previous pain on urination (urin-; -ation) and urinary frequency have resolved. She has major depressive disorder (dis-) and osteoarthritis (osteo-; arthr-; -itis). Current medications are venlafaxine and acetaminophen (acet-; amin-; -ophen). Temperature is 37.0°C (98.6°F), pulse is 66/min, respirations (re-; spir-; -ation) are 18/min, and blood pressure is 122/66 mmHg. The patient appears physically fit. Examination discloses no abnormalities. Repeat urinalysis (urin-; -lysis) is shown:

Specific gravity 1.015 (N=1.003–1.029)

pH 6.0 (N=4.5–7.8)

Protein negative

Blood negative

Leukocyte (leuk-; -cyte) esterase (-ase) negative

Nitrite negative

WBCs 3/hpf

RBCs 1/hpf

Which of the following is the most appropriate additional diagnostic study at this time?

(A) Determination of urine albumin (album-) :creatinine ratio

(B) 24-Hour urine collection for measurement of protein concentration

(C) Ultrasonography (ultra-; sono-; -graphy) of the kidneys

(D) Urine sulfosalicylic (sulfo-; salicyl-) acid method

(E) No additional testing is indicated

中文翻译

一名 68 岁女性来门诊复查。一个月前，因怀疑尿路感染而进行的尿液分析显示尿蛋白阳性。当时，患者接受了3天的口服头孢氨苄治疗。今天，她表示之前的排尿疼痛和尿频已消退。她患有重度抑郁症和骨关节炎。目前服用的药物包括文拉法辛和对乙酰氨基酚。体温37.0℃（98.6℉），脉搏66次/分钟，呼吸18次/分钟，血压122/66 mmHg。患者体型健康。体检未发现异常。复查尿常规结果如下：

比重 1.015（正常范围：1.003 ～ 1.029）

pH 6.0（正常范围：4.5 ～ 7.8）

蛋白 阴性

血液 阴性

白细胞酯酶 阴性

亚硝酸盐 阴性

白细胞 3/ 高倍视野

红细胞 1/ 高倍视野

此时最适当的额外检查是以下哪项？

(A) 测定尿液白蛋白：肌酐比率

(B) 24 小时尿液收集以测量蛋白浓度

(C) 肾脏超声检查

(D) 尿液磺基水杨酸法

(E) 无须额外检查

题目和答案中出现的词根

urin：尿的

-lysis：分解

cephal-：脑

-ation：表示动作的状态

dis-：表示离开

osteo-：骨

arthr-：关节

-itis：炎症

acet-：乙酰基

amin-：胺

-ophen：芳香环

re-：重新；反复

spir：呼吸

-ation：表示动作的状态

leuk-：白色的

-cyte：细胞

-ase：酶

album-：白色的

ultra-：超

sono-：声音的

-graphy：图像

sulfo-：磺酸

salicyl-：柳树

mono-（一个）

monosaccharide 单糖

词根 mono-（一个）+ saccharide（糖）

例句 Glucose and fructose are examples of monosaccharides, the simplest form of carbohydrates. 葡萄糖和果糖是单糖，单糖是碳水化合物的最简单形式。

monochromatic 单色的

词根 mono-（一个）+ chromatic（颜色的）

例句 A monochromatic light source emits light of a single wavelength and color. 单色光源发出波长和颜色单一的光。

mononuclear 单核的

词根 mono-（单）+ nuclear（核的）

例句 Mononuclear cells, such as lymphocytes, have a single, large nucleus. 单核细胞（如淋巴细胞）具有单个较大的细胞核。

monosomy 单体性

词根 mono-（一个）+ somy（染色体）

例句 Monosomy is a chromosomal disorder in which one chromosome of a pair is missing. 单体性是染色体异常的一种形式，指一对染色体中缺失一个。

monoclonal 单克隆的

词根 mono-（单）+ clonal（克隆的）

例句 Monoclonal antibodies are laboratory-made molecules that target specific cells. 单克隆抗体是实验室制造的分子，专门针对特定细胞。

monocyte 单核细胞

词根 mono-（单）+ -cyte（细胞）

例句 Monocytes are a type of white blood cell involved in immune defense and inflammation control. 单核细胞是参与免疫防御和炎症控制的一类白细胞。

morph-（形态）

morphology 形态学

词根 morph-（形态）+ -logy（学科）

例句 Morphology is the study of the form and structure of organisms and their specific structural features. 形态学是研究生物体的形式、结构及其特定结构特征的学科。

polymorphism 多形性

词根 poly-（多）+ morph-（形态）+ -ism（状态）

例句 Polymorphism is common in nature, allowing species to adapt to various environmental conditions. 多形性在自然界中很常见，使物种能够适应各种环境条件。

morphogenesis 形态发生

词根 morph-（形态）+ -genesis（形成）

例句 Morphogenesis is the biological process that causes an organism to develop its shape. 形态发生是引导生物体发育成特定形状的生物学过程。

dimorphic 双形的

词根 di-（双）+ morph-（形态）+ -ic（形容词后缀）

例句 Dimorphic fungi can exist in two different forms depending on environmental conditions. 双形态真菌可以根据环境条件以两种不同的形式存在。

morphometry 形态测量学

词根 morph-（形态）+ -metry（测量）

例句 Morphometry involves measuring the shape, size, and structure of organisms or their parts. 形态测量学指对生物体或其部分的形状、大小和结构的测量。

amorphous 无定形的

词根 a-（无）+ morph-（形态）+ -ous（形容词后缀）

例句 Amorphous materials lack a clear, defined structure or shape, such as glass. 无定形材料没有明确的结构或形状，例如玻璃。

morphotype 形态型

词根 morph-（形态）+ -type（类型）

例句 A morphotype refers to the distinct form or structure exhibited by an organism or cell. 形态型是指生物体或细胞表现出的特定形态或结构。

morphogen 形态发生素

词根 morph-（形态）+ -gen（产生）

例句 Morphogens are substances that govern the pattern of tissue development during morphogenesis. 形态发生素是指导组织发育模式的重要物质。

USMLE Step 2 CK 样题

A 70-year-old woman comes to the office because of three episodes (epi-; -sode) of rectal bleeding during the past 4 days. During each episode, she had the sudden urge to have a bowel movement and then passed a bright red, bloody stool. She has not had chest, abdominal, or rectal pain, palpitations (palpit-; -ation), dizziness, light-headedness, or black stools. Her most recent colonoscopy (colon-; -scopy) 8 years ago showed no abnormalities. She has osteoarthritis (osteo-; arthr-; -itis) treated with daily ibuprofen. She takes no other medications. She is 168 cm tall and weighs 69 kg; BMI is 25 kg/m^2. Temperature is 37.0°C (98.6°F), and respirations (re-; spir-; ation) are 16/min. While sitting, her pulse is 80/min and blood pressure is 130/76 mmHg. While standing, her pulse is 88/min and blood pressure is 126/74 mmHg. On examination, mucous membranes are moist. The abdomen is soft, nontender (non-), and nondistended (non-). There is no rebound (re-) tenderness or guarding. Bowel sounds are normal. Rectal examination shows no stool in the vault; there are no masses. Which of the following is the most likely diagnosis?

(A) Anal fissure

(B) Colonic polyp

(C) Diverticulosis (diverticul-; -osis)

(D) Duodenal ulcer

(E) Gastritis (gastr-; -itis)

(F) Ulcerative colitis (col-; -itis)

中文翻译

一名 70 岁女性来就诊，因过去 4 天内发生 3 次直肠出血。每次出血时，她均突然感到便意迫切，随后排出鲜红色血便。她没有胸痛、腹痛、直肠痛、心悸、头晕或黑便。她最近一次结肠镜检查是在 8 年前，结果正常。她患有骨关节炎，每日服用布洛芬治疗。她未服用其他药物。她身高 168 cm，体重 69 kg；BMI 为 25 kg/m²。体温 37.0℃（98.6℉），呼吸 16 次 / 分钟。坐位时脉搏 80 次 / 分钟，血压 130/76 mmHg；站立时脉搏 88 次 / 分钟，血压 126/74 mmHg。检查显示黏膜湿润。腹部柔软，无压痛，无膨隆。无反跳痛或腹肌紧张。肠鸣音正常。直肠检查显示直肠内无粪便，无肿块。以下哪项是最可能的诊断？

(A) 肛裂

(B) 结肠息肉

(C) 憩室病

(D) 十二指肠溃疡

(E) 胃炎

(F) 溃疡性结肠炎

题目和答案中出现的词根

epi-：在……上（或旁）

-sode：道路

palpit-：快速敲击

-ation：表示动作的状态

colon-：结肠

-scopy：镜

osteo-：骨

arthr-：关节

-itis：炎症

re-：重新；反复

spir：呼吸

non-：表示否定

re-：再次

diverticul-：袋状

-osis：病理状态

gastr-：胃

col-：结肠

-morphy（形态）

M

polymorphy 多形性

词根 poly-（多）+ -morphy（形态）

例句 Polymorphy is common in minerals where the same chemical composition can form different crystal structures. 多形性在矿物中很常见，相同的化学成分可以形成不同的晶体结构。

dimorphy 双形性

词根 di-（二）+ -morphy（形态）

例句 Dimorphy describes organisms or substances that can exist in two distinct forms. 双形性描述的是可以存在两种不同形态的生物或物质。

isomorphy 同形性

词根 iso-（相同）+ -morphy（形态）

例句 Isomorphy occurs when compounds have the same crystal structure but different compositions. 同形性指的是化合物具有相同的晶体结构但成分不同。

monomorphy 单形性

词根 mono-（单一）+ -morphy（形态）

例句 Monomorphy is seen in organisms that maintain a single, consistent form throughout their lifecycle. 单形性在整个生命周期中保持单一稳定形态的生物中可见。

homeomorphy 相似形态

词根 homeo-（相似）+ -morphy（形态）

例句 Homeomorphy is observed in unrelated species that develop similar structures due to convergent evolution. 相似形态见于无亲

缘关系的物种中，这些物种因趋同进化而发育出相似的结构。

trimorphy 三形性

词根 tri-（三）+ -morphy（形态）

例句 Trimorphy describes materials that can exist in three different crystal or molecular forms. 三形性描述的是物质可以以三种不同的晶体或分子形态存在。

heteromorphy 异形性

词根 hetero-（不同）+ -morphy（形态）

例句 Heteromorphy is seen in plants and animals where different life stages exhibit varying forms. 异形性可见于植物和动物，指在不同的生命阶段表现出不同的形态。

amorphy 无形性

词根 a-（无）+ -morphy（形态）

例句 Amorphy refers to the lack of a defined shape or structure, commonly seen in amorphous solids. 无形性指的是缺乏明确形状或结构，常见于无定形固体中。

mort-（死亡）

mortality 死亡率

词根 mort-（死亡）+ -ality（性质）

例句 Mortality rates are used to assess the frequency of deaths within a given population. 死亡率用于评估特定人群中的死亡概率。

immortal 不朽的

词根 im-（否定）+ mort-（死亡）+ -al（形容词后缀）

例句 Many ancient legends describe gods and heroes as immortal beings. 许多古老传说中描述了神和英雄是不朽的存在。

mortician 殡葬师

词根 mort-（死亡）+ -ician（从事某职业的人）

例句 The mortician is responsible for preparing the body and conducting funeral services. 殡葬师负责准备遗体并主持葬礼。

postmortem 死后的

词根 post-（后）+ mort-（死亡）

例句 A postmortem examination is conducted to determine the cause of death. 死后检查用于确定死亡原因。

mortal 凡人

词根 mort-（死亡）+ -al（形容词或名词后缀）

例句 Unlike the gods of mythology, humans are mortal and face death eventually. 与神话中的神不同，人类是凡人，最终会面临死亡。

mortuary 停尸房

词根 mort-（死亡）+ -uary（场所）

例句 The body was taken to the mortuary for identification and postmortem analysis. 遗体被送往停尸房进行身份确认和死后分析。

moribund 濒死的

词根 mort-（死亡）+ -bund（接近）

例句 The patient was moribund and required immediate medical attention. 患者处于濒死状态，需要立即接受医疗救助。

mortiferous 致命的

词根 mort-（死亡）+ -ferous（产生的）

例句 Certain snake species possess mortiferous venom capable of causing death. 某些蛇类具有致命的毒液，可能引发死亡。

-myces（真菌）

actinomyces 放线菌

词根 actino-（射线）+ -myces（真菌）

例句 Actinomyces are bacteria that resemble fungi and are commonly found in soil and decaying organic material. 放线菌是一种类似真菌的细菌，常见于土壤和腐烂的有机物中。

ascomycetes 子囊菌

词根 asco-（囊）+ -mycetes（真菌）

例句 Ascomycetes are a large group of fungi that produce spores in sac-like structures. 子囊菌是产生孢子于囊状结构中的一大类真菌。

basidiomycetes 担子菌

词根 basidio-（基部）+ -mycetes（真菌）

例句 Basidiomycetes include mushrooms and other fungi that produce spores on a basidium. 担子菌包括蘑菇和其他在担子上产生孢子的真菌。

deuteromyces 半知菌

词根 deutero-（第二）+ -myces（真菌）

例句 Deuteromyces are fungi classified based on asexual reproduction as their sexual stage is unknown. 半知菌是根据无性繁殖分类的真菌，其有性阶段尚不明确。

oomycetes 水霉菌

词根 oo-（卵）+ -myces（真菌）

例句 Oomycetes are water molds that can cause serious plant diseases, such as late blight in potatoes. 水霉菌是可引起严重植物疾病的水生霉菌，如马铃薯晚疫病。

zygomyces 接合菌

词根 zygo-（接合）+ -myces（真菌）

例句 Zygomyces are fungi characterized by the formation of zygospores during reproduction. 接合菌是以繁殖过程中形成接合孢子为特征的真菌。

eumycetes 真菌纲

词根 eu-（真正的）+ -myces（真菌）

例句 Eumycetes refer to the true fungi, which include yeasts, molds, and mushrooms. 真菌纲指真核真菌，包括酵母、霉菌和蘑菇。

saccharomyces 酵母菌

词根 saccharo-（糖）+ -myces（真菌）

例句 Saccharomyces is a genus of yeast used in baking, brewing, and fermentation processes. 酵母菌用于烘焙、酿造和发酵过程。

geomyces 地真菌

词根 geo-（地）+ -myces（真菌）

例句 Geomyces are fungi found in soil and known for causing diseases in plants and animals. 地真菌是生活在土壤中的真菌，会引起植物和动物患病。

dermatophytes 皮肤真菌

词根 dermato-（皮肤）+ -myces（真菌）

例句 Dermatophytes are fungi that infect the skin, hair, and nails, leading to conditions such as ringworm. 皮肤真菌是感染皮肤、头发和指甲的真菌，可导致癣等疾病。

-mycin（抗生素）

erythromycin 红霉素

词根 erythro-（红色）+ -mycin（抗生素后缀）

例句 Erythromycin is an antibiotic used to treat a variety of bacterial infections, especially for those allergic to penicillin. 红霉素是一种用于治疗多种细菌感染的抗生素，特别用于对青霉素过敏的患者。

streptomycin 链霉素

词根 strepto-（链状）+ -mycin（抗生素后缀）
例句 Streptomycin is an antibiotic commonly used in the treatment of tuberculosis. 链霉素是治疗结核病的常用抗生素。

clindamycin 克林霉素

词根 clinda-（临床）+ -mycin（抗生素后缀）
例句 Clindamycin is used to treat bacterial infections, particularly those involving anaerobic bacteria. 克林霉素用于治疗细菌感染，特别是厌氧菌的感染。

vancomycin 万古霉素

词根 vancomycin（万古霉素）
例句 Vancomycin is an antibiotic used to treat severe bacterial infections, especially those caused by Gram-positive bacteria. 万古霉素是一种用于治疗严重细菌感染的抗生素，特别是由革兰氏阳性菌引起的感染。

azithromycin 阿奇霉素

词根 azithro-（类阿奇霉素）+ -mycin（抗生素后缀）
例句 Azithromycin is a broad-spectrum antibiotic used to treat respiratory infections and sexually transmitted diseases. 阿奇霉素是一种广谱抗生素，用于治疗呼吸道感染和性传播疾病。

gentamycin 庆大霉素

词根 gent-（庆大）+ -mycin（抗生素后缀）
例句 Gentamicin is an aminoglycoside antibiotic used to treat a variety of serious bacterial infections. 庆大霉素是一种氨基糖苷类抗

生素，用于治疗多种严重的细菌感染。

tobramycin 托布霉素

词根 tobra-（托布霉素）+ -mycin（抗生素后缀）
例句 Tobramycin is an antibiotic used to treat infections caused by Gram-negative bacteria. 托布霉素是一种用于治疗革兰氏阴性细菌感染的抗生素。

neomycin 新霉素

词根 neo-（新的）+ -mycin（抗生素后缀）
例句 Neomycin is an antibiotic used to treat bacterial infections and as a topical treatment for skin infections. 新霉素是一种用于治疗细菌感染的抗生素，也用于治疗局部的皮肤感染。

myco-（真菌）

mycology 真菌学

词根 myco-（真菌）+ -logy（学科）
例句 Mycology is the branch of biology that deals with the study of fungi, including molds and yeasts. 真菌学是研究真菌（包括霉菌和酵母菌）的生物学分支。

mycosis 真菌病

词根 myco-（真菌）+ -osis（病症）
例句 Athlete's foot is a common form of mycosis affecting the skin of the feet. 足癣是真菌病的一种常见形式，影响足部皮肤。

mycotoxin 真菌毒素

词根 myco-（真菌）+ toxin（毒素）
例句 Mycotoxins produced by molds can contaminate food and cause serious health issues. 霉菌产生的真菌毒素会污染食物并引发严重的健康问题。

mycophagous 食真菌的

词根 myco-（真菌）+ -phagous（食）

例句 Certain species of insects are mycophagous, feeding exclusively on fungi. 某些昆虫种类以真菌为食。

mycotoxinogenesis 真菌毒素生成

词根 myco-（真菌）+ toxin（毒素）+ -genesis（生成）

例句 Mycotoxinogenesis is a process by which fungi produce toxic compounds that can be harmful to humans. 真菌毒素生成是指真菌产生对人体有害的毒性化合物的过程。

mycotherapy 真菌疗法

词根 myco-（真菌）+ -therapy（治疗）

例句 Mycotherapy uses medicinal mushrooms to improve immune function and treat various diseases. 真菌疗法利用药用蘑菇来增强免疫功能并治疗各种疾病。

mycogenic 由真菌引起的

词根 myco-（真菌）+ -genic（引起）

例句 Mycogenic infections can affect the skin, lungs, or bloodstream depending on the type of fungus. 由真菌引起的感染可能影响皮肤、肺部或血液。

mycorrhiza 菌根

词根 myco-（真菌）+ rhiza（根）

例句 Mycorrhizae are beneficial associations between fungi and plant roots that enhance nutrient absorption. 菌根是真菌与植物根部之间的有益共生关系，增强了养分的吸收。

myo-（肌肉）

myopathy 肌病

词根 myo-（肌肉）+ -pathy（病）

例句 Myopathy refers to diseases that affect the muscles, leading to weakness or dysfunction. 肌病是指影响肌肉的疾病，导致肌肉无力或功能障碍。

myocardium 心肌

词根 myo-（肌肉）+ -cardium（心脏）

例句 The myocardium is the muscular layer of the heart responsible for pumping blood. 心肌是心脏的肌肉层，负责泵送血液。

myalgia 肌痛

词根 myo-（肌肉）+ -algia（疼痛）

例句 Myalgia is common after intense physical activity or muscle strain. 剧烈运动或肌肉拉伤后，肌肉疼痛很常见。

myositis 肌炎

词根 myo-（肌肉）+ -itis（炎症）

例句 Myositis involves inflammation of the muscles, which can cause pain and weakness. 肌炎是指肌肉的炎症，可引起疼痛和无力。

myomectomy 肌瘤切除术

词根 myo-（肌肉）+ -ectomy（切除）

例句 A myomectomy is performed to remove fibroids from the uterine muscle. 肌瘤切除术是切除子宫肌瘤的手术。

myotonia 肌强直

词根 myo-（肌肉）+ -tonia（紧张）

例句 Myotonia is characterized by delayed muscle relaxation after contraction. 肌强直的特征是肌肉收缩后松弛延迟。

myogenesis 肌生成

词根 myo-（肌肉）+ -genesis（生成）

例句 Myogenesis is the process by which muscle tissue forms during embryonic development. 肌生成是在胚胎发育过程中形成肌肉组织的过程。

myoclonic 肌阵挛的

词根 myo-（肌肉）+ -clonic（阵发性）

例句 Myoclonic seizures involve sudden, brief muscle jerks and are common in epilepsy. 肌阵挛发作表现为突然短暂的肌肉抽搐，在癫痫中较常见。

myocyte 肌细胞

词根 myo-（肌肉）+ -cyte（细胞）

例句 Myocytes are specialized cells that make up muscle tissue and contribute to contraction. 肌细胞是构成肌肉组织并参与收缩的特化细胞。

myoclonus 肌阵挛

词根 myo-（肌肉）+ -clonus（抽搐）

例句 Myoclonus refers to sudden, involuntary muscle contractions that can occur in various neurological disorders. 肌阵挛是指突然、不自主的肌肉收缩，可见于多种神经系统疾病中。

myxo-（黏液的）

myxoma 黏液瘤

词根 myxo-（黏液）+ -oma（肿瘤）

例句 A myxoma is a rare, usually benign tumor that often develops in the heart. 黏液瘤是一种罕见且通常是良性的肿瘤，常见于心脏中。

M

myxomatosis 黏液瘤病

词根 myxo-（黏液）+ -matosis（病症）

例句 Myxomatosis is a viral disease affecting rabbits, causing skin lesions and swelling. 黏液瘤病是一种影响兔子的病毒性疾病，引起皮肤损伤和肿胀。

myxovirus 黏液病毒

词根 myxo-（黏液）+ virus（病毒）

例句 Myxoviruses are a family of viruses that include influenza viruses. 黏液病毒是包括流感病毒在内的一类病毒。

myxocyte 黏液细胞

词根 myxo-（黏液）+ -cyte（细胞）

例句 Myxocytes are found in mucous tissues and secrete mucopolysaccharides. 黏液细胞存在于黏液组织中，分泌黏多糖。

myxodema 黏液性水肿

词根 myxo-（黏液）+ -edema（水肿）

例句 Myxodema is associated with hypothyroidism and involves the accumulation of mucopolysaccharides in tissues. 黏液性水肿与甲状腺功能减退有关，表现为组织中黏多糖的积累。

myxofibroma 黏液纤维瘤

词根 myxo-（黏液）+ fibroma（纤维瘤）

例句 Myxofibroma is a rare benign tumor composed of fibrous and mucous tissue. 黏液纤维瘤是一种由纤维组织和黏液组织构成的罕见良性肿瘤。

myxopapilloma 黏液乳头状瘤

词根 myxo-（黏液）+ papilloma（乳头状瘤）

例句 Myxopapillomas are uncommon tumors that primarily occur in mucous-secreting tissues. 黏液乳头状瘤是一种主要发生在分泌黏液的组织中的罕见肿瘤。

myxofibrosarcoma 黏液纤维肉瘤

词根 myxo-（黏液）+ fibro-（纤维）+ sarcoma（肉瘤）

例句 Myxofibrosarcoma is a type of soft tissue cancer with mucous and fibrous characteristics. 黏液纤维肉瘤是一种具有黏液和纤维特征的软组织癌。

myxomycetes 黏菌

词根 myxo-（黏液）+ mycetes（真菌）

例句 Myxomycetes, or slime molds, are organisms that exhibit characteristics of both fungi and amoebas. 黏菌是具有真菌和变形虫特征的生物。

myxosarcoma 黏液肉瘤

词根 myxo-（黏液）+ sarcoma（肉瘤）

例句 Myxosarcoma is a rare malignant tumor characterized by mucous-producing cancer cells. 黏液肉瘤是一种罕见的恶性肿瘤，其癌细胞会分泌黏液。

USMLE Step 2 CK　样题

A 6-year-old boy is brought to the emergency department by his mother because of the acute onset 1 hour ago of severe rightsided lumbar pain and three episodes of emesis. The pain is sharp and causes him to double over and cry. Medical and family histories are unremarkable (un-) . The patient takes no medications. Temperature is 36.7°C (98.0°F), pulse is 150/min, respirations (re-; spir-; -ation) are 30/min, and blood pressure is 110/70 mmHg. He appears to be in severe pain. Abdominal examination discloses right upper quadrant (quad-) tenderness to palpation. The remainder of the examination discloses no abnormalities. Intravenous (intra-; veno-) morphine is administered and results in improvement in the patient's pain. Results of dipstick urinalysis (urin-; -lysis) are shown:

Specific gravity 1.035 (N=1.003–1.029)

pH 5.5

Protein 30 mg/dL

Glucose Negative

Bilirubin (bili-; -rubin) Negative

Blood 4+

Leukocyte (leuk-; -cyte) esterase 1+

Nitrite Negative

Urobilinogen (uro-; bili-) Negative

WBCs 5–10/hpf

RBCs 50–100/hpf

Renal ultrasonography (ultra-; sono-; -graphy) shows severe right-sided hydronephrosis (hydro-; nephr-; -osis) with moderate hydroureter (hydro-) to the bladder. Which of the following is the most appropriate next step in evaluation?

(A) Captopril renography (reno-; -graphy)

(B) CT scan of the abdomen and pelvis

(C) MAG-3 renal scan with furosemide (-semide)

(D) Radionuclide (radio-; nuclide) cystography (cysto-; -graphy)

(E) Retrograde (retro-; -grade) pyelography (pyelo-; -graphy)

(F) Ultrasonography (ultra-; sono-; -graphy) of the spinal column

(G) Voiding cystourethrography (cysto-; urethro-; -graphy)

中文翻译

一名 6 岁男孩由其母亲带到急诊科，因 1 小时前突然出现右侧腰部剧烈疼痛，并伴有 3 次呕吐。疼痛剧烈且尖锐，导致他蜷缩身体并哭泣。病史和家族史无特殊。患者未服用任何药物。体温 36.7℃（98.0℉），脉搏 150 次 / 分钟，呼吸 30 次 / 分钟，血压 110/70 mmHg。患者表现为剧烈疼痛。腹部检查显示右上腹触诊有压痛。其余体检未发现异常。静脉注射吗啡后，患者疼痛有所缓解。尿液试纸分析结果如下：

比重 1.035（正常范围：1.003 ～ 1.029）

pH 5.5

蛋白 30 mg/dL

葡萄糖 阴性

胆红素 阴性

血液 4+

白细胞酯酶 1+

亚硝酸盐 阴性

尿胆原 阴性

白细胞 5 ～ 0/ 高倍视野

红细胞 50 ～ 100/ 高倍视野

肾脏超声显示右侧严重肾盂积水，伴有中度输尿管积水至膀胱。以下哪项是评估中最适当的下一步？

(A) 卡托普利肾显像

(B) 腹部和骨盆 CT 扫描

(C) MAG-3 肾扫描结合呋塞米

(D) 放射性核素膀胱造影

(E) 逆行肾盂造影

(F) 脊柱超声检查

(G) 排尿性膀胱尿道造影

题目和答案中出现的词根

un-：表否定

re-：重新；反复

spir：呼吸

-ation：表示动作的状态

quad-：四个

intra-：在……内

veno-：静脉

urin-：尿

-lysis：分解

bili-：胆

-rubin：红色

leuk-：白色的

-cyte：细胞

uro-：尿的

ultra-：超

sono-：声音的

-graphy：图像

hydro-：水

nephr-：肾

-osis：病理状态

reno-：肾脏

-semide：表示袢部利尿剂

radio-：放射性

nuclide：元素

cysto-：膀胱的

retro-：反向

-grade：等级；台阶

pyelo-：肾盂

urethro-：尿道的

narco-（睡觉；麻醉）

narcolepsy 嗜睡症

词根 narco-（睡觉）+ -lepsy（发作）

例句 Narcolepsy is a sleep disorder characterized by excessive daytime sleepiness and sudden sleep attacks. 嗜睡症是一种睡眠障碍，其特征是白天过度嗜睡和突然入睡。

narcotic 麻醉药

词根 narco-（麻醉）+ -tic（形容词后缀）

例句 Narcotics are drugs that relieve pain and induce sleep but can be addictive. 麻醉药是一种缓解疼痛并引起睡眠的药物，但可能导致成瘾。

narcosis 麻醉状态

词根 narco-（麻醉）+ -sis（状态）

例句 Narcosis refers to a state of stupor or unconsciousness induced by drugs or anesthesia. 麻醉状态是指由药物或麻醉引起的昏迷或意识丧失状态。

narcotherapy 催眠疗法

词根 narco-（睡觉）+ -therapy（治疗）

例句 Narcotherapy is used in psychiatry to help patients through prolonged sleep therapy. 催眠疗法用于精神病学中，通过长时间睡眠帮助患者恢复。

narcodilation 麻醉扩张

词根 narco-（麻醉）+ dilation（扩张）

例句 Narcodilation is the widening of blood vessels induced by narcotic drugs. 麻醉扩张是由麻醉药物引起的血管扩张。

narcogenesis 麻醉发生

词根 narco-（麻醉）+ -genesis（生成）

例句 Narcogenesis refers to the induction of a state of unconsciousness through the use of anesthetics. 麻醉发生是指使用麻醉剂引发的昏迷状态。

narcomania 麻醉成瘾

词根 narco-（麻醉）+ -mania（狂热）

例句 Narcomania is a psychological condition characterized by an uncontrollable addiction to narcotics. 麻醉成瘾是一种表现为对麻醉药物无法控制依赖的心理疾病。

narcoanesthesia 全身麻醉

词根 narco-（麻醉）+ anesthesia（无感觉）

例句 Narcoanesthesia involves the use of narcotics to induce a temporary loss of sensation or consciousness. 全身麻醉是通过麻醉药物引起的暂时性感觉或意识丧失。

narcodermal 麻醉皮肤的

词根 narco-（麻醉）+ dermal（皮肤的）

例句 Narcodermal patches are used to provide localized pain relief by releasing anesthetics through the skin. 皮肤麻醉贴片通过接触皮肤释放麻醉剂，提供局部止痛效果。

natr-（钠）

natriuretic 促钠尿排泄的

词根 natr-（钠）+ -uretic（尿的）

例句 Natriuretic peptides help regulate blood pressure by promoting sodium excretion through urine. 促钠尿排泄肽通过促进尿液中钠的排泄来调节血压。

hyponatremia 低钠血症

词根 hypo-（不足）+ natr-（钠）+ -emia（血液）

例句 Hyponatremia occurs when the sodium level in the blood is abnormally low. 低钠血症是指血液中的钠含量异常低。

hypernatremia 高钠血症

词根 hyper-（过多）+ natr-（钠）+ -emia（血液）

例句 Hypernatremia can cause dehydration and neurological symptoms due to excessive sodium levels. 高钠血症可能因钠含量过高引起脱水和神经症状。

natriuresis 钠排泄

词根 natr-（钠）+ -uresis（排尿）

例句 Natriuresis is a natural process in which the kidneys excrete excess sodium through urine. 钠排泄是指肾脏通过尿液排出体内多余钠的自然过程。

natriferous 含钠的

词根 natr-（钠）+ -ferous（含有）

例句 Natriferous minerals are important for maintaining sodium balance in the body. 含钠矿物质对于维持体内钠平衡非常重要。

natriphobia 对钠的恐惧

词根 natr-（钠）+ -phobia（恐惧）

例句 Natriphobia is a rare condition where individuals avoid sodium intake due to fear of its effects. 对钠的恐惧是一种罕见现象，患者因害怕钠的影响而避免摄入钠。

natrogenic 钠生成的

词根 natr-（钠）+ -genic（产生）

例句 Natrogenic conditions are caused by an imbalance in sodium metabolism. 钠生成性病症是由钠代谢失衡引起的。

natrioclasia 钠破坏

词根 natr-（钠）+ -clasia（破坏）

例句 Natrioclasia refers to conditions involving the breakdown of sodium in the body. 钠破坏是指体内钠分解的病症。

natriokinetic 钠流动的

词根 natr-（钠）+ kinetic（运动的）

例句 Natriokinetic drugs help regulate sodium movement within the body's fluid compartments. 钠流动药物有助于调节体液中钠的移动。

natriostasis 钠停滞

词根 natr-（钠）+ -stasis（停滞）

例句 Natriostasis can lead to an accumulation of sodium in tissues, causing edema. 钠停滞可能导致组织中钠积累，引起水肿。

nema-（线状）

nematode 线虫

词根 nema-（线）+ -tode（类）

例句 Nematodes are roundworms that can affect plants, animals, and humans. 线虫是一类圆形虫，能够影响植物、动物和人类。

nematoid 线虫状的

词根 nema-（线）+ -oid（类似）

例句 The nematoid appearance refers to an object or organism resembling a nematode in shape. 线虫状的外观指的是物体或生物在形态上类似线虫。

nematocyst 刺丝胞

词根 nema-（线）+ -cyst（囊）

例句 Nematocysts are specialized cells in jellyfish that release toxins when triggered. 刺丝胞是水母中的特化细胞，在受到刺激时释放毒素。

nematology 线虫学

词根 nema-（线）+ -logy（学科）

例句 Nematology is the scientific study of nematodes, including their biology and impact on agriculture. 线虫学是研究线虫及其对农业影响的科学。

nematogenesis 线虫发生

词根 nema-（线）+ -genesis（生成）

例句 Nematogenesis is the process of the reproduction and development of nematodes. 线虫发生是线虫的繁殖和发育过程。

nematocidal 杀线虫的

词根 nema-（线）+ -cidal（杀死的）

例句 Nematocidal treatments are used in agriculture to control nematode infestations in crops. 杀线虫的治疗用于农业中控制作物中的线虫侵害。

nematopathogenic 线虫致病的

词根 nema-（线）+ -pathogenic（致病的）

例句 Nematopathogenic fungi infect nematodes and can be used as a biological control agent. 线虫致病真菌感染线虫，并可用作生物防治剂。

nematophagous 食线虫的

词根 nema-（线）+ -phagous（食）

例句 Nematophagous organisms, like certain bacteria, feed on nematodes in soil. 食线虫的生物，如某些细菌，食用土壤中的线虫。

nematode infection 线虫感染

词根 nema-（线）+ -tode（类）

例句 Nematode infections can cause damage to the digestive system in both humans and animals. 线虫感染可引起人类和动物消化系统的损害。

neo-（新）

neoplasm 新生物；肿瘤

词根 neo-（新）+ -plasm（形成物）

例句 A neoplasm is an abnormal growth of tissue that may form a tumor. 肿瘤是指组织异常增生，可能形成肿块。

neonatal 新生儿的

词根 neo-（新）+ -natal（出生的）

例句 Neonatal care focuses on the medical needs of newborn infants. 新生儿护理专注于新生婴儿的医疗需求。

neogenesis 新生；重新生成

词根 neo-（新）+ -genesis（生成；起源）

例句 Neogenesis refers to the formation of new cells or tissues. 新生是指新细胞或组织的形成。

neurogenesis 神经发生

词根 neo-（新）+ neuro-（神经）+ -genesis（生成）

例句 Neurogenesis is the process by which new neurons are formed in the brain. 神经发生是新神经元在大脑中的形成过程。

neuroplasticity 神经可塑性

词根 neo-（新）+ neuro-（神经）+ -plasticity（可塑性）

例句 Neuroplasticity is the brain's ability to reorganize itself by forming new neural connections. 神经可塑性是大脑通过形成新的神经连接来重新组织自己的能力。

neocortex 新皮层

词根 neo-（新）+ cortex（皮层）

例句 The neocortex is the part of the brain responsible for higher-order functions such as sensory perception, cognition, and motor control. 新皮层是大脑中负责高级功能如感觉感知、认知和运动控制的部分。

neomorphism 新形态

词根 neo-（新）+ -morphism（形态）
例句 Neomorphism refers to the appearance of new morphological traits in an organism. 新形态是指生物体中出现新的形态特征。

USMLE Step 2 CK　样题

A 55-year-old woman comes to the office for a follow-up examination 3 months after sustaining an uncomplicated (un-) myocardial (myo-; cardi-) infarction in the distribution (dis-; tribut-) of the left anterior descending artery. She has participated in an outpatient rehabilitation (re-; habilit-) program since discharge from the hospital 6 weeks ago, but her attendance in the program has become irregular (ir-) during the past 4 weeks. When questioned about this, she reports a 4-week history of depressed mood, inability (in-) to enjoy activities she previously (pre-) found pleasurable, loss of appetite, and insomnia (in-; -somn). She also has hyperlipidemia (hyper-; lipid-; -emia) and hypertension (hyper-; -tension). Medications are aspirin, atorvastatin (-statin), and metoprolol (-lol). She is 163 cm tall and weighs 68 kg; BMI is 26 kg/m^2 . Vital signs are within normal limits. Lungs are clear to auscultation (auscult-; -ation). Cardiac examination discloses a normal rhythm. There is no peripheral edema. Results of serum studies are within the reference ranges. Which of the following is the most likely effect of this patient's depression on her overall health?

(A) It is likely to decrease her perceived (per-; -ceive) quality of life but have no impact on her mortality (-mortal)

(B) It is likely to double her risk for death during the next 3 months

(C) It is likely to decrease her risk for ischemia because she is likely to rest and avoid socializing

(D) It likely will have no significant effect on her physical health

中文翻译

一名 55 岁女性来到门诊复查，她在 3 个月前因左前降支动脉分布区的心肌梗死住院，病情无并发症。自 6 周前出院以来，她一直参加门诊康复计划，但在过去 4 周内，她的参与变得不规律。当被问及此事时，她自述 4 周来情绪低落，无法享受以前觉得愉悦的活动，食欲减退并且失眠。她还患有高脂血症和高血压。目前服用的药物包括阿司匹林、阿托伐他汀和美托洛尔。她身高 163 cm，体重 68 kg；BMI 为 26 kg/m^2。生命体征正常。肺部听诊清晰。心脏检查显示节律正常。无周围水肿。血清检查结果在参考范围内。以下哪项是该患者抑郁情绪对其整体健康最可能的影响？

(A) 可能会降低她的感知生活质量，但对死亡率无影响

(B) 可能会使她在未来 3 个月内的死亡风险翻倍

(C) 可能会降低她的心脏缺血风险，因为她可能会休息并避免社交

(D) 可能对她的身体健康无显著影响

题目和答案中出现的词根

un-：表否定

myo-：肌肉

cardi-：心脏

dis-：离开

tribut-：排列

re-：重新，反复

habilit-：健康

ir-：表否定

in-：表否定

pre-：在……之前

-somn：睡眠

hyper-：高

lipid-：脂肪

-emia：血症

-tension：张力；压力

-statin：静止。

-lol：β受体阻滞剂类的药物

auscult-：听

-ation：表示动作

per-：经过

-ceive：抓住

-mortal：死亡

nephr-（肾）

nephritis 肾炎

词根 nephr-（肾）+ -itis（炎症）

例句 Nephritis is an inflammation of the kidneys, often caused by infection or autoimmune diseases. 肾炎是肾脏的炎症，通常由感染或自身免疫性疾病引起。

nephrectomy 肾切除术

词根 nephr-（肾）+ -ectomy（切除）

例句 A nephrectomy is the surgical removal of one or both kidneys. 肾切除术是切除单侧或双侧肾脏的手术。

nephrology 肾脏学

词根 nephr-（肾）+ -logy（学科）

例句 Nephrology is the medical specialty that focuses on the study and treatment of kidney diseases. 肾脏学是研究和治疗肾脏疾病的医学专业。

nephrosis 肾病

词根 nephr-（肾）+ -osis（病症）

例句 Nephrosis is a general term for kidney disease that does not involve inflammation. 肾病是指不涉及炎症的肾脏疾病的总称。

nephromegaly 肾肿大

词根 nephr-（肾）+ -megaly（肿大）

例句 Nephromegaly refers to the enlargement of the kidneys, which can be caused by various conditions. 肾肿大是指肾脏的增大，可能由各种疾病引起。

nephropathy 肾病

词根 nephr-（肾）+ -pathy（病）

例句 Diabetic nephropathy is a complication of diabetes that damages the kidneys. 糖尿病肾病是糖尿病的一种并发症，导致肾脏受损。

nephrostomy 肾造口术

词根 nephr-（肾）+ -stomy（造口术）

例句 Nephrostomy is a surgical procedure that involves creating an opening in the kidney to drain urine. 肾造口术是一种手术，指在肾脏中开口以引流尿液。

nephrolithiasis 肾结石症

词根 nephr-（肾）+ -lithiasis（结石形成）

例句 Nephrolithiasis is the formation of kidney stones, which can cause severe pain and urinary obstruction. 肾结石症是肾脏结石的形成，可能导致剧烈的疼痛和尿道堵塞。

nephrotoxin 肾毒素

词根 nephr-（肾）+ toxin（毒素）

例句 Nephrotoxins are substances that damage the kidneys, often as a side effect of certain medications. 肾毒素是损害肾脏的物质，通常产生于某些药物的副作用。

nephrostogram 肾造口影像

词根 nephr-（肾）+ -stogram（影像）

例句 A nephrostogram is an imaging technique used to visualize the kidneys and urinary system. 肾造口影像是一种影像学检查，用于观察肾脏和尿道系统。

neuro-（神经）

neurogenic 神经性的

词根 neuro-（神经）+ -genic（产生的）

例句 Neurogenic pain arises from nerve damage or dysfunction. 神经性疼痛是由神经损伤或功能障碍引起的。

neurotoxin 神经毒素

词根 neuro-（神经）+ toxin（毒素）

例句 Certain snakes produce neurotoxins that can paralyze or kill their prey. 某些蛇产生的神经毒素可以使猎物瘫痪或死亡。

neuroanatomy 神经解剖学

词根 neuro-（神经）+ anatomy（解剖学）

例句 Neuroanatomy focuses on the structure and organization of the nervous system. 神经解剖学研究神经系统的结构和组织。

neurolysis 神经松解术

词根 neuro-（神经）+ -lysis（松解；分解）

例句 Neurolysis is a surgical procedure to relieve nerve pain by freeing compressed nerves. 神经松解术是一种通过释放受压神经来缓解疼痛的手术。

neurology 神经学

词根 neuro-（神经）+ -logy（学科）

例句 Neurology is the branch of medicine that deals with disorders of the nervous system. 神经学是研究神经系统疾病的医学分支。

neurosurgery 神经外科手术

词根 neuro-（神经）+ surgery（外科手术）

例句 Neurosurgery involves the surgical treatment of conditions affecting the brain and spinal cord. 神经外科手术指治疗大脑和脊髓相关疾病的外科手术。

neurodegenerative 神经退行性

词根 neuro-（神经）+ degenerative（退行性）
例 句 Alzheimer's disease is a neurodegenerative disorder characterized by progressive memory loss. 阿尔茨海默病是一种以逐步记忆丧失为特征的神经退行性疾病。

neurotransmitter 神经递质

词根 neuro-（神经）+ transmitter（传递者）
例句 Dopamine is a key neurotransmitter involved in regulating mood and movement. 多巴胺是调节情绪和运动的关键神经递质。

neuroimaging 神经影像学

词根 neuro-（神经）+ imaging（影像学）
例句 Neuroimaging techniques, such as MRI, are used to visualize the structure and function of the brain. 神经影像学技术如 MRI，被用于观察大脑的结构。

neuropsychology 神经心理学

词根 neuro-（神经）+ psychology（心理学）
例句 Neuropsychology studies how brain injuries affect cognitive functions and behavior. 神经心理学研究脑损伤如何影响认知功能和行为。

neurosis 神经症

词根 neuro-（神经）+ -osis（病态）
例句 Neurosis refers to a group of mental disorders that involve anxiety and irrational fears. 神经症是指一组涉及焦虑和不合理恐惧的心理障碍。

neurofibromatosis 神经纤维瘤病

词根 neuro-（神经）+ fibroma（纤维瘤）+ -osis（病态）

例句 Neurofibromatosis is a genetic disorder characterized by the growth of tumors along the nerves. 神经纤维瘤病是一种遗传性疾病，其特征是神经沿线肿瘤的生长。

neuroblastoma 神经母细胞瘤

词根 neuro-（神经）+ blastoma（芽肿）

例句 Neuroblastoma is a cancer that develops from immature nerve cells, usually in children. 神经母细胞瘤是一种源自未成熟神经细胞的癌症，通常发生在儿童中。

neurotherapy 神经治疗

词根 neuro-（神经）+ therapy（治疗）

例句 Neurotherapy is a treatment aimed at improving brain function and reducing symptoms of neurological disorders. 神经治疗是一种旨在改善大脑功能并减少神经系统疾病症状的治疗方法。

neuroticism 神经质

词根 neuro-（神经）+ -ism（主义；倾向）

例句 High levels of neuroticism can lead to anxiety and emotional instability. 高水平的神经质可能导致焦虑和情绪不稳定。

noci-（疼痛的）

nociception 伤害感受

词根 noci-（疼痛）+ -ception（感知）

例句 Nociception is the process by which the nervous system detects harmful stimuli. 伤害感受是指神经系统检测有害刺激的过程。

nociceptor 伤害感受器

词根 noci-（疼痛）+ -ceptor（感受器）

例句 Nociceptors are sensory neurons that respond to damaging stimuli. 伤害感受器是对损伤性刺激做出反应的感觉神经元。

nociceptive pain 伤害性感痛

词根 noci-（疼痛）+ -ceptive（感知的）
例句 Nociceptive pain results from actual tissue damage or inflammation. 伤害性感痛是由实际的组织损伤或炎症引起的。

nociperception 痛觉感知

词根 noci-（疼痛）+ -perception（感知）
例句 Nociperception involves the recognition and transmission of pain signals to the brain. 痛觉感知指将疼痛信号传递至大脑并加以识别。

nocigenic 引起疼痛的

词根 noci-（疼痛）+ -genic（产生的）
例句 Nocigenic stimuli trigger pain by activating nociceptors. 引起疼痛的刺激通过激活伤害感受器引发疼痛。

nocifensive response 疼痛防御反应

词根 noci-（疼痛）+ -fensive（防御）
例句 The nocifensive response is a reflex mechanism to protect the body from further injury. 疼痛防御反应是一种保护身体免受进一步伤害的反射机制。

nocistatic 抑制疼痛的

词根 noci-（疼痛）+ -static（抑制）
例句 Certain medications have nocistatic effects, reducing pain perception. 某些药物具有抑制疼痛的效果，可降低痛觉感知。

nocigenesis 疼痛发生

词根 noci-（疼痛）+ -genesis（生成）
例句 Nocigenesis is the process of pain development and propaga-

tion. 疼痛发生是指疼痛的产生和传播过程。

nociphobia 对疼痛的恐惧

词根 noci-（疼痛）+ -phobia（恐惧）
例句 Nociphobia is a psychological condition characterized by an uncontrollable addiction to narcotics. 对疼痛的恐惧是一种心理状态，其特征是对疼痛有强烈的恐惧感。

nocireaction 疼痛反应

词根 noci-（疼痛）+ -reaction（反应）
例句 A nocireaction occurs when the body responds to painful stimuli through reflexes or behavioral responses. 疼痛反应是指身体通过反射或行为对疼痛刺激做出反应。

nocimotor 引起疼痛的运动

词根 noci-（疼痛）+ -motor（运动）
例句 Nocimotor responses are involuntary movements caused by painful stimuli. 引起疼痛的运动是由疼痛刺激引发的非自主运动。

nocifactor 痛觉因素

词根 noci-（疼痛）+ -factor（因素）
例句 Nocifactors are agents or conditions that induce pain sensations. 痛觉因素是引发痛觉的物质或条件。

nociperceptive 痛觉感知的

词根 noci-（疼痛）+ -perceptive（感知的）
例句 Nociperceptive pain is the perception of pain by the body when nociceptors are activated. 痛觉感知性疼痛是当伤害感受器被激活时，身体感知的疼痛。

nociceptive reflex 伤害性感觉反射

词根 noci-（疼痛）+ -ceptive（感知）+ reflex（反射）
例句 The nociceptive reflex is a protective mechanism that helps

the body react quickly to painful stimuli. 伤害性感觉反射是一种保护机制，有助于身体迅速对疼痛刺激做出反应。

nociceptive transmission 伤害性感觉传导

词根 noci-（疼痛）+ -ceptive（感知）+ transmission（传导）
例句 Nociceptive transmission refers to the way pain signals are carried from the site of injury to the brain. 伤害性感觉传导是指疼痛信号从受伤部位传送到大脑的过程。

nociceptive modulation 伤害性感觉调节

词根 noci-（疼痛）+ -ceptive（感知）+ modulation（调节）
例句 Nociceptive modulation involves the regulation of pain signals within the nervous system. 伤害性感觉调节是指在神经系统内对疼痛信号的调节。

nocimodulation 痛觉调节

词根 noci-（疼痛）+ modulation（调节）
例句 Nocimodulation involves altering the intensity of pain by either enhancing or inhibiting pain signals. 痛觉调节是通过增强或抑制疼痛信号来改变疼痛强度的过程。

nociceptive inhibition 伤害性感觉抑制

词根 noci-（疼痛）+ -ceptive（感知）+ inhibition（抑制）
例句 Nociceptive inhibition is the process of decreasing the perception of pain through the nervous system. 伤害性感觉抑制是通过神经系统减少疼痛感知的过程。

nociceptor-mediated pain 伤害感受器介导的疼痛

词根 noci-（疼痛）+ -ceptor（感受器）+ mediated（介导的）
例句 Nociceptor-mediated pain occurs when the pain receptors in the body are activated by harmful stimuli. 伤害感受器介导的疼痛发生在身体的痛觉受体被有害刺激激活时。

noct-（夜）

nocturnal 夜间的

词根 noct-（夜）+ -urnal（的）

例句 Nocturnal animals, such as owls, are active during the night and rest during the day. 夜行性动物，如猫头鹰，在夜间活跃，白天休息。

nocturia 夜尿症

词根 noct-（夜）+ -uria（尿）

例句 Nocturia is the condition of waking up at night to urinate frequently. 夜尿症是指夜间频繁起床排尿的情况。

noctambulation 夜游症

词根 noct-（夜）+ ambul-（走动）+ -ation（名词后缀）

例句 Noctambulation is the act of walking or performing other activities while asleep, also known as sleepwalking. 夜游症是指在睡眠中行走或进行其他活动，也叫作梦游。

noctophobia 夜间恐惧症

词根 noct-（夜）+ phobia（恐惧）

例句 Noctophobia is the fear of the night or darkness, often leading to anxiety and restlessness. 夜间恐惧症是对夜晚或黑暗的恐惧，常常引发焦虑和不安。

noctovision 夜视

词根 noct-（夜）+ vision（视力）

例句 Noctovision refers to the ability to see in low-light conditions, often enhanced by night vision technology. 夜视是指在低光环境下的视力，通常通过夜视技术增强。

noctanuria 夜尿

词根 noct-（夜）+ -anuria（无尿症）

例句 Noctanuria is a condition where there is reduced urine production during the day and increased production at night. 夜尿症是白天尿液产生减少，夜间尿液产生增加的情况。

noctivagant 夜间徘徊的

词根 noct-（夜）+ vagant（漫游的）

例句 A noctivagant person may wander the streets at night, sometimes due to sleep disorders. 夜间徘徊者可能在晚上游荡在街头，通常是由睡眠障碍引起的。

normo-（正常的）

normotension 正常血压

词根 normo-（正常的）+ tension（血压）

例句 Normotension refers to the condition of having normal blood pressure levels. 正常血压指的是血压水平处于正常范围的状态。

normoglycemia 正常血糖

词根 normo-（正常的）+ glycemia（血糖）

例句 Normoglycemia refers to normal levels of glucose in the blood, typically ranging between 70 and 100 mg/dL. 正常血糖指的是血液中葡萄糖的正常水平，通常为 70 ～ 100 mg/dL。

normocardia 正常心律

词根 normo-（正常的）+ cardia（心脏）

例句 Normocardia is the term used to describe a normal heart rate and rhythm. 正常心律是用来描述正常心率和心脏节律的术语。

normocytic 正常细胞的

词根 normo-（正常的）+ cytic（细胞的）

例句 Normocytic refers to red blood cells that are of normal size, often used to describe blood cell morphology in conditions like anemia. 正常细胞指的是正常大小的红细胞，常用于描述贫血等病症中的血细胞形态。

normochromic 正常色素的

词根 normo-（正常的）+ chromic（色素的）

例句 Normochromic anemia is a type of anemia where red blood cells have a normal amount of hemoglobin but are low in number. 正常色素性贫血是一种红细胞血红蛋白含量正常但数量减少的贫血类型。

normothermia 正常体温

词根 normo-（正常的）+ thermia（体温）

例句 Normothermia is the condition of having a normal body temperature, typically around 37℃（98. 6°F）. 正常体温是指体温在正常范围内，通常约为 37℃（98. 6°F）。

normokalemia 正常血钾水平

词根 normo-（正常的）+ kalemia（血钾水平）

例句 Normokalemia refers to having normal potassium levels in the blood, typically between 3. 5 to 5. 0 mEq/L. 正常血钾水平指的是血液中钾的正常水平，通常为 3.5 ～ 5.0 mg/dL。

normoalbuminemia 正常白蛋白血症

词根 normo-（正常的）+ albuminemia（血液中的白蛋白）

例句 Normoalbuminemia is the presence of normal levels of albumin in the blood, which is important for maintaining osmotic pres sure. 正常白蛋白血症是指血液中白蛋白水平正常，这对于维持渗透压至关重要。

normocalcemia 正常血钙水平

词根 normo-（正常的）+ calcemia（血钙水平）

例句 Normocalcemia refers to normal levels of calcium in the blood, which are necessary for bone health and muscle function. 正常血钙水平是指血液中钙的正常水平，对于骨骼健康和肌肉功能是必需的。

normocholesterolemia 正常血胆固醇水平

词根 normo-（正常的）+ cholesterol（胆固醇）+ -emia（血液中的）
例句 Normocholesterolemia refers to the condition in which cholesterol levels in the blood are within the normal range. 正常血胆固醇水平指的是血液中胆固醇水平在正常范围内的状态。

normophagia 正常进食

词根 normo-（正常的）+ phagia（进食）
例句 Normophagia refers to the process of eating in a typical or normal manner without difficulties. 正常进食指的是没有困难的进食过程。

normotrophy 正常营养状态

词根 normo-（正常的）+ troph-（营养）
例句 Normotrophy refers to a state of adequate nutritional status, where the body has the right balance of nutrients. 正常营养状态指的是身体具有适当营养平衡的状态。

normorexia 正常食欲

词根 normo-（正常的）+ orexia（食欲）
例句 Normorexia refers to having a normal appetite and desire for food. 正常食欲指的是对食物有正常的渴望。

normokinesia 正常运动

词根 normo-（正常的）+ kinesia（运动）
例句 Normokinesia refers to normal, unimpeded movement, as seen in healthy individuals. 正常运动指的是健康个体无障碍的运动。

USMLE Step 2 CK　样题

A 2-year-old girl is brought to the clinic by her parents for an initial examination. Medical records show that she has a cleft palate and ventriculoseptal (ventriculo-; sept) defects that have not been repaired. During the past 18 months, she has had two episodes of pneumonia (pneumo-) and at least 10 episodes of otitis (ot-; -itis) media treated with antibiotic (anti-; bio-) therapy. The patient's parents recently adopted her from China. She is at the 10th percentile for length and 5th percentile for weight. Vital signs are within normal limits. Examination shows middle ear effusions bilaterally (bi-; -lateral) and a cleft palate. Lungs are clear to auscultation (auscult-; -ation). A grade 3/6 holosystolic (holo-; systol-) murmur is heard on cardiac examination. There is no hepatosplenomegaly (hepato-; spleno-; mega). Chest X-ray is shown. A complete blood count is most likely to show which of the following leukocyte (leuk-; -cyte) findings in this patient?

(A) Eosinophilia (eosino-; -phil)

(B) Lymphocytosis (lymph-; cyt-; -osis)

(C) Lymphopenia (lymph-; -penia)

(D) Neutropenia (neutro-; -penia)

(E) Neutrophilia (neutro-; -phil)

中文翻译

一名 2 岁女孩由其父母带到诊室进行初次检查。病历显示她患有腭裂和未修复的心室中隔缺损。在过去 18 个月中，她曾有两次肺炎和至少 10 次中耳炎，均通过抗生素治疗。患者的父母最近从中国收养了她。她的身高处于第 10 百分位，体重处于第 5 百分位。生命体征正常。检查显示双侧中耳积液和腭裂。肺部听诊清晰。心脏检查听到 3/6 级全收缩期杂音。无肝脾肿大。全血细胞计数最可能显示该患者的以下哪种白细胞异常？

(A) 嗜酸性粒细胞增多
(B) 淋巴细胞增多
(C) 淋巴细胞减少
(D) 中性粒细胞减少
(E) 中性粒细胞增多

题目和答案中出现的词根

ventriculo-：室（这里指心室，也可以指代脑室）
sept：隔
pneumo-：肺的
ot-：耳朵，是 oto- 的同义变异
-itis：炎症
anti-：抗
bio-：生物
bi-：双
-lateral：侧
auscult-：听
-ation：表示动作
holo-：全
systol-：收缩的
hepato-：肝脏的

spleno-：脾脏的

mega-：大

leuk-：白色的

-cyte：细胞

eosino-：酸性的

-phil：嗜

lymph-：淋巴

cyt-：细胞

-osis：病理状态

-penia：缺少

neutro-：中性的

noso-（医院的；疾病的）

nosocomial 医院获得的

词根 noso-（疾病）+ -comial（来自……的）

例句 Nosocomial infections are those acquired during a hospital stay, often caused by pathogens that are resistant to treatment. 医院获得性感染是在住院期间获得的感染，通常由对治疗具有耐药性的病原体引起。

nosology 疾病学

词根 noso-（疾病）+ -logy（学科）

例句 Nosology is the branch of medicine that deals with the classification of diseases. 疾病学是医学的一个分支，研究疾病的分类。

nosocomial infection 医院感染

词根 noso-（疾病）+ comial（来自……的）+ infection（感染）

例句 Nosocomial infections are a major concern in healthcare settings and can be spread through contaminated medical equipment. 医院感染是医疗环境中的一个主要问题，通常通过污染的医疗设备传播。

nososymptomatology 疾病症状学

词根 noso-（疾病）+ symptomatology（症状学）

例句 Nososymptomatology refers to the study of the symptoms associated with specific diseases. 疾病症状学指的是研究与特定疾病相关的症状。

nosophobia 恐病症

词根 noso-（疾病）+ -phobia（恐惧症）

例句 Nosophobia is the fear of developing a disease, especially a serious or life-threatening condition. 恐病症是对患上疾病的恐惧，尤其是对严重或威胁生命的疾病的恐惧。

nosogenic 致病的

词根 noso-（疾病）+ -genic（产生的）

例句 Nosogenic factors are those that promote or cause disease, such as environmental conditions or genetics. 致病因素是促进或引起疾病的因素，如环境条件或遗传。

ocu（lo）-（眼）

O

oculus 眼睛

词根 ocu-（眼）+ -lus（名词后缀）
例句 The oculus is a central opening in architecture, often found in domes to let in light. 眼状窗是建筑中的中央开口，通常出现在穹顶中，以便让光线进入。

oculist 眼科医生

词根 ocu-（眼）+ -list（从事某职业的人）
例句 An oculist is a medical professional who specializes in the diagnosis and treatment of eye diseases. 眼科医生是专门从事眼病诊断和治疗的医疗专业人员。

ocular 眼睛的

词根 ocu-（眼）+ -ar（形容词后缀）
例句 Ocular health is essential for maintaining good vision and preventing eye diseases. 眼睛健康对于维持良好的视力和预防眼病至关重要。

oculomotor 动眼的

词根 oculo-（眼）+ motor（运动的）
例句 The oculomotor nerve controls most of the eye's movements and pupil constriction. 动眼神经控制大部分眼睛的运动和瞳孔收缩。

oculopathy 眼病

词根 oculo-（眼）+ -pathy（病）
例句 Oculopathy refers to any disease or disorder of the eye, ranging from mild conditions to severe diseases. 眼病指的是眼睛的疾

病或障碍，包括从轻微的情况到严重的疾病。

oculography 眼部影像

词根 oculo-（眼）+ -graphy（记录；图）

例句 An oculography is a type of eye scan that captures images of the retina and other parts of the eye. 眼部影像是一种眼部扫描，能够捕捉到视网膜和眼睛其他部分的图像。

oculocardiac 眼心脏的

词根 oculo-（眼）+ cardi-（心脏）+ -ac（形容词后缀）

例句 Oculocardiac reflex is a physiological phenomenon in which pressure on the eyes causes a slowing of the heart rate. 眼心脏反射是一种生理现象，眼睛受压会导致心率减慢。

oculovestibular 眼 - 前庭的

词根 oculo-（眼）+ vestibul-（前庭）+ -ar（形容词后缀）

例句 The oculovestibular reflex test checks for balance problems by stimulating the vestibular system and observing eye movements. 眼 - 前庭反射测试通过刺激前庭系统并观察眼球运动来检查平衡问题。

oculomotor nerve 动眼神经

词根 oculo-（眼）+ motor（运动）+ nerve（神经）

例句 The oculomotor nerve is responsible for controlling most of the movements of the eye, including the constriction of the pupil. 动眼神经负责控制眼睛的大部分运动，包括瞳孔的收缩。

oculocutaneous 眼 - 皮肤的

词根 oculo-（眼）+ cutan-（皮肤）+ -ous（形容词后缀）

例句 Oculocutaneous albinism is a genetic condition where there is a lack of pigmentation in both the eyes and skin. 眼皮肤白化病是一种遗传性疾病，导致眼睛和皮肤缺乏色素。

odyno-（疼痛）

odynophagia 疼痛性吞咽

词根 odyno-（疼痛）+ -phagia（吞咽）

例句 Odynophagia is a condition where swallowing causes pain, often associated with throat infections or lesions. 疼痛性吞咽是吞咽时引起疼痛的情况，通常与喉咙感染或病变有关。

odynodysphagia 疼痛性吞咽困难

词根 odyno-（疼痛）+ dysphagia（吞咽困难）

例句 Odynodysphagia occurs when swallowing is both painful and difficult, often due to esophageal conditions. 疼痛性吞咽困难是吞咽既疼痛又困难的情况，通常与食管疾病有关。

odynalgia 疼痛

词根 odyno-（疼痛）+ -algia（痛）

例句 Odynalgia refers to localized pain that may result from nerve compression or inflammation. 疼痛是指由于神经压迫或炎症引起的局部疼痛。

odynesthesia 疼痛感知

词根 odyno-（疼痛）+ -esthesia（感觉）

例句 Odynesthesia is the perception of pain, often heightened in cases of nerve damage or sensitivity disorders. 疼痛感知是指疼痛的感觉，在神经损伤或敏感性疾病中通常更加明显。

odynoparalysis 疼痛性麻痹

词根 odyno-（疼痛）+ paralysis（麻痹）

例句 Odynoparalysis is a condition where pain and partial paralysis occur together, often seen in nerve-related injuries. 疼痛性麻痹是

指疼痛和部分麻痹同时出现的情况，常见于神经损伤。

odynodystrophy 疼痛性营养障碍

词根 odyno-（疼痛）+ dystrophy（营养障碍）

例句 Odynodystrophy is a disorder in which pain and tissue degeneration coexist, commonly linked to chronic conditions like diabetes. 疼痛性营养障碍是一种疼痛与组织退化并存的疾病，通常与糖尿病等慢性病相关。

odynophobia 疼痛恐惧症

词根 odyno-（疼痛）+ phobia（恐惧）

例句 Odynophobia is an extreme fear of experiencing pain, often associated with anxiety disorders. 疼痛恐惧症是指对疼痛的极端恐惧，通常与焦虑障碍有关。

odynogeny 疼痛生成

词根 odyno-（疼痛）+ -geny（生成）

例句 Odynogeny refers to the process or origin of pain, often linked to inflammatory responses or trauma. 疼痛生成是指疼痛的产生过程，通常与炎症反应或创伤有关。

odynosis 疼痛性疾病

词根 odyno-（疼痛）+ -osis（病态）

例句 Odynosis is a general term for pain-related medical conditions, including chronic or acute pain syndromes. 疼痛性疾病是指与疼痛相关的医学状况，包括慢性或急性疼痛综合征。

USMLE Step 3 样题

A 30-year-old man comes to the emergency department because of an acute episode of renal colic. Medical history is remarkable for episodes of painful urination (urin-) and passing of what he calls "gravel in my urine". Urinalysis (urin-; -lysis) demonstrates microscopic (micro-; scop-) hematuria (hemat-; -uria) with some crystalluria (crystal-; -uria) and no casts. Supine X-ray of the abdomen shows no abnormalities. A 4-mm renal calculus is detected in the distal right ureter on ultrasonography (ultra-; sono-; -graphy). There is no evidence of dilation of the collecting system. The patient's pain is responsive to narcotic medication. In addition to administering intravenous (intra-; veno-) fluids, which of the following is the most appropriate next step?

(A) Acidification of urine by drinking cranberry juice

(B) Cystoscopic (cysto-; scop-) removal of the calculus

(C) Cystoscopic (cysto-; scop-) ureteral lavage

(D) Shock wave lithotripsy (litho-; -tripsy)

(E) Straining of the urine

中文翻译

一名 30 岁男性因急性肾绞痛来到急诊科。病史包括排尿疼痛和尿液中排出他称为“尿中碎石”的物质。尿液分析显示显微镜下血尿，伴有少量晶体尿，无管型。腹部仰卧位 X 线检查无异常。超声检查发现右侧输尿管远端有一个 4 mm 肾结石。无集合系统扩张的迹象。患者的疼痛对麻醉药物有反应。除了给予静脉补液外，以下哪项是最适当的下一步？

(A) 通过饮用蔓越莓汁酸化尿液

(B) 膀胱镜下取石

(C) 膀胱镜下输尿管冲洗

(D) 体外冲击波碎石术

(E) 过滤尿液

题目和答案中出现的词根

urin-：尿

-lysis：分解

micro-：微小的

scop-：视野

hemat-：血，hemato- 的同义变异

-uria：尿症

crystal-：晶体

ultra-：超

sono-：声音的

-graphy：图像

intra-：在……内

veno-：静脉

cysto-：膀胱

litho-：石头

-tripsy：压碎

-oid（类似）

lipoid 类脂的

词根 lip-（脂肪）+ -oid（类似）

例句 Lipoid substances are similar to lipids and have fat-like properties. 类脂物质类似脂质，具有脂肪样的性质。

spheroid 球状的

词根 spher-（球）+ -oid（类似）

例句 Spheroids are cell aggregates that resemble spherical shapes. 球状体是聚集在一起的细胞，呈现球形。

thyroid 甲状腺的

词根 thyr-（盾）+ -oid（类似）

例句 The thyroid gland plays a crucial role in regulating metabolism. 甲状腺在调节新陈代谢中起着至关重要的作用。

fibroid 纤维状的；纤维瘤

词根 fibr-（纤维）+ -oid（类似）

例句 Fibroid tumors are non-cancerous growths composed of fibrous tissue. 纤维瘤是由纤维组织构成的良性肿瘤。

cardioid 心形的

词根 cardi-（心脏）+ -oid（类似）

例句 A cardioid shape is often used to describe the structure of a heart-like object. 心形常用来描述心脏状物体的结构。

amyloid 类淀粉的；淀粉样物质

词根 amyl-（淀粉）+ -oid（类似）

例句 Amyloid plaques are abnormal deposits of protein found in the brains of Alzheimer's patients. 淀粉样斑块是阿尔茨海默病患者大脑中异常的蛋白质沉积物。

lymphoid 淋巴的

词根 lymph-（淋巴）+ -oid（类似）

例句 Lymphoid tissue is involved in the production and maturation of immune cells. 淋巴组织参与免疫细胞的产生和成熟。

cystoid 囊肿状的

词根 cyst-（囊肿）+ -oid（类似）

例句 Cystoid structures in the eye resemble cysts and may be indicative of certain eye conditions. 眼睛中的囊肿状结构类似囊肿，可能提示某些眼科疾病。

oligo-（少）

oligodendrocyte 少突胶质细胞

词根 oligo-（少）+ dendro-（树状）+ -cyte（细胞）

例句 Oligodendrocytes are glial cells responsible for producing myelin in the central nervous system. 少突胶质细胞是负责在中枢神经系统中产生髓鞘的胶质细胞。

oliguria 少尿

词根 olig-（少）+ -uria（尿）

例句 Oliguria is a clinical condition in which there is reduced urine output, often indicating kidney problems. 少尿是一种临床状况，尿液排出量减少，通常表明肾脏问题。

oligomenorrhea 少月经

词根 oligo-（少）+ men-（月经）+ -rrhea（流出）

例句 Oligomenorrhea is characterized by infrequent or very light menstrual periods. 少月经的特征是月经周期较短或月经量过少。

oligospermia 少精症

词根 oligo-（少）+ sperm-（精子）+ -ia（病症）

例句 Oligospermia is a condition in which there is a low concentration of sperm in the semen, leading to infertility. 少精症是一种精液中精子浓度较低的病症，可能导致不育。

oligopeptide 寡肽

词根 oligo-（少）+ peptide（肽）

例句 Oligopeptides consist of a small number of amino acids linked by peptide bonds. 寡肽是由少量氨基酸通过肽键连接而成的分子。

oligoclonal bands 少克隆带

词根 oligo-（少）+ clonal（克隆的）+ bands（带）

例句 Oligoclonal bands are frequently found in the cerebrospinal fluid of patients with multiple sclerosis. 少克隆带常见于多发性硬化症患者的脑脊液中。

oligosaccharide 寡糖

词根 oligo-（少）+ saccharide（糖）

例句 Oligosaccharides are carbohydrates composed of a few simple sugars, often found in plant fibers. 寡糖是由少量单糖组成的碳水化合物，通常存在于植物纤维中。

oligogenic 少基因的

词根 oligo-（少）+ genic（产生的）

例句 Oligogenic disorders are conditions caused by mutations in a small number of genes. 少基因病是由少量基因突变引起的疾病。

oligophrenia 寡智症

词根 oligo-（少）+ phren-（心灵；智力）+ -ia（病症）

例句 Oligophrenia is a medical term used to describe different degrees of intellectual disability. 寡智症是用于描述不同程度智力障碍的医学术语。

oligotrophic 少营养的

词根 oligo-（少）+ trophic（营养的）

例句 Oligotrophic conditions often refer to environments or biological systems that have low levels of nutrients. 少营养状况通常指的是营养物质含量较低的环境或生物系统。

oligodactyly 少指症

词根 oligo-（少）+ dactyl-（手指）+ -y（病症）

例句 Oligodactyly is a congenital condition characterized by fewer than five fingers or toes on a hand or foot. 少指症是一种先天性疾

病，表现为手或脚上少于五根手指或脚趾。

oligodontia 少牙症

词根 oligo-（少）+ odont-（牙齿）+ -ia（病症）

例句 Oligodontia is a developmental condition in which multiple teeth fail to develop. 少牙症是一种发育异常，表现为多颗牙齿未能正常发育。

oligomyositis 少肌炎

词根 oligo-（少）+ myositis（肌肉炎症）

例句 Oligomyositis refers to inflammation affecting a small number of muscle groups, leading to muscle weakness. 少肌炎是指影响少量肌肉群的炎症，导致肌肉无力。

oligotrichia 少毛症

词根 oligo-（少）+ trich-（毛发）+ -ia（病症）

例句 Oligotrichia is a condition characterized by sparse or reduced hair growth, often due to genetic causes. 少毛症是一种以毛发稀疏或减少为特征的病症，通常由遗传因素引起。

oligoamnios 羊水过少

词根 oligo-（少）+ amnios（羊水）

例句 Oligoamnios is a condition characterized by an insufficient amount of amniotic fluid surrounding the fetus. 羊水过少是指围绕胎儿的羊水量不足的情况。

oligometastasis 寡转移

词根 oligo-（少）+ metastasis（转移）

例句 Oligometastasis refers to a limited number of metastatic cancer sites, which may allow for targeted treatment. 寡转移是指少量的癌症转移部位，可能允许进行靶向治疗。

oligothemia 低血容量

词根 oligo-（少）+ -hemia（血液）

例句 Oligothemia is a condition characterized by reduced blood volume, often due to dehydration or hemorrhage. 低血容量是指血容量减少的病症，通常由脱水或出血引起。

oligoanuria 少无尿症

词根 oligo-（少）+ anuria（无尿）

例句 Oligoanuria occurs when a patient's urine output is severely reduced or completely absent. 少无尿症是指患者的尿量严重减少或完全无尿。

oligocholia 胆汁分泌减少

词根 oligo-（少）+ cholia（胆汁）

例句 Oligocholia is characterized by reduced bile secretion, which can impair digestion. 胆汁分泌减少会影响消化功能。

oligocarbia 低二氧化碳血症

词根 oligo-（少）+ carbia（碳）

例句 Oligocarbia is a condition in which the carbon dioxide levels in the blood are abnormally low, often due to hyperventilation. 低二氧化碳血症是指血液中的二氧化碳水平异常低，通常由过度换气引起。

-ology（学科）

biology 生物学

词根 bio-（生命）+ -ology（学科）

例句 Biology is the scientific study of life and living organisms, including their structure, function, growth, and evolution. 生物学是研究生命和生物体的科学，包括它们的结构、功能、成长和进化。

psychology 心理学

词根 psych-（自然；身体）+ -ology（学科）

例句 Psychology is the study of the human mind, behavior, and mental processes. 心理学是研究人类心灵、行为和心理过程的学科。

sociology 社会学

词根 socio-（社会）+ -ology（学科）
例句 Sociology is the study of society, social behaviors, and the structures that govern them. 社会学是研究社会、社会行为以及支配这些行为的结构的学科。

zoology 动物学

词根 zo-（动物）+ -ology（学科）
例句 Zoology is the branch of biology concerned with the study of animals and their classification. 动物学是生物学的一个分支，专门研究动物及其分类。

anthropology 人类学

词根 anthrop-（人类）+ -ology（学科）
例句 Anthropology is the study of humans, their societies, cultures, and physical characteristics. 人类学是研究人类及其社会、文化和生理特征的学科。

physiology 生理学

词根 physi-（自然；身体）+ -ology（学科）
例句 Physiology is the scientific study of the functions and processes of living organisms. 生理学是研究生物体功能的科学。

epidemiology 流行病学

词根 epi-（在……之上）+ dem-（人群）+ -ology（学科）
例句 Epidemiology is the study of how diseases spread and affect populations. 流行病学是研究疾病如何传播并影响人群的学科。

USMLE Step 2 CK　样题

A hospitalized 37-year-old woman has a 2-hour history of

severe chest pain and blood-streaked sputum 4 days after undergoing hysterectomy (hyster-; -ectomy) and oophorectomy (oophor-; ectomy) for ovarian cancer. Current medications are oxycodone (oxy-; -codone), prophylactic (pro-; phylac-) low-molecular-weight heparin (hepa-; -rin), and a multivitamin (multi-). Temperature is 37.0°C (98.6°F), pulse is 90/min, respirations (re-; spir-; -ation) are 22/min, and blood pressure is 110/70 mmHg. Examination shows a left pleural rub. An X-ray and CT scan of the chest show a triangular (tri-) pleural-based density in the lower lobe of the left lung. No pulmonary (pulmon-) emboli are seen in the major branches. Venous duplex ultrasonography (ultra-; sono-; -graphy) of the lower extremities shows no deep venous thrombosis (thromb-; -osis). Which of the following is the most likely diagnosis?

(A) Air embolism (embol-; -ism)

(B) Empyema (empye-; -ema)

(C) Hemothorax (hemo-; -thorax)

(D) Pericarditis (peri-; cardi-; -itis)

(E) Pneumonia (pneumon-)

(F) Pulmonary hemorrhage (hemo-; -rrhage)

(G) Pulmonary hypertension (hyper-; -tension)

(H) Pulmonary infarction

中文翻译

一名 37 岁住院女性在接受子宫切除术和卵巢切除术治疗卵巢癌 4 天后，出现 2 小时的严重胸痛和血丝痰。目前服用的药物包括羟考酮、预防性低分子量肝素和多种维生素。体温

37.0℃（98.6℉），脉搏 90 次 / 分钟，呼吸 22 次 / 分钟，血压 110/70 mmHg。检查显示左侧胸膜摩擦音。胸部 X 线和 CT 扫描显示左肺下叶有一个基于胸膜的三角形密度影。主要分支未见肺栓塞。下肢静脉双多普勒超声显示无深静脉血栓形成。以下哪项是最可能的诊断？

(A) 空气栓塞
(B) 脓胸
(C) 血胸
(D) 心包炎
(E) 肺炎
(F) 肺出血
(G) 肺动脉高压
(H) 肺梗死

题目和答案中出现的词根

hyster-：子宫
-ectomy：切除术
oophor-：卵巢
oxy-：氧的
-codone：可待因类药物
pro-：在……之前
phylac-：预防
hepa-：肝脏的
-rin：蛋白分子
multi-：多
re-：重新；反复

spir：呼吸

-ation：表示动作的状态

tri-：三个

pulmon-：肺的

ultra-：超

sono-：声音的

-graphy：图像

thromb-：凝血的

-osis：病理状态

embol-：栓子的

-ism：表示状态

empye-：脓的

-ema：病理状态

hemo-：血

-thorax：胸腔

peri-：外周

cardi-：心脏

-itis：炎症

pneumon-：肺

-rrhag(e)：流出，是 rrhea 的同义变异

hyper-：高

-tension：张力；压力

-oma（肿瘤）

carcinoma 癌症

词根 carcin-（癌症）+ -oma（肿瘤）

例句 Carcinoma is a type of cancer that originates in the epithelial cells of tissues. 癌是一种起源于组织上皮细胞的癌变。

melanoma 黑色素瘤

词根 melan-（黑色素）+ -oma（肿瘤）

例句 Melanoma is a serious form of skin cancer that develops in pigment-producing cells. 黑色素瘤是一种严重的皮肤癌，起源于产生色素的细胞。

lymphoma 淋巴瘤

词根 lymph-（淋巴）+ -oma（肿瘤）

例句 Lymphoma is a type of cancer that begins in the lymphatic system. 淋巴瘤是一种始于淋巴系统的癌症。

sarcoma 肉瘤

词根 sarco-（肉）+ -oma（肿瘤）

例句 Sarcoma is a malignant tumor that arises from connective tissues, such as bones and muscles. 肉瘤是一种恶性肿瘤，起源于结缔组织，如骨骼和肌肉。

glioma 胶质瘤

词根 gli-（胶质）+ -oma（肿瘤）

例句 Glioma is a type of tumor that originates in the glial cells of the brain or spinal cord. 胶质瘤是一种起源于大脑或脊髓胶质细胞的肿瘤。

O

adenoma 腺瘤

词根 aden-（腺体）+ -oma（肿瘤）
例句 Adenomas are benign tumors that form in glandular tissue. 腺瘤是形成于腺体组织中的良性肿瘤。

fibroma 纤维瘤

词根 fibr-（纤维）+ -oma（肿瘤）
例句 Fibromas are benign tumors composed of fibrous tissue. 纤维瘤是由纤维组织组成的良性肿瘤。

osteoma 骨瘤

词根 oste-（骨）+ -oma（肿瘤）
例句 Osteomas are benign bone tumors that are usually asymptomatic. 骨瘤是良性的骨肿瘤，通常没有症状。

myeloma 骨髓瘤

词根 myel-（骨髓）+ -oma（肿瘤）
例句 Myeloma is a cancer of the plasma cells in the bone marrow. 骨髓瘤是骨髓中浆细胞的癌症。

chondroma 软骨瘤

词根 chondr-（软骨）+ -oma（肿瘤）
例句 Chondromas are benign tumors that develop in cartilage tissue. 软骨瘤是发生在软骨组织中的良性肿瘤。

-ome（基本单位）

phenome 表型

词根 phen-（表现）+ -ome（基本单位）
例句 Phenome refers to the set of observable characteristics or traits of an organism, including its morphology, development, biochemical properties, and behavior. 表型是指有机体可观察到的特征，包括

形态、发育、生化特性和行为。

genome 基因组

词根 gen-（产生）+ -ome（基本单位）

例句 The genome is the complete set of genes or genetic material present in a cell or organism. 基因组是细胞或有机体内存在的完整基因或遗传物质集合。

proteome 蛋白质组

词根 prote-（蛋白质）+ -ome（基本单位）

例句 The proteome refers to the entire set of proteins expressed by a genome in a particular organism or under specific conditions. 蛋白质组指的是在特定有机体或特定条件下由基因组表达的所有蛋白质集合。

lipidome 脂质组

词根 lipid-（脂质）+ -ome（基本单位）

例句 Lipidome refers to the entire profile of lipids in a cell, tissue, or organism. 脂质组指的是细胞、组织或有机体中所有脂质的集合。

metabolome 代谢组

词根 metabol-（代谢）+ -ome（基本单位）

例句 The metabolome encompasses all metabolites in a biological cell, tissue, or organism, and it is an essential component of metabolic studies. 代谢组包括生物细胞、组织或有机体中的所有代谢物，它是代谢研究的重要组成部分。

microbiome 微生物组

词根 micro-（微小）+ -ome（基本单位）

例句 The microbiome consists of all the microorganisms living in a particular environment, such as the human gut or skin. 微生物组由生活在特定环境（如人体肠道或皮肤）中的所有微生物构成。

transcriptome 转录组

词根 transcript-（转录）+ -ome（基本单位）

例句 The transcriptome refers to all RNA molecules that are transcribed from DNA, reflecting the genes that are actively expressed in a cell. 转录组是指所有从 DNA 转录来的 RNA 分子，反映了细胞中积极表达的基因。

exposome 暴露组

词根 expos-（暴露）+ -ome（基本单位）

例句 The exposome encompasses the totality of environmental exposures that an individual experiences over a lifetime and their impact on health. 暴露组包括个体一生中经历的所有环境暴露及其对健康的影响。

immunome 免疫组

词根 immun-（免疫）+ -ome（基本单位）

例句 The immunome refers to the entire immune system's response to pathogens, including antibodies and immune cells. 免疫组是指免疫系统对病原体的全部反应，包括抗体和免疫细胞。

omphalo-（脐）

omphalocele 脐膨出

词根 omphalo-（脐）+ -cele（肿胀；膨出）

例句 Omphalocele is a birth defect where an infant's intestines or other abdominal organs protrude from the abdomen through the navel. 脐膨出是一种出生缺陷，婴儿的肠道或其他腹部器官通过脐部突出。

omphalitis 脐炎

词根 omphalo-（脐）+ -itis（炎症）

例句 Omphalitis is an infection of the navel area, commonly seen in newborns. 脐炎是脐部区域的感染，常见于新生儿。

omphalorrhea 脐液流出

词根 omphalo-（脐）+ -rrhea（流出）

例句 Omphalorrhea refers to an abnormal discharge of fluids from the umbilical area. 脐液流出指的是从脐部异常流出的液体。

omphaloplasty 脐部修复术

词根 omphalo-（脐）+ -plasty（修复术）

例句 Omphaloplasty is a surgical procedure used to repair abnormal navel conditions, such as an umbilical hernia. 脐部修复术是一种手术，用于修复异常脐部状况，如脐疝。

omphaloskepsis 脐观念

词根 omphalo-（脐）+ -skepsis（思考）

例句 Omphaloskepsis, or navel-gazing, refers to an excessive focus on oneself and one's own thoughts. 脐观念，或称为自我凝视，是指过度关注自己和自己的思想。

omphalogastric 脐胃的

词根 omphalo-（脐）+ gastr-（胃）+ -ic（形容词后缀）

例句 The omphalogastric artery is an embryological structure involved in fetal development. 脐胃动脉是胚胎发育中的一种结构，参与胎儿的发育。

omphalomelanosis 脐黑变症

词根 omphalo-（脐）+ melan-（黑色素）+ -osis（病态）

例句 Omphalomelanosis is a condition characterized by abnormal pigmentation of the navel area. 脐黑变症是一种特征是脐部区域色素异常的病症。

omphalomesenteric 脐肠系膜的

词根 omphalo-（脐）+ mesenteric（肠系膜的）

例句 The omphalomesenteric duct is a fetal structure that connects the intestine to the umbilical cord. 脐肠系膜管是存在于胎儿的结构，连接肠道和脐带。

omphalopagus 脐联合双胞胎

词根 omphalo-（脐）+ pagus（联合）

例句 Omphalopagus is a condition where conjoined twins are connected at the abdomen, often around the navel. 脐联合双胞胎是指连体双胞胎在腹部（常围绕肚脐部位）相连的一种状况。

omphalocelesis 脐膨出症

词根 omphalo-（脐）+ -cele（肿胀；膨出）

例句 Omphalocelesis is a developmental defect where abdominal organs protrude through the navel. 脐膨出症是一种发育缺陷，腹部器官通过脐部突出。

USMLE Step 2 CK　样题

A 42-year-old woman comes to the office because of a 2-week history of sore throat and fullness in her neck. She has no history of serious illness and takes no medications. She appears anxious. Temperature is 37.8°C (100.0°F), pulse is 102/min, respirations (re-; spir-; -ation) are 22/min, and blood pressure is 146/82 mmHg. The oropharynx (oro-; pharyn-) is clear, and there are no exudates. There is palpable fullness and tenderness of the anterior aspect of the neck. There is no lymphadenopathy (lymph-; aden-; -pathy). Lungs are clear to auscultation (auscult-; -ation). Results of a complete blood count are within the reference ranges. Chest X-ray shows no abnormalities. Which of the following is the most likely diagnosis?

(A) Acute mononucleosis (mono-; nucle-; -osis)

(B) Gastroesophageal (gastro-; esophage-) reflux (re-; flux-)

disease

(C) **Laryngitis** (laryng-; -itis)

(D) **Subacute** (sub-) **thyroiditis** (thyroid-; -itis)

(E) **Tracheitis** (trache-; -itis)

中文翻译

一名42岁女性前来就诊，因2周来咽喉痛和颈部肿胀感。她无严重疾病史，也未服用任何药物。她看起来焦虑。体温37.8℃（100.0℉），脉搏102次/分钟，呼吸22次/分钟，血压146/82 mmHg。口咽部无异常，无渗出物。颈前部可触及肿胀感和压痛。无淋巴结病变。肺部听诊清晰。全血细胞计数结果在参考范围内。胸部X线检查无异常。以下哪项是最可能的诊断？

(A) 急性单核细胞增多症

(B) 胃食管反流病

(C) 喉炎

(D) 亚急性甲状腺炎

(E) 气管炎

题目和答案中出现的词根

re-：重新；反复

spir：呼吸

-ation：表示动作的状态

oro-：口

pharyn-：咽

lymph-：淋巴

aden-：腺体

-pathy：病

auscult-：听

-ation：表示动作

mono-：单个的

nucle-：核

-osis：病理状态

gastro-：胃

esophage-：食管

-flex：弯曲

laryng-：喉

-itis：炎症

sub-：在……下

thyroid-：甲状腺

trache-：气管的

onycho-（指甲）

onychomycosis 甲真菌病

词根 onycho-（指甲）+ mycosis（真菌病）

例句 Onychomycosis is a fungal infection of the nails, commonly caused by dermatophytes. 甲真菌病是指甲的真菌感染，通常由皮肤癣菌引起。

onycholysis 甲分离症

词根 onycho-（指甲）+ -lysis（分解）

例句 Onycholysis is the detachment of the nail from the nail bed, which can be caused by trauma or fungal infections. 甲分离症是指

甲与甲床分离，可能由创伤或真菌感染引起。

onychocryptosis 甲沟炎

词根 onycho-（指甲）+ crypt-（埋藏）+ -osis（病态）

例句 Onychocryptosis, commonly known as ingrown toenail, occurs when the nail grows into the surrounding skin. 甲沟炎，通常称为嵌甲，是指甲生长到周围皮肤内。

onychopathy 甲病

词根 onycho-（指甲）+ -pathy（病）

例句 Onychopathy refers to any disease or condition affecting the nails, including fungal infections and trauma. 甲病是指任何影响指甲的疾病或病症，包括真菌感染和创伤。

onychodynia 甲痛症

词根 onycho-（指甲）+ -dynia（痛）

例句 Onychodynia refers to pain in the nails, often caused by infection, injury, or inflammation. 甲痛症是指指甲的疼痛，通常由感染、伤害或炎症引起。

onychorrhexis 甲裂

词根 onycho-（指甲）+ -rrhexis（破裂）

例句 Onychorrhexis is characterized by brittle nails that split or crack easily. 甲裂是指指甲脆弱，容易裂开或断裂。

onychoplasty 甲修复术

词根 onycho-（指甲）+ -plasty（修复术）

例句 Onychoplasty is a surgical procedure to repair or reconstruct a damaged nail. 甲修复术是一种用于修复或重建受损指甲的外科手术。

onychorrhagia 指甲出血

词根 onycho-（指甲）+ -rrhagia（出血）

例句 Onychorrhagia is a condition where blood collects under the nail, usually due to trauma. 指甲出血是一种血液聚集在指甲下方的情况，通常是由创伤引起的。

onychomadesis 指甲脱落

词根 onycho-（指甲）+ -madesis（脱落）
例句 Onychomadesis refers to the shedding of the nail, often as a result of chemotherapy or systemic illness. 指甲脱落是指指甲的脱落，通常是由化疗或全身性疾病引起的。

onychoschizia 指甲裂开

词根 onycho-（指甲）+ -schizia（裂开）
例句 Onychoschizia refers to splitting or cracking of the nail plate, often caused by trauma or chemical exposure. 指甲裂开是指指甲裂开或断裂，通常由创伤或化学物质暴露引起。

-opia（视觉）

myopia 近视

词根 my-（近）+ -opia（视觉）
例句 Myopia is a refractive error where distant objects appear blurry due to an elongated eyeball. 近视是一种屈光不正，远处物体因眼球过长而显得模糊。

hyperopia 远视

词根 hyper-（过度）+ -opia（视觉）
例句 Hyperopia occurs when the eyeball is too short, causing difficulty seeing nearby objects clearly. 远视发生在眼球过短时，表现为看近物困难。

presbyopia 老花眼

词根 presby-（老年）+ -opia（视觉）
例句 Presbyopia is an age-related condition where the eye loses the

ability to focus on close objects. 老花眼是与年龄相关的眼睛变化，导致眼睛失去聚焦近物的能力。

scotopia 暗适应

词根 scot-（黑暗）+ -opia（视觉）
例句 Scotopia is the ability of the eye to adjust to low-light conditions and improve vision in the dark. 暗适应是眼睛在低光条件下调整并改善夜间视力的能力。

nyctalopia 夜盲症

词根 nyctal-（夜间）+ -opia（视觉）
例句 Nyctalopia, also known as night blindness, is the inability to see well in dim light or darkness. 夜盲症是指在昏暗的光线或黑暗中无法看清物体的病症。

hemianopia 半盲

词根 hemi-（半）+ an-（否定）+ -opia（视觉）
例句 Hemianopia is the loss of vision in half of the visual field, often due to brain injury or stroke. 半盲是指视野一半丧失，通常由脑部损伤或中风引起。

bitemporal hemianopia 双颞性半盲

词根 bi-（双）+ temporal（颞）+ hemi-（半）+ -opia（视觉）
例句 Bitemporal hemianopia is a visual field loss on both sides of the central vision, often due to pituitary tumors. 双颞性半盲是指中心视力两侧的视野丧失，通常由垂体肿瘤引起。

opisth-（后的）

opisthotonos 仰卧后弯症

词根 opisth-（后）+ -tonos（紧张）
例句 Opisthotonos is a condition characterized by extreme backward

arching of the back and neck, often seen in severe neurological disorders. 仰卧后弯症是一种病症，表现为背部和颈部的极度后弯，常见于严重的神经系统疾病。

opisthobranch 后鳃的

词根 opisth-（后）+ branch-（鳃）

例句 Opisthobranchs are a group of marine animals, including sea slugs, that have gills located on the back. 后鳃类是一类海洋动物，包括海蛞蝓，它们的鳃位于背部。

opisthoglyphe 后齿的

词根 opisth-（后）+ -glyphe（齿）

例句 Opisthoglyphe refers to a type of snake with backward-facing teeth that aid in grasping prey. 后齿类是指具有朝后方向齿的蛇，这些齿有助于抓住猎物。

opisthogonic 后源性

词根 opisth-（后）+ -gonic（源性）

例句 Opisthogonic diseases are those that originate in the posterior regions of the body, often referring to certain parasitic infections. 后源性疾病是指起源于身体后部的疾病，通常指某些寄生虫感染。

opisthodontia 后齿类

词根 opisth-（后）+ -odontia（齿类）

例句 Opisthodontia refers to animals that have teeth located toward the rear of the mouth. 后齿类指的是那些牙齿位于口腔后部的动物。

opisthoglossal 后舌的

词根 opisth-（后）+ gloss-（舌）+ -al（形容词后缀）

例句 Opisthoglossal species of amphibians have a tongue structure located at the back of the mouth. 后舌类的两栖动物具有位于口腔后部的舌头结构。

opisthoreal 后腔的

词根 opisth-（后）+ -oreal（腔）

例句 Opisthoreal cavities are found in certain species, such as fish, where the body cavity is located toward the posterior region. 后腔结构在某些物种中存在，如鱼类，其身体腔位于后部区域。

opisthocentric 后中心的

词根 opisth-（后）+ centric（中心的）

例句 Opisthocentric configurations refer to a setup where the main focus or center is located toward the back. 后中心结构指的是主焦点或中心位于后部的设置。

opisthodromic 后向奔跑的

词根 opisth-（后）+ -dromic（奔跑）

例句 Opisthodromic movement refers to movement that occurs in a backward direction, such as in certain animals or insects. 后向奔跑运动指的是朝后进行的运动，见于某些动物。

opisthotonus 仰背弯曲症

词根 opisth-（后）+ -tonus（张力）

例句 Opisthotonus is an extreme form of muscle spasm where the body arches backward, often seen in severe illnesses. 仰背弯曲症是肌肉痉挛的极端形式，身体向后弯曲，常见于重病患者。

opthal-（眼的）

ophthalmology 眼科学

词根 ophthalm-（眼）+ -ology（学科）

例句 Ophthalmology is the branch of medicine that deals with the diagnosis, treatment, and prevention of eye diseases. 眼科学是医学的一个分支，专门处理眼睛疾病的诊断、治疗和预防。

ophthalmologist 眼科医生

词根 ophthalm-（眼）+ -ologist（学者；专业人士）

例句 An ophthalmologist is a medical professional who specializes in the diagnosis and treatment of eye conditions. 眼科医生是专门从事眼睛疾病诊断和治疗的医疗专业人员。

ophthalmic 眼科的

词根 ophthalm-（眼）+ -ic（形容词后缀）

例句 Ophthalmic surgeons perform operations on the eyes, such as cataract surgery. 眼科外科医生进行眼部手术，如白内障手术。

ophthalmoscope 眼底镜

词根 ophthalm-（眼）+ -scope（仪器）

例句 An ophthalmoscope is an instrument used to examine the inside of the eyes, including the retina and optic nerve. 眼底镜是一种用于检查眼睛内部（包括视网膜和视神经）的仪器。

ophthalmoscopy 眼底检查

词根 ophthalm-（眼）+ -oscopy（检查）

例句 Ophthalmoscopy is the procedure used to examine the retina and other structures of the eye. 眼底检查是用于检查视网膜和眼睛其他结构的方法。

ophthalmopathy 眼病

词根 ophthalm-（眼）+ -pathy（病）

例句 Ophthalmopathy refers to diseases of the eye, such as glaucoma and diabetic retinopathy. 眼病是指眼睛的疾病，如青光眼和糖尿病视网膜病变。

ophthalmoplegia 眼肌麻痹

词根 ophthalm-（眼）+ -plegia（麻痹）

例句 Ophthalmoplegia is paralysis of the eye muscles, which can lead to double vision or difficulty moving the eye. 眼肌麻痹是眼部

肌肉的麻痹，可能导致双视或眼球运动困难。

ophthalmic artery 眼动脉

词根 ophthalm-（眼）+ artery（动脉）

例句 The ophthalmic artery supplies blood to the eyes and surrounding structures. 眼动脉为眼睛及其周围结构提供血液。

ophthalmic nerve 眼神经

词根 ophthalm-（眼）+ nerve（神经）

例句 The ophthalmic nerve is a branch of the trigeminal nerve that provides sensation to the eye and surrounding areas. 眼神经是三叉神经的一个分支，负责提供眼睛及其周围区域的感觉。

ophthalmotoxic 眼毒性的

词根 ophthalm-（眼）+ toxic（毒性）

例句 Certain medications can be ophthalmotoxic, meaning they may cause damage to the eyes or vision. 某些药物可能具有眼毒性，意味着它们可能对眼睛或视力造成损害。

ophthalmic lens 眼镜镜片

词根 ophthalm-（眼）+ lens（镜片）

例句 Ophthalmic lenses are used in glasses to correct vision problems such as nearsightedness or farsightedness. 眼镜镜片用于矫正视力问题，如近视或远视。

ophthalmia 眼炎

词根 ophthalm-（眼）+ -ia（病）

例句 Ophthalmia refers to inflammation of the eye, often due to infection or injury. 眼炎是指眼睛的炎症，通常由感染或伤害引起。

ophthalmocele 眼球膨出

词根 ophthalm-（眼）+ -cele（膨出）

例句 Ophthalmocele is a condition in which the eye bulges outward, often as a result of injury or disease. 眼球膨出是指眼睛向外

突出，通常是由受伤或疾病引起的。

ophthalmic examination 眼科检查

词根 ophthalm-（眼）+ examination（检查）

例句 An ophthalmic examination includes tests to check for vision problems, eye diseases, and conditions affecting the eyes. 眼科检查包括检查视力问题、眼科疾病和影响眼睛的病症。

ophthalmic surgery 眼科手术

词根 ophthalm-（眼）+ surgery（手术）

例句 Ophthalmic surgery involves surgical procedures to treat eye diseases or conditions, such as cataract removal or LASIK surgery. 眼科手术指治疗眼科疾病的手术，如白内障切除或LASIK手术。

ophthalmography 眼底摄影

词根 ophthalm-（眼）+ -graphy（摄影）

例句 Ophthalmography is a diagnostic technique used to capture detailed images of the retina and optic nerve. 眼底摄影是一种诊断技术，用于捕捉视网膜和视神经的详细图像。

ophthalmic drug 眼药

词根 ophthalm-（眼）+ drug（药物）

例句 Ophthalmic drugs are medications used to treat eye infections, inflammation, or glaucoma. 眼药是用于治疗眼部感染、炎症或青光眼的药物。

ophthalmoplasty 眼科修复手术

词根 ophthalm-（眼）+ -plasty（修复）

例句 Ophthalmoplasty is a surgical procedure that involves repairing or reconstructing eye tissue or structures. 眼科修复手术是一种修复或重建眼部组织或结构的外科手术。

ophthalmitis 眼部炎症

词根 ophthalm-（眼）+ -itis（炎症）

例句 Ophthalmitis is an inflammation of the eye, often caused by bacterial or viral infections. 眼部炎症是眼睛的炎症，通常由细菌或病毒感染引起。

ophthalmosynesis 眼部合成

词根 ophthalm-（眼）+ -synesis（合成）
例句 Ophthalmosynesis is a term used to describe the fusion of eye components in the treatment of certain eye conditions. 眼部合成是在治疗某些眼病时眼部组件的融合过程。

-or（执行者）

receptor 受体

词根 re-（反）+ -ceptor（接受者）
例句 The receptor proteins on the cell membrane bind to signaling molecules to initiate cellular responses. 细胞膜上的受体蛋白质与信号分子结合，启动细胞反应。

effector 效应器

词根 ef-（向外）+ -fector（做；执行）
例句 Effectors in the immune system are responsible for carrying out the immune response after activation. 免疫系统中的效应器负责在激活后执行免疫反应。

inhibitor 抑制因子

词根 in-（不）+ -hibitor（阻止者）
例句 An enzyme inhibitor prevents the enzyme from catalyzing a reaction. 酶抑制剂阻止酶催化反应。

activator 激活因子

词根 act-（做；推动）+ -ivator（使得）
例句 The activator binds to the gene's promoter region to stimulate transcription. 激活因子与基因的启动子区域结合，刺激转录。

protease inhibitor 蛋白酶抑制剂

词根 prote-（蛋白）+ -ase（酶）+ in-（不）+ -hibitor（抑制者）
例句 Protease inhibitors are commonly used to treat viral infections by blocking viral enzymes. 蛋白酶抑制剂常用于通过阻止病毒酶来治疗病毒感染。

transporter 转运蛋白

词根 trans-（跨）+ -porter（运输者）
例句 Transporters in the cell membrane help move ions and molecules across the cell boundary. 细胞膜中的转运蛋白帮助离子和分子穿过细胞边界。

connector 连接蛋白

词根 con-（共同）+ -nector（连接者）
例句 Connector proteins link different cellular structures to form functional complexes. 连接蛋白将不同的细胞结构连接起来，形成功能性复合物。

mediator 介导因子

词根 med-（中间）+ -ator（做；执行）
例句 The mediator proteins play a critical role in transmitting signals between cells during immune responses. 介导因子在免疫反应中传递细胞间信号，发挥着关键作用。

orchi-（睾丸，强调解剖结构）

orchiectomy 睾丸切除术

词根 orchi-（睾丸）+ -ectomy（切除术）
例句 Orchiectomy is a surgical procedure used to remove one or both testicles, often performed in cases of testicular cancer. 睾丸切除术是一种手术，用于切除单侧或双侧睾丸，通常用于治疗睾丸癌。

orchitis 睾丸炎

词根 orchi-（睾丸）+ -itis（炎症）

例句 Orchitis is inflammation of the testicles, often caused by bacterial or viral infections such as mumps. 睾丸炎是指睾丸的炎症，通常由细菌或病毒感染（如腮腺炎）引起。

orchiopathy 睾丸病

词根 orchi-（睾丸）+ -pathy（疾病）

例句 Orchiopathy refers to any disease or disorder affecting the testicles, including infections and trauma. 睾丸病是指任何影响睾丸的疾病或障碍，包括感染和创伤。

orchialgia 睾丸痛

词根 orchi-（睾丸）+ -algia（痛）

例句 Orchialgia is characterized by persistent or intermittent pain in one or both testicles, often caused by trauma or infections. 睾丸痛是指单侧或双侧睾丸持续或间歇性疼痛，通常由创伤或感染引起。

orchioplasty 睾丸修复术

词根 orchi-（睾丸）+ -plasty（修复术）

例句 Orchioplasty is a surgical procedure to repair or reconstruct a damaged testicle. 睾丸修复术是一种修复或重建受损睾丸的外科手术。

orchiectomy with prosthesis 带假体的睾丸切除术

词根 orchi-（睾丸）+ -ectomy（切除术）+ prosthesis（假体）

例句 Following orchiectomy, some patients opt for prosthetic testicle implants to restore cosmetic appearance. 在睾丸切除术后，一些患者选择假体植入以恢复外观。

orchiopexy 睾丸固定术

词根 orchi-（睾丸）+ -pexy（固定术）

例句 Orchiopexy is commonly performed in children with undescended testicles to move the testicle into its proper position. 睾丸固定术通常用于治疗隐睾症儿童，将睾丸移至正确位置。

orchidometer 睾丸测量器

词根 orchi-（睾丸）+ -meter（测量器）

例句 An orchidometer is a device used to measure the size of testicles, often in the evaluation of delayed puberty. 睾丸测量器是一种用于测量睾丸大小的装置，通常用于评估青春期延迟。

orchiodynia 睾丸疼痛

词根 orchi-（睾丸）+ -dynia（痛）

例句 Orchiodynia can occur due to trauma, infection, or conditions like varicocele. 睾丸疼痛可能由创伤、感染或静脉曲张等疾病引起。

orchiocarcinoma 睾丸癌

词根 orchi-（睾丸）+ carcinoma（癌）

例句 Orchiocarcinoma is a type of testicular cancer that can spread rapidly if not treated early. 睾丸癌如果不及时治疗，可能迅速扩散。

orchiocele 睾丸突出

词根 orchi-（睾丸）+ -cele（膨出）

例句 Orchiocele refers to a protrusion of the testicle, often associated with inguinal hernia. 睾丸突出是指睾丸的膨出，通常与腹股沟疝有关。

orchioepididymitis 睾丸附睾炎

词根 orchi-（睾丸）+ epididymitis（附睾炎）

例句 Orchioepididymitis is an infection involving both the testicle and epididymis, often requiring antibiotic treatment. 睾丸附睾炎是一种同时影响睾丸和附睾的感染，通常需要抗生素治疗。

orchidolysis 睾丸松解术

词根 orchi-（睾丸）+ -lysis（松解）

例句 Orchidolysis is a procedure performed to release adhesions around the testicles, often to relieve pain. 睾丸松解术是一种用于松解睾丸周围粘连以缓解疼痛的手术。

orchiectomy for hormone control 激素控制的睾丸切除术

词根 orchi-（睾丸）+ -ectomy（切除术）

例句 Bilateral orchiectomy may be performed to control hormone production in prostate cancer patients. 双侧睾丸切除术可能用于控制前列腺癌患者的激素分泌。

orchiectomy for gender reassignment 变性手术中的睾丸切除

词根 orchi-（睾丸）+ -ectomy（切除术）

例句 Orchiectomy is an essential step in gender-affirming surgery for transgender women. 睾丸切除术是变性手术的重要步骤。

orchiectomy with chemotherapy 化疗后的睾丸切除术

词根 orchi-（睾丸）+ -ectomy（切除术）

例句 In cases of advanced testicular cancer, orchiectomy is often combined with chemotherapy for better outcomes. 在晚期睾丸癌病例中，睾丸切除术通常与化疗联合进行以取得更好的效果。

orchiectomy with radiation therapy 放疗结合的睾丸切除术

词根 orchi-（睾丸）+ -ectomy（切除术）

例句 Patients undergoing orchiectomy for seminoma often receive additional radiation therapy to prevent recurrence. 进行睾丸切除术治疗精原细胞瘤的患者通常接受额外的放疗以防止复发。

orchiectomy for testicular torsion 睾丸扭转的睾丸切除术

词根 orchi-（睾丸）+ -ectomy（切除术）

例句 In severe cases of testicular torsion where blood flow cannot be restored, orchiectomy may be necessary. 在严重的睾丸扭转情

况下，无法恢复血流时，可能需要进行睾丸切除术。

orchioatrophy 睾丸萎缩

词根 orchi-（睾丸）+ atrophy（萎缩）

例句 Orchioatrophy is often seen in patients with untreated cryptorchidism or testicular trauma. 睾丸萎缩通常见于未治疗的隐睾症或睾丸创伤患者。

orchioneuralgia 睾丸神经痛

词根 orchi-（睾丸）+ neuro-（神经）+ -algia（疼痛）

例句 Orchioneuralgia involves chronic testicular pain due to nerve irritation or damage. 睾丸神经痛是由于神经刺激或损伤引起的慢性睾丸疼痛。

orexi-（食欲的）

orexis 食欲

词根 orexi-（食欲）

例句 Orexis refers to the desire or appetite for food. 食欲指的是对食物的渴望。

anorexia 食欲缺乏症

词根 an-（无）+ orexi-（食欲）

例句 Anorexia is an eating disorder characterized by an intense fear of gaining weight, leading to severe food restriction. 食欲缺乏症是一种进食障碍，特点是对增加体重的强烈恐惧，导致极度限制食物摄入。

hyperorexia 食欲亢进症

词根 hyper-（过度）+ orexi-（食欲）

例句 Hyperorexia is characterized by excessive hunger and is sometimes seen in conditions like bulimia. 食欲亢进症的特点是过度饥

饿，某些情况下如贪食症中可见。

orexigenic 促食欲的

词根 orexi-（食欲）+ -genic（产生的）

例句 Orexigenic drugs are used to stimulate appetite in patients who are experiencing severe weight loss. 促食欲药物用于刺激那些经历严重体重减轻的患者的食欲。

anorexigenic 抑制食欲的

词根 an-（无）+ orexi-（食欲）+ -genic（产生的）

例句 Anorexigenic medications help suppress appetite, and are often used for weight management. 抑制食欲药物帮助抑制食欲，通常用于体重管理。

ortho-（正；直）

orthopedics 骨科

词根 ortho-（正）+ ped-（脚；骨骼）+ -ics（学科）

例句 Orthopedics deals with the prevention, diagnosis, and treatment of skeletal and muscular disorders. 骨科处理骨骼和肌肉疾病的预防、诊断和治疗。

orthodontics 牙齿矫正学

词根 ortho-（正）+ dont-（牙齿）+ -ics（学科）

例句 Orthodontics specializes in the alignment of teeth and jaws, particularly through the use of braces. 牙齿矫正学专注于牙齿和颌骨的排列矫正，尤其通过使用牙套来实现。

orthostatic hypotension 直立性低血压

词根 ortho-（直）+ static（站立）+ hypo-（低）+ tension（血压）

例句 Orthostatic hypotension is a form of low blood pressure that occurs when standing up quickly. 直立性低血压是在快速站立时

出现的一种低血压类型。

orthognathic surgery 正颌手术

词根 ortho-（正）+ gnath-（下巴）+ -ic（形容词后缀）

例句 Orthognathic surgery is performed to correct jaw misalignments and improve facial aesthetics and function. 正颌手术用于矫正下颌错位，改善面部美学和功能。

orthopnea 端坐呼吸

词根 ortho-（直）+ -pnea（呼吸）

例句 Orthopnea is a condition in which a person has difficulty breathing when lying flat and must sit up to breathe comfortably. 端坐呼吸是一种患者平躺时呼吸困难，必须坐起才能舒适呼吸的病症。

orthotic 矫形的

词根 ortho-（正）+ -ic（形容词后缀）

例句 Orthotic devices are used to support or align bones, joints, or muscles, often to correct deformities. 矫形器是用来支撑或对齐骨骼、关节或肌肉的设备，通常用于矫正畸形。

orthosomnia 正睡症

词根 ortho-（正）+ somnia（睡眠）

例句 Orthosomnia refers to the obsession with achieving perfect sleep, often leading to sleep disturbances. 正睡症是指对完美睡眠的执念，常常导致睡眠障碍。

orthogenesis 正向进化

词根 ortho-（正）+ -genesis（生成）

例句 Orthogenesis refers to the theory of evolution in which organisms evolve in a straight-line direction, rather than by natural selection. 正向进化是指一种进化理论，认为有机体沿直线方向进化，而不是通过自然选择。

orthochromic 正色的

词根 ortho-（正）+ chromic（颜色的）

例句 Orthochromic refers to a standard or true color, often used in reference to imaging technologies. 正色指的是标准色或真实色，通常用于成像技术中。

orthotropic growth 正向生长

词根 ortho-（正）+ tropic（生长方向）

例句 Orthotropic growth describes the development of cells or tissues in a directed, upright manner. 正向生长描述了细胞或组织朝着特定方向、直立生长的过程。

USMLE Step 3 样题

A 2-year-old girl is brought to the office by her mother for evaluation of fever. You have been the girl's physician since birth. While in the office, the girl stiffens and then has bilateral (bi-; -lateral), symmetrical shaking of her upper and lower extremities; she becomes mildly cyanotic (cyan-). The episode lasts for approximately 45 seconds, after which she becomes relaxed and appears to fall asleep (a-). Vital signs at this time are temperature 40.0°C (104.0°F), pulse 120/min, and respirations (re-; spir-; -ation) 40/min. On physical examination she has a generally pink complexion and flushed cheeks. She is limp and somnolent (somn-) and responds with a cry to noxious (nox-) stimulus. Tympanic (tympan-) membranes are inflamed bilaterally (bi-; -lateral), nose has a scant, clear discharge (dis-; -charge), and throat is mildly erythematous (eryth-; -ema) . Lungs are clear to auscultation (auscult-;-ation) except for transmitted (trans-) upper airway sounds. Heart has rapid rate with a grade 1/6 systolic murmur at the left sternal border. Complete blood count, blood culture, lumbar puncture, and catheterized urine specimen are obtained and sent for stat analysis. Acetaminophen (acet-; amin-; -ophen) is administered by rectal suppository. Thirty minutes later the patient awakens and is smiling. She is afebrile (a-; febr-). Additional history discloses that she was born at term, she had an uneventful (un-) neonatal (neo-; -natal) course, she has normal growth and development, and vaccinations are up-to-date. She has never had an episode similar to this. Initial laboratory results are shown:

Blood

WBC 10,400/mm^3

Neutrophils (neutro-; -phil), segmented 25%

Neutrophils (neutro-; -phil), bands 5%

Lymphocytes (lymph-; -cyte) 65%

Monocytes (mono-; -cyte) 5%

Cerebrospinal (cerebro-; -spin) fluid 0 RBC/mm^3

Urinalysis (urin-; -lysis) Normal

Other laboratory studies are pending.

In addition to ampicillin (-cilin) for otitis (ot-; -itis) media and acetaminophen (acet-; amin-; -ophen), this child also should receive which of the following?

(A) Oral ethosuximide (etho-; suxim-)

(B) Oral phenobarbital (pheno-; barb-)

(C) Oral phenytoin (pheny-; -toin)

(D) Rectal diazepam (-zepam)

(E) No additional medications

Two weeks later the patient is brought to the office for a follow-up visit. Her mother says that she is doing well and she has had no recurrence (re-; curr-; -ence) of her symptoms. Examination of the ears shows resolution (re-; solut-) of the otitis (ot-; -itis) media. Which of the following is the most important diagnostic step at this time?

(A) Audiology (audi-; -ology) testing

(B) Cognitive testing

(C) CT scan of the head

(D) EEG

(E) No additional testing

中文翻译

一名 2 岁女孩由其母亲带到诊室对其发热进行评估。你自她出生以来一直是她的医生。在就诊期间，女孩身体突然僵硬，随后出现双侧、对称性的上肢和下肢抖动，并伴有轻度发绀。发作持续约 45 秒，之后她放松下来，似乎睡着了。此时的生命体征为体温 40.0°C（104.0°F），脉搏 120 次 / 分钟，呼吸 40 次 / 分钟。体检显示她肤色整体偏粉红，双颊潮红。她四肢松弛，嗜睡，对疼痛刺激有哭泣反应。双侧鼓膜发炎，鼻腔有少量透明分泌物，咽部轻度红斑。肺部听诊清晰，仅有上呼吸道传导音。心脏节律快，在左侧胸骨旁听到 1/6 级收缩期杂音。采集了全血细胞计数、血培养、腰椎穿刺和导尿尿液样本，并送往实验室进行紧急分析。通过直肠栓剂给予了对乙酰氨基酚。30 分钟后，患者醒来，情绪稳定，体温恢复正常。进一步病史显示，她足月出生，新生儿期无异常，生长发育正常，疫苗接种齐全。

她从未有过类似发作。初步实验室结果如下：

白细胞计数 10,400/mm³

分叶核中性粒细胞 25%

带状核中性粒细胞 5%

淋巴细胞 65%

单核细胞 5%

脑脊液红细胞 0/mm³

尿液分析正常

其他实验室检查结果待定。

除了用于治疗中耳炎的氨苄西林和对乙酰氨基酚外，该患儿还应接受以下哪项治疗？

(A) 口服乙琥胺

(B) 口服苯巴比妥

(C) 口服苯妥英

(D) 直肠给药地西泮

(E) 无须额外药物

两周后，患者被带到门诊进行随访。她的母亲表示她恢复良好，未再次出现症状。耳部检查显示中耳炎已消退。此时最重要的诊断步骤是以下哪项？

(A) 听力测试

(B) 认知测试

(C) 头部 CT 扫描

(D) 脑电图（EEG）

(E) 无须额外检查

题目和答案中出现的词根

bi-：双

-lateral：侧

cyan-：蓝色

a-：表示否定

re-：重新；反复

spir：呼吸

-ation：表示动作的状态

somn-：睡眠

nox-：有害的

tympan-：鼓

dis-：离开

-charge：负担

eryth-：红色

-ema：病理状态

auscult-：听

trans-：转；跨

acet-：乙酰基

amin-：胺

-ophen：芳香环

un-：表否定

neo-：新的

-natal：出生

neutro-：中性的

-phil：嗜

lymph-：淋巴

-cyte：细胞

mono-：单个的

cerebro-：大脑的

spin-：脊髓

urin-：尿

-lysis：分解

-cilin：青霉素衍生药物

ot-：耳的，是 oto- 的同义变异

-itis：炎症

etho-：乙酰基

suxim-：琥珀酸

pheno-：苯环

barb-：巴比妥类药物的衍生物

pheny-：苯环的

-toin：抗癫痫类药物

-zepam：通过提升 γ- 氨基丁酸（γ-GABA）抗焦虑等作用的药物

curr-：跑

-ence：表示状态

audi-：听力

-ology：学科

-ose（糖）

glucose 葡萄糖

词根 gluc-（糖）+ -ose（糖）

例句 Glucose is a simple sugar that serves as the primary source of energy for the body. 葡萄糖是一种简单的糖类，作为身体的主要能量来源。

fructose 果糖

词根 fruct-（果）+ -ose（糖）

例句 Fructose is a monosaccharide found in fruits and honey, often used as a sweetener. 果糖是一种单糖，存在于水果和蜂蜜中，常用作甜味剂。

sucrose 蔗糖

词根 suc-（糖）+ -ose（糖）

例句 Sucrose, also known as table sugar, is a disaccharide made up of glucose and fructose. 蔗糖，也称为食糖，是由葡萄糖和果糖组成的二糖。

maltose 麦芽糖

词根 malt-（麦芽）+ -ose（糖）

例句 Maltose is a sugar formed from two glucose units and is commonly found in malted beverages and beer. 麦芽糖是由两个葡萄糖单元组成的糖，常见于麦芽饮料和啤酒中。

cellulose 纤维素

词根 cellul-（细胞）+ -ose（糖）

例句 Cellulose is a complex carbohydrate that forms the structural component of plant cell walls. 纤维素是一种复杂的碳水化合物，是植物细胞壁的结构成分。

lactulose 乳果糖

词根 lact-（乳）+ -ulose（糖）

例句 Lactulose is a synthetic sugar used as a laxative to treat constipation. 乳果糖是一种合成糖，用作泻药治疗便秘。

arabinose 阿拉伯糖

词根 arabin-（阿拉伯）+ -ose（糖）

例句 Arabinose is a sugar found in plants, particularly in the polysaccharides of plant cell walls. 阿拉伯糖是一种存在于植物中的糖，尤其是在植物细胞壁的多糖中。

xylose 木糖

词根 xylo-（木）+ -ose（糖）
例句 Xylose is a sugar derived from wood and other plant materials, used in various industrial applications. 木糖是一种从木材和其他植物材料中提取的糖，广泛应用于各种工业。

sorbose 山梨糖

词根 sorb-（山梨）+ -ose（糖）
例句 Sorbose is a sugar used in the production of vitamin C and as a sweetener. 山梨糖是一种用于生产维生素 C 和作为甜味剂的糖。

mannose 甘露糖

词根 mann-（甘露）+ -ose（糖）
例句 Mannose is a simple sugar found in some fruits and vegetables, involved in various biological processes. 甘露糖是一种存在于某些水果和蔬菜中的单糖，参与多种生物学过程。

USMLE Step 3　样题

A 55-year-old woman, gravida 4, para 4, comes to the office because of vaginal spotting that has occurred once monthly for the past 2 months. Menopause (meno-; -pause) occurred 1 year ago, and this is the patient's first postmenopausal (post-; meno-; -pause) examination. Medical history is significant for elevated blood pressure readings during the past 2 years and diabetes mellitus for which she follows an 1,800-calorie diet. She takes no medications. Her most recent cervical cytology (cyt-; -ology) and mammography (mamm-; -graphy) obtained 1 year ago disclosed no abnormalities. Family history is significant for hypertension (hyper-; -tension) in her mother who died at age 58 years from an unknown cancer. The patient has smoked one pack of cigarettes (cigar-; -ette) daily for the past 30 years and drinks beer occasionally. BMI is 42 kg/m^2. Temperature is 36.7°C (98.0°F), pulse is 90/min, respirations (re-; spir-; -ation) are 16/min, and blood pressure is 136/84 mmHg. Bimanual (bi-) examination discloses a firm, smooth, mobile, nontender (non-) uterus that is consistent in size with a 6-week gestation (gest-; -ation). The remainder of the physical examination discloses no abnormalities. Results of dipstick urinalysis (urin-;-lysis) are within the reference ranges; fingerstick hematocrit (hemato-; -crit) is 35% and 2-hour postprandial (post-; prand-) serum glucose concentration is 188 mg/dL. Which of the following is the most appropriate diagnostic study at this time?

(A) Complete blood count
(B) CT scan of the pelvis
(C) Endometrial (endo-; metr-) biopsy
(D) Hysterosalpingography (hystero-; salpingo-; -graphy)
(E) Serum CA 125 concentration

中文翻译

一名 55 岁女性，孕 4 产 4，因过去 2 个月每月一次的阴道点滴出血前来就诊。她在 1 年前进入更年期，这是她首次进行绝经后检查。病史包括过去 2 年血压升高和糖尿病，她为此遵循 1,800 kcal（约 7,500 kJ）的饮食控制。她未服用任何药物。

她最近一次宫颈细胞学检查和乳腺X线检查是在1年前，均无异常。家族史显示其母亲患有高血压，并于58岁时死于未知癌症。患者有30年每天吸一包烟的吸烟史，偶尔饮啤酒。BMI为42 kg/m²。体温36.7℃（98.0°F），脉搏90次/分钟，呼吸16次/分钟，血压136/84 mmHg。双合诊显示子宫坚实、光滑、可移动、无压痛，大小与妊娠6周相当。其余体检未发现异常。尿液试纸分析结果在参考范围内；指尖血细胞比容为35%，餐后2小时血清葡萄糖浓度为188 mg/dL。此时最适当的诊断检查是以下哪项？

(A) 全血细胞计数
(B) 骨盆CT扫描
(C) 子宫内膜活检
(D) 子宫输卵管造影
(E) 血清CA 125浓度

题目和答案中出现的词根

meno-：每个月
-pause：停止
post-：在……之后
cyt-：细胞
-ology：学科
mamm-：乳房
-graphy：图像
hyper-：高
-tension：张力；压力
cigar-：雪茄

-ette：小的

re-：重新；反复

spir：呼吸

-ation：表示动作的状态

bi-：双

non-：表示否定

gest-：携带

urin-：尿

-lysis：分解

hemato-：血

-crit：分离法

prand-：吃饭

endo-：内

metr-：子宫

hystero-：子宫的

salpingo-：输卵管的

-osis（病态）

neurosis 神经症

词根 neuro-（神经）+ -osis（病态）

例句 Neurosis refers to a range of mental health conditions that involve distress but do not impair reality testing. 神经症是指一系列精神健康问题，痛苦但不影响现实能力。

psoriasis 银屑病

词根 psor-（皮肤屑）+ -iasis（病态）

例句 Psoriasis is a chronic autoimmune condition that leads to the rapid growth of skin cells. 银屑病是一种慢性自身免疫性疾病，导致皮肤细胞快速生长。

cirrhosis 肝硬化

词根 cirrh-（黄色）+ -osis（病态）

例句 Cirrhosis is a condition where the liver becomes severely scarred, often due to alcohol abuse or chronic hepatitis. 肝硬化是肝脏严重受损的病症，通常由酗酒或慢性肝炎引起。

tuberculosis 结核病

词根 tubercul-（小肿块）+ -osis（病态）

例句 Tuberculosis is a bacterial infection that primarily affects the lungs but can spread to other parts of the body. 结核病是一种主要影响肺部的细菌感染，但也可以传播到身体其他部位。

scoliosis 脊柱侧弯

词根 scoli-（弯曲）+ -osis（病态）

例句 Scoliosis is a condition characterized by an abnormal curvature of the spine. 脊柱侧弯是指脊柱的异常弯曲。

leukocytosis 白细胞增多

词根 leuk-（白）+ cyt-（细胞）+ -osis（病态）

例句 Leukocytosis refers to an increase in white blood cell count, often indicating infection or inflammation. 白细胞增多是指白细胞数量的增加，通常表示感染或炎症。

osteoporosis 骨质疏松症

词根 oste-（骨）+ por-（孔）+ -osis（病态）

例句 Osteoporosis is a condition in which bones become brittle and fragile, leading to an increased risk of fractures. 骨质疏松症是指骨骼变得脆弱和易碎，导致骨折风险增加。

fibrosis 纤维化

词根 fibr-（纤维）+ -osis（病态）

例句 Fibrosis occurs when excess fibrous connective tissue forms as a result of injury or inflammation. 纤维化发生在因伤害或炎症导致过多的纤维结缔组织形成时。

psychosis 精神病

词根 psych-（心理）+ -osis（病态）

例句 Psychosis is a mental disorder characterized by a disconnection from reality, often involving hallucinations or delusions. 精神病是一种精神障碍，表现为与现实的脱节，通常伴随幻觉或妄想。

USMLE Step 2 CK　样题

A 1-week-old male newborn is evaluated in the hospital nursery 4 days after undergoing operative repair of a myelomeningocele (myelo-; meningo-; -cele). He was born at 37 weeks' gestation (gest-; -ation) via uncomplicated (un-), spontaneous vaginal delivery to an 18-year-old primigravid (primi-; -gravid) woman. The defect was diagnosed prenatally (pre-; -natal) by ultrasonography (ultra-; sono-; -graphy), and the repair was done 72 hours after delivery. He is at the 5th percentile for length, 10th percentile for weight, and 25th percentile for head circumference (circum-; fer-; -ence). Temperature is 36.9°C (98.4°F), pulse is 138/min, and respirations (re-; spir-; -ation) are 42/min. Pulse oximetry (oxi-; -metry) on room air shows an oxygen saturation of 98%. The newborn appears comfortable. Physical examination shows a soft, flat, anterior fontanel (fontan-). Red reflexes (re-; -flex) are normal. Moro reflex is symmetric in the upper extremities; there is no movement in the lower extremities. Ultrasonography (ultra-; sono-; -graphy) of the brain shows mildly enlarged ventricles.

Which of the following is the most likely associated finding in this patient?

(A) Congenital heart malformation (mal-)

(B) Cryptorchidism (crypt-; orchid-)

(C) Impaired folate metabolism

(D) Neurogenic (neuro-) bladder

(E) Severe cognitive impairment

中文翻译

一名 1 周岁男婴在医院新生儿室接受评估，他在出生后 4 天接受了脊髓脊膜膨出修复手术。他由一名 18 岁初孕妇在妊娠 37 周通过无并发症的自然阴道分娩出生。胎儿期通过超声检查确诊该缺陷，并在分娩后 72 小时进行了修复手术。他的身长处于第 5 百分位，体重处于第 10 百分位，头围处于第 25 百分位。体温 36.9℃（98.4℉），脉搏 138 次 / 分钟，呼吸 42 次 / 分钟。在室温空气下的脉搏血氧饱和度为 98%。新生儿看起来舒适。体检显示前囟门柔软平坦。红光反射正常。莫罗反射在上肢对称；下肢无运动。脑部超声显示脑室轻度扩大。以下哪项是该患者最可能相关的发现？

(A) 先天性心脏畸形

(B) 隐睾症

(C) 叶酸代谢障碍

(D) 神经源性膀胱

(E) 严重认知障碍

题目和答案中出现的词根

myelo-：脊髓的

meningo-：脑膜的

-cele：凸出

gest-：携带

-ation：表示动作

un-：表否定

primi-：第一次

-gravid：怀孕

pre-：在……之前

-natal：出生

ultra-：超

sono-：声音的

-graphy：图像

circum-：环状的

fer-：携带

-ence：状态（在医学上，环状携带状态指的是解剖结构的周长）

re-：重新；反复

spir：呼吸

oxi-：氧气的

-metry：测量仪

-flex：弯曲

mal-：错误的

crypt-：隐性的

orchid-：睾丸

neuro-: 神经的

oste-/osteo-（骨）

osteoporosis 骨质疏松

词根 osteo-（骨）+ por-（孔隙）+ -osis（病态）

例句 Osteoporosis is a condition characterized by weakened bones, increasing the risk of fractures. 骨质疏松是一种骨骼变弱、骨折风险增加的疾病。

osteoarthritis 骨关节炎

词根 osteo-（骨）+ arthr-（关节）+ -itis（炎症）

例句 Osteoarthritis is a degenerative joint disease that commonly affects older adults. 骨关节炎是一种常见于老年人的退行性关节疾病。

osteomalacia 骨软化症

词根 osteo-（骨）+ -malacia（软化）

例句 Osteomalacia is caused by a deficiency of vitamin D, leading to soft and weakened bones. 骨软化症是维生素 D 缺乏导致骨骼软化和脆弱的疾病。

osteogenesis 骨生成

词根 osteo-（骨）+ -genesis（生成）

例句 Osteogenesis is the process of bone formation, crucial during growth and healing of fractures. 骨生成是骨骼形成的过程，在生长和骨折愈合中至关重要。

osteopathy 整骨疗法

词根 osteo-（骨）+ -pathy（病；疗法）

例句 Osteopathy focuses on the treatment of musculoskeletal disorders through manipulation and physical therapy. 整骨疗法通过手

法和物理治疗来治疗肌肉骨骼系统的疾病。

osteomyelitis 骨髓炎

词根 osteo-（骨）+ myel-（骨髓）+ -itis（炎症）

例句 Osteomyelitis is a serious infection of the bone or bone marrow, often requiring antibiotic treatment. 骨髓炎是骨或骨髓的严重感染，通常需要抗生素治疗。

osteosarcoma 骨肉瘤

词根 osteo-（骨）+ sarc-（肉）+ -oma（肿瘤）

例句 Osteosarcoma is a type of cancer that starts in the bones, most commonly affecting teenagers. 骨肉瘤是一种起源于骨骼的癌症，最常见于青少年。

osteodystrophy 骨营养不良

词根 osteo-（骨）+ dys-（异常）+ -trophy（营养）

例句 Osteodystrophy is commonly seen in patients with chronic kidney disease, affecting bone mineralization. 骨营养不良常见于慢性肾病患者，影响骨骼矿化。

osteonecrosis 骨坏死

词根 osteo-（骨）+ -necrosis（坏死）

例句 Osteonecrosis occurs when the blood supply to the bone is disrupted, leading to bone death. 骨坏死是指骨骼的血液供应中断，导致骨组织死亡。

osteoblast 成骨细胞

词根 osteo-（骨）+ -blast（未成熟细胞）

例句 Osteoblasts are responsible for forming new bone tissue during growth and healing. 成骨细胞在生长和愈合期间负责形成新的骨组织。

osteoclast 破骨细胞

词根 osteo-（骨）+ -clast（破坏细胞）

例句 Osteoclasts play a key role in bone remodeling by breaking down old or damaged bone tissue. 破骨细胞在骨骼重塑中起关键作用，分解旧的或受损的骨组织。

osteopenia 骨密度降低

词根 osteo-（骨）+ -penia（缺乏）
例句 Osteopenia refers to lower-than-normal bone density, which is often a precursor to osteoporosis. 骨密度降低是指骨密度低于正常水平，通常是骨质疏松的前兆。

osteotomy 截骨术

词根 osteo-（骨）+ -tomy（切开）
例句 Osteotomy is a surgical procedure used to cut and realign bones to correct deformities. 截骨术是一种用于切割和重新排列骨骼以矫正畸形的手术。

osteochondritis 骨软骨炎

词根 osteo-（骨）+ chondr-（软骨）+ -itis（炎症）
例句 Osteochondritis is the inflammation of the bone and cartilage, often caused by repetitive trauma. 骨软骨炎是骨骼和软骨的炎症，通常由反复创伤引起。

osteolysis 骨溶解

词根 osteo-（骨）+ -lysis（分解）
例句 Osteolysis is a process in which bone tissue is broken down, commonly seen in metastatic bone disease. 骨溶解是指骨组织被分解的过程，常见于骨转移疾病。

osteophyte 骨赘

词根 osteo-（骨）+ -phyte（生长物）
例句 Osteophytes, or bone spurs, are bony outgrowths that develop along joint margins, often due to arthritis. 骨赘，也称骨刺，是沿关节边缘生长的骨质增生物，通常由关节炎引起。

osteochondroma 骨软骨瘤

词根 osteo-（骨）+ chondro-（软骨）+ -oma（肿瘤）

例句 Osteochondroma is a benign bone tumor that often occurs near growth plates. 骨软骨瘤是一种良性骨肿瘤，通常发生在生长板附近。

osteosclerosis 骨硬化

词根 osteo-（骨）+ -sclerosis（硬化）

例句 Osteosclerosis is characterized by abnormal hardening of the bone, often seen in conditions such as Paget's disease. 骨硬化是指骨骼异常硬化，常见于佩吉特病等疾病。

osteofibroma 骨纤维瘤

词根 osteo-（骨）+ fibr-（纤维）+ -oma（瘤）

例句 Osteofibroma is a benign tumor made of fibrous tissue and bone, often found in the jaw or long bones. 骨纤维瘤是一种由纤维组织和骨组成的良性肿瘤，常见于下颌骨或长骨。

osteoarthritis deformans 变形性骨关节炎

词根 osteo-（骨）+ arthr-（关节）+ -itis（炎症）

例句 Osteoarthritis deformans leads to joint deformity and pain, commonly affecting the knees and hips. 变形性骨关节炎导致关节畸形和疼痛，常见于膝盖和髋部。

oto-（耳）

otolaryngology 耳鼻喉科学

词根 oto-（耳）+ laryng-（喉）+ -ology（学科）

例句 Otolaryngology is the medical specialty focused on diagnosing and treating disorders of the ear, nose, and throat. 耳鼻喉科学是专注于诊断和治疗耳、鼻、喉疾病的医学专业。

otitis media 中耳炎

词根 oto-（耳）+ -itis（炎症）+ media（中部）

例句 Otitis media is a common condition in children and is characterized by inflammation and infection of the middle ear. 中耳炎是儿童中常见的疾病，其特点是中耳部位的炎症和感染。

otosclerosis 耳硬化症

词根 oto-（耳）+ -sclerosis（硬化）

例句 Otosclerosis leads to abnormal bone growth in the middle ear, causing hearing loss. 耳硬化症导致中耳内异常骨质生长，引起听力损失。

otalgia 耳痛

词根 oto-（耳）+ -algia（痛）

例句 Otalgia can be caused by infections, trauma, or referred pain from nearby structures like the throat. 耳痛可能由感染、创伤或邻近结构（如喉咙）引起的牵涉痛导致。

otorrhea 耳漏

词根 oto-（耳）+ -rrhea（流出）

例句 Otorrhea refers to the discharge of fluid from the ear, often associated with infections or trauma. 耳漏是指从耳朵流出液体，通常与感染或创伤有关。

ototoxicity 耳毒性

词根 oto-（耳）+ toxic（毒性）+ -ity（状态）

例句 Ototoxicity is a side effect of certain medications, leading to damage to the ear and potential hearing loss. 耳毒性是某些药物的副作用，会损害耳朵并可能导致听力损失。

otorrhagia 耳出血

词根 oto-（耳）+ -rrhagia（出血）

例句 Otorrhagia occurs when there is bleeding from the ear, often due to trauma or infection. 耳出血是指耳朵出血，通常由创伤或感染引起。

otoacoustic emissions 耳声发射

词根 oto-（耳）+ acoustic（声音）+ emissions（发射）

例句 Otoacoustic emissions are sounds produced by the inner ear and are used to assess hearing function in newborns. 耳声发射是内耳产生的声音，用于评估新生儿的听力功能。

otoconia 耳石

词根 oto-（耳）+ conia（小颗粒）

例句 Displacement of otoconia within the inner ear is a common cause of benign paroxysmal positional vertigo（BPPV）. 内耳中的耳石移位是良性阵发性位置性眩晕（BPPV）的常见原因。

otitis externa 外耳炎

词根 oto-（耳）+ -itis（炎症）+ externa（外部）

例句 Otitis externa, also known as swimmer's ear, is an infection of the ear canal caused by moisture buildup. 外耳炎，也称游泳者耳，是由于耳道积水引起的感染。

otoplasty 耳整形术

词根 oto-（耳）+ -plasty（修复术）

例句 Otoplasty is a surgical procedure to reshape or reposition the ears, often for cosmetic or reconstructive purposes. 耳整形术是一种手术，用于重新塑造或调整耳朵的位置，通常出于美容或修复目的。

otoscopic examination 耳镜检查

词根 oto-（耳）+ scopic（观察）+ examination（检查）

例句 Otoscopic examination is routinely performed to inspect the ear canal and eardrum for signs of infection or damage. 耳镜检查是常规操作，用于检查耳道和耳膜是否有感染或损伤的迹象。

otology 耳科学

词根 oto-（耳）+ -logy（学科）

例句 Otology is the branch of medicine that deals with the anatomy, function, and diseases of the ear. 耳科学是研究耳朵解剖结构、功能及疾病的医学分支。

otomastoiditis 耳乳突炎

词根 oto-（耳）+ mastoid-（乳突）+ -itis（炎症）

例句 Otomastoiditis is the inflammation of the mastoid process of the temporal bone, often secondary to middle ear infections. 耳乳突炎是颞骨乳突部位的炎症，通常继发于中耳感染。

ototomy 耳切开术

词根 oto-（耳）+ -tomy（切开）

例句 Ototomy is a surgical procedure in which an incision is made into the ear, often to relieve pressure or drain fluid. 耳切开术是一种手术，在耳部切开以缓解压力或引流液体。

otoencephalitis 耳脑炎

词根 oto-（耳）+ encephal-（脑）+ -itis（炎症）

例句 Otoencephalitis is an inflammatory condition that involves both the ear and the brain, often resulting from infections. 耳脑炎是同时涉及耳部和大脑的炎症，通常由感染引起。

otosyphilis 耳梅毒

词根 oto-（耳）+ syphilis（梅毒）

例句 Otosyphilis is a complication of syphilis that can lead to hearing loss and balance issues. 耳梅毒是梅毒的一种并发症，可导致听力丧失和平衡问题。

otopathy 耳病

词根 oto-（耳）+ -pathy（疾病）

例句 Otopathy refers to any disease or disorder affecting the ear, including infections and structural abnormalities. 耳病是指任何影响耳部的疾病或障碍，包括感染和结构异常。

otolithiasis 耳石症

词根 oto-（耳）+ -lithiasis（结石）
例句 Otolithiasis is a condition where small crystals in the inner ear become dislodged, causing vertigo. 耳石症是指内耳中的小晶体移位，引起眩晕的病症。

otoporosis 耳骨疏松

词根 oto-（耳）+ -porosis（孔隙增加）
例句 Otoporosis refers to the loss of bone density in the auditory ossicles, potentially affecting hearing. 耳骨疏松是指听小骨的骨密度下降，可能影响听力。

-otomy（切开）

laparotomy 腹部切开术

词根 laparo-（腹部）+ -otomy（切开）
例句 Laparotomy is a surgical procedure in which the abdomen is opened to diagnose or treat conditions inside the abdominal cavity. 腹部切开术是一种外科手术，打开腹部以诊断或治疗腹腔内的疾病。

tracheotomy 气管切开术

词根 tracheo-（气管）+ -otomy（切开）
例句 Tracheotomy is performed when an obstruction in the upper airway requires direct access to the trachea for breathing. 气管切开术是当上气道阻塞需要直接进入气管以供呼吸时进行的手术。

phlebotomy 静脉切开术

词根 phleb-（静脉）+ -otomy（切开）

例句 Phlebotomy is the practice of making an incision into a vein to withdraw blood for medical tests or treatments. 静脉切开术是指对静脉进行切开以取血进行医学检测或治疗的操作。

thoracotomy 胸腔切开术

词根 thoraco-（胸腔）+ -otomy（切开）
例句 Thoracotomy is a surgery that involves making an incision in the chest to access the organs within the thoracic cavity. 胸腔切开术是一种手术，通过在胸部做切口以进入胸腔内器官。

craniotomy 颅骨切开术

词根 crani-（颅骨）+ -otomy（切开）
例句 Craniotomy is performed to access the brain in order to treat conditions like tumors or brain injuries. 颅骨切开术是为了治疗肿瘤或脑部损伤等病症而进行的颅脑手术。

cystotomy 膀胱切开术

词根 cyst-（膀胱）+ -otomy（切开）
例句 Cystotomy is a procedure in which the bladder is surgically opened, often to remove stones or repair damage. 膀胱切开术是一种手术，通常用于去除膀胱结石或修复损伤。

gastrotomy 胃切开术

词根 gastro-（胃）+ -otomy（切开）
例句 Gastrotomy is a surgical procedure where the stomach is opened to treat ulcers, tumors, or other conditions. 胃切开术是对胃进行开刀治疗溃疡、肿瘤或其他疾病的手术。

enterotomy 肠切开术

词根 enter-（肠）+ -otomy（切开）
例句 Enterotomy involves making an incision into the intestine to remove obstructions or treat other bowel conditions. 肠切开术是对肠道进行切开以去除阻塞物或治疗其他肠道病症的手术。

herniotomy 疝气切开术

词根 hernio-（疝气）+ -otomy（切开）

例句 Herniotomy is a surgical procedure to repair a hernia, involving the incision of the area affected by the hernia. 疝气切开术是修复疝气的手术，指对疝气部位进行切开。

rhizotomy 根切开术

词根 rhiz-（根）+ -otomy（切开）

例句 Rhizotomy is a surgical procedure used to cut the nerve roots in the spine to relieve chronic pain. 根切开术是一种手术，用于切断脊柱中的神经根以缓解慢性疼痛。

lobotomy 脑叶切开术

词根 lob-（脑叶）+ -otomy（切开）

例句 Lobotomy is a controversial procedure that involves severing connections in the brain's frontal lobe to treat severe mental disorders. 脑叶切开术是一种争议性手术，指切断大脑前额叶的连接，用于治疗严重的精神障碍。

colotomy 结肠切开术

词根 col-（结肠）+ -otomy（切开）

例句 Colotomy is a procedure in which an incision is made in the colon for diagnostic or therapeutic purposes. 结肠切开术是一种在结肠上做切口以用于诊断或治疗的手术。

pericardiotomy 心包切开术

词根 peri-（周围）+ cardi-（心脏）+ -otomy（切开）

例句 Pericardiotomy is the surgical incision into the pericardium, often performed to drain fluid or relieve pressure on the heart. 心包切开术是对心包的切开手术，常用于引流液体或缓解心脏的压力。

gingivotomy 牙龈切开术

词根 gingiv-（牙龈）+ -otomy（切开）

例句 Gingivotomy is a surgical procedure to make an incision in the gum tissue to treat gum disease. 牙龈切开术是一种手术，用于对牙龈组织进行切开以治疗牙龈病。

urethrotomy 尿道切开术

词根 urethr-（尿道）+ -otomy（切开）
例句 Urethrotomy is a surgical procedure used to relieve blockages in the urethra. 尿道切开术是一种手术，用于缓解尿道的阻塞。

ox-（氧）

hypoxia 缺氧

词根 hypo-（低）+ ox-（氧）+ -ia（状态）
例句 Hypoxia occurs when tissues do not receive sufficient oxygen, leading to cell damage or death. 缺氧是指组织未能获得足够的氧气，可能导致细胞损伤或死亡。

hyperoxia 高氧症

词根 hyper-（过度）+ ox-（氧）+ -ia（状态）
例句 Prolonged hyperoxia can cause oxidative stress and damage to lung tissues. 长期高氧可能引起氧化应激和肺组织损伤。

oxidation 氧化

词根 ox-（氧）+ -idation（过程）
例句 Oxidation is a chemical reaction where a substance loses electrons, often producing free radicals. 氧化是指物质失去电子的化学反应，通常会产生自由基。

oxidative stress 氧化应激

词根 ox-（氧）+ -ative（形容词后缀）+ stress（压力）
例句 Oxidative stress occurs when the body's antioxidant defense system is overwhelmed by free radicals. 氧化应激是指当体内抗氧

化防御系统无法应对自由基时出现的情况。

oxygenation 氧合

词根 ox-（氧）+ -genation（生成）

例句 Oxygenation of blood is critical during surgery to ensure proper tissue perfusion. 在手术中，血液的氧合对于确保组织灌注至关重要。

anoxia 无氧症

词根 an-（无）+ ox-（氧）+ -ia（状态）

例句 Anoxia occurs when oxygen supply to the tissues is completely cut off, often leading to severe organ damage. 无氧症是指组织的氧气供应完全中断，通常导致严重的器官损伤。

oxymetry 血氧测定

词根 ox-（氧）+ -metry（测量）

例句 Pulse oximetry is commonly used to monitor blood oxygen saturation in patients during surgery. 脉搏血氧仪常用于手术期间监测患者的血氧饱和度。

oxytocin 催产素

词根 ox-（氧）+ toc-（分娩）+ -in（物质）

例句 Oxytocin plays a key role in childbirth and bonding between mother and infant. 催产素在分娩和母婴之间的情感联系中起着关键作用。

oximeter 血氧计

词根 ox-（氧）+ -meter（测量器）

例句 An oximeter is used to measure the level of oxygen saturation in the blood. 血氧计用于测量血液中的氧饱和度。

oxalate 草酸盐

词根 ox-（氧）+ -alate（盐）

例句 High levels of oxalate in the body can lead to the formation of kidney stones. 体内高水平的草酸盐可能导致肾结石的形成。

oxidoreductase 氧化还原酶

词根 ox-（氧）+ reductase（还原酶）
例句 Oxidoreductases are enzymes involved in oxidation-reduction reactions in cells. 氧化还原酶是细胞中参与氧化还原反应的酶类。

hypoxemia 低氧血症

词根 hypo-（低）+ ox-（氧）+ -emia（血液）
例句 Hypoxemia occurs when the oxygen level in the blood is abnormally low, often indicating respiratory issues. 低氧血症是指血液中的氧含量异常偏低，通常预示着呼吸系统问题。

oxidant 氧化剂

词根 ox-（氧）+ -ant（物质）
例句 Oxidants, such as hydrogen peroxide, play an important role in cellular defense mechanisms. 氧化剂（如过氧化氢）在细胞防御机制中起重要作用。

oxalosuccinate 草酰琥珀酸

词根 ox-（氧）+ succinate（琥珀酸）
例句 Oxalosuccinate is an intermediate in the citric acid cycle, crucial for cellular respiration. 草酰琥珀酸是三羧酸循环中的中间体，对于细胞呼吸至关重要。

oxidative phosphorylation 氧化磷酸化

词根 ox-（氧）+ phosph-（磷）+ -orylation（过程）
例句 Oxidative phosphorylation is the primary method by which cells generate ATP. 氧化磷酸化是细胞产生 ATP 的主要方式。

oxidizable 可氧化的

词根 ox-（氧）+ -izable（能够）
例句 Fatty acids are highly oxidizable, making them an important energy source during metabolism. 脂肪酸易于氧化，使其成为代

谢过程中重要的能量来源。

oxidopathy 氧化病变

词根 ox-（氧）+ -pathy（病）

例句 Oxidopathy refers to tissue damage caused by oxidative stress, often associated with aging and chronic diseases. 氧化病变是指由氧化应激引起的组织损伤，通常与衰老和慢性疾病有关。

pan-（全）

pandemic 大流行病

词根 pan-（全）+ -demic（流行的）

例句 The COVID-19 pandemic affected millions of people worldwide. COVID-19 大流行病影响了全球数百万人。

pancreas 胰腺

词根 pan-（全）+ -creas（腺体）

例句 The pancreas is a gland that produces insulin to regulate blood sugar levels. 胰腺是分泌胰岛素以调节血糖水平的腺体。

panhypopituitarism（全垂体功能减退症）

词根 pan-（全）+ hypo-（不足）+ pituitarism（垂体功能）

例句 Panhypopituitarism is a condition in which the pituitary gland fails to secrete all of its hormones. 全垂体功能减退症是一种垂体腺无法分泌所有激素的疾病。

panacea 万灵药

词根 pan-（全）+ -acea（药物）

例句 A panacea is a remedy that is believed to cure all diseases, though such a cure doesn't actually exist. 万灵药是一种被认为能治愈所有疾病的疗法，尽管实际上并不存在这种疗法。

panophthalmitis 全眼炎

词根 pan-（全）+ ophthalm-（眼睛）+ -itis（炎症）

例句 Panophthalmitis refers to a severe inflammation of the entire eye, including the sclera, cornea, and retina. 全眼炎是指整个眼球的严重炎症，包括巩膜、角膜和视网膜。

pancytopenia 全血细胞减少症

词根 pan-（全）+ cyt-（细胞）+ -penia（减少）

例句 Pancytopenia is a condition in which all blood cell types are reduced in number. 全血细胞减少症是一种所有类型血细胞数量减少的疾病。

pancreatitis 胰腺炎

词根 pancreat-（胰腺）+ -itis（炎症）

例句 Pancreatitis is an inflammation of the pancreas, which can cause severe abdominal pain. 胰腺炎是胰腺发生的一种炎症反应，可能引起严重的腹痛。

panhypogammaglobulinemia 全免疫球蛋白低下症

词根 pan-(全)+ hypo-(不足)+ gammaglobulinemia(免疫球蛋白)

例句 Panhypogammaglobulinemia is a condition in which all immunoglobulin levels are abnormally low. 全免疫球蛋白低下症是一种所有免疫球蛋白水平异常低的病症。

panenteritis 全肠炎

词根 pan-（全）+ enter-（肠）+ -itis（炎症）

例句 Panenteritis refers to inflammation of the entire intestine, which may be caused by infections or autoimmune diseases. 全肠炎是指整个肠道的炎症，可能由感染或自身免疫性疾病引起。

papill-（乳头状的）

papilloma 乳头状瘤

词根 papill-（乳头）+ -oma（肿瘤）

例句 Papilloma is a benign tumor often found on the skin or mucous membranes. 乳头状瘤是一种良性肿瘤，通常发生在皮肤或黏膜上。

papillitis 乳头炎

词根 papill-（乳头）+ -itis（炎症）

例句 Papillitis refers to the inflammation of the optic nerve head, often caused by infection or autoimmune diseases. 乳头炎指视神经头的炎症，通常由感染或自身免疫性疾病引起。

papillary 乳头状的

词根 papill-（乳头）+ -ary（形容词后缀，表示“的”）

例句 Papillary tumors are characterized by finger-like projections from the surface of the tissue. 乳头状肿瘤的特点是从组织表面伸出的指状突起。

papillomavirus 乳头状瘤病毒

词根 papill-（乳头）+ -virus（病毒）

例句 Human papillomavirus（HPV）is known to cause warts and is linked to certain cancers. 人乳头状瘤病毒（HPV）已知可引起疣，并与某些癌症相关。

papillary carcinoma 乳头状癌

词根 papill-（乳头）+ -ary（形容词后缀）+ carcinoma（癌）

例句 Papillary carcinoma is a type of cancer that arises in glandular tissues and has a papillary structure. 乳头状癌是一种源自腺体组织并具有乳头状结构的癌症。

papillomatosis 乳头状瘤病

词根 papill-（乳头）+ -omatosis（肿瘤形成）

例句 Papillomatosis refers to a condition in which multiple papillomas develop in different parts of the body. 乳头状瘤病是指在身体多个部位出现多个乳头状瘤的病症。

papillosclerosis 乳头硬化症

词根 papill-（乳头）+ -sclerosis（硬化）

例句 Papillosclerosis involves thickening or scarring of the optic disc, often due to high blood pressure. 乳头硬化症涉及视神经盘的增厚或疤痕化，通常由高血压引起。

papillomatosis laryngis 喉部乳头状瘤病

词根 papill-（乳头）+ -omatosis（肿瘤形成）+ laryngis（喉部）
例句 Papillomatosis laryngis refers to the presence of papillomas in the larynx, which can cause hoarseness and breathing difficulties. 喉部乳头状瘤病是指喉部出现乳头状瘤，可能引起声音沙哑和呼吸困难。

papillary thyroid cancer 乳头状甲状腺癌

词根 papill-（乳头）+ -ary（形容词后缀）+ thyroid（甲状腺）+ cancer（癌症）
例句 Papillary thyroid cancer is the most common type of thyroid cancer and generally has a good prognosis. 乳头状甲状腺癌是最常见的甲状腺癌类型，通常预后较好。

papillary muscular rupture 乳头状肌肉断裂

词根 papill-（乳头）+ -ary（形容词后缀）+ muscular（肌肉的）+ rupture（断裂）
例句 Papillary muscular rupture is a condition where the muscle responsible for closing the heart valves ruptures, often leading to valve dysfunction. 乳头状肌肉断裂是一种病症，负责关闭心脏瓣膜的肌肉发生断裂，通常导致瓣膜功能障碍。

para-（旁）

paralysis 麻痹

词根 para-（旁）+ -lysis（分解）
例句 Paralysis is the loss of the ability to move one or more muscles, often caused by nerve damage. 麻痹是指一个或多个肌肉失去运动能力，通常由神经损伤引起。

paroxysm 阵发；突发

词根 para-（旁）+ -oxysm（发作）

例句 A paroxysm of coughing often occurs during respiratory infections. 阵发性咳嗽通常在呼吸道感染期间发生。

parasympathetic 副交感神经的

词根 para-（旁）+ sympathetic（交感神经的）

例句 The parasympathetic nervous system is responsible for rest and digestion functions. 副交感神经系统负责休息和消化功能。

parainfluenza 副流感

词根 para-（旁）+ influenza（流感）

例句 Parainfluenza viruses cause respiratory infections, especially in young children. 副流感病毒引起呼吸道感染，特别是在年幼儿童中。

parenteral 非肠道的

词根 para-（旁）+ enteral（肠道的）

例句 Parenteral nutrition is administered through veins, bypassing the digestive system. 非肠道营养通过静脉给予，绕过消化系统。

paraclinical 临床旁证的

词根 para-（旁）+ clinical（临床的）

例句 Paraclinical tests are diagnostic tools used to support clinical examination findings. 临床旁证测试是用来支持临床检查结果的诊断工具。

paracellular 细胞旁的

词根 para-（旁）+ cellular（细胞的）

例句 Paracellular transport refers to the movement of substances between cells rather than through them. 细胞旁转运指物质在细胞之间而非穿过细胞进行的移动。

paravertebral 脊椎旁的

词根 para-（旁）+ vertebral（脊椎的）
例句 Paravertebral muscles are located alongside the vertebral column and are important for movement. 脊椎旁肌肉位于脊柱两侧，对运动非常重要。

paracentesis 腹腔侧穿术

词根 para-（旁）+ -centesis（穿刺）
例句 Paracentesis is a procedure in which fluid is removed from the peritoneal cavity using a needle. 腹腔侧穿术是一种通过针头从腹膜腔中抽取液体的手术。

parasite 寄生虫

词根 para-（旁）+ site（栖息地）
例句 A parasite is an organism that lives in or on another organism, deriving nourishment at the host's expense. 寄生虫是一种生活在或寄生于其他生物体上的有机体，从宿主的营养中获益。

-pathy（病态）

neuropathy 神经病

词根 neur-（神经）+ -pathy（病态）
例句 Diabetic neuropathy is a common complication of diabetes, affecting the nerves. 糖尿病神经病是糖尿病的一种常见并发症，影响神经。

cardiomyopathy 心肌病

词根 cardio-（心脏）+ myo-（肌肉）+ -pathy（病态）
例句 Cardiomyopathy refers to diseases of the heart muscle that affect its ability to pump blood. 心肌病是指影响心脏肌肉的疾病，导致其泵血能力下降。

osteopathy 整骨疗法

词根 oste-（骨）+ -pathy（病态）

例句 Osteopathy is a treatment method that emphasizes the role of the musculoskeletal system in health and disease. 整骨疗法是一种治疗方法，强调肌肉骨骼系统在健康和疾病中的作用。

hepatopathy 肝病

词根 hepat-（肝脏）+ -pathy（病态）

例句 Hepatopathy is a general term for liver diseases, including cirrhosis and hepatitis. 肝病是指一类肝脏疾病，包括肝硬化和肝炎。

retinopathy 视网膜病变

词根 retino-（视网膜）+ -pathy（病态）

例句 Diabetic retinopathy is a complication of diabetes that affects the blood vessels in the retina. 糖尿病视网膜病变是糖尿病的一种并发症，影响视网膜的血管。

myopathy 肌病

词根 myo-（肌肉）+ -pathy（病态）

例句 Myopathy refers to a variety of diseases that affect the muscles, leading to weakness and pain. 肌病是指一类影响肌肉的疾病，导致肌肉无力和疼痛。

nephropathy 肾病

词根 nephr-（肾脏）+ -pathy（病态）

例句 Chronic nephropathy is a long-term kidney condition that can lead to kidney failure. 慢性肾病是一种长期肾脏疾病，可以导致肾衰竭。

encephalopathy 脑病

词根 encephal-（脑）+ -pathy（病态）

例句 Encephalopathy can result from a variety of causes, including infections, toxins, and head trauma. 脑病可能由多种原因引起，包括感染、毒素和头部创伤。

arthropathy 关节病

词根 arthr-（关节）+ -pathy（病态）
例句 Arthropathy involves the inflammation or degeneration of the joints, often leading to pain and disability. 关节病涉及关节的炎症或退化，常导致疼痛和功能障碍。

vasopathy 血管病

词根 vaso-（血管）+ -pathy（病态）
例句 Vasopathy refers to disorders of the blood vessels, which can affect circulation and organ function. 血管病是指血管的病变，可能影响血液循环和器官功能。

pectin-（齿状的）

pectinate 齿状的

词根 pectin-（齿状）+ -ate（形容词后缀）
例句 The pectinate muscles in the heart's atria have a comb-like, tooth-like structure. 心房中的齿状肌具有类似梳子或牙齿的结构。

pectinate ligament 齿状韧带

词根 pectin-（齿状）+ ligament（韧带）
例句 The pectinate ligament is a fibrous band in the eye, important for stabilizing the iris. 齿状韧带是眼睛中的一条纤维带，对稳定虹膜非常重要。

pectinate gyrus 齿状回

词根 pectin-（齿状）+ gyrus（回）
例句 The pectinate gyrus is a part of the brain involved in process-

ing emotions. 齿状回是大脑的一部分，参与情绪处理。

pectinate structure 齿状结构

词根 pectin-（齿状）+ structure（结构）

例句 Pectinate structure refers to any arrangement that resembles a comb or teeth. 齿状结构指的是任何类似梳子或牙齿的排列方式。

pectinate muscle 齿状肌肉

词根 pectin-（齿状）+ muscle（肌肉）

例句 The pectinate muscle is a comb-like muscle found in the atria of the heart, aiding in the contraction of the atrial walls. 齿状肌肉是位于心脏心房内的一种梳状肌肉，可辅助心房壁的收缩。

pectinate process 齿状突起

词根 pectin-（齿状）+ process（突起）

例句 The pectinate process in some fish species helps in attachment to surfaces and offers protection. 一些鱼类物种中的齿状突起有助于附着于表面并提供保护。

–penia（少）

leukopenia 白细胞减少症

词根 leuko-（白）+ -penia（减少）

例句 Leukopenia is a condition characterized by a low white blood cell count, making the body more vulnerable to infections. 白细胞减少症是指白细胞计数低，使身体更容易受到感染。

thrombocytopenia 血小板减少症

词根 thrombocyto-（血小板）+ -penia（减少）

例句 Thrombocytopenia occurs when there is a reduced number of platelets in the blood, leading to increased bleeding risk. 血小板减少症是指血液中血小板数量减少，增加出血风险。

neutropenia 中性粒细胞减少症

词根 neutro-（中性）+ -penia（减少）

例句 Neutropenia is a condition where there is a decrease in neutrophils, a type of white blood cell, which can impair the immune response. 中性粒细胞减少症是中性粒细胞（一种白细胞）的减少，这可能损害免疫反应。

erythropenia 红细胞减少症

词根 erythro-（红）+ -penia（减少）

例句 Erythropenia refers to a decrease in red blood cells, which can lead to anemia and fatigue. 红细胞减少症是指红细胞减少，可以导致贫血和疲劳。

lymphopenia 淋巴细胞减少症

词根 lympho-（淋巴）+ -penia（减少）

例句 Lymphopenia is a condition where there is a decrease in lymphocytes, which may compromise immune function. 淋巴细胞减少症是指淋巴细胞减少，可能削弱免疫功能。

granulocytopenia 粒细胞减少症

词根 granulocyto-（粒细胞）+ -penia（减少）

例句 Granulocytopenia is a disorder characterized by a reduced number of granulocytes, increasing the risk of infections. 粒细胞减少症是一以粒细胞数量减少为特征的疾病，会增加感染风险。

monocytopenia 单核细胞减少症

词根 mono-（单）+ cyto-（细胞）+ -penia（减少）

例句 Monocytopenia is a condition where the number of monocytes is abnormally low, potentially impairing the body's ability to fight infections. 单核细胞减少症是单核细胞数量异常低的情况，可能损害身体抵抗感染的能力。

P

penta-（五个）

pentose 五碳糖

词根 penta-（五个）+ ose（糖）

例句 Pentose refers to a type of sugar molecule that contains five carbon atoms. 五碳糖是指含有五个碳原子的糖分子。

pentamer 五聚体

词根 penta-（五个）+ mer（单位）

例句 A pentamer is a molecule that consists of five monomer units joined together. 五聚体是由五个单体单位连接在一起的分子。

pentavalent 五价的

词根 penta-（五个）+ valent（价）

例句 A pentavalent vaccine is one that contains five different strains of a virus or bacteria to provide immunity. 五价疫苗是指含有五种不同病毒或细菌株的疫苗，以提供免疫力。

pentaerythritol 五氯乙醇

词根 penta-（五个）+ erythritol（赤藓糖醇）

例句 Pentaerythritol is a chemical compound used in the production of explosives and synthetic resins. 五氯乙醇是一种用于生产炸药和合成树脂的化学化合物。

pentachrome stain 五色染色

词根 penta-（五个）+ chrome（色）

例句 Pentachrome stain is a histological staining method that uses five colors to differentiate tissue components. 五色染色是一种组织学染色方法，使用五种颜色区分组织成分。

USMLE Step 3　样题

A 38-year-old woman is brought to the emergency department because of a 4-hour history of confusion (con-; fus-) and lethargy. Medical history is remarkable for major depressive disorder and a 6-month history of moderate low back pain that began after she lifted heavy boxes during a move. Her medications are fluoxetine (-xetine) daily and acetaminophen (acet-; amin-; -ophen) with codeine as needed. Family history is remarkable for hypertension (hyper-; -tension) and congestive (con-; gest-) heart failure in her mother. The patient lives with her husband and her mother. The patient drinks two glasses of wine on weekends. On arrival, she is somnolent (somn-) but arousable to sternal rub. Temperature is 36.4°C (97.5°F), pulse is 32/min, respirations (re-; spir-; -ation) are 16/min, and blood pressure is 74/36 mmHg. Oxygen saturation is 100% on room air. Pupils measure 6 mm in diameter. Examination shows no other abnormalities. Results of laboratory studies are shown:

Serum Blood

ALT 180 U/L

Hemoglobin (hemo-; -globin)12 g/dL

AST 150 U/L

WBC 12,000/mm^3

Creatinine 2.5 mg/dL

Platelet (plate-; -let) count 400,000/mm^3

Acetaminophen (acet-; amin-; -ophen) negative

Urine toxicology (toxic-; -ology)

Opiates positive

An overdose (over-) of a drug with which of the following mechanisms of action is the most likely cause of this patient's condition?

(A) Agonism of μ-opioid receptors (-or)

(B) Inhibition of aldosterone (aldo-; ster-; -one)

(C) Inhibition of angiotensin (angio-; -tens)-converting enzyme

(D) Inhibition of β1-adrenergic receptors (-or)

(E) Inhibition of central nervous system neuron serotonin (sero-) reuptake (re-)

(F) Inhibition of prostaglandin (prosta-; gland-; -in) synthesis

(G) Inhibition of renal sodium and chloride resorption (re-; sorp-)

中文翻译

一名 38 岁女性被送至急诊科，其表现为持续 4 小时的意识混乱和嗜睡症状。既往病史方面，她患有重度抑郁症，且 6 个月前在搬家搬运重物后开始出现中度腰痛，此后一直未愈。目前服用的药物包括每日氟西汀和按需服用的对乙酰氨基酚与可待因。家族史显示其母亲患有高血压和充血性心力衰竭。患者与丈夫和母亲同住。她在周末饮用两杯葡萄酒。到达时，她嗜睡，但对胸骨摩擦刺激可被唤醒。体温 36.4℃（97.5℉），脉搏 32 次 / 分钟，呼吸 16 次 / 分钟，血压 74/36 mmHg。室温空气下的氧饱和度为 100%。瞳孔直径 6 mm。检查未发现其他异常。实验室检查结果如下：

血清

丙氨酸氨基转移酶（ALT） 180 U/L

天门冬氨酸氨基转移酶（AST） 150 U/L

肌酐 2.5 mg/dL

对乙酰氨基酚 阴性

血液

血红蛋白 12 g/dL

白细胞计数 12,000/mm^3

血小板计数 400,000/mm^3

尿液毒理学

阿片类 阳性

以下哪种作用机制的药物过量是最可能导致该患者病情的原因？

(A) μ- 阿片受体激动

(B) 醛固酮抑制

(C) 血管紧张素转换酶抑制

(D) β_1- 肾上腺素受体抑制

(E) 中枢神经系统神经元 5- 羟色胺再摄取抑制

(F) 前列腺素合成抑制

(G) 肾脏钠和氯重吸收抑制

题目和答案中出现的词根

con-：共同

fus-：倾泻（共同倾泻指的是混淆，即脑子里被很多东西同时倾泻引起认识的迷惑和混淆）

-xetine：SSRI（选择性 5- 羟色胺重吸收抑制剂）类抗抑郁药的后缀

acet-：乙酰基

amin-：胺

-ophen：芳香环（乙酰基—胺—芳香环加一起指代对乙酰基酚，即扑热息痛）

hyper-：高

-tension：张力；压力

con-：一起

gest-：携带（一起携带医学上指的是充血，即部分血管内一起携带了过多的红细胞）

somn-：睡眠

re-：重新；反复

spir：呼吸

-ation：表示动作的状态（重复呼吸的状态指代呼吸这个动作）

P

hemo-：血

-globin：球蛋白

plate-：板状的

-lets：小

toxic-：毒性的

-ology：学科

over-：超过

-or：执行者

aldo-：乙醛相关的

ster-：固体的（这里指胆固醇）

-one：酮（乙醛相关的胆固醇酮，即醛固酮）

angio-：血管

-tens：紧张

sero-：血清

prosta-：前列腺的

gland-：腺体

-in：化合物（前列腺体的化合物就是前列腺素）

sorp-：吸

per-（通过）

percutaneous 经皮的

词根 per-（通过）+ cutaneous（皮肤的）

例句 Percutaneous procedures are performed through the skin, such as inserting a needle or catheter. 经皮手术是通过皮肤进行的，例如插入针头或导管。

peritoneal 腹膜的

词根 per-（通过）+ -itoneal（腹膜的）

例句 Peritoneal dialysis involves the use of the peritoneum to filter waste from the blood. 腹膜透析利用腹膜从血液中过滤废物。

pericardial 心包的

词根 per-（通过）+ -cardial（心脏的）

例句 Pericardial effusion occurs when fluid builds up in the pericardial sac around the heart. 心包积液是指围绕心脏的心包腔中液体积聚。

perforation（穿孔）

词根 per-（通过）+ -foration（穿孔）

例句 A perforation of the intestine can lead to a serious infection if not treated promptly. 如果不及时治疗，肠道穿孔可能导致严重感染。

perfusion 灌注

词根 per-（通过）+ -fusion（流动）

例句 Perfusion refers to the process of delivering blood to the organs and tissues of the body. 灌注是指将血液输送到身体器官和组织的过程。

permeability 渗透性

词根 per-（通过）+ -meability（可渗透性）

例句 Cell membrane permeability determines the movement of substances in and out of the cell. 细胞膜的渗透性决定了物质在细胞内外的流动。

peroneal 腓骨的

词根 per-（通过）+ -oneal（腓骨的）

例句 The peroneal nerve is located along the outer side of the leg and controls foot movement. 腓神经位于小腿外侧，控制脚部运动。

periapical 根尖周围的

词根 per-（通过）+ -apical（顶端的）

例句 Periapical radiographs are used in dentistry to assess the condition of the root tips of teeth. 根尖片在牙科中用于评估牙根尖端的状况。

perioperative 围手术期的

词根 per-（通过）+ -operative（手术的）

例句 Perioperative care is crucial in ensuring the success of surgical procedures and preventing complications. 围手术期护理在确保手术成功和防止并发症中至关重要。

perinatal 围产期的

词根 per-（通过）+ -natal（出生的）

例句 Perinatal care focuses on the health of both the mother and the newborn around the time of birth. 围产期护理关注母亲和新生儿在分娩时的健康。

peri-（周围）

periosteum 骨膜

词根 peri-（周围）+ osteum（骨）

例句 The periosteum is a membrane that covers the surface of bones except at the joints. 骨膜是覆盖骨骼表面的膜，关节处除外。

pericardium 心包

词根 peri-（周围）+ cardium（心脏）

例句 The pericardium is a double-layered membrane surrounding the heart. 心包是环绕心脏的双层膜。

peritoneum 腹膜

词根 peri-（周围）+ toneum（膜）

例句 The peritoneum is a membrane that lines the abdominal cavity and covers most of the abdominal organs. 腹膜是覆盖腹腔并包裹大部分腹部器官的膜。

periphlebitis 静脉周围炎

词根 peri-（周围）+ phlebitis（静脉炎）

例句 Periphlebitis refers to inflammation of the tissues surrounding a vein. 静脉周围炎指的是围绕静脉的组织发生炎症。

pericranial 头骨的

词根 peri-（周围）+ cranial（头骨的）

例句 Pericranial swelling can occur due to trauma or infection in the skull area. 头骨周围的肿胀可能是由于创伤或感染引起的。

perimysium 肌膜

词根 peri-（周围）+ mysium（肌肉）

例句 The perimysium is the connective tissue that surrounds muscle fibers. 肌膜是包裹肌肉纤维的结缔组织。

periventricular 脑室周围的

词根 peri-（周围）+ ventricular（脑室的）
例句 Periventricular white matter is often affected in conditions like multiple sclerosis. 脑室周围的白质常在多发性硬化症等病症中受影响。

peripartum 围产期的

词根 peri-（周围）+ partum（分娩）
例句 Peripartum depression refers to depression that occurs during or shortly after childbirth. 围产期抑郁是指在分娩期间或分娩后不久发生的抑郁症。

perioperative 围手术期的

词根 peri-（周围）+ operative（手术的）
例句 Perioperative care is essential to prevent complications during and after surgery. 围手术期护理对于预防手术期间及术后并发症至关重要。

perineal 会阴的

词根 peri-（周围）+ neal（会阴的）
例句 Perineal tears can occur during childbirth when the baby's head passes through the birth canal. 会阴撕裂是分娩时婴儿头部通过产道时可能发生的情况。

periorbital 眼眶周围的

词根 peri-（周围）+ orbital（眼眶的）
例句 Periorbital edema refers to swelling around the eyes, often caused by allergies or infection. 眼眶周围水肿是指眼睛周围的肿胀，通常由过敏或感染引起。

perivascular 血管周围的

词根 peri-（周围）+ vascular（血管的）

例句 Perivascular inflammation is the inflammation around blood vessels, often seen in autoimmune diseases. 血管周围炎是指围绕血管的炎症，通常出现在自身免疫性疾病中。

peridontal 牙周的

词根 peri-（周围）+ dental（牙齿的）

例句 Periodontal disease involves inflammation of the tissues surrounding the teeth. 牙周病涉及牙齿周围组织的炎症。

pericardial effusion 心包积液

词根 peri-（周围）+ cardial（心脏的）+ effusion（积液）

例句 Pericardial effusion is the accumulation of fluid in the pericardial sac, which can lead to heart compression. 心包积液是指心包腔内液体的积聚，可能导致心脏压迫。

perinatal 围产期的

词根 peri-（周围）+ natal（出生的）

例句 Perinatal care is the medical care provided to both the mother and the newborn around the time of birth. 围产期护理是指在分娩时为母亲和新生儿提供的医疗护理。

periscope 窥镜

词根 peri-（周围）+ scope（镜）

例句 A periscope is used to view surroundings from a concealed position, typically in submarines. 窥镜用于从隐蔽位置观察周围环境，通常用于潜水艇中。

peripharyngeal 咽周的

词根 peri-（周围）+ pharyngeal（咽的）

例句 Peripharyngeal abscesses can cause difficulty in swallowing and may require surgical drainage. 咽周脓肿可能引起吞咽困难，

可能需要外科引流。

perilunar 月周围的

词根 peri-（周围）+ lunar（月亮的）
例句 Perilunar fractures affect the area around the lunate bone in the wrist. 月骨周围骨折影响腕部月骨周围的区域。

periventricular leukomalacia 脑室周围白质软化

词根 peri-（周围）+ ventricular（脑室的）+ leuko-（白质的）+ malacia（软化）
例句 Periventricular leukomalacia is a type of brain injury that occurs near the ventricles, often affecting preterm infants. 脑室周围白质软化是一种发生在脑室附近的脑损伤，常见于早产儿。

peritonsillar 扁桃体周围的

词根 peri-（周围）+ tonsillar（扁桃体的）
例句 Peritonsillar abscesses occur near the tonsils and can cause severe throat pain and swelling. 扁桃体周围脓肿发生在扁桃体附近，可引起严重的喉咙痛和肿胀。

pes（足）

pes anserinus 鹅足部

词根 pes（足）+ anserinus（鹅的）
例句 Pes anserinus refers to the area on the medial side of the knee where three tendons insert, resembling a goose's foot. 鹅足部指的是膝盖内侧的区域，三个肌腱插入的地方，形状像鹅的脚。

pes planus 扁平足

词根 pes（足）+ planus（平的）
例句 Pes planus, commonly known as flat feet, occurs when the arches of the feet collapse. 扁平足，俗称平足，是指足弓塌陷的情况。

pes cavus 高足弓

词根 pes（足）+ cavus（凹陷的）
例句 Pes cavus refers to a condition in which the foot has a very high arch, leading to discomfort. 高足弓是指足弓非常高，可能导致不适的情况。

pes valgus 外翻足

词根 pes（足）+ valgus（外翻）
例句 Pes valgus is a condition where the foot turns outward, causing abnormal foot alignment. 外翻足是指足部向外翻转，导致不正常的脚部对齐。

pes rectus 正足

词根 pes（足）+ rectus（直的）
例句 Pes rectus is a term used to describe a normal, well-aligned foot with a neutral arch. 正足用于描述足部形态正常、排列良好且具有中性足弓的脚形。

pes equinus 马足

词根 pes（足）+ equinus（马的）
例句 Pes equinus refers to a condition where the foot is held in a downward position, often seen in patients with neurological disorders. 马足是指脚被保持在下垂位置的状况，通常见于神经系统疾病患者。

pes falciform 镰状足

词根 pes（足）+ falciform（镰刀状的）
例句 Pes falciform is a term used when the foot has a shape resembling a sickle. 镰状足指的是足部形状像镰刀的情况。

pes pedis 足部

词根 pes（足）+ pedis（的）
例句 Pes pedis refers to the anatomical structure of the human foot.

足部指的是人类脚的解剖结构。

pes dorsiflexion 足背屈

词根 pes（足）+ dorsiflexion（背屈）

例句 Pes dorsiflexion involves the upward movement of the foot, flexing the ankle joint. 足背屈是指脚的上升运动，弯曲踝关节。

pes adductus 足内翻

词根 pes（足）+ adductus（内收）

例句 Pes adductus is a deformity where the foot is turned inward, often seen in congenital conditions. 足内翻是一种畸形，足部向内转动，通常出现在先天性疾病中。

-pexy（固定）

hysteropexy 子宫固定术

词根 hyster-（子宫）+ -pexy（固定）

例句 Hysteropexy is a surgical procedure used to fix the uterus in place, often performed in cases of uterine prolapse. 子宫固定术是一种用于固定子宫的位置的手术，通常用于治疗子宫脱垂。

mammopexy 乳房固定术

词根 mamm-（乳房）+ -pexy（固定）

例句 Mammopexy is a surgical procedure to lift and fix the breast tissue, often done for cosmetic reasons. 乳房固定术是一种提拉并固定乳腺组织的手术，通常出于美容目的。

gastropexy 胃固定术

词根 gastro-（胃）+ -pexy（固定）

例句 Gastropexy is a surgical procedure used to attach the stomach to the abdominal wall, often done in cases of gastric volvulus. 胃固定术是一种将胃固定在腹壁上的手术，通常用于胃扭转的病例。

nephropexy 肾脏固定术

词根 nephr-（肾脏）+ -pexy（固定）

例句 Nephropexy is a procedure used to surgically attach a kidney that has dropped or moved out of its normal position. 肾脏固定术是一种用于外科固定下垂或移位的肾脏，使其恢复至正常位置的手术。

cystopexy 膀胱固定术

词根 cyst-（膀胱）+ -pexy（固定）

例句 Cystopexy is a surgical procedure to fix the bladder in place, often performed to treat bladder prolapse. 膀胱固定术是一种将膀胱固定在适当位置的手术，常用于治疗膀胱脱垂。

retinopexy 视网膜固定术

词根 retin-（视网膜）+ -pexy（固定）

例句 Retinopexy is a procedure used to treat retinal detachment by reattaching the retina to the back of the eye. 视网膜固定术是一种治疗视网膜脱落的手术，通过将视网膜重新附着到眼后部。

orchiopexy 睾丸固定术

词根 orchio-（睾丸）+ -pexy（固定）

例句 Orchiopexy is a surgical procedure used to correct undescended testicles in children. 睾丸固定术是一种治疗儿童隐睾症的手术。

urethropexy 尿道固定术

词根 urethr-（尿道）+ -pexy（固定）

例句 Urethropexy is a surgery used to fix the urethra in place, often used in cases of urinary incontinence. 尿道固定术是一种将尿道固定的手术，通常用于治疗尿失禁。

prostatopexy 前列腺固定术

词根 prostat-（前列腺）+ -pexy（固定）

例句 Prostatopexy is a surgical procedure that involves the fixation of the prostate gland, typically in cases of prostate cancer. 前列腺固定术是一种涉及前列腺固定的手术，通常用于治疗前列腺癌。

colpopexy 阴道固定术

词根 colp-（阴道）+ -pexy（固定）
例句 Colpopexy is a surgical procedure to support the vaginal wall, often performed in cases of vaginal prolapse. 阴道固定术是一种支持阴道壁的手术，常用于治疗阴道脱垂。

phag-（吃）

phagocytosis 吞噬作用

词根 phag-（吃）+ -cytosis（细胞作用）
例句 Phagocytosis is the process by which certain cells engulf and digest foreign particles or pathogens. 吞噬作用是某些细胞吞噬并消化外来颗粒或病原体的过程。

phagocyte 吞噬细胞

词根 phag-（吃）+ -cyte（细胞）
例句 Phagocytes, such as neutrophils and macrophages, are essential for the immune response. 吞噬细胞，如中性粒细胞和巨噬细胞，对于免疫反应至关重要。

phagolysosome 吞噬溶酶体

词根 phag-（吃）+ -lysosome（溶酶体）
例句 The phagolysosome is formed when a phagocyte engulfs a pathogen and merges with a lysosome to digest it. 当吞噬细胞吞噬病原体并与溶酶体合并以消化病原体时，便形成了吞噬溶酶体。

phagomembrane 吞噬膜

词根 phag-（吃）+ membrane（膜）
例句 The phagomembrane is the membrane that surrounds the in-

gested material inside a phagocyte. 吞噬膜是吞噬细胞内包裹被吞噬物质的膜结构。

bacteriophagy 细菌吞噬

词根 bacterio-（细菌）+ phag-（吃）
例句 Bacteriophagy is the process where bacteria are ingested and digested by phagocytes. 细菌吞噬是细菌被吞噬细胞摄入并消化的过程。

phagolysis 吞噬溶解作用

词根 phag-（吃）+ -lysis（溶解）
例句 Phagolysis refers to the dissolution of a pathogen inside a phagocyte. 吞噬溶解作用指的是病原体在吞噬细胞内的溶解过程。

autophagy 自噬作用

词根 auto-（自）+ phag-（吃）
例句 Autophagy is a process in which cells digest their own damaged or unnecessary components. 自噬作用是细胞消化自己损坏或不必要的成分的过程。

phagostimulant 摄食刺激物

词根 phago-（吞噬）+ stimulant（刺激物）
例句 Phagostimulants are substances that trigger or enhance the process of phagocytosis in organisms. 摄食刺激物是能够触发或增强生物体吞噬作用的物质。

heterophagy 异噬作用

词根 hetero-（异）+ phag-（吃）
例句 Heterophagy is the ingestion of foreign materials by a cell or organism. 异噬作用是细胞或有机体吞噬外来物质的过程。

phagocytosis inhibition 吞噬作用抑制

词根 phag-（吃）+ cytosis（细胞作用）+ inhibition（抑制）

例句 Phagocytosis inhibition can occur when pathogens produce substances that prevent phagocytes from engulfing them. 吞噬作用抑制是指病原体产生物质，阻止吞噬细胞吞噬它们。

phalang-（指）

phalanx 指骨

词根 phalang-（指）
例句 A phalanx is one of the bones that make up a finger or toe. 指骨是构成手指或脚趾的骨骼之一。

polyphalanx 多指骨

词根 poly-（多）+ phalang-（指）
例句 Polyphalanx describes a condition where there are multiple phalanges in a finger. 多指骨描述的是手指中存在多个指骨的情况。

phalangectomy 指骨切除术

词根 phalang-（指）+ -ectomy（切除）
例句 Phalangectomy is a surgical procedure to remove a damaged or diseased finger bone. 指骨切除术是一种去除受损或患病指骨的外科手术。

phalangeal 指骨的

词根 phalang-（指）+ -eal（形容词后缀）
例句 Phalangeal fractures are common in traumatic hand injuries. 指骨骨折在创伤性手部损伤中很常见。

brachyphalanx 短指骨

词根 brachy-（短）+ phalang-（指）
例句 Brachyphalanx refers to abnormally short phalanges, which can affect hand function. 短指骨是指指骨异常短小，可能影响手部功能。

biphalangeal 双指骨的

词根 bi-（双）+ phalang-（指）

例句 Biphalangeal syndactyly occurs when two fingers fuse together, sharing a common phalanx. 双指骨并指畸形指两根手指融合在一起，共享一个指骨。

phalangeal amputation 指骨截肢

词根 phalang-（指）+ -ectomy（切除）

例句 Phalangeal amputation may be necessary when a finger is severely damaged or diseased. 当手指严重受损或患病时，可能需要进行指骨截肢手术。

USMLE Step 3 样题

An 8-year-old girl is brought to the emergency department via ambulance 1 hour after the onset of a generalized tonic-clonic seizure. Paramedics (para-; -medics) noted a pulse of 50/min followed by a 30-minute period of asystole (a-; systo-). En route, the patient was intubated (in-; tub-) and oxygen therapy and an epinephrine (epi-; nephr-; -ine) inotropic (ino-; trop-) drip were initiated. On arrival, the patient is unconscious (un-). Temperature is 36.7℃ (98.0°F), pulse is 40/min, respirations (re-; spir-; -ation) are 16/min, and blood pressure cannot be obtained. Oxygen saturation is 99% on an FIO_2 of 1.0. Physical examination shows mildly dysmorphic (dys-; morph-) facies. Pupils are sluggish in response to light. Lungs are clear to auscultation (auscult-; -ation) with ventilated (ventil-) sounds. Cardiac examination discloses a regular rhythm and sinus bradycardia (brady-; -cardia). Abdomen is soft and nontender (non-). Neurologic (neuro-) examination discloses paralysis (para-; -lysis). Distal pulses are 1+ and weak. Echocardiography (echo-; cardi-; -graphy) shows global hypokinesis (hypo-; kine-; -sis) with lateral inferior wall and septal akinesis (a-; kine-; -sis). Left ventricular (ventricul-) function is 20%. The patient is admitted to the hospital. Four days later, there has been no improvement in her condition. Life support is withdrawn, and the patient dies. At autopsy (auto-; -opsy), examination of the heart shows evidence of an acute myocardial (myo-; cardi-) infarction. Which of the following is the most likely underlying cause of this patient's death?

(A) Cardiac conduction abnormality

(B) Coronary (coron-) artery plaque rupture

(C) Increased pulmonary (pulmon-) vascular resistance

(D) Systolic (systo-) prolapse (pro-; -lapse) of mitral valve

(E) Thickened left ventricular (ventricul-) wall and contractile dysfunction (dys-)

中文翻译

一名 8 岁女孩在发生全身强直—阵挛性癫痫发作 1 小时后，由救护车送往急诊科。急救人员记录到脉搏 50 次 / 分钟，随后出现 30 分钟的心跳停止。在途中，患者被插管并开始氧疗和肾上腺素强心滴注。到达时，患者处于昏迷状态。体温 36.7℃（98.0℉），脉搏 40 次 / 分钟，呼吸 16 次 / 分钟，无法测得血压。在氧气浓度（FIO_2）为 1.0 时，氧饱和度为 99%。体检显示轻度面部畸形。瞳孔对光反应迟钝。肺部听诊清晰，伴有通气音。心脏检查显示节律规则，伴窦性心动过缓。腹部柔软，无压痛。神经系统检查显示瘫痪。远端脉搏 1+ 且微弱。心脏超声显示整体心肌运动减弱，侧下壁和间隔无运动。左心室功能为 20%。患者被转入医院。4 天后，病情无改善。撤除生命支持后，患者死亡。尸检时，心脏检查显示急性心肌梗死的证据。以下哪项是导致该患者死亡的最可能根本原因？

(A) 心脏传导异常
(B) 冠状动脉斑块破裂
(C) 肺血管阻力增加
(D) 二尖瓣收缩期脱垂
(E) 左心室壁增厚和收缩功能障碍

题目和答案中出现的词根

para-：旁边

medic-：医生（医生旁边指医生助理，即和医生并肩工作的职业）

a-：表示否定

systo-：收缩

in-：向内

tub-：管（向内管道指的是气管插管，即把管道插到气管里）

epi-：在……上（或旁）

nephr：肾脏

-ine：化合物（在肾脏上面的化合物指的是肾上腺素）

ino-：肌肉纤维

trop-：变化（肌肉纤维变化即影响肌肉收缩的）

un-：表示否定

re-：重新；反复

spir：呼吸

-ation：表示动作的状态

dys-：困难的；错误的

morph-：形状

auscult-：听

-ation：表示动作（听的动作指的是听诊）

ventil-：通气

brady-：缓慢的

-cardia：心脏（缓慢的心脏指的是心率变缓）

non-：表示否定

neuro-：神经的

para-：旁边

-lysis-：分解（由于肌肉或神经分解引起的不正常，指代瘫痪）

echo-：回声

cardi-：心脏

-graphy：图像

hypo- 低

kine-：动力

-sis：状态

a-：表示否定

ventricul-：室的（这里指心室，也可以表示脑室）

auto-：自我

-opsy：检查（自我检查指尸检，即通过检查死者自己的身体发现死者死亡的原因）

myo-：肌肉

cardi-：心脏

coron-：冠状

pulmon-：肺的（指的是解剖意义上的肺）

systo-：收缩

pro-：在……之前

-lapse：滑倒（向前滑倒指的是脱垂）

dys-：困难的；异常的

phas-（语言；说）

aphasia 失语症

词根 a-（无）+ phas-（语言）

例句 Aphasia is a language disorder that affects a person's ability to speak, understand, read, or write. 失语症是一种语言障碍，影响一个人说话、理解、阅读或写作的能力。

dysphasia 语言障碍

词根 dys-（困难）+ phas-（语言）

例句 Dysphasia refers to partial impairment of language abilities, often due to brain injury or stroke. 语言障碍是指语言能力的部分受损，通常由脑损伤或中风引起。

paraphasia 错语症

词根 para-（旁边）+ phas-（语言）

例句 Paraphasia is a speech disorder in which words are substituted with incorrect ones, often seen in stroke patients. 错语症是一种语言障碍，其表现为用错误词汇替代正确词汇，常见于中风患者。

bradyphasia 言语迟缓症

词根 brady-（迟缓）+ phas-（语言）

例句 Bradyphasia is characterized by slow and delayed speech, often caused by neurological conditions. 言语迟缓症的特征是言语缓慢和延迟，通常由神经系统疾病引起。

USMLE Step 3 样题

A 72-year-old man is admitted to the hospital through the emergency department because of a 12-hour history of fever, chills, increasingly severe abdominal pain, nausea, and vomiting. Medical history includes hypertension (hyper-; -tension), hypercholesterolemia (hyper-; chole-; ster-; -emia), and atherosclerotic (ather-; sclero-) heart disease with placement of a coronary (coron-) artery stent 3 years ago. Current medications are atorvastatin (-statin) and lisinopril (-pril). He appears anxious and pale. BMI is 30 kg/m^2. Temperature is 40.0°C (104.0°F), pulse is 116/min, respirations (re-; spir-; -ation) are 20/min, and blood pressure is 100/65 mmHg. Oxygen saturation is 94% on room air. A bruit is heard over the right carotid (carot-) artery. Cardiac examination discloses no murmurs; an S4 is present. Lungs are clear to auscultation (auscult-; -ation). Abdominal examination discloses decreased bowel sounds and diffuse tenderness with guarding that is most severe in the left upper quadrant (quad-). Both lower extremities are cool to touch with weak pedal pulses. Abdominal X-ray shows dilation of the proximal colon. Results of serum laboratory studies are shown:

Amylase 230 U/L

Urea nitrogen 20 mg/dL

Creatinine 1.0 mg/dL

Na^+ 138 mEq/L

K^+ 3.5 mEq/L

Cl^- 101 mEq/L

HCO_3^- 12 mEq/L

Glucose 180 mg/dL

Surgical resection (re-; -sect) of the colon is done. Which of the following histopathologic (histo-; patho-) changes will most likely be identified in the resected (re-; sect-) colon?

(A) Caseating granulomatous (granul-; -omatous) inflammation with serosal (sero-) fibrous (fibro-) adhesions (ad-; -hesion)

(B) Coagulative (coagul-) necrosis involving mucosa and submucosa (sub-)

(C) Neutrophilic (neutro-; -phil) infiltrates in the mucosa with venous congestion and edema

(D) Patchy mucopurulent (muco-) exudate with exploding glandular (gland-) crypts

(E) Transmural (trans-; -mural) chronic inflammation with ulcerations extending into submucosa (sub-)

中文翻译

一名 72 岁男性因发热、寒战、腹痛逐渐加剧、恶心及呕吐，且症状已持续 12 小时，经急诊科收治入院。病史包括高血压、高胆固醇血症和动脉粥样硬化性心脏病，3 年前置入冠状动脉支架。目前服用的药物为阿托伐他汀和赖诺普利。他看起来焦虑且面色苍白。BMI 为 30 kg/m²。体温 40.0°C（104.0°F），脉搏 116 次 / 分钟，呼吸 20 次 / 分钟，血压 100/65 mmHg。室温空气下的氧饱和度为 94%。右侧颈动脉可闻及杂音。心脏检查未发现杂音，存在 S4 音。肺部听诊清晰。腹部检查显示肠鸣音减弱，弥漫性压痛伴腹部防护，左上腹最为严重。双下肢触之冰凉，足部脉搏微弱。腹部 X 线显示近端结肠扩张。血清实验室检查结果如下：

淀粉酶 230 U/L

尿素氮 20 mg/dL

肌酐 1.0 mg/dL

钠 138 mEq/L

钾 3.5 mEq/L

氯 101 mEq/L

碳酸氢根 12 mEq/L

葡萄糖 180 mg/dL

进行了结肠手术切除。在切除的结肠中，最可能发现以下哪种组织病理学变化？

(A) 伴有浆膜纤维粘连的干酪样肉芽肿性炎症

(B) 累及黏膜和黏膜下层的凝固性坏死

(C) 黏膜中性粒细胞浸润伴静脉充血和水肿

(D) 伴有腺体隐窝爆裂的斑片状黏液脓性渗出物

(E) 累及全层的慢性炎症伴溃疡延伸至黏膜下层

题目和答案中出现的词根

hyper-：高

-tension：张力；压力

chole-：胆

ster-：固体的（这里指胆固醇）

-emia：血症

athero-：斑块

sclero-：硬化

coron：冠状

-statin：静止（这里指把合成胆固醇的关键酶 HMG-CoA 还原酶静止，通常为降脂药物）

-pril：普利（血管紧张素转换酶抑制剂的通用后缀）

re-：重新，反复

spir：呼吸

-ation：表示动作的状态（重复呼吸的状态指代呼吸这个动作）

auscult-：听

-ation：表示动作（表示听的动作就是听诊）

quad-：四个

re-：重新；反复

sect-：切（再次切指代切除）

histo-：组织的

patho-：病理的

granul-：小颗粒

-omatous：类似的

sero-：血清

fibro-：纤维的

ad-：向上

-hesion：黏附

coagul-：凝血的

sub-：在……下（在种类的下面指的是亚分类，即在一层分类的下级再分类）

neutro-：中性的

-phil：嗜

muco-：黏液

gland-：腺体的

trans-：跨；转

mural：壁

pheo-（暗色）

pheochromocytoma 嗜铬细胞瘤

词根 pheo-（暗色）+ chromo-（颜色）+ cytoma（肿瘤）

例句 Pheochromocytoma is a rare tumor of the adrenal glands that produces excessive hormones. 嗜铬细胞瘤是一种罕见的肾上腺肿瘤，产生过多的激素。

pheomelanin 黄黑色素

词根 pheo-（暗色）+ melanin（黑色素）

例句 Pheomelanin is a type of melanin that gives hair its yellow or red color. 黄黑色素是一种使头发呈黄色或红色的黑色素类型。

Pheomelanogenesis 黄黑色素生成

词根 pheo-（暗色）+ melanogenesis（黑色素生成）

例句 Pheomelanogenesis is the process by which pheomelanin is produced in the body. 黄黑色素生成是体内产生黄黑色素的过程。

pheochromoblastoma 嗜铬细胞母细胞瘤

词根 pheo-（暗色）+ chromo-（颜色）+ blastoma（胚胎肿瘤）

例句 Pheochromoblastoma is a type of cancerous tumor that arises from pheochromocytes. 嗜铬细胞母细胞瘤是一种源自嗜铬细胞的癌性肿瘤。

pheochromocytosis 嗜铬细胞增生

词根 pheo-（暗色）+ chromo-（颜色）+ cytosis（细胞）

例句 Pheochromocytosis refers to the abnormal growth of pheochromocytes in the adrenal glands. 嗜铬细胞增生是指肾上腺中嗜铬细胞的异常增生。

pheomelanotic 黄黑色素的

词根 pheo-（暗色）+ melanotic（黑色素的）
例句 Pheomelanotic skin pigmentation is associated with a reddish or yellowish hue. 黄黑色素的皮肤色素沉着与红色或黄色的色调相关。

pheomelanins 黄黑色素类物质

词根 pheo-（暗色）+ melanins（黑色素类物质）
例句 Pheomelanins are a group of pigments responsible for red and yellow hues in hair and skin. 黄黑色素类物质是一组负责头发和皮肤红色及黄色的色素。

pheomelaninogenic 黄黑色素生成的

词根 pheo-（暗色）+ melaninogenic（黑色素生成的）
例句 Pheomelaninogenic pathways are responsible for producing lighter pigments in the skin. 黄黑色素生成途径负责产生皮肤中的浅色素。

pheohypomelanosis 黄黑色素缺乏症

词根 pheo-（暗色）+ hypo-（低）+ melanosis（黑色素沉积症）
例句 Pheohypomelanosis is a condition characterized by a lack of pheomelanin in the skin. 黄黑色素缺乏症是一种皮肤中缺乏黄黑色素的疾病。

Pheopigmentation 黄黑色素沉积

词根 pheo-（暗色）+ pigmentation（色素沉积）
例句 Pheopigmentation can lead to a distinct color pattern in the hair or skin. 黄黑色素沉积可导致头发或皮肤中出现独特的颜色模式。

-phil（嗜）

acidophil 嗜酸性细胞

词根 acid-（酸）+ -phil（嗜）

例句 Acidophils are cells that are attracted to acidic environments and are typically found in certain endocrine glands. 嗜酸性细胞是倾向于聚集在酸性环境中的细胞，通常在某些内分泌腺中发现。

basophil 嗜碱性粒细胞

词根 baso-（碱）+ -phil（嗜）

例句 Basophils release histamine during allergic reactions and play a role in inflammatory processes. 嗜碱性粒细胞在过敏反应中释放组胺，并在炎症过程中发挥作用。

eosinophil 嗜酸性粒细胞

词根 eosino-（酸）+ -phil（嗜）

例句 Eosinophils are a type of white blood cell involved in allergic reactions and parasitic infections. 嗜酸性粒细胞是一种白细胞，参与过敏反应和寄生虫感染。

neutrophil 中性粒细胞

词根 neutro-（中性）+ -phil（嗜）

例句 Neutrophils are the most abundant type of white blood cells and play a critical role in the body's immune response to infection. 中性粒细胞是最常见的白细胞类型，在身体对感染的免疫反应中起着关键作用。

monophilous 单核细胞的

词根 mono-（单）+ -phil（嗜）

例句 Monophilous cells specialize in attacking pathogens and debris within the immune system. 单核细胞专门在免疫系统中攻击

病原体和残骸。

hydrophilic 亲水的

词根 hydro-（水）+ -phil（嗜）

例句 Hydrophilic substances readily absorb water, which is important for many biological processes. 亲水物质能够轻易吸水，这对许多生物学过程至关重要。

lipophilic 亲脂的

词根 lipo-（脂肪）+ -phil（嗜）

例句 Lipophilic substances, such as certain medications, dissolve in fats and lipids. 亲脂物质，例如某些药物，能溶解于脂肪和脂类中。

bacteriophilous 嗜细菌的

词根 bacterio-（细菌）+ -phil（嗜）

例句 Bacteriophilous organisms thrive in environments with abundant bacteria and often feed on them. 嗜细菌生物在细菌丰富的环境中茁壮成长，通常以其为食。

xerophilous 耐旱的

词根 xero-（干旱）+ -phil（嗜）

例句 Xerophilous plants are capable of surviving in extremely dry conditions. 耐旱植物能够在极干燥的环境中生存。

thermophilic 嗜热的

词根 thermo-（热）+ -phil（嗜）

例句 Thermophilic organisms thrive in high-temperature environments, such as hot springs and deep-sea vents. 嗜热生物在高温环境中茁壮成长，例如温泉和深海喷口。

psychrophilic 嗜冷的

词根 psycho-（冷）+ -phil（嗜）

例句 Psychrophilic organisms are adapted to live in cold environments such as the polar regions and glaciers. 嗜冷生物适应在寒冷环境中生存，如极地地区和冰川。

phim-（包皮的）

phimosis 包茎

词根 phim-（包皮的）+ -osis（病理状态）

例句 Phimosis is a condition where the foreskin of the penis cannot be fully retracted. 包茎是指阴茎的包皮无法完全翻转。

postphismosis 包皮后缩

词根 post-（后）+ phim-（包皮的）+ -osis（病理状态）

例句 Postphismosis refers to a condition where the foreskin is unable to return to its normal position after being retracted. 包皮后缩是指包皮被翻转后无法恢复到原来的位置。

phimotic 包茎的

词根 phim-（包皮的）+ -otic（形容词后缀）

例句 Phimotic conditions require medical intervention to prevent discomfort or infection. 包茎的情况需要医疗干预，以防止不适或感染。

phimocyst 包皮囊肿

词根 phim-（包皮的）+ cyst（囊肿）

例句 A phimocyst is a cyst that forms under the foreskin. 包皮囊肿是形成在包皮下的囊肿。

phimolysis 包皮松解术

词根 phim-（包皮的）+ -lysis（溶解；分解）

例句 Phimolysis is a surgical procedure that involves the removal or loosening of the tight foreskin. 包皮松解术是一种通过切除或松解过紧包皮的手术操作。

phimectomy 包皮切除术

词根 phim-（包皮的）+ -ectomy（切除术）

例句 Phimectomy is the surgical removal of the foreskin to treat phimosis. 包皮切除术是治疗包茎的外科手术，涉及切除包皮。

phimosectomy 包茎切除术

词根 phim-（包皮的）+ -osectomy（切除术）

例句 Phimosectomy is performed when the foreskin cannot be retracted, causing pain or infection. 包茎切除术是在包皮无法翻转，导致疼痛或感染时进行的手术。

phimositis 包皮炎

词根 phim-（包皮的）+ -itis（炎症）

例句 Phimositis is the inflammation of the foreskin, often caused by infection. 包皮炎是包皮的炎症，通常由感染引起。

phimosomatosis 包皮性病变

词根 phim-（包皮的）+ -somatosis（病变）

例句 Phimosomatosis refers to the pathological changes or disorders of the foreskin. 包皮性病变指包皮的病理变化或紊乱。

phimogenesis 包皮生成

词根 phim-（包皮的）+ -genesis（生成；起源）

例句 Phimogenesis refers to the development of the foreskin during fetal development. 包皮生成是指在胎儿发育过程中包皮的形成。

phlebo-（静脉的）

phlebectomy 静脉切除术

词根 phlebo-（静脉）+ -ectomy（切除术）

例句 Phlebectomy is the surgical removal of a vein, typically to treat varicose veins. 静脉切除术是通过手术去除静脉，通常用于

治疗静脉曲张。

phlebology 静脉学

词根 phlebo-（静脉）+ -ology（学科）

例句 Phlebology is the branch of medicine that focuses on the diagnosis and treatment of vein disorders. 静脉学是医学的一个分支，专注于静脉疾病的诊断和治疗。

phlebitis 静脉炎

词根 phlebo-（静脉）+ -itis（炎症）

例句 Phlebitis is the inflammation of a vein, often caused by an infection or injury. 静脉炎是静脉的炎症，通常由感染或损伤引起。

phlebotomy 静脉切开术

词根 phlebo-（静脉）+ -tomy（切开术）

例句 Phlebotomy is the practice of making an incision in a vein to draw blood. 静脉切开术是通过切开静脉来抽取血液的做法。

phlebosclerosis 静脉硬化

词根 phlebo-（静脉）+ sclerosis（硬化）

例句 Phlebosclerosis refers to the thickening and hardening of the veins. 静脉硬化是指静脉的增厚和硬化。

phlebospasm 静脉痉挛

词根 phlebo-（静脉）+ spasm（痉挛）

例句 Phlebospasm occurs when the veins contract abnormally, often causing pain. 静脉痉挛是指静脉异常收缩，通常会引起疼痛。

phlebectasia 静脉扩张

词根 phlebo-（静脉）+ ectasia（扩张）

例句 Phlebectasia refers to the dilation or enlargement of a vein. 静脉扩张是指静脉的扩张或增大。

phlebosclerotic 静脉硬化的

词根 phlebo-（静脉）+ sclerotic（硬化的）

例句 Phlebosclerotic conditions can lead to poor blood circulation. 静脉硬化性疾病可导致血液循环不良。

phlebothrombosis 静脉血栓形成

词根 phlebo-（静脉）+ thrombosis（血栓形成）

例句 Phlebothrombosis is the formation of a blood clot within a vein. 静脉血栓形成是指静脉内形成血栓。

phlebomelanosis 静脉黑色素沉积症

词根 phlebo-（静脉）+ melanosis（黑色素沉积症）

例句 Phlebomelanosis is a rare condition involving the deposition of melanin in the veins. 静脉黑色素沉积症是一种罕见的病症，涉及静脉内黑色素的沉积。

USMLE Step 3　样题

Age: 19 years

Gender: M, self-identified

Race/Ethnicity: unspecified (un-)

Site of Care: hospital

The patient who is a college student is admitted because of fever, chills, intense headache (-ache), nonproductive (non-) cough, and generalized weakness for the past 3 days. Medical history is unremarkable (un-) and he takes no medications. He does not use any substances. He works as a greenskeeper at a local golf course in western North Carolina. On admission, he appears acutely ill. He is somnolent (somn-) but arousable. Temperature is 39.0°C (102.2°F), pulse is 106/min, respirations (re-; spir-; -ation) are 22/min, and blood pressure is 90/56 mmHg. Oxygen saturation is 98% on room air. Examination of the skin shows an erythematous (eryth-; -ema), macular rash with superimposed (super-) petechiae on the palms, soles, legs, and thighs. Funduscopic (fundu-; scop-) examination discloses no abnormalities. Neck is supple with no adenopathy (aden-; -pathy). The remainder of the physical examination, including neurologic (neuro-) examination, discloses no abnormalities. Intravenous (intra-; ven-) access is established. Lumbar puncture for examination of cerebrospinal (cerebro-; -spinal) fluid discloses an opening pressure of 210 mmH_2O; the cerebrospinal (cerebro-; -spinal) fluid is slightly turbid. ECG shows nonspecific (non-) ST-segment and T-wave abnormalities. Portable chest X-ray shows no abnormalities. Results of laboratory studies are shown:

Serum Blood

Urea nitrogen 23 mg/dL

Hemoglobin (hemo-; -globin) 11.5 g/dL

Creatinine 1.3 mg/dL

WBC 11,600/mm^3

Glucose 99 mg/dL

Neutrophils (neutro-; -phil), segmented 75%

Na^+ 134 mEq/L

Neutrophils (neutro-; -phil), bands 15%

K^+ 4.5 mEq/L

Lymphocytes (lymph-; -cyte) 10%

Cl^- 104 mEq/L

Platelet (plate-; -let) count 43,000/mm^3

HCO_3^- 22 mEq/L

INR 1.3

Cerebrospinal (cerebro-; -spinal) fluid

Cell count 20 cells/mm^3

Glucose 70 mg/dL

Lymphocytes (lymph-; -cyte) 95%

Proteins 75 mg/dL

Gram stain Negative

India ink preparation Negative

Appropriate therapy is initiated and the patient's condition improves during the next week. Cultures of the blood and cerebrospinal (cerebro-; -spinal) fluid are negative. Which of the following is the most likely source of this patient's illness?

(A) Inhaling (in-; -hal) contaminated droplets (-let)

(B) Insecticide (-cide) from the golf course

(C) Kissing

(D) Mosquito bite

(E) Tick bite

中文翻译

年龄：19 岁

性别：男性，自认性别

种族 / 民族：未指定

就诊地点：医院

该患者是一名大学生，因过去 3 天出现发热、寒战、剧烈头痛、干咳和全身无力等症状被送往医院。无特殊病史，未服用任何药物。他不使用任何物质。他在北卡罗来纳州西部一家高尔夫球场担任草坪管理员。入院时，他看起来病情严重，嗜睡但可被唤醒。体温 39.0℃（102.2℉），脉搏 106 次 / 分钟，呼吸 22 次 / 分钟，血压 90/56 mmHg。室温空气下的氧饱和度为98%。皮肤检查显示手掌、足底、腿部和大腿有红斑状斑丘疹，伴有叠加的瘀点。眼底检查未见异常。颈部柔软，无淋巴结肿大。其余体检，包括神经系统检查，未发现异常。已建立静脉通路。腰椎穿刺检查脑脊液显示开放压为210 mmH_2O，脑脊液略浑浊。心电图显示非特异性 ST 段和 T 波异常。便携式胸部 X 线检查无异常。实验室检查结果如下：

血清

尿素氮 23 mg/dL

肌酐 1.3 mg/dL

葡萄糖 99 mg/dL

钠 134 mEq/L

钾 4.5 mEq/L

氯 104 mEq/L

碳酸氢根 22 mEq/L

血液

血红蛋白 11.5 g/dL

白细胞计数 11,600/mm^3

分叶核中性粒细胞 75%

带状核中性粒细胞 15%

淋巴细胞 10%

血小板计数 43,000/mm^3

国际标准化比值（INR） 1.3

脑脊液

细胞计数 20 /mm³

葡萄糖 70 mg/dL

淋巴细胞 95%

蛋白 75 mg/dL

革兰氏染色 阴性

印度墨汁染色 阴性

适当治疗已开始，患者在接下来的一周内病情好转。血培养和脑脊液培养均为阴性。以下哪项是该患者疾病的最可能来源？

(A) 吸入受污染的飞沫

(B) 高尔夫球场使用的杀虫剂

(C) 接吻

(D) 蚊虫叮咬

(E) 蜱虫叮咬

题目和答案中出现的词根

un-：表示否定

-ache：疼痛

non-：表示否定

somn-：睡眠

re-：重新；反复

spir：呼吸

-ation：表示动作的状态（重复呼吸的状态指代呼吸这个动作）

eryth-：红色

-ema：病理状态

super：在……上面

fundu-：底

scop-：视野

aden-：腺体

-pathy：病

neuro-：神经的

intra-：在……内

ven(o)-：静脉的

cerebro-：大脑

-spinal：脊髓

hemo-：血

-globin：球蛋白

neutro-：中性的

-phil：嗜

lympho-：淋巴

-cyte：细胞

plate-：板状的

-lets：小

in-：向内

-hal：吸气

-let：小的

-cide：杀

-phobia（恐惧）

claustrophobia 幽闭恐惧症

词根 claustro-（封闭空间）+ -phobia（恐惧）

例句 Claustrophobia is characterized by an intense fear of being trapped in enclosed or narrow spaces. 幽闭恐惧症的特征是对被困在封闭或狭小空间中产生极度恐惧。

acrophobia 恐高症

词根 acro-（高处）+ -phobia（恐惧）

例句 Acrophobia is an extreme fear of heights, which can cause dizziness and anxiety. 恐高症是对高处的极度恐惧，可能引起眩晕和焦虑。

hydrophobia 恐水症

词根 hydro-（水）+ -phobia（恐惧）

例句 Hydrophobia is a symptom commonly associated with rabies, where the patient has difficulty swallowing liquids. 恐水症是狂犬病的常见症状，患者对吞咽液体有困难。

thanatophobia 死亡恐惧症

词根 thanato-（死亡）+ -phobia（恐惧）

例句 Thanatophobia is the fear of death or dying, which can interfere with daily activities. 死亡恐惧症是对死亡或濒死的恐惧，可影响日常生活。

nosophobia 疾病恐惧症

词根 noso-（疾病）+ -phobia（恐惧）

例句 Nosophobia is the fear of contracting a specific disease, such as cancer or COVID-19. 疾病恐惧症是对感染特定疾病（如癌症

或新冠病毒）的恐惧。

nyctophobia 黑暗恐惧症

词根 nycto-（夜晚、黑暗）+ -phobia（恐惧）

例句 Nyctophobia is a fear of darkness, often experienced by children but can persist into adulthood. 黑暗恐惧症是对黑暗的恐惧，儿童中常见，但也可能延续到成年。

ophidiophobia 蛇恐惧症

词根 ophidio-（蛇）+ -phobia（恐惧）

例句 Ophidiophobia is an irrational fear of snakes, which can cause severe anxiety even when seeing pictures of snakes. 蛇恐惧症是对蛇的非理性恐惧，即使看到蛇的图片也可能引起严重的焦虑。

aerophobia 飞行恐惧症

词根 aero-（空气、飞行）+ -phobia（恐惧）

例句 Aerophobia is a fear of flying, which can prevent people from traveling by plane. 飞行恐惧症是对乘飞机飞行的恐惧，可能阻碍人们乘坐飞机旅行。

hemophobia 血液恐惧症

词根 hemo-（血）+ -phobia（恐惧）

例句 Hemophobia is a fear of blood, which can cause fainting or nausea when seeing blood. 血液恐惧症是对血液的恐惧，看到血液时可能引起晕厥或恶心。

agoraphobia 广场恐惧症

词根 agora-（公共场所）+ -phobia（恐惧）

例句 Agoraphobia is a fear of being in open or crowded places, making it difficult to leave home. 广场恐惧症是对开放或拥挤场所的恐惧，使患者难以离开家。

cynophobia 犬恐惧症

词根 cyno-（犬）+ -phobia（恐惧）

例句 Cynophobia is an extreme fear of dogs, which can develop after a traumatic experience. 犬恐惧症是对狗的极度恐惧，可能源于创伤性经历。

trypanophobia 针刺恐惧症

词根 trypano-（钻刺）+ -phobia（恐惧）

例句 Trypanophobia is the fear of needles and injections, which can lead to avoidance of medical procedures. 针刺恐惧症是对针头和注射的恐惧，可导致回避医疗程序。

pyrophobia 火恐惧症

词根 pyro-（火）+ -phobia（恐惧）

例句 Pyrophobia is a fear of fire, which can cause anxiety even when seeing controlled fires like candles. 火恐惧症是对火的恐惧，即使看到蜡烛等可控火源也可引起焦虑。

hypnophobia 睡眠恐惧症

词根 hypno-（睡眠）+ -phobia（恐惧）

例句 Hypnophobia is the fear of falling asleep, often due to nightmares or a fear of losing control. 睡眠恐惧症是对入睡的恐惧，通常是由于噩梦或害怕失去控制而引起的。

ailurophobia 猫恐惧症

词根 ailuro-（猫）+ -phobia（恐惧）

例句 Ailurophobia is an irrational fear of cats, which can lead to avoidance of places where cats are present. 猫恐惧症是对猫的非理性恐惧，可能导致患者回避有猫的地方。

pharmacophobia 药物恐惧症

词根 pharmaco-（药物）+ -phobia（恐惧）

例句 Pharmacophobia involves an irrational fear of taking medications, even when prescribed by a doctor. 药物恐惧症是对服用药物的非理性恐惧，即使医生开具处方也不敢服用。

musophobia 鼠恐惧症

词根 muso-（鼠）+ -phobia（恐惧）

例句 Musophobia is an extreme fear of mice and rats, often triggered by past negative experiences. 鼠恐惧症是对老鼠和鼠类的极度恐惧，通常是由过去的负面经历引发的。

carcinophobia 癌症恐惧症

词根 carcino-（癌症）+ -phobia（恐惧）

例句 Carcinophobia is the fear of developing cancer, which can lead to obsessive health monitoring. 癌症恐惧症是对罹患癌症的恐惧，可能导致强迫性健康监测。

autophobia 孤独恐惧症

词根 auto-（自己）+ -phobia（恐惧）

例句 Autophobia is the fear of being alone, which can result in severe anxiety and panic attacks. 孤独恐惧症是对独处的恐惧，可能导致严重的焦虑和惊恐发作。

phon-（声音的）

phonology 音韵学

词根 phon-（声音）+ -logy（学科）

例句 Phonology studies the systematic organization of sounds in languages. 音韵学研究语言中声音的系统组织。

dysphonia 发声困难

词根 dys-（异常）+ phon-（声音）+ -ia（病态）

例句 Dysphonia is characterized by difficulty or discomfort in speaking due to problems with the vocal cords. 发声困难是由声带问题导致的说话困难或不适。

aphonia 失声症

词根 a-（无）+ phon-（声音）+ -ia（病态）

例句 Aphonia is a condition in which a person loses their voice completely, often due to damage to the vocal cords. 失声症是指由声带损伤导致的完全失声。

phonocardiogram 心音图

词根 phon-（声音）+ cardio-（心脏）+ -gram（记录）

例句 A phonocardiogram is a graphic record of heart sounds used to detect abnormalities. 心音图是一种记录心音的图形，用于检测心脏异常。

phonetics 语音学

词根 phon-（声音）+ -etics（学科）

例句 Phonetics studies the production and perception of speech sounds. 语音学研究语音的产生和感知。

phonometer 声强计

词根 phon-（声音）+ -meter（测量仪）

例句 A phonometer is an instrument used to measure the intensity of sound waves. 声强计是一种用于测量声波强度的仪器。

cacophony 刺耳的声音

词根 caco-（不和谐）+ phon-（声音）+ -y（名词后缀）

例句 The cacophony of car horns during rush hour can be overwhelming. 高峰时段汽车喇叭声的嘈杂刺耳令人不堪其扰。

euphony 悦耳的声音

词根 eu-（良好）+ phon-（声音）+ -y（名词后缀）

例句 The choir's performance created a beautiful euphony that captivated the audience. 合唱团的演出创造出一种悦耳的声音，吸引了观众。

symphony 交响乐

词根 sym-（共同）+ phon-（声音）+ -y（名词后缀）
例句 A symphony is an extended musical composition for an orchestra, combining various instruments in harmony. 交响乐是为管弦乐队创作的长篇音乐作品，将各种乐器和谐地融合在一起。

microphone 麦克风

词根 micro-（小）+ phon-（声音）
例句 A microphone converts sound waves into electrical signals for amplification or recording. 麦克风将声波转化为电信号用于放大或记录。

polyphonic 多声部的

词根 poly-（多）+ phon-（声音）+ -ic（形容词后缀）
例句 Polyphonic music involves multiple independent melodies played simultaneously. 多声部音乐涉及多个独立旋律同时演奏。

homophony 同音异义

词根 homo-（相同）+ phon-（声音）+ -y（名词后缀）
例句 In linguistics, homophony refers to words that sound the same but have different meanings. 在语言学中，同音异义指的是发音相同但意思不同的词语。

phonophobia 声音恐惧症

词根 phon-（声音）+ -phobia（恐惧）
例句 Phonophobia is an extreme sensitivity or fear of loud sounds, often associated with migraines. 声音恐惧症是对响亮声音的极度敏感或恐惧，通常与偏头痛有关。

phonopathy 语音疾病

词根 phon-（声音）+ -pathy（疾病）
例句 Phonopathy refers to any disease or disorder affecting the vocal cords or sound production. 语音疾病是指任何影响声带或语音

产生的疾病或障碍。

stereophonic 立体声的

词根 stereo-（立体）+ phon-（声音）+ -ic（形容词后缀）
例句 Stereophonic sound systems create a three-dimensional audio effect by using two or more speakers. 立体声系统通过使用两个或多个扬声器来创造三维音效。

antiphony 对唱

词根 anti-（相对）+ phon-（声音）+ -y（名词后缀）
例句 Antiphony is a form of music where two groups of singers or musicians alternate or respond to each other. 对唱是一种音乐形式，即两组歌唱或演奏团体轮流演唱或相互呼应。

phonautograph 声波记录器

词根 phon-（声音）+ auto-（自动）+ graph（记录）
例句 The phonautograph was one of the earliest devices used to visually record sound waves. 声波记录器是最早用于可视化记录声波的设备之一。

phonosurgery 语音手术

词根 phon-（声音）+ surgery（手术）
例句 Phonosurgery is a surgical procedure to correct vocal cord disorders and improve speech quality. 语音手术是一种用于矫正声带疾病并改善语音质量的手术。

USMLE Step 3 样题

A 52-year-old man comes to the emergency department because of fever and nonpruritic (non-; prurit-) lesions that suddenly developed over his legs 2 hours ago. He has not had any gastrointestinal (gastro-; intestin-) symptoms. Medical history is significant for type 2 diabetes mellitus and cirrhosis (cirrh-; -osis) secondary to hemochromatosis (hemo-; chrom-; -osis). Medications include insulin and spironolactone (spir-; -lactone). Vaccinations (vaccin-; -ation) are up-to-date. The patient returned home 1 day ago from a vacation in a southeastern state. He has had no known contact with anyone who has been ill. On arrival, temperature is 38.6°C (101.5°F), pulse is 118/min, respirations (re-; spir-; -ation) are 22/min, and blood pressure is 84/50 mmHg. Oxygen saturation is 93% on room air. Lungs are clear to auscultation (auscult-; -ation). Cardiac examination discloses a grade 2/6 systolic (systo-) murmur heard best along the left sternal border. Spider angiomas (angio-; -oma) are present over the torso. Abdomen is distended and diffusely dull to percussion (per-; -cuss). Palpation (palp-; -ation) of the abdomen does not disclose tenderness. The liver and spleen are not palpated. The lower extremities are erythematous (eryth-; -ema) and warm to the touch; hemorrhagic (hemo-; -rrhag) bullae are present from the dorsum of the feet to the knees bilaterally (bi-; -lateral). Results of laboratory studies are shown:

Serum Blood

ALT 68 U/L

Hematocrit (hemato-; -crit) 33%

AST 61 U/L

Hemoglobin (hemo-; -globin) 11.0 g/dL

Urea nitrogen 31 mg/dL

WBC 16,000/mm^3

Creatinine 2.1 mg/dL

Neutrophils (neutro-; -phil), segmented 85%

Na^+ 127 mEq/L

Neutrophils (neutro-; -phil), bands 4%

K^+ 5.0 mEq/L

Lymphocytes (lymph-; -cyte) 7%

Cl^- 95 mEq/L

Monocytes (mono-; -cyte) 4%

HCO_3^- 16 mEq/L

Platelet (plate-; -let) count 83,000/mm^3

Lactate dehydrogenase (de-; hydrogen-; -ase) 166 U/L

Glucose 354 mg/dL

Which of the following microorganisms (micro-) is the most likely causal agent of this patient's condition?

(A) Enterobacter (entero-; -bacter) aerogenes (aero-; -gen)

(B) Enterococcus (entero-; -coccus) faecalis (faec-)

(C) Mycobacterium (myco-) marinum (marin-)

(D) Vibrio vulnificus (vulni-; -ficus)

中文翻译

一名 52 岁男性因发热和 2 小时前突然出现在腿部的非瘙痒性皮损来到急诊科。他没有胃肠道症状。病史包括 2 型糖尿病和血色病继发的肝硬化。目前服用的药物包括胰岛素和螺内酯。疫苗接种情况齐全。患者 1 天前从东南部某州度假归来。他没有与任何生病患者的接触史。到达时，体温 38.6℃（101.5℉），脉搏 118 次 / 分钟，呼吸 22 次 / 分钟，血压 84/50 mmHg。室温空气下的氧饱和度为 93%。肺部听诊清晰。心脏检查显示沿左侧胸骨旁最佳听诊点的 2/6 级收缩期杂音。

躯干上有蜘蛛痣。腹部膨隆，叩诊呈弥漫性浊音。腹部触诊无压痛。未触及肝脾。双下肢红斑，触之温热；双侧足背至膝部有出血性大疱。实验室检查结果如下：

血清

丙氨酸氨基转移酶（ALT） 68 U/L

天门冬氨酸氨基转移酶（AST） 61 U/L

尿素氮 31 mg/dL

肌酐 2.1 mg/dL

钠 127 mEq/L

钾 5.0 mEq/L

氯 95 mEq/L

碳酸氢根 16 mEq/L

乳酸脱氢酶 166 U/L

葡萄糖 354 mg/dL

血液

血细胞比容 33%

血红蛋白 11.0 g/dL

白细胞计数 16,000/mm³

分叶核中性粒细胞 85%

带状核中性粒细胞 4%

淋巴细胞 7%

单核细胞 4%

血小板计数 83,000/mm³

以下哪种微生物是最可能导致该患者病情的病原体？

(A) 产气肠杆菌

(B) 粪肠球菌

(C) 海分枝杆菌

(D) 创伤弧菌

题目和答案中出现的词根

non-：表示否定

prurit-：瘙痒

gastro-：胃

intestin-：肠

cirrh-：橘黄色（这里表示肝，因为肝病引起皮肤和黏膜的黄染）

-osis：病理状态（肝脏的病理状态这里指肝硬化）

hemo-：血

chrom-：颜色

-osis：病理状态（血液颜色的病理状态这里指代血色素病）

spir-：呼吸

-lactone：含有七环酯类的药物

vaccin-：牛

-ation：表示动作（牛的动作，指疫苗引起第一个疫苗是牛痘预防天花）

re-：重新；反复

spir：呼吸

-ation：表示动作的状态（重复呼吸的状态指代呼吸这个动作）

auscult-：听

-ation：表示动作（听的动作表示听诊）

systo-：收缩

angio-：血管

-oma：瘤

palp-：触摸（触摸的动作表示触诊）

eryth-：红色

-ema：病理状态

-rrhag（e）：流出，是 rrhea 的同义变异

bi-：双

-lateral：侧

hemato-：血

-crit：分离法（血液分离法指代红细胞比容，即血清和红细胞的分离）

-globin：球蛋白

neutro-：中性的

-phil：嗜

lymph- 淋巴

-cyte：细胞

mono-：单个的

plate-：板状的

-lets：小

de-：去掉

hydrogen-：氢

-ase：酶

micro-：微小的

entero-：肠道的

aero-：气体的

-gen：产生

-bacter：杆菌

-coccus：浆果状

faec：粪便

myco-：真菌的

marin-：海洋的

vulni-：创伤的

-ficus：引起

phospha-（磷）

phosphaturia 磷尿症

词根 phospha-（磷）+ -uria（尿）

例句 Phosphaturia is the excessive excretion of phosphate in the urine, commonly associated with kidney disorders. 磷尿症是尿中磷酸盐排泄过多，通常与肾病有关。

hypophosphatemia 低磷血症

词根 hypo-（低）+ phospha-（磷）+ -emia（血液状况）

例句 Hypophosphatemia occurs when phosphate levels in the blood are abnormally low, often due to malnutrition or kidney disease. 低磷血症是指血液中磷酸盐水平异常偏低，通常由营养不良或肾病引起。

hyperphosphatemia 高磷血症

词根 hyper-（高）+ phospha-（磷）+ -emia（血液状况）

例句 Hyperphosphatemia is a condition characterized by elevated phosphate levels in the blood, often seen in chronic kidney disease. 高磷血症是指血液中磷酸盐水平升高，常见于慢性肾病患者。

phospholipid 磷脂

词根 phospha-（磷）+ lipid（脂肪）

例句 Phospholipids are essential components of cell membranes, forming lipid bilayers. 磷脂是细胞膜的重要组成部分，可形成脂质双层结构。

phosphorylation 磷酸化

词根 phospha-（磷）+ -ylation（过程）
例句 Phosphorylation is a key regulatory mechanism in cells, affecting enzyme activity and signal transduction. 磷酸化是细胞中的关键调控机制，影响酶的活性和信号传递。

phosphatase 磷酸酶

词根 phospha-（磷）+ -ase（酶）
例句 Phosphatase enzymes remove phosphate groups from proteins, playing a role in many metabolic pathways. 磷酸酶通过从蛋白质上去除磷酸基团，在许多代谢途径中发挥作用。

phosphoenolpyruvate 磷酸烯醇丙酮酸

词根 phospha-（磷）+ enol（烯醇）+ pyruvate（丙酮酸）
例句 Phosphoenolpyruvate is an important intermediate in glycolysis, involved in ATP generation. 磷酸烯醇丙酮酸是糖酵解中的重要中间体，参与 ATP 的生成。

phosphocreatine 磷酸肌酸

词根 phospha-（磷）+ creatine（肌酸）
例句 Phosphocreatine serves as an energy reserve in muscles by quickly regenerating ATP during high-intensity activity. 磷酸肌酸在高强度活动中通过快速再生 ATP，为肌肉提供能量储备。

phosphoprotein 磷蛋白

词根 phospha-（磷）+ protein（蛋白质）
例句 Phosphoproteins are proteins that have phosphate groups attached, regulating various cellular processes. 磷蛋白是附着有磷酸基团的蛋白质，可调控多种细胞过程。

phosphoglycerate 磷酸甘油酸

词根 phospha-（磷）+ glycerate（甘油酸）

例句 Phosphoglycerate is an intermediate in metabolic pathways, including glycolysis and gluconeogenesis. 磷酸甘油酸是代谢途径中的中间产物，包括糖酵解和糖异生。

phosphomycin 磷霉素

词根 phospha-（磷）+ mycin（抗生素）

例句 Phosphomycin is an antibiotic used to treat bacterial infections by inhibiting cell wall synthesis. 磷霉素是一种抗生素，通过抑制细菌细胞壁的合成来治疗细菌感染。

phosphite 亚磷酸盐

词根 phospha-（磷）+ -ite（化学名词后缀）

例句 Phosphite compounds are used in agriculture as fertilizers and fungicides. 亚磷酸盐化合物在农业中被用作肥料和杀菌剂。

phosphate buffer 磷酸盐缓冲液

词根 phospha-（磷）+ buffer（缓冲）

例句 Phosphate buffers help maintain a stable pH in biological systems. 磷酸盐缓冲液有助于维持生物系统中的稳定 pH 值。

phosphocarnitine 磷酸肉碱

词根 phospha-（磷）+ carnitine（肉碱）

例句 Phosphocarnitine is involved in fatty acid metabolism and energy production in cells. 磷酸肉碱参与脂肪酸代谢和细胞内的能量生产。

phosphoglycolate 磷酸乙醇酸

词根 phospha-（磷）+ glycolate（乙醇酸）

例句 Phosphoglycolate is a byproduct of photorespiration and is recycled in metabolic processes. 磷酸乙醇酸是光呼吸的副产物，在代谢过程中被回收利用。

phosphoribosyl pyrophosphate 磷酸核糖焦磷酸

词根 phospha-（磷）+ ribosyl（核糖）+ pyrophosphate（焦磷酸）
例句 Phosphoribosyl pyrophosphate is a critical intermediate in the synthesis of nucleotides and amino acids. 磷酸核糖焦磷酸是核苷酸和氨基酸合成中的关键中间体。

phosphoenolpyruvate carboxykinase 磷酸烯醇丙酮酸羧化激酶

词根 phospha-（磷）+ enol（烯醇）+ pyruvate（丙酮酸）
例句 This enzyme plays a key role in gluconeogenesis, converting oxaloacetate to phosphoenolpyruvate. 该酶在糖异生中起关键作用，将草酰乙酸转化为磷酸烯醇丙酮酸。

phosphatide 磷脂类

词根 phospha-（磷）+ -ide（化学后缀）
例句 Phosphatides are a group of lipids containing phosphoric acid, essential for cell membrane structure. 磷脂类是一类含有磷酸的脂质，是细胞膜结构的重要成分。

phosphomolybdate 磷钼酸盐

词根 phospha-（磷）+ molybdate（钼酸盐）
例句 Phosphomolybdate compounds are commonly used in chemical analysis to detect phosphate levels. 磷钼酸盐化合物常用于化学分析中检测磷酸盐含量。

-phylaxis（保护）

prophylaxis 预防

词根 pro-（前）+ -phylaxis（保护）
例句 Prophylaxis refers to preventive treatments aimed at reducing the risk of disease. 预防是指旨在降低疾病风险的预防性治疗。

anaphylaxis 过敏性反应

词根 ana-（过度）+ -phylaxis（保护）

例句 Anaphylaxis is a severe allergic reaction that requires immediate medical attention. 过敏性反应是一种严重的过敏反应，需要立即进行医疗处理。

immunoprophylaxis 免疫预防

词根 immuno-（免疫）+ -phylaxis（保护）

例句 Immunoprophylaxis involves the use of vaccines or immune therapies to prevent infections. 免疫预防是通过疫苗或免疫疗法来预防感染。

chemoprophylaxis 化学预防

词根 chemo-（化学）+ -phylaxis（保护）

例句 Chemoprophylaxis is commonly used to prevent infections in people traveling to high-risk regions. 化学预防常用于防止前往高风险地区的人群感染疾病。

radioprophylaxis 辐射预防

词根 radio-（辐射）+ -phylaxis（保护）

例句 Radioprophylaxis involves measures taken to protect individuals from harmful radiation exposure. 辐射预防是指采取措施保护个体免受有害辐射的影响。

-physeal（生长板）

epiphyseal plate 骺板

词根 epi-（上）+ -physeal（生长板）

例句 The epiphyseal plate is responsible for longitudinal growth of long bones in children. 骺板负责儿童长骨的纵向生长。

metaphyseal fracture 干骺端骨折

词根 meta-（中间）+ -physeal（生长板）

例句 A metaphyseal fracture commonly occurs in children and is often related to growth plate injuries. 干骺端骨折在儿童中常见，通常与生长板损伤有关。

diaphyseal growth 骨干生长

词根 dia-（贯穿）+ -physeal（生长板）

例句 Diaphyseal growth occurs as the bone shaft lengthens during skeletal development. 骨干生长发生在骨干随着骨骼发育而延长的过程中。

physeal arrest 生长板闭合

词根 physeal（生长板）+ arrest（停止）

例句 Physeal arrest occurs when the growth plate closes prematurely, affecting bone development. 生长板闭合是指生长板过早关闭，影响骨骼发育。

epiphyseal fusion 骺板融合

词根 epi-（上）+ -physeal（生长板）+ fusion（融合）

例句 Epiphyseal fusion marks the end of bone growth and occurs after puberty. 骺板融合标志着骨骼生长的结束，通常发生在青春期后。

USMLE Step 3 样题

A 79-year-old retired executive schedules an urgent office visit. When you see him, he says that he had difficulty walking upon getting out of bed this morning because of dizziness, which started last week and worsened last night. He has a 20-year history of hypertension (hyper-; -tension), for which he was treated, but for the past 10 years his blood pressure has been normal without treatment. At his most recent visit 3 weeks ago, his blood pressure was 150/90 mmHg and he was instructed to adhere to a low-salt diet.

He drank a moderate amount of alcoholic beverages in the past and smoked about 16 cigarettes (cigar-; -ette) daily from age 20 years to age 50 years. He has not smoked cigarettes (cigar-; -ette) during the past 29 years. He is taking no medication at present. All his close relatives have lived to be at least in their 80s. This morning, pulse is 78/min and regular and blood pressure is 160/90 mmHg. Neurologic (neuro-) examination shows instability (in-) when the patient is turning and horizontal nystagmus with change in position. Funduscopic (fundu-; scop-) examination shows no abnormalities. Which of the following is the most likely diagnosis?

(A) Cardiac arrhythmia (a-; -rhythm)

(B) Cerebellar ataxia (a-; -taxia) due to alcohol abuse

(C) Labyrinthitis (labyrinth-; -itis)

(D) Orthostatic (ortho-; -stat) hypotension (hypo-; -tension)

(E) Stroke

中文翻译

一名 79 岁退休高管预约了紧急门诊就诊。他表示，今天早上起床后因头晕而行走困难，头晕从上周开始，昨晚加重。他有 20 年高血压病史，曾接受治疗，但过去 10 年未治疗血压仍正常。在 3 周前的最近一次就诊中，他的血压为 150/90 mmHg，被嘱咐遵循低盐饮食。他过去饮酒适量，从 20 岁到 50 岁每天吸烟约 16 支，过去 29 年未吸烟。目前未服用任何药物。他的近亲均活到至少 80 岁。今天早上，脉搏 78 次 / 分钟且规律，血压 160/90 mmHg。神经系统检查显示患者转身时不稳定，体位变化时出现水平眼震。眼底检查未见异常。以下哪项是最可能的诊断？

(A) 心律失常

(B) 酒精滥用导致的小脑共济失调

(C) 迷路炎

(D) 体位性低血压

(E) 中风

题目和答案中出现的词根

hyper-：高

-tension：张力；压力

cigar-：雪茄

-ette：小的（小的雪茄即普通香烟）

neuro-：神经的

in-：表示否定

fundu-：底（这里指眼底）

scop-：视野

a-：表示否定

-rhythm：节律

-taxia：协调

labyrinth-：迷路（这里指内耳的解剖结构）

-itis：炎症

ortho-：正（这里指站立正）

-stat：静止（站立正并保持静止，这里指从平躺到站立过程）

hypo-：低

-plasia（生长）

hyperplasia 增生

词根 hyper-（过度）+ -plasia（生长）

例句 Endometrial hyperplasia is a condition where the lining of the uterus thickens excessively. 子宫内膜增生是子宫内膜过度增厚的病症。

hypoplasia 发育不全

词根 hypo-（不足）+ -plasia（生长）

例句 Hypoplasia of the lung can lead to respiratory distress due to underdeveloped lung tissue. 肺发育不全可能因肺组织发育不足而引发呼吸窘迫。

aplasia 发育缺失

词根 a-（无）+ -plasia（生长）

例句 Bone marrow aplasia occurs when the bone marrow fails to produce enough blood cells. 骨髓发育缺失指骨髓未能产生足够的血细胞。

metaplasia 化生

词根 meta-（转变）+ -plasia（生长）

例句 Metaplasia is the reversible transformation of one cell type into another, often in response to chronic irritation. 化生是指细胞类型的可逆性转变，通常是对慢性刺激的反应。

neoplasia 新生物，肿瘤

词根 neo-（新）+ -plasia（生长）

例句 Neoplasia refers to abnormal and excessive tissue growth, which can be benign or malignant. 新生物是指组织异常过度生长，

可以是良性或恶性。

dysplasia 发育异常

词根 dys-（异常）+ -plasia（生长）

例句 Cervical dysplasia is a precancerous condition characterized by abnormal cell growth on the cervix. 宫颈发育异常是一种癌前状态，表现为宫颈上的细胞生长异常。

fibroplasia 纤维增生

词根 fibro-（纤维）+ -plasia（生长）

例句 Fibroplasia is a normal part of wound healing, involving the growth of fibrous tissue. 纤维增生是伤口愈合的正常部分，涉及纤维组织的生长。

chondroplasia 软骨发育

词根 chondro-（软骨）+ -plasia（生长）

例句 Achondroplasia is a genetic disorder characterized by abnormal cartilage development and short stature. 软骨发育不全是一种遗传性疾病，以软骨发育异常和身材矮小为特征。

myelodysplasia 骨髓发育异常

词根 myelo-（骨髓）+ dys-（异常）+ -plasia（生长）

例句 Myelodysplasia is a group of disorders in which the bone marrow produces defective or insufficient blood cells. 骨髓发育异常是一组疾病，骨髓产生的血细胞有缺陷或不足。

anaplasia 去分化

词根 ana-（向后；退化）+ -plasia（生长）

例句 Anaplasia is often seen in aggressive cancers, where cells lose their normal structure and function. 去分化常见于侵袭性癌症中，此时细胞丧失正常结构和功能。

osteoplasia 骨生成

词根 osteo-（骨）+ -plasia（生长）

例句 Osteoplasia involves the formation of new bone tissue, which is crucial during growth and fracture repair. 骨生成是指新骨组织的形成，对于生长和骨折修复至关重要。

angioplasia 血管生成

词根 angio-（血管）+ -plasia（生长）
例句 Angioplasia is the formation of new blood vessels, which can occur during wound healing or tumor development. 血管生成是指新血管的形成，可以发生在伤口愈合或肿瘤发展过程中。

neuroplasia 神经再生

词根 neuro-（神经）+ -plasia（生长）
例句 Neuroplasia involves the regeneration of nerve cells, which is limited in the central nervous system. 神经再生涉及神经细胞的再生，在中枢神经系统中受限。

retinoplasia 视网膜增生

词根 retino-（视网膜）+ -plasia（生长）
例句 Retinoplasia can lead to retinal tumors if abnormal cell growth occurs. 视网膜增生如果出现异常细胞生长，可能会导致视网膜肿瘤。

adenoplasia 腺体增生

词根 adeno-（腺体）+ -plasia（生长）
例句 Adenoplasia can be observed in glandular tissues, often as a response to hormonal stimulation. 腺体增生可在腺体组织中观察到，通常是对激素刺激的反应。

craniofacial dysplasia 颅面发育异常

词根 cranio-（颅骨）+ facial（面部）+ dys-（异常）+ -plasia（生长）
例句 Craniofacial dysplasia affects the growth and development of the skull and face, leading to deformities. 颅面发育异常影响颅骨和面部的生长发育，导致畸形。

sideroblastic anemia with erythroid hyperplasia 伴红系增生的铁粒幼细胞性贫血

词根 sidero-（铁）+ -plasia（生长）

例句 In this condition, the bone marrow shows erythroid hyperplasia while iron metabolism is impaired. 在这种病症中，骨髓显示红系增生，同时铁代谢受损。

fibrous dysplasia 纤维性发育异常

词根 fibro-（纤维）+ dys-（异常）+ -plasia（生长）

例句 Fibrous dysplasia causes normal bone to be replaced by fibrous tissue, leading to deformities and fractures. 纤维性发育异常导致正常骨组织被纤维组织取代，引起畸形和骨折。

bronchopulmonary dysplasia 支气管肺发育不良

词根 broncho-（支气管）+ pulmonary（肺）+ dys-（异常）+ -plasia（生长）

P

例句 Bronchopulmonary dysplasia is a chronic lung condition affecting premature infants who require mechanical ventilation. 支气管肺发育不良是一种影响早产儿的慢性肺病，他们通常需要机械通气。

hematopoietic hyperplasia 造血组织增生

词根 hemato-（血）+ poietic（生成）+ -plasia（生长）

例句 Hematopoietic hyperplasia is seen in conditions where the body needs increased production of blood cells. 当机体需要增加血细胞生成时，可见造血组织增生。

-plasty（塑形的）

rhinoplasty 鼻整形术

词根 rhino-（鼻）+ -plasty（塑形）

例句 Rhinoplasty is a surgical procedure performed to change the shape of the nose. 鼻整形术是一种用于改变鼻子形状的手术。

angioplasty 血管成形术

词根 angio-（血管）+ -plasty（塑形）

例句 Angioplasty is used to restore blood flow by widening narrowed or blocked blood vessels. 血管成形术用于通过扩张狭窄或堵塞的血管来恢复血流。

arthroplasty 关节成形术

词根 arthro-（关节）+ -plasty（塑形）

例句 Arthroplasty is often recommended for patients with severe joint arthritis. 关节成形术通常推荐给关节炎严重的患者。

mammoplasty 乳房成形术

词根 mammo-（乳房）+ -plasty（塑形）

例句 Mammoplasty can be performed for cosmetic or reconstructive purposes. 乳房成形术可以用于美容或重建目的。

otoplasty 耳部整形术

词根 oto-（耳）+ -plasty（塑形）

例句 Otoplasty is commonly used to correct prominent or misshapen ears. 耳部整形术通常用于矫正突出的或畸形的耳朵。

cranioplasty 颅骨修复术

词根 cranio-（颅骨）+ -plasty（塑形）

例句 Cranioplasty is performed to repair defects in the skull caused by trauma or surgery. 颅骨修复术用于修复由创伤或手术引起的颅骨缺损。

phalloplasty 阴茎成形术

词根 phallo-（阴茎）+ -plasty（塑形）

例句 Phalloplasty is a surgical procedure to reconstruct or enhance the penis. 阴茎成形术是一种用于重建或增强阴茎的手术。

vaginoplasty 阴道成形术

词根 vagino-（阴道）+ -plasty（塑形）

例句 Vaginoplasty is performed to reconstruct or tighten the vaginal canal. 阴道成形术用于重建或收紧阴道通道。

gingivoplasty 牙龈成形术

词根 gingivo-（牙龈）+ -plasty（塑形）

例句 Gingivoplasty reshapes the gums to improve aesthetics or treat periodontal disease. 牙龈成形术通过重塑牙龈改善美观或治疗牙周病。

blepharoplasty 眼睑成形术

词根 blepharo-（眼睑）+ -plasty（塑形）

例句 Blepharoplasty is a surgical procedure to remove excess skin or fat from the eyelids. 眼睑成形术是一种去除眼睑多余皮肤或脂肪的手术。

-plegia（瘫）

hemiplegia 半身不遂

词根 hemi-（半）+ -plegia（瘫）

例句 Hemiplegia is commonly seen in stroke patients, affecting one side of the body. 半身不遂常见于中风患者，影响身体的一侧。

paraplegia 下身瘫痪

词根 para-（旁）+ -plegia（瘫）

例句 Paraplegia results from spinal cord injuries affecting the lower limbs. 下身瘫痪是由脊髓损伤引起的，影响下肢。

quadriplegia 四肢瘫痪

词根 quadri-（四）+ -plegia（瘫）

例句 Quadriplegia affects both the arms and legs, often caused by severe spinal injuries. 四肢瘫痪影响手臂和腿部，通常由严重的脊髓损伤引起。

monoplegia 单肢瘫痪

词根 mono-（单一）+ -plegia（瘫）

例句 Monoplegia usually results from brain injuries affecting specific motor areas. 单肢瘫痪通常由影响特定运动区域的脑损伤引起。

facial plegia 面部瘫痪

词根 facial（面部）+ -plegia（瘫）

例句 Facial plegia is commonly associated with Bell's palsy, causing weakness or paralysis on one side of the face. 面部瘫痪通常与贝尔麻痹有关，导致面部一侧无力或瘫痪。

ophthalmoplegia 眼肌瘫痪

词根 ophthalmo-（眼睛）+ -plegia（瘫）

例句 Ophthalmoplegia results in the inability to move the eyes due to nerve or muscle dysfunction. 眼肌瘫痪是由神经或肌肉功能障碍引起的眼睛无法移动。

diplegia 双侧瘫痪

词根 di-（双）+ -plegia（瘫）

例句 Diplegia often affects both legs and is common in cerebral palsy patients. 双侧瘫痪通常影响双腿，常见于脑瘫患者。

pseudoplegia 假性瘫痪

词根 pseudo-（假）+ -plegia（瘫）

例句 Pseudoplegia mimics paralysis without actual nerve or muscle damage. 假性瘫痪表现出瘫痪症状，但并没有真正的神经或肌肉损伤。

-ploid（倍体，特指染色体）

haploid 单倍体

词根 haplo-（单）+ -ploid（倍体）

例句 Haploid cells contain one set of chromosomes, as seen in gametes. 单倍体细胞含有一组染色体，例如配子。

diploid 二倍体

词根 di-（二）+ -ploid（倍体）

例句 Most human cells are diploid, containing two sets of chromosomes. 大多数人体细胞是二倍体，含有两组染色体。

triploid 三倍体

词根 tri-（三）+ -ploid（倍体）

例句 Triploidy is a chromosomal disorder that results in developmental abnormalities. 三倍体是一种导致发育异常的染色体病。

tetraploid 四倍体

词根 tetra-（四）+ -ploid（倍体）

例句 Tetraploidy can occur in certain plants and some animal cells. 四倍体可以在某些植物和动物细胞中出现。

polyploid 多倍体

词根 poly-（多）+ -ploid（倍体）

例句 Polyploidy is common in plants and contributes to species diversity. 多倍体在植物中很常见，有助于物种多样性。

aneuploid 非整倍体

词根 an-（无）+ eu-（正常）+ -ploid（倍体）

例句 Aneuploidy is a common feature in cancer cells and can lead to genetic instability. 非整倍体是癌细胞中的常见特征，会导致

遗传不稳定。

autopolyploid 自源多倍体

词根 auto-（自身）+ poly-（多）+ -ploid（倍体）

例句 Autopolyploid plants arise from chromosome duplication within a single species. 自源多倍体植物是由单一物种的染色体复制形成的。

allopolyploid 异源多倍体

词根 allo-（异）+ poly-（多）+ -ploid（倍体）

例句 Allopolyploid plants result from hybridization between different species. 异源多倍体植物是不同物种杂交的结果。

endopolyploidy 内倍体增倍

词根 endo-（内部）+ poly-（多）+ -ploid（倍体）

例句 Endopolyploidy occurs when cells replicate their DNA without undergoing cell division. 内倍体增倍是指细胞在不分裂的情况下复制其 DNA。

hypertetraploidy 高四倍体

词根 hyper-（高）+ tetra-（四）+ -ploid（倍体）

例句 Hypertetraploidy is often seen in certain cancer types and can lead to chromosomal instability. 高四倍体常见于某些癌症类型，可能导致染色体不稳定。

USMLE Step 3 样题

A 78-year-old woman who resides in a nursing care facility has had increasing confusion and drowsiness during the past 10 days. The head nurse says, “The patient is usually alert, talkative, and outgoing, but during the past several days she has become increasingly confused and withdrawn. She drifts off to sleep even during activities that she enjoys." Vital signs have remained normal, and she has been eating well. There has been no change in her medication regimen, which includes pravastatin (-statin) for hypercholesterolemia (hyper-; chole-; ster-; -emia), amlodipine (-dipine) for hypertension (hyper-; -tension), a daily 81-mg aspirin, and periodic sublingual (sub-; lingu-) nitroglycerin (nitro-; glycer-) for stable angina pectoris. On interview, the patient says she does not have any symptoms. The patient identifies as White. Temperature is 37.0°C (98.6°F), pulse is 80/min, respirations (re-; spir-; -ation) are 16/min, and blood pressure is 117/84 mmHg. The patient appears to be drifting in and out of sleep during the physical examination, but she is arousable and not in distress (dis-; -tress). She is oriented only to person and place. There is a 5-cm ecchymosis (ec-; chym-; -osis) without hematoma (hemat-; -oma) on the right parietal scalp. Pupils are equal, round, and reactive to light and accommodation. Ocular movements are intact. Optic discs are poorly visualized due to bilateral (bi-; -lateral) cataracts. The remainder of the physical examination, including neurologic (neuro-) examination, shows no abnormalities.

Results of laboratory studies are shown:

Serum Blood

Urea nitrogen 15 mg/dL

Hemoglobin (hemo-; -globin) 13.0 g/dL

Creatinine 1.0 mg/dL

WBC 8,000/mm^3

Na^+ 136 mEq/L

Platelet (plate-; -let) count 160,000/mm^3

K^+ 3.9 mEq/L

Cl^- 95 mEq/L

HCO_3^- 25 mEq/L

Glucose 98 mg/dL

Urine

Specific gravity 1.015

pH 6.5

Protein Negative

Glucose Negative

Occult blood Negative

Leukocyte (leuk-; -cyte) esterase (-ase) Negative

Nitrite Negative

Which of the following is the most likely explanation for the patient's worsening condition?

(A) Drug-drug interaction

(B) Head trauma

(C) Hypothyroidism (hypo-; thyroid-; -ism)

(D) Major depressive episode

(E) Viral encephalitis (encephal-; -itis)

中文翻译

一名 78 岁居住在养老院的女性在过去 10 天内出现逐渐加重的意识模糊和嗜睡。护士长表示：“患者通常警觉、健谈且外向，但过去几天她变得越来越困惑和孤僻。即使在参与她喜欢的活动时，她也会昏昏欲睡。”生命体征一直正常，饮食良好。

她的药物治疗方案未发生变化，包括用于高胆固醇血症的普伐他汀、用于高血压的氨氯地平、每日 81 mg 的阿司匹林，以及用于稳定型心绞痛的按需舌下含服硝酸甘油。在访谈中，患者表示她没有任何症状。患者自认为是白人。体温 37.0℃（98.6℉），脉搏 80 次 / 分钟，呼吸 16 次 / 分钟，血压 117/84 mmHg。

在体检期间，患者似乎时而入睡时而清醒，但可被唤醒且无痛苦表现。她仅能辨认人物和地点。右侧顶骨头皮有 5 cm 瘀斑，无血肿。瞳孔等大、圆形，对光和调节反应正常。眼球运动完整。由于双侧白内障，眼底盘难以看清。其余体检，包括神经系统检查，未发现异常。

实验室检查结果如下：

血清

尿素氮 15 mg/dL

肌酐 1.0 mg/dL

钠 136 mEq/L

钾 3.9 mEq/L

氯 95 mEq/L

碳酸氢根 25 mEq/L

葡萄糖 98 mg/dL

血液

血红蛋白 13.0 g/dL

白细胞计数 8000/mm^3

血小板计数 160,000/mm^3

尿液

比重 1.015

pH 6.5
蛋白 阴性
葡萄糖 阴性
隐血 阴性
白细胞酯酶 阴性
亚硝酸盐 阴性
以下哪项是患者病情恶化的最可能原因？

(A) 药物相互作用
(B) 头部外伤
(C) 甲状腺功能减退症
(D) 重性抑郁发作
(E) 病毒性脑炎

题目和答案中出现的词根

-statin：静止，这里指把合成胆固醇的关键酶 HMG-CoA 还原酶静止，通常为降脂药物。

hyper-：高

chole-：胆

ster-：固体的（这里指胆固醇）

-emia：血症

-dipine：钙离子通路抑制剂类的降压药

-tension：张力；压力

sub-：在……下（在种类的下面指的是亚分类，即在一层分类的下级再分类）

lingu-：舌头

nitro-：硝基

glycer-：甘油

re-：重新；反复

spir：呼吸

-ation 表示动作的状态（重复呼吸的状态指代呼吸这个动作）

dis-：分开

-tress：用力（用力分开表示非常难受，英文里用 being torn apart “被撕成碎片”表示难受）

ec-：向外

chym-：液体

-osis：病理状态（液体向外的病理状态指的是血液这个液体向外，指代皮下的血管外的流出，即淤斑）

hemat-：血，hemato- 的同义变异

-oma：瘤（血液的瘤，即血肿）

bi-：双

-lateral：侧

neuro-：神经的

hemo-：血

-globin：球蛋白

plate-：板状的

-lets：小

leuk-：白色的

-cyte：细胞

hypo-：低

thyroid-：甲状腺

-ism：表示状态

encephal-：脑

-itis：炎症

-pnea（呼吸）

apnea 呼吸暂停

词根 a-（无）+ -pnea（呼吸）

例句 Apnea is a condition characterized by the temporary cessation of breathing during sleep. 呼吸暂停是一种在睡眠中暂时停止呼吸的情况。

dyspnea 呼吸困难

词根 dys-（困难）+ -pnea（呼吸）

例句 Dyspnea is commonly experienced by individuals with heart or lung conditions. 呼吸困难通常是心脏或肺部疾病患者的症状。

tachypnea 呼吸急促

词根 tachy-（快速）+ -pnea（呼吸）

例句 Tachypnea is an abnormally rapid breathing rate often seen in fever or anxiety. 呼吸急促是指呼吸速率异常加快，通常见于发热或焦虑的情况。

bradypnea 呼吸缓慢

词根 brady-（缓慢）+ -pnea（呼吸）

例句 Bradypnea refers to abnormally slow breathing, often seen in neurological disorders. 呼吸缓慢是指呼吸异常缓慢，通常见于神经系统疾病。

orthopnea 直立呼吸困难

词根 ortho-（直立）+ -pnea（呼吸）

例句 Orthopnea occurs when a person has difficulty breathing while lying flat. 直立呼吸困难是指人在平躺时呼吸困难。

hyperpnea 过度呼吸

词根 hyper-（过度）+ -pnea（呼吸）

例句 Hyperpnea is excessive breathing, typically associated with physical exertion or metabolic conditions. 过度呼吸是指异常强烈的呼吸，通常与身体运动或代谢异常相关。

hypopnea 呼吸浅表

词根 hypo-（不足）+ -pnea（呼吸）

例句 Hypopnea is characterized by abnormally shallow breathing, often seen in sleep apnea syndrome. 呼吸浅表是指异常浅的呼吸，通常见于睡眠呼吸暂停综合征。

pneumo-（气）

pneumonia 肺炎

词根 pneumo-（气）+ -ia（病理状态）

例句 Pneumonia is an infection of the lungs that causes inflammation and fluid buildup. 肺炎是一种肺部感染，导致炎症和液体积聚。

pneumothorax 气胸

词根 pneumo-（气）+ thorax（胸）

例句 Pneumothorax occurs when air accumulates in the pleural cavity, causing the lung to collapse. 气胸发生在空气积聚在胸膜腔内，导致肺部塌陷。

pneumonectomy 肺切除术

词根 pneumo-（气）+ -ectomy（切除术）

例句 Pneumonectomy is the surgical removal of one lung, often due to lung cancer. 肺切除术是指由于肺癌而切除一侧肺部的手术。

pneumoconiosis 尘肺病

词根 pneumo-（气）+ coniosis（尘土）

例句 Pneumoconiosis is a lung disease caused by the inhalation of dust particles. 尘肺病是由吸入尘土颗粒引起的肺部疾病。

pneumoperitoneum 腹膜气肿

词根 pneumo-（气）+ peritoneum（腹膜）

例句 Pneumoperitoneum refers to the presence of air within the peritoneal cavity, often seen in abdominal surgeries. 腹膜气肿是指腹膜腔内存在空气，通常在腹部手术中见到。

pneumomediastinum 纵隔气肿

词根 pneumo-（气）+ mediastinum（纵隔）

例句 Pneumomediastinum occurs when air accumulates in the mediastinum, often due to trauma. 纵隔气肿是指空气积聚在纵隔内，通常由创伤引起。

pneumothoracic 气胸的

词根 pneumo-（气）+ thoracic（胸的）

例句 Pneumothoracic conditions can cause chest pain and difficulty breathing. 气胸病症可引起胸痛和呼吸困难。

pneumonitis 肺炎症

词根 pneumo-（气）+ -itis（炎症）

例句 Pneumonitis is the inflammation of lung tissue often caused by infection or inhalation of irritants. 肺炎症是指肺组织的炎症，通常由感染或吸入刺激物引起。

pneumocystis 肺囊虫病

词根 pneumo-（气）+ cystis（囊肿）

例句 Pneumocystis carinii pneumonia is an opportunistic infection commonly seen in immunocompromised patients. 肺囊虫病肺炎是免疫受损患者中常见的一种机会性感染。

pneumogastric 胃气的

词根 pneumo-（气）+ gastric（胃的）

例句 The pneumogastric nerve controls functions in both the lungs and the stomach. 胃气神经控制着肺部和胃部的功能。

pod-（足）

podiatry 足病学

词根 pod（足）+ iatry（医学）
例句 Podiatry is a branch of medicine dedicated to the diagnosis and treatment of foot disorders. 足病学是医学的一个分支，专门诊断和治疗足部疾病。

podiatrist 足病医生

词根 pod（足）+ iatrist（医生）
例句 A podiatrist specializes in treating conditions such as bunions, plantar fasciitis, and foot injuries. 足病医生专门治疗如拇外翻、足底筋膜炎和足部伤害等疾病。

podagra 痛风

词根 pod（足）+ agra（痛苦）
例句 Podagra is a form of gout that specifically affects the big toe. 痛风是一种特别影响大脚趾的痛风类型。

podiatric 足病的

词根 pod（足）+ iatric（医学的）
例句 Podiatric medicine focuses on treating foot and ankle disorders. 足病医学专注于治疗足部和踝部疾病。

podocyte 足细胞

词根 pod（足）+ cyte（细胞）
例句 Podocytes are specialized cells in the kidneys that help filter blood. 足细胞是肾脏中的专门细胞，帮助过滤血液。

pododermatitis 足部皮炎

词根 pod（足）+ dermat-（皮肤）+ itis（炎症）

例句 Pododermatitis is the inflammation of the skin on the foot, often due to infection. 足部皮炎是足部皮肤的炎症，通常由感染引起。

podocyst 足囊肿

词根 pod（足）+ cyst（囊肿）

例句 A podocyst is a cyst that forms in the foot, often causing pain. 足囊肿是形成在足部的囊肿，通常会引起疼痛。

podology 足科学

词根 pod（足）+ -ology（学科）

例句 Podology is the study of the feet and their medical conditions. 足科学是研究足部及其医学病症的学科。

podomotor 足部运动的

词根 pod（足）+ motor（运动的）

例句 Podomotor functions refer to the movement and control of the foot during walking. 足部运动功能是指在行走过程中足部的运动和控制。

podophyllum 足叶草

词根 pod（足）+ phyllum（叶）

例句 Podophyllum is a plant used in medicine to treat certain types of warts. 足叶草是一种用于治疗某些类型疣的植物。

-poiesis（生成）

hematopoiesis 造血

词根 hemato-（血液）+ -poiesis（生成）

例句 Hematopoiesis is the process of blood cell formation in the bone marrow. 造血是血细胞在骨髓中形成的过程。

erythropoiesis 红细胞生成

词根 erythro-（红）+ -poiesis（生成）

例句 Erythropoiesis is the process by which red blood cells are produced in the bone marrow. 红细胞生成是红细胞在骨髓中生成的过程。

leukopoiesis 白细胞生成

词根 leuko-（白）+ -poiesis（生成）

例句 Leukopoiesis refers to the production of white blood cells. 白细胞生成是指白细胞的产生。

thrombopoiesis 血小板生成

词根 thrombo-（血栓）+ -poiesis（生成）

例句 Thrombopoiesis is the production of platelets from megakaryocytes in the bone marrow. 血小板生成是血小板在骨髓中的生成过程。

myelopoiesis 骨髓生成

词根 myelo-（骨髓）+ -poiesis（生成）

例句 Myelopoiesis is the formation of blood cells in the bone marrow. 骨髓生成是指血细胞在骨髓中的形成。

neutropoiesis 中性粒细胞生成

词根 neutro-（中性）+ -poiesis（生成）

例句 Neutropoiesis involves the generation of neutrophils in the bone marrow. 中性粒细胞生成是指中性粒细胞在骨髓中的生成过程。

lymphopoiesis 淋巴细胞生成

词根 lympho-（淋巴）+ -poiesis（生成）

例句 Lymphopoiesis is the process by which lymphocytes are generated. 淋巴细胞生成是指淋巴细胞的生成过程。

spermatopoiesis 精子生成

词根 spermato-（精子）+ -poiesis（生成）

例句 Spermatopoiesis is the process of sperm cell production. 精子生成是精子细胞产生的过程。

oogenesis 卵子生成

词根 o-（卵子）+ -poiesis（生成）

例句 Oogenesis refers to the process of egg cell formation in females. 卵子生成是指女性卵细胞的形成过程。

poikilo-（形状不同的）

poikilocytosis 红细胞形态异常

词根 poikilo-（不规则的）+ cytosis（细胞状态）

例句 Poikilocytosis is often observed in patients with severe anemia. 红细胞形态异常通常见于严重贫血患者。

poikiloderma 皮肤色素异常

词根 poikilo-（不规则的）+ derma（皮肤）

例句 Poikiloderma can be caused by chronic sun exposure or genetic conditions. 皮肤色素异常可能由长期日晒或遗传因素引起。

poikilothermia 变温性

词根 poikilo-（变化的）+ thermia（体温）

例句 Patients with spinal cord injuries may develop poikilothermia due to autonomic dysfunction. 脊髓损伤患者可能因自主神经功能障碍而出现变温现象。

poikiloblast 不规则幼稚细胞

词根 poikilo-（不规则的）+ blast（幼稚细胞）

例句 The presence of poikiloblasts in bone marrow can indicate a hematologic malignancy. 骨髓中存在不规则幼稚细胞可能提示血

液系统恶性疾病。

poikiloderma congenitale 先天性色素异常皮肤病

词根 poikilo-（不规则的）+ derma（皮肤）+ congenitale（先天的）

例句 Poikiloderma congenitale is a rare genetic disorder affecting skin pigmentation and structure. 先天性色素异常皮肤病是一种影响皮肤色素和结构的罕见遗传病。

USMLE Step 3 样题

A 68-year-old woman was admitted to the intensive care unit 36 hours ago after becoming obtunded (ob-; -tund) due to respiratory (re-; spir-) distress (dis-; -tress). She is now intubated (in-; tub-) and chest X-ray is consistent with congestive heart failure and pneumonia (pneumon-). She has a long history of morbid obesity, chronic bronchitis (bronch-; -itis), schizoaffective (schizo-) disorder (dis-) , and cigarette (cigar-; -ette) smoking. She is reported to have been relatively stable on haloperidol (halo-; -ridol), benztropine (benz-; -tropine), and lithium carbonate (carbon). Her present medication regimen includes acetaminophen (acet-; amin-; -ophen), methylprednisolone (methy-; -olone) ciprofloxacin (flo-; -xacin), haloperidol (halo-; -ridol), benztropine (benz-; -tropine), and lithium carbonate (carbon-). She also requires intravenous (intra-ven-) lorazepam (-zepam) every 2 hours for agitation that caused her to fight the ventilator (vent-). Vital signs now show a spike in temperature to 38.9°C (102.0°F). Physical examination discloses lead pipe rigidity. Serum creatine kinase (-ase) concentration is 846 U/L and serum lithium concentration is 0.86 mEq/L. Arterial (arter-) blood gas analysis while breathing 40% oxygen is shown:

PO_2 68 mmHg

PCO_2 36 mmHg

pH 7.46

O_2 saturation 91%

At this time it is most important to discontinue (dis-) which of the following medications?

(A) Benztropine (benz-; -tropine)

(B) Ciprofloxacin (flo-; -xacin)

(C) Haloperidol (halo-; -ridol)

(D) Lorazepam (-zepam)

(E) Methylprednisolone (methy-; -olone)

中文翻译

一名 68 岁女性在 36 小时前因呼吸窘迫导致意识迟钝而被送入重症监护室。她目前已插管，胸部 X 线显示与充血性心力衰竭和肺炎一致。她有长期病态肥胖、慢性支气管炎、精神分裂情感障碍和吸烟史。据报道，她在服用氟哌啶醇、苯托品和碳酸锂时病情相对稳定。她目前的药物治疗方案包括对乙酰氨基酚、甲泼尼龙、环丙沙星、氟哌啶醇、苯托品和碳酸锂。她还需每 2 小时静脉注射劳拉西泮，以控制因躁动而反抗呼吸机的行为。目前生命体征显示体温突然升至 38.9°C（102.0°F）。体检显示铅管样僵直。血清肌酸激酶浓度为 846 U/L，血清锂浓度为 0.86 mEq/L。在吸入 40% 氧气时的动脉血气分析结果如下：

氧分压 68 mmHg

二氧化碳分压 36 mmHg

pH 7.46

氧饱和度 91%

此时最重要的是停止以下哪种药物?

(A) 苯托品

(B) 环丙沙星

(C) 氟哌啶醇

(D) 劳拉西泮

(E) 甲泼尼龙

题目和答案中出现的词根

ob-：朝向

-tund：不明亮（朝向不明亮指的是迟钝，即头脑意识朝向不明亮变化）

re-：重新；反复

spir：呼吸

dis-：离开

-tress：用力（用力分开表示非常难受，英文里用 being torn apart “被撕成碎片”表示难受）

in-：向内

tub-：管（向内的管这里指代气管插管，即向气管内插管）

pneumon-：肺（病理意义上的肺）

bronch-：支气管

-itis：炎症

schizo-：分裂

dis-：离开

cigar-：雪茄

-ette：小的（小的雪茄即普通香烟）

halo-：卤化物

-ridol：治疗精神错乱类药物

benz-：苯环

-tropine：抗胆碱能神经类的药物

carbon-：碳

acet-：乙酰基

amin-：胺

-ophen：芳香环（乙酰基—胺—芳香环加一起指代对乙酰基酚，即扑热息痛）

methy-：甲基

-olone：皮质醇类的药物

flo-：氟

-xacin：喹诺酮类抗生素（即抑制拓扑异构酶 II 的抗生素）

intra-：在……内

ven(o)-：静脉

vent-：通气

-ase：酶

arter-：动脉的

-zepam：通过提升 γ- 氨基丁酸（γ-GABA) 抗焦虑等作用的药物

poly-（多）

polyuria 多尿

词根 poly-（多）+ uria（尿）

例句 Polyuria is a condition characterized by the production of an abnormally large volume of urine. 多尿是指产生异常大量尿液的病症。

polyphagia 多食症

词根 poly-（多）+ phagia（吃）
例句 Polyphagia is an abnormal increase in hunger and food intake. 多食症是指食欲和食物摄入异常增加。

polycythemia 多血症

词根 poly-（多）+ cythemia（血液）
例句 Polycythemia is a condition in which the body produces too many red blood cells. 多血症是一种体内产生过多红细胞的病症。

polyarthritis 多关节炎

词根 poly-（多）+ arthritis（关节炎）
例句 Polyarthritis refers to inflammation in multiple joints. 多关节炎是指多处关节的炎症。

polydipsia 多饮症

词根 poly-（多）+ dipsia（口渴）
例句 Polydipsia is characterized by excessive thirst and fluid intake. 多饮症表现为过度口渴和液体摄入。

polyneuropathy 多发性神经病

词根 poly-（多）+ neuropathy（神经病）
例句 Polyneuropathy involves damage to multiple peripheral nerves throughout the body. 多发性神经病是指全身多个外周神经的损伤。

polygenic 多基因的

词根 poly-（多）+ genic（基因的）
例句 Polygenic traits are determined by the combined effects of multiple genes. 多基因特征由多个基因的综合效应决定。

polyploidy 多倍体

词根 poly-（多）+ ploidy（倍体）
例句 Polyploidy refers to organisms that have more than two complete sets of chromosomes. 多倍体指的是具有两个以上完整染色体组的生物。

polyneuropathy 多神经病

词根 poly-（多）+ neuro-（神经）+ pathy（病）
例句 Polyneuropathy affects multiple nerves and can result in pain, numbness, and weakness. 多神经病影响多个神经，可能导致疼痛、麻木和无力。

polymorphism 多态性

词根 poly-（多）+ morph（形态）+ ism（状态）
例句 Polymorphism in genetics refers to the occurrence of two or more distinct forms in the population. 遗传学中的多态性指的是在人群中出现两种或更多不同形式的现象。

por-（孔）

pore 孔

词根 por-（孔）
例句 Skin pores allow sweat and oils to reach the surface of the skin. 皮肤毛孔允许汗水和油脂到达皮肤表面。

porous 多孔的

词根 por-（孔）+ -ous（形容词后缀，表示……的）
例句 Porous materials are often used in filters due to their ability to allow liquids or gases to pass through. 多孔材料因其能让液体或气体通过而常用于过滤器。

porencephaly 脑孔病

词根 por-（孔）+ encephaly（脑部）
例句 Porencephaly is a rare condition where cysts or cavities form in the brain. 脑孔病是一种罕见的疾病，脑中形成囊肿或空腔。

porosity 孔隙性

词根 por-（孔）+ osity（性质）
例句 Bone porosity refers to the condition where the bones have increased holes or spaces, often associated with diseases like osteoporosis. 骨孔隙性是指骨骼中孔洞或空隙增多的情况，通常与骨质疏松等疾病相关。

porokeratosis 孔角化症

词根 por-（孔）+ keratosis（角化症）
例句 Porokeratosis is a skin disorder characterized by abnormal ke ratinization and the formation of pores in the skin. 孔角化症是一种皮肤病，特点是角化异常，皮肤上形成孔洞。

prandi-（和餐相关的）

prandial 餐时的

词根 prandi-（餐）+ -al（形容词后缀）
例句 Prandial insulin is administered at mealtime to control blood glucose levels. 餐时胰岛素是在进餐时使用的，用于控制血糖水平。

postprandial 餐后

词根 post-（后）+ prandi-（餐）
例句 Postprandial blood sugar levels are measured to assess how well the body processes glucose after a meal. 餐后血糖水平用于评估身体在进餐后如何处理葡萄糖。

preprandial 餐前

词根 pre-（前）+ prandi-（餐）

例句 Preprandial blood sugar levels should be checked before eating, especially for diabetics. 餐前血糖水平应在进餐前检测，特别是对糖尿病患者。

prandial hyperglycemia 餐后高血糖

词根 prandi-（餐）+ hyperglycemia（高血糖）

例句 Prandial hyperglycemia occurs when blood glucose levels rise excessively after a meal. 餐后高血糖是指餐后血糖水平过度升高的情况。

hyperprandial 餐时高血糖的

词根 hyper-（高）+ prandi-（餐）+ -al（形容词后缀）

例句 Hyperprandial conditions may result from overeating or poor glucose metabolism after meals. 餐时高血糖可能是过量进食或餐后糖代谢不良引起的。

-prax（行为能力）

apraxia 失用症

词根 a-（无）+ -prax（行为能力）

例句 Apraxia is a neurological disorder where patients are unable to perform movements despite having the desire and ability. 失用症是一种神经系统疾病，患者尽管有意愿和能力，却无法执行动作。

dyspraxia 运动协调障碍

词根 dys-（困难）+ -prax（行为能力）

例句 Dyspraxia is a developmental disorder that causes difficulty with motor coordination and planning. 运动协调障碍是一种发育障碍，导致运动协调和规划的困难。

ideomotor apraxia 意象运动性失用症

词根 ideo-（思想）+ motor（运动）+ -prax（行为能力）

例句 Ideomotor apraxia affects the ability to perform tasks that require motor planning. 意象运动性失用症影响需要运动规划的任务执行能力。

constructional apraxia 构建性失用症

词根 construct-（构建）+ -prax（行为能力）

例句 Constructional apraxia involves difficulty in drawing or assembling objects despite having the ability to perform individual tasks. 构建性失用症是指尽管具备执行单个任务的能力，却难以画出或组合物体。

buccofacial Apraxia 口面失用症

词根 bucco-（口腔）+ -faci-（面部）+ -prax（行为能力）

例句 Buccofacial apraxia involves difficulty with facial movements such as smiling or blowing. 口面失用症表现为面部动作困难，如微笑或吹气。

pre-（前）

premature 早产的

词根 pre-（前）+ mature（成熟的）

例句 Premature babies require special medical care to support their development. 早产婴儿需要特殊的医疗护理来支持其发育。

preoperative 术前的

词根 pre-（前）+ operative（手术的）

例句 A preoperative assessment is conducted to evaluate a patient's health before surgery. 术前评估是为了在手术前评估患者的健康状况。

prenatal 产前的

词根 pre-（前）+ natal（出生的）

例句 Prenatal care is essential for monitoring the health of both the mother and the baby. 产前护理对监测母婴健康至关重要。

prehypertension 前期高血压

词根 pre-（前）+ hypertension（高血压）

例句 Prehypertension is a condition where blood pressure is elevated but not yet in the hypertensive range. 前期高血压是指血压升高但尚未达到高血压范围的状态。

precordial 心前区的

词根 pre-（前）+ cordis（心脏）

例句 Precordial pain is often associated with cardiac conditions. 心前区疼痛通常与心脏疾病有关。

preclinical 临床前的

词根 pre-（前）+ clinical（临床的）

例句 Preclinical studies are conducted before a drug is tested on humans. 临床前研究是在药物进入人体试验之前进行的。

prepubertal 青春期前的

词根 pre-（前）+ pubertal（青春期的）

例句 Prepubertal children experience different hormonal changes than those in puberty. 青春期前的儿童经历的激素变化与青春期的儿童不同。

prebiotics 益生元

词根 pre-（前）+ biotics（生命的）

例句 Prebiotics are dietary fibers that promote the growth of beneficial gut bacteria. 益生元是一种膳食纤维，促进有益肠道细菌的生长。

prefrontal 额叶前部的

词根 pre-（前）+ frontal（额叶的）

例句 The prefrontal cortex is responsible for complex cognitive behavior and decision-making. 额叶前部皮层负责复杂的认知行为和决策制定。

preemptive 预防性的

词根 pre-（前）+ emptive（夺取的）

例句 Preemptive pain management helps reduce post-surgical discomfort. 预防性疼痛管理有助于减少术后不适。

presby-（老年的）

presbyopia 老花眼

词根 presby-（老年）+ -opia（视力）

例句 Presbyopia is the age-related loss of the ability to focus on close objects. 老花眼是与年龄相关的失去聚焦近处物体的能力。

presbycusis 老年性耳聋

词根 presby-（老年）+ -cusis（听觉）

例句 Presbycusis is the gradual loss of hearing that occurs with age. 老年性耳聋是随着年龄增长而逐渐失去听力的情况。

presbylarynx 老年性喉病变

词根 presby-（老年）+ larynx（喉部）

例句 Presbylarynx refers to age-related changes in the larynx that may affect voice quality. 老年性喉病变指的是与年龄相关的喉部变化，这些变化可能会影响音质。

presbydentia 老年痴呆

词根 presby-（老年）+ dementia（痴呆）

例句 Presbydentia is the cognitive decline associated with aging, leading to memory loss and confusion. 老年痴呆是与年龄相关的认知下降，导致记忆丧失和混乱。

presbyterian 长老会的

词根 presby-（老年）+ -terian（会员）
例句 The Presbyterian church organization includes elders, or presbyters, who are leaders within the community. 长老会的教会组织包括长老，他们是社区中的领导者。

presbyphonia 老年性声音改变

词根 presby-（老年）+ phonia（声音）
例句 Presbyphonia is the alteration of voice quality with aging, often characterized by hoarseness. 老年性声音改变是随着年龄增长，声音质量的变化，通常表现为沙哑。

presbycardia 老年性心脏病

词根 presby-（老年）+ -cardia（心脏）
例句 Presbycardia is the age-related weakening of the heart's function. 老年性心脏病是心脏功能随年龄衰退的现象。

pro-（支持）

probiotic 益生菌

词根 pro-（支持）+ biotic（生命的）
例句 Probiotics help maintain a healthy balance of gut bacteria. 益生菌有助于维持肠道细菌的健康平衡。

prophylaxis 预防

词根 pro-（支持）+ phylaxis（保护）
例句 Vaccination is a form of prophylaxis against infectious diseases. 接种疫苗是一种预防传染病的方法。

P

prothrombin 凝血酶原

词根 pro-（前）+ thrombin（凝血酶）

例句 Prothrombin is a protein in the blood that is essential for clotting. 凝血酶原是一种血液中的蛋白质，对血液凝固至关重要。

progenitor 祖细胞

词根 pro-（支持）+ genitor（产生）

例句 Progenitor cells are early descendants of stem cells that can differentiate into specific cell types. 祖细胞是干细胞的早期后代，可以分化为特定的细胞类型。

prokinetic 促动力的

词根 pro-（支持）+ kinetic（运动的）

例句 Prokinetic drugs help improve gastrointestinal motility. 促动力药物有助于改善胃肠道运动。

proinflammatory 促炎的

词根 pro-（支持）+ inflammatory（炎症的）

例句 Proinflammatory cytokines contribute to immune responses but can also cause tissue damage. 促炎细胞因子有助于免疫反应，但也可能导致组织损伤。

prohormone 激素原

词根 pro-（支持）+ hormone（激素）

例句 A prohormone is a precursor to an active hormone. 激素原是活性激素的前体。

proenzyme 酶原

词根 pro-（支持）+ enzyme（酶）

例句 A proenzyme must be activated before it can perform its enzymatic function. 酶原在发挥酶功能之前必须被激活。

procoagulant 促凝剂

词根 pro-（支持）+ coagulant（凝血的）

例句 Procoagulant factors promote blood clotting to prevent excessive bleeding. 促凝剂促进血液凝固，以防止过度出血。

probiotic therapy 益生菌疗法

词根 pro-（支持）+ biotic（生命的）
例句 Probiotic therapy is used to restore gut microbiota balance in patients with digestive disorders. 益生菌疗法用于恢复消化系统疾病患者的肠道微生物平衡。

procto-（直肠）

proctology 肛门直肠学

词根 procto-（直肠）+ -logy（学科）
例句 Proctology is the medical specialty that deals with disorders of the rectum and anus. 肛门直肠学是研究直肠和肛门疾病的医学分科。

proctitis 直肠炎

词根 procto-（直肠）+ -itis（炎症）
例句 Proctitis is the inflammation of the rectal lining, often caused by infection or autoimmune diseases. 直肠炎是直肠黏膜的炎症，通常由感染或自身免疫疾病引起。

proctoscopy 直肠镜检查

词根 procto-（直肠）+ -scopy（镜检）
例句 A proctoscopy is performed to examine the rectum for abnormalities or diseases. 直肠镜检查用于检查直肠是否存在异常或疾病。

proctectomy 直肠切除术

词根 procto-（直肠）+ -ectomy（切除术）
例句 Proctectomy is a surgical procedure to remove all or part of the rectum. 直肠切除术是一种切除全部或部分直肠的手术。

proctalgia 直肠痛

词根 procto-（直肠）+ -algia（疼痛）

例句 Proctalgia refers to unexplained pain in the rectal area. 直肠痛指的是直肠区域的不明原因疼痛。

proctoplasty 直肠成形术

词根 procto-（直肠）+ -plasty（成形术）

例句 Proctoplasty is performed to reconstruct or repair a damaged rectum. 直肠成形术用于重建或修复受损的直肠。

proctocele 直肠膨出

词根 procto-（直肠）+ -cele（突出）

例句 Proctocele is a condition where the rectal wall protrudes into the vaginal canal. 直肠膨出是指直肠壁向阴道管突出的一种情况。

proctodynia 直肠神经痛

词根 procto-（直肠）+ -dynia（疼痛）

例句 Proctodynia is characterized by severe episodic rectal pain without an apparent cause. 直肠神经痛的特征是间歇性的严重直肠疼痛，但没有明显病因。

proctospasm 直肠痉挛

词根 procto-（直肠）+ -spasm（痉挛）

例句 Proctospasm can cause discomfort and difficulty during bowel movements. 直肠痉挛可能导致不适并影响排便。

proctodermatitis 直肠皮炎

词根 procto-（直肠）+ dermatitis（皮炎）

例句 Proctodermatitis is inflammation of the skin around the anus and rectum. 直肠皮炎是肛门和直肠周围皮肤的炎症。

USMLE Step 3 样题

A 67-year-old woman with osteopenia (osteo-; -penia) comes to the office because of a 6-month history of increasingly severe, constant pain in her left hip and thigh. Before her symptoms began, she walked 1 mile daily. She now walks with a limp and must use a walker. Medical history also is remarkable for hypertension (hyper-; -tension). Medications are hydrochlorothiazide (hydro-; chloro-), ibuprofen (-fen), and calcium and vitamin D supplementation. Her DEXA scan T-score was –1.8 1 year ago. Vital signs are within normal limits. Examination of the left lower extremity produces mild groin tenderness. Passive range of motion of the left hip is limited by pain. Serum studies show a calcium concentration of 8.6 mg/dL, intact parathyroid (para-; thyr-; -oid) hormone concentration of 55 pg/mL, and 25-hydroxyvitamin (hydro-; oxy-) D concentration of 30 ng/mL (N>20). X-rays of the left hip and femur show cortical thickening of the subtrochanteric (sub-; trochanter-) region. MRI of the left hip and femur shows moderate edema of the bone marrow and soft tissue in the subtrochanteric (sub-; trochanter-) region; there is cortical discontinuity (dis-) laterally. Which of the following is the most appropriate next step in management?

(A) Bisphosphonate (bis-; phosphon-) therapy

(B) Brace stabilization

(C) Calcitonin (calci-) therapy

(D) Cast immobilization (im-; mobil-)

(E) Intra-articular (intra-; articul-) dexamethasone (-sone) injection

(F) Surgical fixation

(G) Observation only

中文翻译

一名 67 岁患有骨量减少的女性前来就诊，因 6 个月来左髋部和大腿持续加重的剧烈疼痛。她在症状开始前每天步行 1 英里。现在她走路时跛行，必须使用助行器。病史还包括高血压。目前服用的药物为氢氯噻嗪、布洛芬以及钙和维生素 D 补充剂。她 1 年前的 DEXA 扫描 T 值为−1.8。生命体征正常。左下肢检查显示轻度腹股沟压痛。左髋关节被动活动范围因疼痛受限。血清检查显示钙浓度为 8.6 mg/dL，完整甲状旁腺激素浓度为 55 pg/mL，25- 羟基维生素 D 浓度为 30 ng/mL（正常值 >20）。左髋部和股骨 X 光显示转子下区域皮质增厚。左髋部和股骨 MRI 显示转子下区域骨髓和软组织中度水肿，侧方皮质不连续。以下哪一项是后续处理中最合适的措施？

(A) 双膦酸盐治疗

(B) 支具固定

(C) 降钙素治疗

(D) 石膏固定

(E) 关节内注射地塞米松

(F) 手术固定

(G) 仅观察

题目和答案中出现的词根

osteo-：骨

-penia：缺少

hyper-：高

-tension：张力；压力

hydro-：氢

chloro-：氯

-fen：部分非甾体类抗炎药的后缀

para-：旁边

thyr-：盾

-oid：类似的（类盾状的指代甲状腺）

oxy-：氧

sub-：在……下（在种类的下面指的是亚分类，即在一层分类的下级再分类

trochanter-：转子

dis-：离开

bis-：两

phosphon-：磷酸

calci-：钙

im-：表否定

mobil-：移动

intra-：在……内

articul-：关节

-sone：糖皮质激素类的药物

proprio-（自身）

proprioception 本体感觉

词根 proprio-（自身）+ -ception（感知）

例句 Proprioception refers to the body's ability to sense its position in space. 本体感觉指的是身体感知自己在空间中的位置的能力。

proprioceptor 本体感受器

词根 proprio-（自身）+ -ceptor（感受器）

例句 Proprioceptors are sensory receptors that detect changes in body position and movement. 本体感受器是检测身体位置和运动变化的感受器。

proprioceptive neuromuscular facilitation 本体感知神经肌肉促进法

词根 proprio-（自身）+ -ceptive（感知的）+ neuromuscular（神经肌肉的）+ facilitation（促进）

例句 Proprioceptive neuromuscular facilitation（PNF）is a rehabilitation technique used to improve muscle strength and flexibility. 本体感知神经肌肉促进法（PNF）是一种用于改善肌肉力量和柔韧性的康复技术。

proprioceptive input 本体感知输入

词根 proprio-（自身）+ -ceptive（感知的）+ input（输入）

例句 Proprioceptive input helps the body understand its orientation and movement in space. 本体感知输入有助于身体理解在空间中的定位和运动。

proprioreception 本体感知

词根 proprio-（自身）+ -reception（接收）

例句 Proprioreception is critical for tasks requiring coordination and balance. 本体感知对于需要协调和平衡的任务至关重要。

proprioceptive deficit 本体感知缺失

词根 proprio-（自身）+ -ceptive（感知的）+ deficit（缺失）

例句 Proprioceptive deficit can occur after neurological injuries, leading to difficulties with movement and balance. 本体感知缺失可以在神经损伤后发生，导致运动和平衡困难。

proprioceptive training 本体感知训练

词根 proprio-（自身）+ -ceptive（感知的）+ training（训练）

例句 Proprioceptive training helps improve balance, coordination, and motor control. 本体感知训练有助于提高平衡、协调和运动控制。

proprioreflex 本体反射

词根 proprio-（自身）+ reflex（反射）

例句 The proprioreflex is an automatic response to changes in muscle length or tension. 本体反射是对肌肉长度或张力变化的自动反应。

propriovision 本体视觉

词根 proprio-（自身）+ vision（视觉）

例句 Propriovision refers to the visual processing of the body's position and movement in space. 本体视觉指的是对身体在空间中位置和运动的视觉处理。

propriopathic 本体病学的

词根 proprio-（自身）+ -pathic（疾病的）

例句 Propriopathic disorders affect the nervous system's ability to process proprioceptive information. 本体病学的疾病影响神经系统处理本体感知信息的能力。

USMLE Step 3　样题

A 3-month-old female infant is admitted to the intensive care unit via the emergency department in winter because of respiratory (re-; spir-) distress (dis-; -tress). The infant first became ill 3 days ago with fever and congestion (con-; gest-), but her symptoms have worsened since that time. This morning she developed pallor, lethargy, cough, copious respiratory (re-; spir-) secretions, and tachypnea (tachy-; -pnea). On arrival at the emergency department today, temperature was 37.1°C (98.8°F), pulse was 124/min, respirations (re-; spir-; -ation) were 80/min, and blood pressure was 80/35 mmHg. Oxygen saturation was 78% on room air; after administration of supplemental oxygen, oxygen saturation increased to 94%. The infant's pallor has not subsided, and she is in obvious respiratory (re-; spir-) distress (dis-; -tress). Physical examination discloses head bobbing, nasal flaring, and subcostal (sub-; -costal) retractions (re-;-tract) with each breath. Auscultation (auscult-; -ation) of the lungs discloses crepitant crackles throughout both lung fields with scattered expiratory (ex-; pir-) wheezing. The remainder of the physical examination discloses no abnormalities. The infant is prepared for intubation (in-; tub-; -ation) based on her clinical status.

Results of laboratory studies are shown:

Capillary (capill-) blood gas analysis on oxygen at 2 L/min

Blood

PO_2 55 mmHg

Hematocrit (hemato-; -crit) 30%

PCO_2 64 mmHg

Hemoglobin (hemo-; -globin) 10.1 g/dL

pH 7.22

WBC 9,800/mm^3

HCO_3^- 26 mEq/L

Neutrophils (neutro-; -phil), segmented 18%

Lymphocytes (lymph-; -cyte) 80%

Platelet (plate-; -let) count 220,000/mm^3

Chest X-ray is shown. Which of the following is the most likely cause of this infant's illness?

(A) Haemophilus (haemo-; -phil) influenzae

(B) Herpes virus

(C) Mycoplasma (myco-; -plasm) pneumoniae (pneumon-)

(D) Respiratory (re-; spir-) syncytial (syn-; cyt-) virus

(E) Streptococcus (strepto-; -coccus) pneumoniae (pneumon-)

中文翻译

一名 3 个月大的女婴因呼吸窘迫（冬季发病），经急诊科转送至重症监护室。3 天前，婴儿开始出现发热和鼻塞，但此后症状加重。今天早晨，她出现面色苍白、嗜睡、咳嗽、大量呼吸道分泌物和呼吸急促。今天到达急诊科时，体温 37.1℃（98.8°F），脉搏 124 次 / 分钟，呼吸 80 次 / 分钟，血压 80/35 mmHg。室温空气下的氧饱和度为 78%；给予补充氧气后，氧饱和度升至 94%。婴儿的苍白未消退，且明显处于呼吸窘迫状态。体检显示每次呼吸伴有头部摆动、鼻翼扇动和肋下凹陷。肺部听诊显示双肺遍布爆裂音，伴有散在的呼气性哮鸣音。其余体检未发现异常。根据她的临床状况，准备进行插管。实验室检查结果如下：

毛细血管血气分析（氧气 2 L/min）

氧分压 55 mmHg

二氧化碳分压 64 mmHg

pH 7.22

碳酸氢根 26 mEq/L

血液

血细胞比容 30%

血红蛋白 10.1 g/dL

白细胞计数 9,800/mm³

分叶核中性粒细胞 18%

淋巴细胞 80%

血小板计数 220,000/mm³

以下哪项是该婴儿疾病的最可能原因？

(A) 流感嗜血杆菌

(B) 疱疹病毒

(C) 支原体肺炎

(D) 呼吸道合胞病毒

(E) 肺炎链球菌

题目和答案中出现的词根

re-：重新；反复

spir：呼吸

dis-：分开

-tress：用力（用力分开表示非常难受，英文里有用 being torn apart“被撕成碎片”表示难受）

con-：一起

gest-：携带（“一起携带”医学上指的是充血，即部分血管内一起携带了过多的红细胞）

tachy-：快速的

-pnea：呼吸

sub-：在……下（在种类的下面指的是亚分类，即在一层分类的下级再分类）

-costal：肋骨

auscult-：听

-ation：表示动作（听的动作就是听诊）

ex-：向外

pir-：呼吸（向外呼吸就是呼气）

in-：向内

tub-：管

-ation：表示动作（向内的管指的是气管插管，即向气管内插管）

capill-：毛发

hemato-：血

-crit：分离法（血液分离法指代红细胞比容，即血清和红细胞的分离）

hemo-：血

-globin：球蛋白

neutro-：中性的

-phil：嗜

lymph：淋巴

-cyte：细胞

plate-：板状的

-lets：小

heamo-：血（是 hemato-，hemo- 的同义变异）

pneumon-：肺（病理意义上的肺）

syn-：合 （合细胞指的是合胞体）

strepto-：链状的

cocc-：浆果状的（链状的浆果状的指的是链球菌的形状）

prosta-（前列腺的）

prostatitis 前列腺炎

词根 prosta-（前列腺）+ -itis（炎症）

例句 Prostatitis is an inflammation of the prostate gland, often caused by infection. 前列腺炎是前列腺的炎症，通常由感染引起。

prostatectomy 前列腺切除术

词根 prosta-（前列腺）+ -ectomy（切除术）

例句 Prostatectomy is a surgical procedure to remove part or all of the prostate gland. 前列腺切除术是切除部分或全部前列腺的手术。

prostatomegaly 前列腺肥大

词根 prosta-（前列腺）+ -megaly（肿大）

例句 Prostatomegaly is the abnormal enlargement of the prostate gland. 前列腺肥大是前列腺异常增大的情况。

prostatosis 前列腺病

词根 prosta-（前列腺）+ -osis（病理状态）

例句 Prostatosis refers to any non-inflammatory disorder of the prostate gland. 前列腺病指的是任何非炎症性的前列腺疾病。

prostatodynia 前列腺疼痛

词根 prosta-（前列腺）+ -dynia（疼痛）

例句 Prostatodynia is characterized by chronic pelvic pain without infection. 前列腺疼痛的特点是慢性骨盆疼痛，但没有感染。

prostatorrhea 前列腺溢液

词根 prosta-（前列腺）+ -rrhea（流出）

例句 Prostatorrhea is the abnormal discharge of prostatic fluid without ejaculation. 前列腺溢液是指在没有射精的情况下，前列

腺液异常流出。

prostatalgia 前列腺痛

词根 prosta-（前列腺）+ -algia（疼痛）

例句 Prostatalgia is a condition where patients experience chronic prostate pain. 前列腺痛是一种患者持续感到前列腺疼痛的疾病。

prostatovesiculitis 前列腺及精囊炎

词根 prosta-（前列腺）+ vesicul-（精囊）+ -itis（炎症）

例句 Prostatovesiculitis is the inflammation of both the prostate and seminal vesicles. 前列腺及精囊炎是前列腺和精囊的炎症。

prostatolithiasis 前列腺结石

词根 prosta-（前列腺）+ -lithiasis（结石病）

例句 Prostatolithiasis is the formation of stones within the prostate gland. 前列腺结石是指前列腺内形成结石。

prostatography 前列腺造影术

词根 prosta-（前列腺）+ -graphy（影像记录）

例句 Prostatography is a radiographic imaging technique used to assess prostate abnormalities. 前列腺造影术是一种用于评估前列腺异常的放射成像技术。

proto-（原）

protozoa 原生动物

词根 proto-（原）+ zoa（动物）

例句 Protozoa are single-celled microorganisms that can cause infectious diseases. 原生动物是单细胞微生物，可能引起传染病。

protoplasm 原生质

词根 proto-（原）+ plasm（物质）

例句 Protoplasm is the living substance inside a cell, including the cytoplasm and nucleus. 原生质是细胞内部的活性物质，包括细胞质和细胞核。

protooncogene 原癌基因

词根 proto-（原）+ oncogene（癌基因）
例句 A protooncogene is a normal gene that can become an oncogene due to mutations. 原癌基因是一种正常基因，因突变可能转变为癌基因。

protoderm 原表皮

词根 proto-（原）+ derm（皮肤）
例句 The protoderm is the outermost layer of cells in a developing embryo. 原表皮是发育中胚胎的最外层细胞。

protogyny 原雌性

词根 proto-（原）+ gyny（雌性）
例句 Protogyny is a type of sequential hermaphroditism where an organism starts as female and later changes to male. 原雌性是一种连续性雌雄同体现象，生物先为雌性，后转变为雄性。

protohematin 原卟啉血红素

词根 proto-（原）+ hematin（血红素）
例句 Protohematin is an intermediate in the biosynthesis of heme. 原卟啉血红素是血红素生物合成的中间产物。

protostome 原口动物

词根 proto-（原）+ stome（口）
例句 Protostomes are a group of animals in which the mouth develops before the anus in embryonic development. 原口动物是一类动物，在胚胎发育过程中，口先于肛门形成。

protoporphyrin 原卟啉

词根 proto-（原）+ porphyrin（卟啉）
例句 Protoporphyrin is a precursor to heme, essential for oxygen

transport in blood. 原卟啉是血红素的前体，对血液中的氧运输至关重要。

protonephridium 原肾管

词根 proto-（原）+ nephridium（肾管）

例句 Protonephridia are excretory structures found in some invertebrates. 原肾管是某些无脊椎动物的排泄结构。

pseudo-（假）

pseudotumor 假瘤

词根 pseudo-（假）+ tumor（肿瘤）

例句 Pseudotumor cerebri is a condition that mimics the symptoms of a brain tumor. 假瘤性脑压升高是一种模拟脑瘤症状的疾病。

pseudomembranous colitis 假膜性结肠炎

词根 pseudo-（假）+ membranous（膜状的）+ colitis（结肠炎）

例句 Pseudomembranous colitis is an inflammation of the colon often caused by Clostridioides difficile infection. 假膜性结肠炎是一种结肠炎症，通常由艰难梭菌感染引起。

pseudocyesis 假孕

词根 pseudo-（假）+ cyesis（妊娠）

例句 Pseudocyesis is a psychological condition where a woman believes she is pregnant despite the absence of a fetus. 假孕是一种心理病症，女性误以为自己怀孕，但实际并无胎儿。

pseudohypertension 假性高血压

词根 pseudo-（假）+ hypertension（高血压）

例句 Pseudohypertension is when blood pressure readings are falsely elevated due to arterial stiffness. 假性高血压是指因动脉僵硬导致血压读数虚高。

pseudocyst 假性囊肿

词根 pseudo-（假）+ cyst（囊肿）

例句 A pancreatic pseudocyst is a fluid-filled sac that forms in the pancreas after inflammation. 胰腺假性囊肿是胰腺炎后形成的充满液体的囊状结构。

pseudogout 假性痛风

词根 pseudo-（假）+ gout（痛风）

例句 Pseudogout is caused by calcium pyrophosphate crystal deposits in the joints. 假性痛风由焦磷酸钙晶体沉积在关节中引起。

pseudodementia 假性痴呆

词根 pseudo-（假）+ dementia（痴呆）

例句 Pseudodementia is a condition where depression mimics the symptoms of dementia. 假性痴呆是一种抑郁症状模拟痴呆的疾病。

pseudocapsule 假囊

词根 pseudo-（假）+ capsule（囊）

例句 A pseudocapsule can form around tumors or cysts as a protective barrier. 假囊可能在肿瘤或囊肿周围形成，作为一种保护屏障。

pseudopregnancy 假妊娠

词根 pseudo-（假）+ pregnancy（妊娠）

例句 Pseudopregnancy occurs in some animals, mimicking the physical changes of pregnancy without conception. 假妊娠在某些动物中出现，表现出类似怀孕的生理变化，但实际并未受孕。

pseudomotor 假性运动

词根 pseudo-（假）+ motor（运动）

例句 Pseudomotor responses can occur in neurological disorders, causing involuntary movements. 假性运动可能出现在神经系统疾病中，导致非自主运动。

-ptosis（下垂）

blepharoptosis 眼睑下垂

词根 blepharo-（眼睑）+ -ptosis（下垂）

例句 Blepharoptosis is a condition in which the upper eyelid droops, sometimes obstructing vision. 眼睑下垂是上眼睑下垂的病症，有时会阻碍视力。

ptosis 器官下垂

词根 -ptosis（下垂）

例句 Ptosis can affect various organs, such as the eyelid, stomach, or bladder. 下垂症可以影响各种器官，如眼睑、胃或膀胱。

gastric ptosis 胃下垂

词根 gastric（胃的）+ -ptosis（下垂）

例句 Gastric ptosis refers to the abnormal downward displacement of the stomach. 胃下垂是指胃部异常下移。

renal ptosis 肾下垂

词根 renal（肾的）+ -ptosis（下垂）

例句 Renal ptosis is the condition where one or both kidneys descend lower than their normal position. 肾下垂是指一个或两个肾脏低于正常位置。

uterine ptosis 子宫下垂

词根 uterine（子宫的）+ -ptosis（下垂）

例句 Uterine ptosis refers to the downward displacement of the uterus, often due to weakness in the pelvic muscles. 子宫下垂是指子宫的下移，通常由于盆底肌肉的无力。

bladder ptosis 膀胱下垂

词根 bladder（膀胱）+ -ptosis（下垂）

例句 Bladder ptosis occurs when the bladder drops from its normal position, often causing urinary problems. 膀胱下垂是膀胱从正常位置下移，通常会引发尿路问题。

mammary ptosis 乳房下垂

词根 mammary（乳房的）+ -ptosis（下垂）

例句 Mammary ptosis is the sagging of the breasts, often due to aging or pregnancy. 乳房下垂是乳房因衰老或怀孕而下垂的情况。

cardiac ptosis 心脏下垂

词根 cardiac（心脏的）+ -ptosis（下垂）

例句 Cardiac ptosis involves the downward displacement of the heart, a rare but serious condition. 心脏下垂是指心脏向下移位，这是一种罕见但严重的病症。

pulmonary ptosis 肺下垂

词根 pulmonary（肺的）+ -ptosis（下垂）

例句 Pulmonary ptosis involves abnormal displacement of the lung, often caused by trauma or disease. 肺下垂是指肺部异常移位，通常由创伤或疾病引起。

USMLE Step 3 样题

A 39-year-old woman comes to the office because of a 1-year history of progressively worsening shortness of breath. She had been generally healthy and says that initially the shortness of breath occurred only after strenuous exercise; however, she now becomes fatigued and short of breath after walking two to three blocks. During the past 2 weeks, she has noted a rapid heart rate and light-headedness. She has not had chest pain, lower extremity edema, orthopnea (ortho-; -pnea), or any nocturnal (noct-; -urnal) symptoms. Medical history is remarkable for Graves disease, which was diagnosed 4 years ago and treated with radioactive (radio-) iodine. Current medications include levothyroxine (levo-; thyro-), a daily multivitamin (multi-), and an oral contraceptive (contra-; cept-). She does not smoke cigarettes (cigar-; -ette) or drink alcoholic beverages. She is 168 cm tall and weighs 57 kg; BMI is 20 kg/m^2 . Temperature is 37.0°C (98.6°F), pulse is 120/min and irregular (ir-), respirations (re-; spir-; -ation) are 16/min, and blood pressure is 110/85 mmHg. Lungs are clear to auscultation (auscult-; -ation). Cardiac examination discloses a rapid rate, a palpable parasternal (para-; -sternal) lift, a normal S1, and a widely split, prominent S2. There is a grade 2/6 systolic (systo-) murmur heard best over the second intercostal (inter-; -costal) space. Examination of the lower extremities discloses trace edema of both feet. The remainder of the physical examination discloses no abnormalities. Results of laboratory studies are shown:

Serum Blood

Na^+ 140 mEq/L

Hemoglobin 13.0 g/dL

K^+ 3.4 mEq/L

Platelet count 155,000/mm^3

Cl^- 100 mEq/L

HCO_3^- 25 mEq/L

Glucose 130 mg/dL

TSH 0.58 μU/mL

ECG shows atrial fibrillation (fibrill-; -ation) with a ventricular (ventricul-) rate of 140/min and right axis deviation (de-; via-; -ation). Chest X-ray shows clear lung fields, no effusion (ef-; fus-), and prominent pulmonary (pulmon-) arteries. Which of the following is the most appropriate additional diagnostic study?

(A) CT scan of the chest

(B) Echocardiography (echo-; cardi-; -graphy)

(C) Perfusion (per-; fus-) lung scan

(D) Pulmonary (pulmon-) function testing

(E) Ultrasonography (ultra-; sono-; -graphy) of the thyroid

中文翻译

一名 39 岁女性因 1 年来呼吸困难症状逐渐加重前来就诊。她原本健康，表示最初仅在剧烈运动后出现呼吸困难；但现在走两到三个街区后就会感到疲劳和呼吸困难。在过去 2 周，她注意到心率加快和头晕。她没有胸痛、下肢水肿、端坐呼吸或夜间症状。病史显著包括 4 年前诊断的格雷夫斯病，通过放射性碘治疗。目前服用的药物包括左甲状腺素、每日多种维生素和口服避孕药。她不吸烟也不饮酒。她身高 168 cm，体重 57 kg；BMI 为 20 kg/m²。体温 37.0℃（98.6℉），脉搏 120 次 / 分钟且不规则，呼吸 16 次 / 分钟，血压 110/85 mmHg。肺部听诊清晰。心脏检查显示心率快，可触及胸骨旁抬举感，S1 正常，S2 明显分裂并增强。第二肋间隙最佳听诊点听到 2/6 级收缩期杂音。下肢检查显示双足轻微水肿。其余体检未发现异常。实验室检查结果如下：

血清

钠 140 mEq/L

钾 3.4 mEq/L

氯 100 mEq/L

碳酸氢根 25 mEq/L

葡萄糖 130 mg/dL

促甲状腺激素（TSH） 0.58 μU/mL

血液

血红蛋白 13.0 g/dL

血小板计数 155,000/mm^3

心电图显示房颤，室率 140 次 / 分钟，伴右轴偏离。胸部 X 线显示肺野清晰，无积液，肺动脉突出。以下哪项是最适当的进一步诊断检查？

(A) 胸部 CT 扫描

(B) 心脏超声检查

(C) 肺灌注扫描

(D) 肺功能测试

(E) 甲状腺超声检查

题目和答案中出现的词根

ortho-：正

-pnea：呼吸（正位呼吸指端坐呼吸，即只能坐正才能呼吸获得足够的氧，而躺着不能）

noct-：夜里的

urnal-：时间段

radio-：放射性

levo-：左的

thyro-：甲状腺的

multi-：多

contra-：反

-cept：获得（反获得指代避孕，即反获得胎儿）

cigar-：雪茄

-ette：小的（小的雪茄即普通香烟）

ir-：表示否定

re-：重新；反复

spir：呼吸

-ation表示动作的状态（重复呼吸的状态指代呼吸这个动作）

auscult-：听

-ation：表示动作（听的动作指听诊）

para-：旁边

-sternal：胸骨

systo-：收缩的

inter-：在……之间

-costal：肋骨

hemo-：血

-globin：球蛋白

plate-：板状的

-lets：小

fibrill-：纤维状的（纤维状的动作这里指代颤动，即只有肌纤维的运动，而非肌肉协同运动带动的大幅度收缩）

ventricul-：室的（这里指的是心室，也可以用于形容脑室）

de-：去掉

via-：路

-ation：表示动作（离开路的动作表示偏离）

ef-：向外

fus-：倾泻（向外倾斜即外溢）

pulmon-：肺的（指的是解剖意义上的肺）

echo-：回声

cardi-：心脏

-graphy：图像

per-：经过

fus-：倾泻（经过倾泻指的是灌注，即经过血管倾泻血液）

ultra-：超

sono-：声音的（表示可听见的声音波段）

pulmon-（肺）

pulmonology 肺病学

词根 pulmon-（肺）+ -ology（学科）

例句 Pulmonology is the medical specialty focused on diseases of the lungs and respiratory system. 肺病学是专门研究肺部和呼吸系统疾病的医学分科。

pulmonary 肺的

词根 pulmon-（肺）+ -ary（形容词后缀）

例句 Pulmonary function tests measure how well the lungs are working. 肺功能测试用于测量肺的工作状况。

pulmonary embolism 肺栓塞

词根 pulmon-（肺）+ -ary（形容词后缀）+ embolism（栓塞）

例句 A pulmonary embolism occurs when a blood clot blocks blood flow to the lungs. 肺栓塞是指血栓阻塞肺部血流的情况。

pulmonectomy 肺切除术

词根 pulmon-（肺）+ -ectomy（切除术）

例句 A pulmonectomy is a surgical procedure to remove a lung. 肺切除术是一种切除肺部的外科手术。

pulmonary edema 肺水肿

词根 pulmon-（肺）+ -ary（形容词后缀）+ edema（水肿）

例句 Pulmonary edema occurs when excess fluid builds up in the lungs. 肺水肿是指肺部积聚过多液体的情况。

pulmonary fibrosis 肺纤维化

词根 pulmon-（肺）+ -ary（形容词后缀）+ fibrosis（纤维化）

例句 Pulmonary fibrosis causes scarring in the lungs, making it harder to breathe. 肺纤维化会导致肺部结疤，使呼吸变得更加困难。

pulmonary hypertension 肺动脉高压

词根 pulmon-（肺）+ -ary（形容词后缀）+ hypertension（高血压）

例句 Pulmonary hypertension is a condition where high blood pressure affects the arteries in the lungs. 肺动脉高压是一种影响肺动脉的高血压疾病。

pulmonic stenosis 肺动脉狭窄

词根 pulmon-（肺）+ -ic（形容词后缀）+ stenosis（狭窄）

例句 Pulmonic stenosis is a congenital heart defect that affects blood flow from the heart to the lungs. 肺动脉狭窄是一种影响心脏向肺输送血流的先天性心脏缺陷。

pulmonary tuberculosis 肺结核

词根 pulmon-（肺）+ -ary（形容词后缀）+ tuberculosis（结核病）

例句 Pulmonary tuberculosis is an infectious disease caused by Mycobacterium tuberculosis. 肺结核是一种由结核分枝杆菌引起的传染病。

pulmectomy 肺切除术

词根 pulmon-（肺）+ -ectomy（切除术）

例句 Pulmectomy is performed to remove a diseased portion of the lung. 肺切除术用于切除病变的肺组织。

USMLE Step 3 样题

A 49-year-old woman is brought to the emergency department by her husband because of a 1-hour history of generalized weakness, dizziness, and palpitations (palpit-; -ation). The patient says she has felt like she is going to faint. She also reports a 3-day history of an upper respiratory (re-; spir-) infection, for which she has taken over-the-counter cold remedies. Medical history is remarkable for hyperthyroidism (hyper-; thyr-; -oid; -ism) diagnosed 1 month ago, for which she was given prescriptions for several medications, none of which she has filled. She is 160 cm tall and weighs 54 kg; BMI is 21 kg/m^2 . She appears anxious. Temperature is 38.9°C (102.0°F), pulse is 168/min and irregular (ir-), respirations (re-; spir-; -ation) are 26/min, and blood pressure is 124/56 mmHg supine. Oxygen saturation is 97% on room air. Physical examination shows mild muscle wasting, mild pharyngeal (pharyn-) erythema (eryth-; -ema) without exudate, and watery nasal discharge (dis-). Examination of the neck discloses (dis-) a goiter, an audible (audi-) bruit, and no jugular venous distention (dis-; tent-). Lungs are clear to auscultation (auscult-; -ation) with good breath sounds. Cardiac examination shows an irregularly (ir-) irregular (ir-) rhythm and a grade 3/6 systolic (systo-) ejection (e-; ject-) murmur heard best along the left sternal border. The abdomen is soft with no tenderness. A tremor of the upper extremities is noted. There is no clubbing, cyanosis (cyan-; -osis), or edema to any of the extremities. Neurologic (neuro-) examination shows no abnormalities. ECG shows atrial fibrillation (fibrill-; -ation) with a rapid ventricular (ventricul-) response. The patient is placed on a cardiac monitor and is given a 1 L bolus of isotonic (iso-) saline. Which of the following is the most appropriate next step?

(A) Cardioversion (cardi-)
(B) Intravenous (intra-; ven-) dexamethasone (-sone)
(C) Intravenous (intra-; ven-) diltiazem
(D) Intravenous (intra-; ven-) propranolol (-lol)
(E) Oral potassium (potass-) iodide (iod-)

中文翻译

一名 49 岁女性由其丈夫带到急诊科，因 1 小时来全身无力、头晕和心悸。她表示感觉自己像是晕厥了。她还报告有 3 天的上呼吸道感染病史，为此她服用了非处方感冒药。病史显著包括 1 个月前诊断的甲状腺功能亢进症，当时开具了几种药物处方，但她均未取药。她身高 160 cm，体重 54 kg；BMI 为 21 kg/m^2。她看起来焦虑。体温 38.9°C（102.0°F），脉搏 168 次 / 分钟且不规则，呼吸 26 次 / 分钟，仰卧位血压 124/56 mmHg。室温空气下的氧饱和度为 97%。体检显示轻度肌肉萎缩，轻度咽部红斑无渗出物，鼻腔有水样分泌物。颈部检查显示甲状腺肿大，可闻及杂音，无颈静脉怒张。肺部听诊清晰，呼吸音良好。心脏检查显示不规则的不规则节律，沿左侧胸骨旁最佳听诊点听到 3/6 级收缩期射血杂音。腹部柔软，无压痛。上肢有震颤。四肢无杵状指、发绀或水肿。神经系统检查未发现异常。心电图显示房颤伴快速室率反应。患者被连接到心脏监护仪，并给予 1 L 等渗盐水快速输注。以下哪项是最适当的后续步骤？

(A) 心脏复律

(B) 静脉注射地塞米松

(C) 静脉注射地尔硫䓬

(D) 静脉注射普萘洛尔

(E) 口服碘化钾

题目和答案中出现的词根

palpit-：快速敲击

-ation：表示动作（快速敲击的动作就是心悸）

re-：重新；反复

spir：呼吸

hyper-：高

thyr-：盾

-oid：类似的（类似盾状的指代甲状腺）

-ism：表示状态

ir-：表示否定

pharyn-：咽

eryth-：红色

-ema：病理状态

dis-：离开

audi-：听力

tent-：拉伸（离开拉伸指的是膨胀，即体积向外拉伸，离

开内部中心位置）

auscult-：听

-ation：动作（听的动作就是听诊）

systo-：收缩

e-：向外的

ject-：流（向外流，即射出）

cyan-：蓝色

-osis：病理状态，是 -ema 的同义变异，蓝色病理状态指的是发绀

neuro-：神经的

fibrill-：纤维状的（纤维状的动作这里指代颤动，即只有肌纤维的运动，而非肌肉协同运动带动的大幅度收缩）

ventricul-：室（这里指心室，也可以指脑室）

iso-：等同

cardi-：心脏

intra-：在……内

ven-：静脉

-sone：糖皮质激素类的药物

-lol：β 受体阻滞剂类药物

potass-：钾

iod-：碘

pyelo-（肾盂）

pyelonephritis 肾盂肾炎

词根 pyelo-（肾盂）+ nephritis（肾炎）

例句 Pyelonephritis is a bacterial infection that affects the kidneys and renal pelvis. 肾盂肾炎是一种影响肾脏和肾盂的细菌感染。

pyelogram 肾盂造影

词根 pyelo-（肾盂）+ -gram（影像）

例句 A pyelogram is an imaging test used to examine the renal pelvis and urinary tract. 肾盂造影是一种用于检查肾盂和尿路的影像学测试。

pyeloplasty 肾盂成形术

词根 pyelo-（肾盂）+ -plasty（成形术）

例句 Pyeloplasty is a surgical procedure to correct a blockage in the renal pelvis. 肾盂成形术是一种用于矫正肾盂阻塞的外科手术。

pyelolithotomy 肾盂取石术

词根 pyelo-（肾盂）+ litho-（结石）+ -tomy（切开术）

例句 Pyelolithotomy is performed to remove kidney stones from the renal pelvis. 肾盂取石术用于从肾盂中取出肾结石。

pyelopathy 肾盂病变

词根 pyelo-（肾盂）+ -pathy（疾病）

例句 Pyelopathy refers to any disease affecting the renal pelvis. 肾盂病变指影响肾盂的任何疾病。

pyeloureteral 肾盂输尿管的

词根 pyelo-（肾盂）+ ureteral（输尿管的）

例句 Pyeloureteral obstruction can lead to kidney dysfunction if left untreated. 若未得到治疗，肾盂输尿管梗阻可能导致肾功能障碍。

pyelotomy 肾盂切开术

词根 pyelo-（肾盂）+ -tomy（切开术）

例句 Pyelotomy is a surgical procedure to open the renal pelvis for stone removal. 肾盂切开术是一种通过切开肾盂以取出结石的手术。

pyelocaliectasis 肾盂肾盏扩张

词根 pyelo-（肾盂）+ caliectasis（肾盏扩张）

例句 Pyelocaliectasis is the dilation of the renal pelvis and calyces. 肾盂肾盏扩张是指肾盂和肾盏的扩张。

pyelovenous reflux 肾盂静脉逆流

词根 pyelo-（肾盂）+ venous（静脉）+ reflux（逆流）

例句 Pyelovenous reflux occurs when urine flows backward from the renal pelvis into the veins. 肾盂静脉逆流是指尿液从肾盂逆流进入静脉。

pyelocystostomy 肾盂膀胱造口术

词根 pyelo-（肾盂）+ cysto-（膀胱）+ -stomy（造口术）

例句 Pyelocystostomy is a procedure that connects the renal pelvis to the bladder. 肾盂膀胱造口术是一种连接肾盂和膀胱的手术。

pyo-（脓）

pyoderma 脓皮病

词根 pyo-（脓）+ derma（皮肤）

例句 Pyoderma is a bacterial skin infection characterized by pus-filled lesions. 脓皮病是一种由细菌感染引起的皮肤病，其特征是脓液填充的皮损。

pyemia 脓毒血症

词根 pyo-（脓）+ -emia（血液疾病）

例句 Pyemia is a severe bloodstream infection caused by pus-forming bacteria. 脓毒血症是一种由化脓细菌引起的严重血液感染。

pyosalpinx 输卵管积脓

词根 pyo-（脓）+ salpinx（输卵管）

例句 Pyosalpinx occurs when pus accumulates in the fallopian tube due to infection. 输卵管积脓是由于感染导致脓液积聚在输卵管内的情况。

pyothorax 脓胸

词根 pyo-（脓）+ thorax（胸腔）
例句 Pyothorax is a condition where pus collects in the pleural cavity surrounding the lungs. 脓胸是指脓液积聚在包围肺部的胸膜腔内。

pyonephritis 脓肾炎

词根 pyo-（脓）+ nephritis（肾炎）
例句 Pyonephritis is a severe kidney infection that results in pus accumulation in the renal tissue. 脓肾炎是一种严重的肾脏感染，导致肾组织内脓液积聚。

pyometra 子宫积脓

词根 pyo-（脓）+ metra（子宫）
例句 Pyometra is a life-threatening uterine infection that often requires surgical intervention. 子宫积脓是一种危及生命的子宫感染，通常需要手术治疗。

pyogenic 化脓性的

词根 pyo-（脓）+ -genic（产生的）
例句 Pyogenic bacteria are responsible for infections that produce pus. 化脓性细菌会导致产生脓液的感染。

pyocyst 脓肿囊

词根 pyo-（脓）+ cyst（囊肿）
例句 A pyocyst is a cyst filled with pus due to bacterial infection. 脓肿囊是一种由于细菌感染导致的充满脓液的囊肿。

pyoarthritis 化脓性关节炎

词根 pyo-（脓）+ arthritis（关节炎）
例句 Pyoarthritis is a bacterial infection of a joint that results in pus formation. 化脓性关节炎是一种关节细菌感染，导致脓液形成。

pyocolpos 阴道积脓

词根 pyo-（脓）+ colpos（阴道）
例句 Pyocolpos is a condition where pus accumulates in the vagina due to an infection. 阴道积脓是由于感染导致脓液积聚在阴道内的情况。

pyogranuloma 化脓性肉芽肿

词根 pyo-（脓）+ granuloma（肉芽肿）
例句 Pyogranuloma is a chronic inflammatory lesion characterized by the presence of pus and granulomas. 化脓性肉芽肿是一种慢性炎性病变，其特征是脓液和肉芽肿的存在。

pyosepsis 化脓性败血症

词根 pyo-（脓）+ sepsis（败血症）
例句 Pyosepsis is a severe systemic infection caused by pus-forming bacteria in the bloodstream. 化脓性败血症是一种由化脓细菌进入血液引起的严重全身性感染。

pyopneumothorax 脓气胸

词根 pyo-（脓）+ pneumo-（气）+ thorax（胸腔）
例句 Pyopneumothorax occurs when both pus and air accumulate in the pleural cavity. 脓气胸是指脓液和空气同时积聚在胸膜腔内的情况。

pyodermatitis 化脓性皮炎

词根 pyo-（脓）+ dermatitis（皮炎）
例句 Pyodermatitis is an inflammatory skin condition caused by pus-forming bacterial infections. 化脓性皮炎是一种由化脓性细菌感染引起的皮肤炎症。

pyocystitis 膀胱积脓

词根 pyo-（脓）+ cystitis（膀胱炎）
例句 Pyocystitis is a condition where pus collects in the bladder

due to infection. 膀胱积脓是指由于感染导致脓液积聚在膀胱内的情况。

pyogaster 腹腔积脓

词根 pyo-（脓）+ gaster（胃；腹部）

例句 Pyogaster is a rare condition where pus accumulates in the abdominal cavity. 腹腔积脓是一种罕见的病症，指腹腔内脓液积聚。

pyorrhea 脓溢症

词根 pyo-（脓）+ -rrhea（流出）

例句 Pyorrhea is a severe gum infection that results in the discharge of pus. 脓溢症是一种严重的牙龈感染，导致脓液流出。

pyocystoma 脓性囊瘤

词根 pyo-（脓）+ cyst（囊肿）+ -oma（瘤）

例句 Pyocystoma is a type of cystic tumor filled with pus. 脓性囊瘤是一种充满脓液的囊性肿瘤。

pyonephrosis 化脓性肾积水

词根 pyo-（脓）+ nephrosis（肾病）

例句 Pyonephrosis is a severe kidney infection leading to pus accumulation in the renal pelvis. 化脓性肾积水是一种严重的肾脏感染，导致脓液积聚在肾盂内。

pyospermatosis 脓性精液病

词根 pyo-（脓）+ spermato-（精液）+ -osis（病理状态）

例句 Pyospermatosis is a condition where pus is present in the semen, indicating an infection. 脓性精液病是指精液中含有脓液，表明存在感染。

radiculo-（神经根）

radiculopathy 神经根病

词根 radiculo-（神经根）+ -pathy（病）

例句 Radiculopathy is a condition where a nerve root is compressed or irritated, leading to pain or weakness. 神经根病是指神经根被压迫或刺激，导致疼痛或无力。

radiculitis 神经根炎

词根 radiculo-（神经根）+ -itis（炎症）

例句 Radiculitis refers to the inflammation of the nerve roots, often caused by infection or injury. 神经根炎指的是神经根的炎症，通常由感染或损伤引起。

radiculalgia 神经根痛

词根 radiculo-（神经根）+ -algia（疼痛）

例句 Radiculalgia is pain that radiates from the nerve root due to compression or irritation. 神经根痛是由神经根压迫或刺激引起的放射性疼痛。

radiculocervical 颈部神经根的

词根 radiculo-（神经根）+ cervical（颈部的）

例句 Radiculocervical pain refers to neck pain caused by a compressed nerve root in the cervical spine. 颈部神经根痛指的是由颈椎中的神经根压迫引起的颈部疼痛。

radiculogram 神经根图

词根 radiculo-（神经根）+ -gram（图；记录）

例句 A radiculogram is an imaging technique used to assess nerve root conditions. 神经根图是一种用来评估神经根状况的成像技术。

radiculoneuropathy 神经根神经病

词根 radiculo-（神经根）+ neuro-（神经）+ -pathy（病）
例句 Radiculoneuropathy involves both the nerve root and the peripheral nerves, leading to a variety of symptoms. 神经根神经病同时涉及神经根和外周神经，导致多种症状。

radiculocutaneus 神经根皮肤的

词根 radiculo-（神经根）+ cutaneus（皮肤的）
例句 Radiculocutaneus fibers transmit sensory information from the skin to the spinal cord. 神经根皮肤纤维将来自皮肤的感觉信息传递至脊髓。

radiculoneuritis 神经根神经炎

词根 radiculo-（神经根）+ neuro-（神经）+ -itis（炎症）
例句 Radiculoneuritis is the inflammation of both the nerve roots and the associated peripheral nerves. 神经根神经炎是指神经根和相关外周神经的炎症。

radiculopathy treatment 神经根病治疗

词根 radiculo-（神经根）+ -pathy（病）+ treatment（治疗）
例句 Treatment for radiculopathy may include physical therapy, medications, and sometimes surgery. 神经根病的治疗可能包括物理治疗、药物治疗，有时还需要手术。

radiculotoxin 神经根毒素

词根 radiculo-（神经根）+ -toxin（毒素）
例句 Radiculotoxin is a substance that can damage nerve roots and cause severe neurological symptoms. 神经根毒素是一种能损害神经根并引起严重神经症状的物质。

radio-（放射的）

radiology 放射学

词根 radio-（射线）+ -logy（学科）

例句 Radiology is the medical field that uses imaging techniques such as X-rays, MRIs, and CT scans to diagnose and treat diseases. 放射学是利用影像学技术（如 X 线、磁共振成像和 CT 扫描）来诊断和治疗疾病的医学领域。

radiotherapy 放射治疗

词根 radio-（射线）+ therapy（治疗）

例句 Radiotherapy is a treatment that uses high-energy radiation to kill cancer cells or shrink tumors. 放射治疗是一种使用高能辐射来杀死癌细胞或缩小肿瘤的治疗方法。

radiographX 光片

词根 radio-（射线）+ -graph（记录）

例句 A radiograph is an image obtained through the use of X-rays to view the inside of the body. X 线片是通过使用 X 射线获得的图像，用于查看身体内部。

radiation 辐射

词根 radio-（射线）+ -ation（名词后缀）

例句 Radiation is the emission of energy in the form of rays or waves, used in various medical treatments and diagnostic tests. 辐射是以射线或波的形式发射的能量，在各种医疗治疗和诊断测试中使用。

radiopaque 不透光的

词根 radio-（射线）+ opaque（不透明的）

例句 A radiopaque substance is one that blocks X-rays and appears white on a radiograph. 不透光物质是指能阻挡 X 射线并在 X 线片上呈现白色的物质。

radioactive 放射性的

词根 radio-（射线）+ active（活跃的）
例句 Radioactive substances emit radiation and are used in medical imaging and cancer treatment. 放射性物质会发射辐射，并用于医学影像和癌症治疗。

radiodermatitis 放射性皮炎

词根 radio-（射线）+ dermat-（皮肤）+ -itis（炎症）
例句 Radiodermatitis is a skin condition that results from exposure to radiation, causing redness and irritation. 放射性皮炎是由于暴露于辐射而引起的皮肤病，表现为发红和刺激。

radioimmunoassay 放射免疫分析

词根 radio-（射线）+ immuno-（免疫）+ assay（分析）
例句 Radioimmunoassay is a laboratory technique used to measure the concentration of antigens or antibodies in a sample. 放射免疫分析是一种实验室技术，用于测定样本中抗原或抗体的浓度。

R

radionuclide 放射性核素

词根 radio-（射线）+ nuclide（核素）
例句 Radionuclides are unstable isotopes that emit radiation and are used in imaging techniques like PET scans. 放射性核素是不稳定的同位素，会释放辐射，并用于如 PET 扫描等影像技术。

radiocystography 放射性膀胱造影

词根 radio-（射线）+ cysto-（膀胱）+ -graphy（成像术）
例句 Radiocystography is an imaging technique used to examine the bladder and its function using contrast and X-rays. 放射性膀胱造影是一种用于检查膀胱及其功能的成像技术，使用对比剂和 X 射线。

radiobiology 放射生物学

词根 radio-（射线）+ bio-（生物）+ -logy（学科）

例句 Radiobiology is the study of the effects of radiation on living organisms and their biological processes. 放射生物学是研究辐射对生物体及其生物过程的影响的学科。

re-（再）

reconstruct 重建

词根 re-（再）+ construct（构建）

例句 The surgeon had to reconstruct the damaged tissue after the accident. 事故发生后，外科医生必须重建受损的组织。

reevaluate 重新评估

词根 re-（再）+ evaluate（评估）

例句 The doctor decided to reevaluate the patient's condition after the new test results came in. 医生决定在新测试结果出来后重新评估患者的病情。

restructure 重组

词根 re-（再）+ structure（结构）

例句 The hospital restructured its internal departments to improve efficiency. 医院重组了内部部门，以提高效率。

reproduce 再生产

词根 re-（再）+ produce（生产）

例句 The laboratory is studying how the virus reproduces within human cells. 实验室正在研究病毒如何在人体细胞内再生产。

reignite 重新点燃

词根 re-（再）+ ignite（点燃）

例句 The doctor was concerned about the possibility that the infection might reignite after treatment. 医生担心治疗后感染可能再次复发。

reestablish 重新建立

词根 re-（再）+ establish（建立）

例句 The goal of rehabilitation is to help patients reestablish their physical function. 康复的目标是帮助患者重新恢复他们的身体功能。

reinterpret 重新解释

词根 re-（再）+ interpret（解释）

例句 After new findings were discovered, the researchers had to reinterpret the data. 在发现新数据后，研究人员不得不重新解释这些数据。

regenerate 再生

词根 re-（再）+ generate（生成）

例句 Regenerative medicine aims to repair or replace damaged tissues or organs. 再生医学旨在修复或替换受损的组织或器官。

reactivate 重新激活

词根 re-（再）+ activate（激活）

例句 The vaccine is designed to reactivate the immune system to protect against the virus. 该疫苗旨在重新激活免疫系统，以保护免受病毒侵害。

reintegrate 再整合

词根 re-（再）+ integrate（整合）

例句 Reintegrating the patient into the community after recovery is an important part of the healing process. 患者康复后重新融入社会是治疗过程中的重要一环。

replenish 补充

词根 re-（再）+ plenish（充实）

例句 The doctor advised the patient to replenish their fluids after the procedure. 医生建议患者在手术后补充液体。

USMLE Step 3 样题

A 40-year-old woman, gravida 2, para 2, comes to the office because of a 1-month history of weakness and intermittent (inter-; mitt-) diarrhea (dia-; -rrhea). She also reports frequent palpitations (palpit-; -ation) and says she has felt shaky and warm during the past 2 weeks. She has lost 9 kg during the past 2 months and was initially excited about the weight loss. Medical history is remarkable for two cesarean deliveries at ages 20 and 22 years. She takes no medications. Family history is remarkable for glaucoma (glauc-; -oma) diagnosed in her maternal (mater-) grandfather at age 65 years. The patient does not smoke cigarettes (cigar-; -ette), drink alcoholic beverages, or use other substances. She is 173 cm tall and weighs 54 kg; BMI is 18 kg/m^2 . She appears anxious and is sweating mildly. Temperature is 37.4°C (99.4°F), pulse is 115/min, respirations (re-; spir-; -ation) are 18/min, and blood pressure is 140/90 mmHg. Physical examination discloses bilateral (bi-; -lateral) lid lag and exophthalmos (ex-; ophthalm-). There is mildly diffuse enlargement of the thyroid (thyr-; -oid) with no discrete palpable (palp-) nodules (nod-; -ule). Cardiac examination discloses a regular rate and rhythm. There is a fine resting tremor of both hands and hyperreflexia (hyper-; re-; flex-) in all extremities. Results of laboratory studies show a serum thyroid (thyr-; -oid) -stimulating hormone concentration of 0.2 μU/mL. Without treatment, which of the following is most likely to develop in this patient?

(A) Chronic kidney disease

(B) Congestive heart failure

(C) Fibromyalgia (fibro-; my-; -algia)

(D) Glaucoma (glauc-; -oma)

(E) Multiple (multi-) sclerosis (scler-; -osis)

中文翻译

一名 40 岁女性，孕 2 产 2，因 1 个月来全身无力、间歇性腹泻来到诊所。她还报告频繁心悸，并表示过去 2 周感到颤抖和发热。她在过去 2 个月内体重减轻了 9 kg，最初对此感到兴奋。病史显著包括在 20 岁和 22 岁时两次剖宫产。她未服用任何药物。家族史显示其外祖父在 65 岁时诊断出青光眼。患者不吸烟、不饮酒，也不使用其他物质。她身高 173 cm，体重 54 kg；BMI 为 18 kg/m²。她看起来焦虑，伴有轻度出汗。体温 37.4℃（99.4℉），脉搏 115 次 / 分钟，呼吸 18 次 / 分钟，血压 140/90 mmHg。体检显示双侧眼睑迟滞和眼球突出。甲状腺轻度弥漫性增大，无明显可触及结节。心脏检查显示心率和节律规则。双手有细微静止性震颤，四肢反射亢进。实验室检查结果显示血清促甲状腺激素浓度为 0.2 μU/mL。如果不进行治疗，该患者最可能出现以下哪种情况？

(A) 慢性肾病

(B) 充血性心力衰竭

(C) 纤维肌痛

(D) 青光眼

(E) 多发性硬化

题目和答案中出现的词根

inter-：在……之间

mitt-：时间区间（在时间区间之间表示间歇性的）

dia-：通过（这里指通过肠道）

-rrhea：流出（通过肠道流出指腹泻）

palpit-：快速敲击

-ation：表示动作

glauc-：蓝灰色

-oma：肿瘤（蓝灰色肿瘤指的是青光眼，即眼内压增高导致角膜水肿看起来像角膜肿瘤，角膜水肿导致其看起来为蓝灰色）

mater-：母亲的

cigar-：雪茄

-ette：小的（小的雪茄即普通香烟）

re-：重新；反复

spir：呼吸

-ation 表示动作的状态（重复呼吸的状态指代呼吸这个动作）

bi-：双

-lateral：侧

ex-：向外

ophthalm-：眼睛的（眼睛向外指的是突眼）

thyr-：盾

-oid：类似的（类似盾状指的是甲状腺）

palp-：触摸

nod-：结节

-ule：小的

hyper-：高

-flex：弯曲（弯曲回指的是反射，指的是电信号在反射弧神经的传导，从中央神经系统传出到外周通常是肌肉，再弯曲返回中央神经系统）

fibro-：纤维的

my-：肌肉

-algia：疼痛

multi-：多

scler-：硬的

-osis：病理状态

rect-（直的）

rectus 直肌

词根 rect-（直的）+ -us（肌肉）

例句 The rectus abdominis is a major muscle of the abdominal wall that helps with trunk movement. 腹直肌是腹壁的重要肌肉，有助于躯干的运动。

rectus abdominis 腹直肌

词根 rect-（直的）+ -us（肌肉）+ abdominis（腹部的）

例句 Rectus abdominis exercises are commonly recommended to strengthen the abdominal region. 腹直肌锻炼通常被推荐用来加强腹部肌肉力量。

rectus sheath 腹直肌鞘

词根 rectus（直的）+ sheath（鞘）

例句 The rectus sheath surrounds the rectus abdominis muscle and helps protect it. 直腹肌鞘包围着直腹肌并有助于保护它。

rectus capitis muscle 头直肌

词根 rectus（直的）+ capitis（头部的）+ muscle（肌肉）
例句 The rectus capitis muscle is involved in the movement of the head, helping in flexion and rotation. 头直肌参与头部运动，帮助头部弯曲和旋转。

rectus spinalis 腹直肌棘肌

词根 rectus（直的）+ spinalis（脊柱的）
例句 The rectus spinalis is a muscle that aids in maintaining posture and stabilizing the spine. 直脊肌有助于维持姿势并稳定脊柱。

reticulo-（网状的）

reticulocyte 网织红细胞

词根 reticulo-（网状的）+ -cyte（细胞）
例句 Reticulocytes are immature red blood cells that are released from the bone marrow into the bloodstream. 网织红细胞是从骨髓释放到血液中的未成熟的红细胞。

reticulopathy 网状结构病

词根 reticulo-（网状的）+ -pathy（病）
例句 Reticulopathy refers to diseases affecting the reticular structure of the tissues or organs. 网状结构病是指影响组织或器官网状结构的疾病。

reticulum 网状结构

词根 reticulo-（网状的）+ -um（名词后缀）
例句 The reticulum is a part of the lymphatic system that helps in filtering pathogens. 网状结构是淋巴系统的一部分，帮助过滤病原体。

reticulin 网状蛋白

词根 reticulo-（网状的）+ -in（蛋白质后缀）

例句 Reticulin is a type of collagen that forms a network-like structure in tissues. 网状蛋白是一种胶原蛋白，形成组织中的网状结构。

reticuloperitoneal 网状腹膜的

词根 reticulo-（网状的）+ peritoneal（腹膜的）
例句 Reticuloperitoneal fibrosis can develop as a result of chronic peritoneal inflammation. 网状腹膜纤维化可能是由慢性腹膜炎引起的。

reticulohistiocytosis 网状组织细胞增生症

词根 reticulo-（网状的）+ histio-（组织）+ -cytosis（细胞增生）
例句 Reticulohistiocytosis involves the abnormal increase of histiocytes and reticulocytes in the tissue. 网状组织细胞增生症涉及组织中组织细胞和网织红细胞的异常增生。

reticulospinal 网状脊髓的

词根 reticulo-（网状的）+ spinal（脊髓的）
例句 The reticulospinal tract plays a role in motor control and maintaining posture. 网状脊髓束在运动控制和维持姿势中发挥作用。

reticuloendothelial 网状内皮的

词根 reticulo-（网状的）+ endo-（内）+ -thelial（上皮的）
例句 The reticuloendothelial system is involved in filtering blood and removing pathogens. 网状内皮系统参与过滤血液并清除病原体。

reticulocyte count 网织红细胞计数

词根 reticulo-（网状的）+ -cyte（细胞）+ count（计数）
例句 The reticulocyte count is often measured to assess bone marrow function. 网织红细胞计数常用于评估骨髓功能。

reticulonodular 网状结节的

词根 reticulo-（网状的）+ nodular（结节的）
例句 Reticulonodular changes in the chest X-ray may indicate inter-

stitial lung disease. 胸部 X 线中的网状结节变化可能表明间质性肺病。

retro-（后面）

retroperitoneal 腹膜后

词根 retro-（后面）+ peritoneal（腹膜的）
例句 Retroperitoneal tumors are located behind the peritoneum, the membrane that lines the abdominal cavity. 腹膜后肿瘤位于腹膜后，即腹腔的衬里。

retroactive 追溯的

词根 retro-（后面）+ active（活跃的）
例句 Retroactive treatments may be applied when previous interventions have failed. 当之前的治疗未能奏效时，可能会采取追溯性治疗。

R

retrograde 逆行的

词根 retro-（后面）+ grade（步伐；程度）
例句 Retrograde amnesia occurs when a person loses memory of events before a brain injury. 逆行性健忘发生在大脑受伤后，患者失去对伤前事件的记忆。

retrospective 回顾的

词根 retro-（后面）+ spect（看）+ -ive（形容词后缀）
例句 A retrospective study of cancer patients helps to evaluate long-term outcomes. 对癌症患者进行回顾性研究有助于评估长期结果。

retrosternal 胸骨后的

词根 retro-（后面）+ sternal（胸骨的）
例句 Retrosternal pain is a common symptom of heartburn or gast-

roesophageal reflux disease. 胸骨后疼痛是胃灼热或胃食管反流病的常见症状。

retropharyngeal 咽后

词根 retro-（后面）+ pharyngeal（咽的）

例句 A retropharyngeal abscess can cause difficulty swallowing and breathing. 咽后脓肿可能导致吞咽和呼吸困难。

retrovirus 逆转录病毒

词根 retro-（后面）+ virus（病毒）

例句 HIV is a retrovirus that integrates its RNA into the host's DNA. HIV 是一种逆转录病毒，它将其 RNA 整合到宿主的 DNA 中。

retroflex 后弯的

词根 retro-（后面）+ flex（弯曲）

例句 A retroflexed uterus is a condition where the uterus tilts backward. 后弯子宫是指子宫向后倾斜的情况。

retroaction 反作用

词根 retro-（后面）+ action（作用）

例句 Retroaction in medicine refers to the effect of a treatment on past symptoms or conditions. 医学中的反作用是指治疗对过去症状或病情的影响。

retro-ocular 眼后部的

词根 retro-（后面）+ ocular（眼的）

例句 Retro-ocular pain can be caused by conditions such as glaucoma or optic neuritis. 眼后部疼痛可能由青光眼或视神经炎等疾病引起。

rhabo-（横纹肌）

rhabdomyolysis 横纹肌溶解

词根 rhabo-（横纹肌）+ -myolysis（肌溶解）
例句 Rhabdomyolysis occurs when muscle tissue breaks down, releasing toxins into the bloodstream. 横纹肌溶解发生在肌肉组织破裂时，毒素释放到血液中。

rhabdomyoma 横纹肌瘤

词根 rhabo-（横纹肌）+ -oma（肿瘤）
例句 A rhabdomyoma is a benign tumor that arises from skeletal muscle tissue. 横纹肌瘤是一种来源于骨骼肌组织的良性肿瘤。

rhabdomyosarcoma 横纹肌肉瘤

词根 rhabo-（横纹肌）+ myo-（肌肉）+ -sarcoma（肉瘤）
例句 Rhabdomyosarcoma is a type of cancer that starts in the skeletal muscle tissue. 横纹肌肉瘤是一种起源于骨骼肌组织的癌症。

rhabdomuscular 横纹肌的

词根 rhabo-（横纹肌）+ muscular（肌肉的）
例句 Rhabdomuscular disorders can lead to muscle weakness and pain. 横纹肌相关疾病可能导致肌肉无力和疼痛。

rhabdotoxin 横纹肌毒素

词根 rhabo-（横纹肌）+ -toxin（毒素）
例句 Rhabdotoxin is a type of toxin that targets skeletal muscle cells. 横纹肌毒素是一种针对骨骼肌细胞的毒素。

rhabdomyopathy 横纹肌病

词根 rhabo-（横纹肌）+ -pathy（病）

例句 Rhabdomyopathy refers to diseases that affect the skeletal muscles, often leading to muscle weakness. 横纹肌病指的是影响骨骼肌的疾病，常导致肌肉无力。

rhabdomotor 横纹肌运动的

词根 rhabo-（横纹肌）+ -motor（运动的）

例句 The rhabdomotor pathway is responsible for controlling voluntary muscle movements. 横纹肌运动通路负责控制随意肌的运动。

rhabdomorphous 具有横纹肌形态的

词根 rhabo-（横纹肌）+ -morphous（形态的）

例句 Rhabdomorphous cells are found in muscle tissue and have a striated appearance. 横纹肌形态的细胞存在于肌肉组织中，具有条纹状外观。

rhabdomastopathy 横纹肌病

词根 rhabo-（横纹肌）+ -pathy（病）

例句 Rhabdomastopathy can cause significant pain and stiffness in affected muscles. 横纹肌病会导致受影响肌肉的剧烈疼痛和僵硬。

rhabdomyelopathy 横纹肌脊髓病

词根 rhabo-（横纹肌）+ myelo-（脊髓）+ -pathy（病）

例句 Rhabdomyelopathy is a rare condition that involves both muscle and spinal cord dysfunction. 横纹肌脊髓病是一种罕见的疾病，涉及肌肉和脊髓功能障碍。

USMLE Step 3　样题

A 63-year-old man is brought to the emergency department by his wife because of a 2-day history of double vision, feeling off-balance, difficulty walking, and leaning to his right side while standing. He also has had sore throat, hoarseness, difficulty swallowing and talking, and fatigue during this time. He had severe stabbing pain on the right side of his face a few minutes before his other symptoms began. The severity of his symptoms has been constant since onset. The patient is right-hand dominant but he has had difficulty accurately using his right arm during this time. When he tries to eat, his right forearm (fore-) and hand do not accurately guide food to his mouth. He has not had a fever. He has hypertension (hyper-; -tension) treated with lisinopril (-pril). Temperature is 37.2°C (99.0°F), pulse is 75/min, respirations (re-; spir-; -ation) are 16/min, and blood pressure is 148/98 mmHg. Oxygen saturation is 98% on room air. On examination, the patient leans to the right while seated. The left pupil measures 6 mm and constricts to 4 mm in response to light; the right pupil measures 4 mm and constricts to 3 mm in response to light. There is no conjunctival icterus. There is horizontal and rotational nystagmus on right gaze. The fast phase of nystagmus is to the left. There is mild right ptosis. The patient can hear finger rubs and whispers bilaterally (bi-; -lateral). The right soft palate does not elevate with phonation (phon-; -ation); the patient's voice is hoarse, and he has dysarthric (dys-; arthr-) speech. Peripheral pulses are 2+ throughout. Muscle strength, bulk, and tone are normal in all extremities. Deep tendon reflexes are 1+ throughout. Babinski sign is absent (a-) bilaterally. Sensation to pain and temperature is decreased over the right side of the face, the left extremities, and the left side of the trunk. Finger-nose testing shows dysmetria (dys-; metr-) on the right only. Gait is broad based, and the patient leans to the right while walking. Based on these findings, this patient is most likely to develop which of the following?

(A) Achalasia (a-; -chalasia) and gastroparesis (gatro-; -paresis)

(B) Angle-closure glaucoma (glauc-; -oma)

(C) Orthostatic (ortho-; stat-) hypertension (hyper-; stat-)

(D) Sleep-related hypoventilation (hypo-; vent-)

(E) Third-degree atrioventricular (atrio-; ventricul-) block

中文翻译

一名 63 岁男性，因持续 2 天出现复视、平衡感丧失、行走困难、站立时向右侧倾斜，被妻子送至急诊科。他同期还出现咽喉痛、声音嘶哑、吞咽和说话困难以及疲劳。症状开始前几分钟，他右侧面部有剧烈的刺痛感。症状自发作以来严重程度未变。患者惯用右手，但在此期间使用右臂时准确性下降。尝试进食时，右前臂和手无法准确将食物送入口中。他未出现发热。他有高血压，服用赖诺普利治疗。体温 37.2℃（99.0℉），脉搏 75 次 / 分钟，呼吸 16 次 / 分钟，血压 148/98 mmHg。室温空气下的氧饱和度为 98%。检查时，患者坐位时向右侧倾斜。左瞳孔直径 6 mm，对光反应收缩至 4 mm；右瞳孔直径 4 mm，对光反应收缩至 3 mm。无结膜黄疸。向右凝视时出现水平和旋转性眼震，眼震快相向左。右侧有轻度眼睑下垂。患者双耳可听到手指摩擦和低语声。发声时右侧软腭未抬高；患者声音嘶哑，伴构音障碍。全身外周脉搏为 2+。四肢肌肉力量、体积和张力正常。深腱反射全身为 1+。双侧巴宾斯基征阴性。右侧面部、左侧肢体和左侧躯干的痛觉和温度觉减退。指鼻试验显示仅右侧有共济失调。步态基底宽，行走时向右侧倾斜。根据临床表现，该患者最可能发展为以下哪种情况？

R

(A) 食管弛缓症和胃轻瘫

(B) 闭角型青光眼

(C) 体位性高血压

(D) 睡眠相关低通气

(E) 三度房室传导阻滞

题目和答案中出现的词根

fore-：在……之前

hyper-：高

-tension：张力；压力

-pril：普利（血管紧张素转换酶抑制剂的通用后缀）

re-：重新；反复

spir：呼吸

-atio 表示动作的状态（重复呼吸的状态指代呼吸这个动作）

bi-：双

-lateral：侧

phon-：音

-ation：表示动作（表示音的动作即为发音）

dys-：困难的

arthr-：关节（这里代指发音，即产生发音的关节和肌肉的协同运动）

a-：表示否定

metr-：测量（测量困难指代测具不准的症状）

-chalasia：松弛

gastro-：胃

-paresis：瘫痪

glau-：蓝灰色

-oma：瘤（蓝灰色肿瘤指的是青光眼，即眼内压增高导致角膜水肿看起来像角膜肿瘤，角膜水肿导致其看起来为蓝灰色）

ortho-：正

stat-：静止

hypo-：低

vent-：通气

atrio-：心房

ventricul-：心室

rhino-（鼻）

rhinoplasty 鼻整形术

词根 rhino-（鼻）+ -plasty（塑形）

例句 Rhinoplasty is a surgical procedure performed to change the shape of the nose. 鼻整形术是一种用于改变鼻子形状的手术。

rhinitis 鼻炎

词根 rhino-（鼻）+ -itis（炎症）

例句 Rhinitis is an inflammation of the nasal mucous membranes, often caused by allergies. 鼻炎是鼻腔黏膜的炎症，通常由过敏引起。

rhinovirus 鼻病毒

词根 rhino-（鼻）+ virus（病毒）

例句 Rhinovirus is a common cause of the common cold. 鼻病毒是感冒的常见病因。

rhinorrhea 鼻溢

词根 rhino-（鼻）+ -rrhea（流出）

例句 Rhinorrhea refers to the discharge of mucus from the nose, commonly seen during colds. 鼻溢是指鼻涕从鼻腔流出，常见于感冒期间。

rhinoscopy 鼻镜检查

词根 rhino-（鼻）+ -scopy（检查）
例句 Rhinoscopy is a diagnostic procedure to examine the inside of the nasal passages. 鼻镜检查是一种用于检查鼻腔内部的诊断程序。

rhinolith 鼻石

词根 rhino-（鼻）+ -lith（石）
例句 A rhinolith is a calcified mass that forms in the nasal cavity, often due to chronic sinusitis. 鼻石是形成在鼻腔内的钙化物，通常由慢性鼻窦炎引起。

rhinocerebral 鼻脑的

词根 rhino-（鼻）+ cerebr-（脑）
例句 Rhinocerebral mucormycosis is a rare fungal infection that affects the nose and brain. 鼻脑型黑曲霉病是一种罕见的真菌感染，影响鼻腔和大脑。

rhinomanometry 鼻腔压力测定

词根 rhino-（鼻）+ -manometry（压力测定）
例句 Rhinomanometry is a test used to measure airflow through the nasal passages and determine obstruction. 鼻腔压力测定是一种用于测量空气通过鼻腔的流量并判断是否有阻塞的测试。

rhinopharyngitis 鼻咽炎

词根 rhino-（鼻）+ pharyng-（咽）+ -itis（炎症）
例句 Rhinopharyngitis is the inflammation of both the nose and the throat, often caused by viral infections. 鼻咽炎是鼻子和咽部的炎症，通常由病毒感染引起。

rhinocondyloma 鼻部赘生物

词根 rhino-（鼻）+ condyl-（赘生物）+ -oma（肿瘤）

例句 Rhinocondyloma is a benign growth that can form on the nasal mucosa. 鼻部赘生物是一种可以在鼻腔黏膜上形成的良性肿瘤。

rhythm-（节律）

arrhythmia 心律不齐

词根 a-（无）+ rhythm-（节律）+ -ia（疾病）

例句 Arrhythmia is a condition where the heart beats irregularly, too fast, or too slow. 心律不齐是心脏跳动不规律、过快或过慢的病症。

dysrhythmia 节律障碍

词根 dys-（异常）+ rhythm-（节律）+ -ia（疾病）

例句 Dysrhythmia refers to abnormal electrical activity in the heart that causes irregular heartbeats. 节律障碍是指心脏内异常的电活动，导致心跳不规律。

sinus rhythm 窦性节律

词根 sinus-（窦）+ rhythm-（节律）

例句 Sinus rhythm is the normal rhythm of the heart, originating from the sinoatrial node. 窦性节律是心脏的正常节律，起源于窦房结。

circadian rhythm 昼夜节律

词根 circa-（大约）+ dian-（天）+ rhythm-（节律）

例句 Circadian rhythm refers to the body's internal clock that regulates sleep and wake cycles. 昼夜节律指的是调节睡眠和觉醒周期的身体内在时钟。

tachyarrhythmia 快速心律不齐

词根 tachy-（快速）+ rhythm-（节律）

例句 Tachyarrhythmia is a type of arrhythmia where the heart rate is abnormally fast. 快速心律不齐是一种心律不齐，心跳异常加速。

bradyarrhythmia 慢性心律不齐

词根 brady-（缓慢）+ rhythm-（节律）

例句 Bradyarrhythmia occurs when the heart rate is abnormally slow. 慢性心律不齐发生在心跳异常缓慢时。

rhythmicity 节奏性

词根 rhythm-（节律）+ -icity（性质）

例句 The rhythmicity of heartbeats is controlled by the sinoatrial node. 心跳的节奏性由窦房结控制。

rhythmos 节奏

词根 rhythm-（节律）+ -os（名词后缀）

例句 In physiology, rhythm refers to the regular pattern of biological functions, like the heartbeat. 在生理学中，节奏指的是生物功能的规律性模式，如心跳。

heart rhythm 心脏节律

词根 heart-（心脏）+ rhythm-（节律）

例句 Heart rhythm disorders can be detected by electrocardiogram（ECG）testing. 心脏节律障碍可以通过心电图（ECG）检测出来。

neurocardiac rhythm 神经心脏节律

词根 neuro-（神经）+ cardiac（心脏的）+ rhythm-（节律）

例句 Neurocardiac rhythm refers to the interaction between the nervous system and the heart's rhythm. 神经心脏节律指的是神经系统与心脏节律之间的相互作用。

ribo-（核糖）

ribonucleic acid 核糖核酸

词根 ribo-（核糖）+ nucleic（核的）

例句 Ribonucleic acid（RNA）plays a crucial role in protein synthesis and gene expression. 核糖核酸（RNA）在蛋白质合成和基因表达中发挥重要作用。

ribosome 核糖体

词根 ribo-（核糖）+ some（体）

例句 The ribosome is the site of protein synthesis in the cell. 核糖体是细胞内蛋白质合成的场所。

ribozymes 核糖酶

词根 ribo-（核糖）+ -zyme（酶）

例句 Ribozymes are RNA molecules that act as enzymes to catalyze chemical reactions. 核糖酶是充当酶的 RNA 分子，能够催化化学反应。

ribonucleoprotein 核糖核蛋白

词根 ribo-（核糖）+ nucleoprotein（核蛋白）

例句 Ribonucleoproteins are complex molecules consisting of RNA and proteins, involved in cellular processes. 核糖核蛋白是由 RNA 和蛋白质组成的复合分子，参与细胞过程。

ribonuclease 核糖核酸酶

词根 ribo-（核糖）+ nuclease（酶）

例句 Ribonuclease is an enzyme that breaks down RNA molecules. 核糖核酸酶是一种分解 RNA 分子的酶。

ribonucleotide 核糖核苷酸

词根 ribo-（核糖）+ nucleotide（核苷酸）

例句 Ribonucleotides are the building blocks of RNA. 核糖核苷酸是 RNA 的基本组成单位。

ribosylation 核糖基化

词根 ribo-（核糖）+ -ylation（化学基团加成）

例句 Ribosylation is a process where a ribose sugar is added to a molecule, altering its function. 核糖基化是将核糖添加到分子中的过程，从而改变其功能。

ribose 核糖

词根 ribo-（核糖）

例句 Ribose is a sugar molecule that is a key component of RNA. 核糖是一种糖分子，是 RNA 的关键组成部分。

ribosomal RNA 核糖体 RNA

词根 ribo-（核糖）+ somal（体的）+ RNA（核糖核酸）

例句 Ribosomal RNA（rRNA）is an essential component of ribosomes, helping in protein synthesis. 核糖体 RNA（rRNA）是核糖体的重要组成部分，帮助蛋白质合成。

ribosome biogenesis 核糖体生物发生

词根 ribo-（核糖）+ some（体）+ biogenesis（生物发生）

例句 Ribosome biogenesis is the process by which cells produce ribosomes from RNA and proteins. 核糖体生物合成是细胞通过 RNA 和蛋白质合成核糖体的过程。

-rrhaphy（修补）

herniorrhaphy 疝修补术

词根 hernio-（疝）+ -rrhaphy（修补术）

例句 Herniorrhaphy is a surgical procedure to repair a hernia. 疝修补术是一种用于修复疝气的外科手术。

neurorrhaphy 神经缝合术

词根 neuro-（神经）+ -rrhaphy（修补术）

例句 Neurorrhaphy is performed to repair a severed nerve. 神经缝合术用于修复断裂的神经。

tenorrhaphy 腱缝合术

词根 teno-（腱）+ -rrhaphy（修补术）

例句 Tenorrhaphy is a surgical procedure used to suture a torn tendon. 腱缝合术是一种用于缝合撕裂腱的外科手术。

perineorrhaphy 会阴缝合术

词根 perineo-（会阴）+ -rrhaphy（修补术）

例句 Perineorrhaphy is a surgical repair of the perineum, often after childbirth. 会阴缝合术是一种用于修复会阴的手术，通常用于分娩后。

colporrhaphy 阴道缝合术

词根 colpo-（阴道）+ -rrhaphy（修补术）

例句 Colporrhaphy is a procedure to repair the vaginal wall. 阴道缝合术是一种用于修复阴道壁的手术。

myorrhaphy 肌肉缝合术

词根 myo-（肌肉）+ -rrhaphy（修补术）

例句 Myorrhaphy is the surgical suturing of a muscle wound. 肌肉缝合术是对肌肉伤口进行外科缝合的手术。

cystorrhaphy 膀胱缝合术

词根 cysto-（膀胱）+ -rrhaphy（修补术）

例句 Cystorrhaphy is performed to repair a tear in the bladder. 膀胱缝合术用于修补膀胱的破裂。

hysterorrhaphy 子宫缝合术

词根 hystero-（子宫）+ -rrhaphy（修补术）

例句 Hysterorrhaphy is a surgical procedure to repair a torn uterus. 子宫缝合术是一种用于修复子宫撕裂的手术。

gastrorrhaphy 胃缝合术

词根 gastro-（胃）+ -rrhaphy（修补术）

例句 Gastrorrhaphy is a surgical repair of a perforated stomach. 胃缝合术是一种修复胃穿孔的外科手术。

angiorrhaphy 血管缝合术

词根 angio-（血管）+ -rrhaphy（修补术）

例句 Angiorrhaphy is used to suture a damaged blood vessel. 血管缝合术用于缝合破损的血管

USMLE Step 3 样题

A 21-year-old man, who is a member of the US Air Force, comes to the emergency department because of a 2-day history of shortness of breath on exertion and when lying down, as well as fever, chills, and swelling of his legs. Medical history is unremarkable (un-) and he takes no medications. Temperature is 38.1°C (100.5°F), pulse is 97/min, respirations (re-; spir-; -ation) are 20/min, and blood pressure is 140/91 mmHg. Oxygen saturation is 92% on room air. The patient is dyspneic (dys-; -pneic) but able to speak in full sentences. Jugular venous pressure is 14 mmHg. Auscultation (auscult-; -ation) of the lungs discloses bilateral (bi-; -lateral) basilar (basil-) crackles. Cardiac examination discloses a regular rhythm with an S3 gallop but no murmur. Abdominal examination discloses no abnormalities. There is 1+ pitting edema of the lower extremities. Results of laboratory studies show a serum B-type natriuretic (natri-; uret-) peptide concentration of 2,000 pg/mL (N<100) and a leukocyte (leuk-; -cyte) count of 13,000/mm^3. Results of serum chemistry profile and remainder of complete blood count are within the reference ranges. ECG shows no abnormalities except for nonspecific (non-) STsegment changes. Echocardiography (echo-; cardi-; -graphy) shows a dilated left ventricle with an ejection (e-; ject-) fraction of 0.40 and no pericardial (peri-; cardi-) effusion (ef-; fus-). Which of the following is the most likely long-term outcome for this patient?

(A) Complete recovery

(B) Mild diastolic (diasto-) dysfunction (dys-)

(C) Pulmonary (pulmon-) embolism (embol-)

(D) Recurrent (re-; curr-) pericarditis (peri-; cardi-; -itis)

(E) Severe systolic (systo-) heart failure requiring cardiac transplant (trans-)

中文翻译

一名 21 岁男性，美国空军成员，因 2 天来运动时和躺下时呼吸困难，以及发热、寒战和双腿肿胀来到急诊科。无病史特殊，未服用任何药物。体温 38.1℃（100.5℉），脉搏 97 次 / 分钟，呼吸 20 次 / 分钟，血压 140/91mmHg。室温空气下的氧饱和度为 92%。患者呼吸困难，但能说完整的句子。颈静脉压为 14 mmHg。肺部听诊显示双侧肺底部湿啰音。心脏检查显示节律规则，伴有 S3 奔马律，但无杂音。腹部检查未发现异常。下肢有 1+ 凹陷性水肿。实验室检查结果显示血清 B 型钠尿肽浓度为 2,000 pg/mL（正常值 <100），白细胞计数为 13,000/mm^3。

血清生化检查和全血细胞计数的其余结果在参考范围内。心电图除非特异性 ST 段改变外无异常。心脏超声显示左心室扩张，射血分数为 0.40，无心包积液。以下哪项是该患者最可能的长期预后结果？

(A) 完全恢复
(B) 轻度舒张功能障碍
(C) 肺栓塞
(D) 复发性心包炎
(E) 严重收缩性心力衰竭需心脏移植

题目和答案中出现的词根

un-：表示否定
re-：重新；反复
spir：呼吸
-ation 表示动作的状态（重复呼吸的状态指代呼吸这个动作）
dys-：困难的
-pneic：呼吸（pnea 的形容词形式）
auscult-：听
-ation：表示动作（表示听的动作就是听诊）
basil-：底
natri-：钠
uret-：尿
leuk-：白色
-cyte：细胞
non-：表示否定
echo-：回声

cardi-：心脏

-graphy：影像

e-：向外

ject-：流（向外流指代喷射）

peri-：外周

cardi-：心脏（心脏周围即为心包）

ef-：向外

fus-：倾泻（向外倾斜，即外溢）

diasto-：舒张的

pulmon-：肺的（指的是解剖意义上的肺）

embol-：栓子的（通常是形成后随血液流动堵在另一个血管位置，而血栓形成是局部形成堵在形成的部位）

curr-：跑

peri-：外周

cardi-：心脏 （心脏周围指的是心包）

-itis：炎症

systo-：收缩

trans-：转；跨

-rrhea（流出）

diarrhea 腹泻

词根 dia-（通过）+ -rrhea（流出）

例句 Diarrhea is characterized by frequent, watery bowel movements. 腹泻的特点是频繁的水样大便。

gonorrhea 淋病

词根 gon-（性腺的）+ -rrhea（流出）

例句 Gonorrhea is a sexually transmitted disease that can cause discharge from the genital tract. 淋病是一种性传播疾病，可引起生殖道分泌物。

leukorrhea 白带

词根 leuko-（白色）+ -rrhea（流出）
例句 Leukorrhea refers to a whitish or yellowish vaginal discharge that is common in women. 白带指的是女性常见的白色或黄色阴道分泌物。

menorrhea 月经

词根 meno-（月经）+ -rrhea（流出）
例句 Menorrhea refers to the normal monthly flow of blood during a woman's menstrual cycle. 月经指的是女性每月的正常经血流动。

pyorrhea 脓漏

词根 py-（脓）+ -rrhea（流出）
例句 Pyorrhea is a condition where pus drains from the gums due to infection. 脓漏是由于感染导致牙龈流脓的病症。

orrhea 漏出

词根 or-（口）+ -rrhea（流出）
例句 Orrhea is a term used for the leaking or flowing of fluids, especially from the mouth. 漏出是指体液从口腔等地方泄漏或流出的现象。

phlegmorrhea 痰流

词根 phlegm-（痰）+ -rrhea（流出）
例句 Phlegmorrhea refers to the excessive flow of mucus or phlegm from the respiratory tract. 痰流指的是呼吸道分泌过多黏液或脓痰的病症。

rhinorrhea 鼻漏

词根 rhino-（鼻）+ -rrhea（流出）

例句 Rhinorrhea is the condition where mucus is discharged from the nose. 鼻漏是指从鼻腔分泌出黏液的症状。

-rrhexis（破裂）

hysterorrhexis 子宫破裂

词根 hystero-（子宫）+ -rrhexis（破裂）

例句 Hysterorrhexis is a rare but life-threatening complication of pregnancy. 子宫破裂是妊娠中的一种罕见但危及生命的并发症。

myorrhexis 肌撕裂

词根 myo-（肌肉）+ -rrhexis（破裂）

例句 Myorrhexis occurs when muscle tissue tears, often due to excessive strain. 肌撕裂是指肌肉组织因过度用力而发生撕裂的状况。

angiorrhexis 血管破裂

词根 angio-（血管）+ -rrhexis（破裂）

例句 Angiorrhexis refers to the rupture of blood vessels, which can lead to internal bleeding. 血管破裂是指血管发生破裂的状况，可能导致内出血。

neurorrhexis 神经破裂

词根 neuro-（神经）+ -rrhexis（破裂）

例句 Neurorrhexis refers to the rupture or tear of a nerve, often resulting in loss of function. 神经破裂指的是神经的破裂或撕裂，通常导致功能丧失。

splenorrhexis 脾破裂

词根 spleno-（脾）+ -rrhexis（破裂）

例句 Splenorrhexis is a medical emergency that occurs when the spleen ruptures. 脾破裂是一种急症，发生在脾脏破裂时。

cardiorrhexis 心脏破裂

词根 cardio-（心脏）+ -rrhexis（破裂）

例句 Cardiorrhexis can result from severe trauma and is typically fatal. 心脏破裂可能由严重创伤引起，通常是致命的。

osteorrhexis 骨破裂

词根 osteo-（骨）+ -rrhexis（破裂）

例句 Osteorrhexis refers to the fracture or rupture of a bone. 骨破裂指的是骨骼的骨折或破裂。

pulmorrhexis 肺破裂

词根 pulmo-（肺）+ -rrhexis（破裂）

例句 Pulmorrhexis refers to the rupture of lung tissue, which may result in a pneumothorax. 肺破裂指的是肺组织的破裂，可能导致气胸。

hepatorrhexis 肝脏破裂

词根 hepato-（肝脏）+ -rrhexis（破裂）

例句 Hepatorrhexis can occur as a result of trauma to the abdomen, leading to bleeding. 肝脏破裂可能由腹部创伤引起，导致出血。

ureterorrhexis 输尿管破裂

词根 uretero-（输尿管）+ -rrhexis（破裂）

例句 Ureterorrhexis is a condition where the ureter ruptures, often due to obstruction or injury. 输尿管破裂是一种病症，通常由阻塞或损伤引起。

rubro-（红色的）

rubrospinal 红核脊髓的

词根 rubro-（红色）+ spinal（脊髓的）

例句 The rubrospinal tract is involved in motor control and coordination of voluntary movements. 红核脊髓束参与运动控制和自愿运动的协调。

rubric 红色的；正式的

词根 rubro-（红色）+ -ic（形容词后缀）
例句 In medical terminology, a rubric is a heading or category for a group of related terms. 在医学术语中，“rubric”是指一组相关术语的标题或类别。

rubrocellular 红核细胞的

词根 rubro-（红色）+ cellular（细胞的）
例句 Rubrocellular neurons are located in the red nucleus and are involved in motor function. 红核细胞神经元位于红核，参与运动功能。

rubrospinal tract 红核脊髓束

词根 rubro-（红色）+ spinal（脊髓的）+ tract（束）
例句 The rubrospinal tract transmits motor signals from the red nucleus to the spinal cord. 红核脊髓束将运动信号从红核传递到脊髓。

rubral 红核的

词根 rubro-（红色）+ -al（形容词后缀）
例句 Rubral nuclei are clusters of neurons in the brainstem involved in movement control. 红核是位于脑干的神经元簇，参与运动控制。

rubrotectal 红核顶盖的

词根 rubro-（红色）+ tectal（顶盖的）
例句 The rubrotectal pathway plays a role in controlling eye movements and visual reflexes. 红核顶盖通路在控制眼动和视觉反射中起作用。

rubrophthalmic 红核眼的

词根 rubro-（红色）+ ophthalmic（眼的）

例句 Rubro-ophthalmic reflexes are related to visual processing in the brain. 红核眼反射与大脑中的视觉处理有关。

rubrization 红核化

词根 rubro-（红色）+ -ization（化）

例句 Rubrization refers to the process in which neurons in the red nucleus become activated. 红核化指的是红核中的神经元被激活的过程。

rubrodentate 红核齿状的

词根 rubro-（红色）+ dentate（齿状的）

例句 The rubrodentate pathway is involved in coordinating motor movements. 红核齿状通路参与协调运动。

rubromotor 红核运动的

词根 rubro-（红色）+ motor（运动的）

例句 The rubromotor system helps to transmit signals for voluntary muscle movement. 红核运动系统帮助传递自愿肌肉运动的信号。

LMCHK Part 1　样题

A 50-year-old woman complains of a tendency to fall when walking. When moving her upper limbs, her hands start to shake and holding a glass of water becomes a problem. When talking, she cannot produce fluent sentences. Her cognitive functions and memory are clear and unaffected (un-). Upon examination, she is found to have hypotonia (hypo-; -ton), pendular knee jerk, mild nystagmus and dysarthria (dys-; arthr-).

Which of the following areas is MOST LIKELY to be affected?

(A) Cerebellum

(B) Cerebral cortex

(C) Diencephalon (di-; encephal-)

(D) Limbic (limb-) system

(E) Substantia (sub-; stant-) nigra

中文翻译

一名 50 岁女性抱怨走路时容易跌倒。移动上肢时，双手开始颤抖，拿一杯水变得困难。说话时，她无法说出流畅的句子。她的认知功能和记忆清晰，未受影响。检查发现她有肌张力减低、膝跳反射呈钟摆样、轻度眼震和构音障碍等症状。

以下哪个区域最可能受到影响？

(A) 小脑

(B) 大脑皮层

(C) 间脑

(D) 边缘系统

(E) 黑质

题目和答案中出现的词根

un-：表示否定

hypo-：低

-ton：张力

dys-：困难的

arthr-：关节（这里代指发音，即产生发音的关节和肌肉的协同运动）

di-：双

encephal-：脑

limb-：四肢，代指边缘

sub-：在……下（在种类的下面指的是亚分类，即在一层分类的下级再分类

stant-：站立

R

salping-/-salpinx（输卵管）

salpingectomy 输卵管切除术

词根 salping-（输卵管）+ -ectomy（切除）

例句 Salpingectomy is a surgical procedure to remove one or both of a woman's fallopian tubes. 输卵管切除术是一种手术，用于切除一侧或双侧输卵管。

salpingitis 输卵管炎

词根 salping-（输卵管）+ -itis（炎症）

例句 Salpingitis is the inflammation of the fallopian tubes, often caused by bacterial infections. 输卵管炎是输卵管的炎症，通常由细菌感染引起。

salpingostomy 输卵管造口术

词根 salping-（输卵管）+ -ostomy（造口）

S

例句 Salpingostomy is a surgical procedure in which a new opening is created in the fallopian tube, often done in cases of ectopic pregnancy. 输卵管造口术是一种外科手术，通过在输卵管中创建一个新开口，常用于异位妊娠的治疗。

salpingoscope 输卵管镜

词根 salping-（输卵管）+ -scope（镜子）

例句 A salpingoscope is an instrument used to view the inside of the fallopian tubes. 输卵管镜是一种用于观察输卵管内部的仪器。

salpingography 输卵管造影术

词根 salping-（输卵管）+ -graphy（影像学）

例句 Salpingography is a diagnostic procedure that uses X-rays to examine the shape and structure of the fallopian tubes. 输卵管造影术是一种使用 X 射线检查输卵管形态和结构的诊断方法。

tubal ligation 输卵管结扎术

词根 salping-（输卵管）+ ligation（结扎）

例句 Tubal ligation is a surgical procedure that permanently closes a woman's fallopian tubes to prevent pregnancy. 输卵管结扎术是一种外科手术，通过永久性关闭女性输卵管来防止怀孕。

salpingectasia 输卵管扩张

词根 salping-（输卵管）+ -ectasia（扩张）

例句 Salpingectasia refers to the abnormal enlargement of the fallopian tube, which can lead to complications. 输卵管扩张是指输卵管的异常增大，可能导致并发症。

salpingectomy with hysterectomy 输卵管联合子宫切除术

词根 salping-（输卵管）+ -ectomy（切除）+ hyster-（子宫）

例句 Salpingectomy with hysterectomy is a surgical procedure where both the fallopian tubes and uterus are removed. 输卵管联合子宫切除术是同时切除输卵管和子宫的手术。

ectopic pregnancy with salpingectomy 异位妊娠伴输卵管切除术

词根 salping-（输卵管）+ -ectomy（切除）

例句 In cases of ectopic pregnancy, a salpingectomy may be performed to remove the embryo from the fallopian tube. 在异位妊娠的情况下，可能需要进行输卵管切除术来移除输卵管中的胚胎。

salpingoconization 输卵管锥形切除术

词根 salping-（输卵管）+ -conization（锥形切除）

例句 Salpingoconization is a surgical procedure that involves removing a portion of the fallopian tube. 输卵管锥形切除术是一种切除部分输卵管的手术。

hydrosalpinx 输卵管积水

词根 hydro-（水）+ salpinx（输卵管）

例句 Hydrosalpinx is a condition in which the fallopian tube is filled with fluid, often caused by infection or previous surgeries. 输卵管积水是指输卵管内充满液体，通常由感染或先前的手术引起。

pyosalpinx 脓性输卵管

词根 pyo-（脓）+ salpinx（输卵管）

例句 Pyosalpinx is a condition where the fallopian tube becomes infected and filled with pus, often due to pelvic inflammatory disease. 脓性输卵管是指输卵管被感染并充满脓液，通常由盆腔炎引起。

salpingitis isthmica nodosa 输卵管峡部结节性炎症

词根 salping-（输卵管）+ -itis（炎症）+ isthmica（峡部的）+ nodosa（结节）

例句 Salpingitis isthmica nodosa is a condition characterized by chronic inflammation and the formation of nodules in the isthmus of the fallopian tubes. 输卵管峡部结节性炎症是一种特征为慢性炎症和在输卵管峡部形成结节的疾病。

salpingophore 输卵管指

词根 salping-（输卵管）+ -phore（携带）

例句 Salpingophore refers to a small finger-like projection from the fallopian tube, often involved in the transport of the egg toward the uterus. 输卵管指是从输卵管伸出的一个小指状突起，通常参与将卵子运输到子宫。

sarco-（肉）

sarcoma 肉瘤

词根 sarco-（肉）+ -oma（肿瘤）

例句 Sarcoma is a type of cancer that arises from connective tissue, such as muscles or bones. 肉瘤是一种源自结缔组织（如肌肉或骨骼）的癌症。

sarcopenia 肌肉萎缩症

词根 sarco-（肉）+ -penia（缺乏）
例句 Sarcopenia is the loss of muscle mass and strength, often associated with aging. 肌肉萎缩症是指肌肉质量和力量的丧失，通常与衰老有关。

sarcosine 肌氨酸

词根 sarco-（肉）+ -ine（化学物质）
例句 Sarcosine is an amino acid derivative found in muscles and is involved in various metabolic processes. 肌氨酸是一种存在于肌肉中的氨基酸衍生物，参与各种代谢过程。

sarcoplasm 肌质

词根 sarco-（肉）+ -plasm（质）
例句 Sarcoplasm is the cytoplasm of muscle cells, where the contractile elements are found. 肌质是肌肉细胞的细胞质，其中包含了收缩元件。

sarcocyst 肉孢子囊

词根 sarco-（肉）+ -cyst（囊）
例句 Sarcocyst is a cyst formed in the muscles of certain animals by the parasite Sarcocystis. 肉孢子囊是由肉孢子虫在特定动物肌肉组织内形成的囊状结构。

sarcomere 肌节

词根 sarco-（肉）+ -mere（部分）
例句 A sarcomere is the basic unit of muscle contraction, found within muscle fibers. 肌节是肌肉收缩的基本单位，存在于肌纤维中。

sarcopenic obesity 肌肉减少性肥胖

词根 sarco-（肉）+ -penic（缺乏）+ obesity（肥胖）

例句 Sarcopenic obesity refers to the combination of muscle loss and increased fat accumulation, commonly seen in older adults. 肌肉减少性肥胖指的是肌肉量减少与脂肪堆积增加并存的一种状态，常见于老年人。

sarcomatous 肉瘤的

词根 sarco-（肉）+ -matous（具有……性质的）

例句 Sarcomatous tumors are characterized by rapid growth and the ability to invade surrounding tissues. 肉瘤性肿瘤的特点是快速生长并能侵入周围组织。

sarcomere shortening 肌节缩短

词根 sarco-（肉）+ -mere（部分）+ shortening（缩短）

例句 Sarcomere shortening occurs when the muscle contracts, reducing the length of the sarcomere and generating force. 肌节缩短发生于肌肉收缩时，表现为肌节长度减少并产生力量。

-schisis（分裂）

gastroschisis 腹壁裂

词根 gastro-（胃）+ -schisis（裂开）

例句 Gastroschisis is a birth defect where the baby's intestines are outside the body. 腹壁裂是一种先天性缺陷，表现为胎儿的肠道在体外。

neuroschisis 神经裂

词根 neuro-（神经）+ -schisis（裂开）

例句 Neuroschisis refers to a developmental defect in the neural tube where the spinal cord fails to close properly. 神经裂是神经管发育缺陷，导致脊髓未能正确闭合。

hernioschisis 疝裂

词根 hernio-（疝）+ -schisis（裂开）

例句 Hernioschisis occurs when part of an organ pushes through a tear or opening in the surrounding tissue. 疝裂是指器官的一部分通过周围组织的撕裂或开口突出。

coloschisis 结肠裂

词根 colo-（结肠）+ -schisis（裂开）

例句 Coloschisis is a rare condition where a gap or fissure appears in the colon. 结肠裂是一种罕见病，指结肠中出现裂缝或裂隙。

lipomatoschisis 脂肪瘤裂

词根 lipo-（脂肪）+ -schisis（裂开）

例句 Lipomatoschisis refers to the splitting of a lipoma, which is a benign tumor made of fat tissue. 脂肪瘤裂指的是脂肪瘤的分裂，脂肪瘤是由脂肪组织组成的良性肿瘤。

osteoschisis 骨裂

词根 osteo-（骨）+ -schisis（裂开）

例句 Osteoschisis is a condition where there is a crack or split in the bone. 骨裂是指骨骼中出现裂缝或断裂。

rhachischisis 脊柱裂

词根 rhachi-（脊柱）+ -schisis（裂开）

例句 Rhachischisis refers to a severe form of spina bifida, where the spinal column fails to close completely. 脊柱裂是脊髓裂的一种严重形式，脊柱未能完全闭合。

splenomesoschisis 脾脏裂

词根 spleno-（脾脏）+ meso-（中间）+ -schisis（裂开）

例句 Splenomesoschisis is a rare anomaly where the spleen splits into two sections due to a mesenteric defect. 脾脏裂是一种罕见畸形，脾脏由于肠系膜缺陷而分裂成两部分。

vasoschisis 血管裂

词根 vaso-（血管）+ -schisis（裂开）

例句 Vasoschisis occurs when there is a rupture or opening in a blood vessel. 血管裂是指血管出现破裂或开口。

craniocerebral schisis 颅脑分裂

词根 cranio-（颅骨）+ cerebr-（大脑）+ -schisis（分裂）

例句 Craniocerebral schisis is a rare condition characterized by the abnormal splitting of the brain and skull. 颅脑分裂是一种罕见的病症，特征是大脑和颅骨的异常分裂。

schisto-（裂）

schistosomiasis 血吸虫病

词根 schisto-（裂）+ -somiasis（感染）

例句 Schistosomiasis is a parasitic disease caused by schistosome worms, leading to tissue damage and fibrosis. 血吸虫病是由血吸虫引起的寄生虫病，导致组织损伤和纤维化。

schistosome 血吸虫

词根 schisto-（裂）+ -some（体）

例句 Schistosomes are parasitic worms that cause schistosomiasis, infecting the urinary or intestinal tract. 血吸虫是引起血吸虫病的寄生虫，主要感染尿道或肠道。

schistocytosis 裂细胞症

词根 schisto-（裂）+ cytosis（细胞）

例句 Schistocytosis refers to the presence of fragmented red blood cells in the blood, often seen in conditions like hemolytic anemia. 裂细胞症是指血液中出现碎裂的红细胞，常见于溶血性贫血等疾病。

schistosomal hepatitis 血吸虫性肝炎

词根 schisto-（裂）+ -somal（与体相关）+ hepatitis（肝炎）

例句 Schistosomal hepatitis is liver inflammation caused by infection with schistosome worms, typically seen in endemic areas. 血吸虫性肝炎是由血吸虫感染引起的肝脏炎症，常见于流行地区。

schistosome dermatitis 血吸虫性皮炎

词根 schisto-（裂）+ -some（体）+ dermatitis（皮炎）

例句 Schistosome dermatitis occurs when the skin reacts to the presence of schistosome larvae, resulting in a rash. 血吸虫性皮炎是当皮肤对血吸虫幼虫的存在产生反应时，导致皮疹。

schistosomiasis japonica 日本血吸虫病

词根 schisto-（裂）+ -somiasis（感染）+ japonica（日本的）

例句 Schistosomiasis japonica is a type of schistosomiasis caused by the Schistosoma japonicum parasite, found mainly in East Asia. 日本血吸虫病是一种由日本血吸虫引起的血吸虫病，主要分布在东亚。

schistosomiasis mansoni 曼氏血吸虫病

词根 schisto-（裂）+ -somiasis（感染）+ mansoni（曼氏的）

例句 Schistosomiasis mansoni is caused by the Schistosoma mansoni parasite and is endemic in parts of Africa, the Middle East, and South America. 曼氏血吸虫病是由曼氏血吸虫引起的，主要流行于非洲、中东和南美的部分地区。

schistosome larvae 血吸虫幼虫

词根 schisto-（裂）+ -some（体）+ larvae（幼虫）

例句 Schistosome larvae are released into the water, where they can penetrate the skin of humans who come into contact with contaminated water. 血吸虫幼虫被释放到水中，当人类接触受污染的水体时，这些幼虫可穿透皮肤侵入人体。

schistosomiasis control 血吸虫病防控

词根 schisto-（裂）+ -somiasis（感染）+ control（控制）

例句 Schistosomiasis control involves strategies such as treatment with anti-parasitic drugs and improving sanitation to reduce the spread of the disease. 血吸虫病防控策略包括使用抗寄生虫药物治疗感染者，并通过改善卫生条件以减少疾病传播途径。

schistosomiasis treatment 血吸虫病治疗

词根 schisto-（裂）+ -somiasis（感染）+ treatment（治疗）

例句 Schistosomiasis treatment usually involves the use of praziquantel, a drug that effectively targets the parasites. 血吸虫病治疗通常使用吡喹酮，这是一种有效针对寄生虫的药物。

scler-（硬化的）

sclerosis 硬化症

词根 scler-（硬）+ -osis（病理状态）

例句 Sclerosis is the abnormal hardening of tissues, often associated with chronic diseases such as multiple sclerosis. 硬化症是指组织异常硬化，通常与慢性疾病如多发性硬化症相关。

scleroderma 硬皮病

词根 scler-（硬）+ -derma（皮肤）

例句 Scleroderma is a group of autoimmune diseases that cause skin and connective tissues to become thick and hard. 硬皮病是一组自身免疫性疾病，导致皮肤和结缔组织变厚和变硬。

atherosclerosis 动脉硬化

词根 ather-（脂肪）+ scler-（硬）+ -osis（病理状态）

例句 Atherosclerosis is the buildup of fatty deposits inside the arteries, leading to hardening and narrowing of the blood vessels. 动脉硬化是脂肪沉积在动脉内，导致血管硬化和变窄的过程。

arteriosclerosis 动脉硬化症

词根 arteri-（动脉）+ scler-（硬）+ -osis（病理状态）

例句 Arteriosclerosis is a condition where the arteries become thickened and stiff, restricting blood flow. 动脉硬化症是一种动脉变厚和变硬的病症，限制了血流。

myosclerosis 肌肉硬化

词根 myo-（肌肉）+ scler-（硬）+ -osis（病理状态）

例句 Myosclerosis refers to the hardening of muscle tissue, which can occur in certain autoimmune diseases. 肌肉硬化是指肌肉组织的硬化，可能发生在某些自身免疫性疾病中。

osteosclerosis 骨硬化

词根 oste-（骨）+ scler-（硬）+ -osis（病理状态）

例句 Osteosclerosis is the abnormal hardening or thickening of bone tissue, often seen in diseases such as osteopetrosis. 骨硬化是骨组织的异常硬化或增厚，常见于如骨质增生症等疾病中。

scleredema 硬皮水肿

词根 scler-（硬）+ -edema（水肿）

例句 Scleredema is a condition characterized by swelling and hardening of the skin, often associated with systemic diseases. 硬皮水肿是一种皮肤肿胀和硬化的病症，通常与全身性疾病有关。

neurodegenerative sclerosis 神经退行性硬化症

词根 neuro-（神经）+ degener-（退行性）+ scler-（硬）+ -osis（病理状态）

例句 Neurodegenerative sclerosis is a condition where nerve cells progressively degenerate and harden, leading to loss of function. 神经退行性硬化症是一种神经细胞逐渐退化和硬化的病症，最终导致功能丧失。

sclerosing cholangitis 硬化性胆管炎

词根 scler-（硬）+ -osing（形容词后缀）+ cholangi-（胆管）+ -itis（炎症）

例句 Sclerosing cholangitis is a chronic liver disease where the bile ducts become inflamed and scarred, leading to liver damage. 硬化性胆管炎是一种慢性肝脏疾病，胆管发炎并疤痕化，导致肝脏损伤。

pulmonary sclerosing 肺硬化

词根 pulmon-（肺）+ scler-（硬）+ -osing（形容词后缀）

例句 Pulmonary sclerosing refers to the hardening of lung tissue, often observed in chronic lung diseases like pulmonary fibrosis. 肺硬化指的是肺组织的硬化，通常见于如肺纤维化等慢性肺部疾病。

scleroedema 硬皮水肿

词根 scler-（硬）+ -edema（水肿）

例句 Scleroedema causes the skin to become thick and hard, often due to systemic conditions. 硬皮水肿导致皮肤增厚和硬化，通常由全身性疾病引起。

sclerosteosis 硬化性骨病

词根 scler-（硬）+ osteo-（骨）+ -osis（病理状态）

例句 Sclerosteosis is a genetic condition that causes abnormal bone growth and hardening. 硬化性骨病是一种遗传性疾病，导致骨骼的异常生长和硬化。

sclerotic plaque 硬化斑块

词根 scler-（硬）+ -otic（形容词后缀）+ plaque（斑块）

例句 Sclerotic plaques are hard deposits found in arteries or tissues, often seen in conditions like atherosclerosis. 硬化斑块是发现于动脉或组织中的硬沉积物，常见于动脉硬化等疾病。

sclerochoroiditis 硬脉络膜炎

词根 scler-（硬）+ choroid-（脉络膜）+ -itis（炎症）

例句 Sclerochoroiditis is an inflammation of the sclera and choroid layer of the eye, often causing vision problems. 硬脉络膜炎是眼球硬膜和脉络膜的炎症，常导致视力问题。

sclerocornea 硬角膜症

词根 scler-（硬）+ corne-（角膜）+ -a（名词后缀）

例句 Sclerocornea is a condition where the cornea becomes abnormally hard, affecting vision. 硬角膜症是角膜异常硬化的病症，影响视力。

LMCHK Part 1　样题

A 2½ -year-old boy was born at 26 weeks gestation (gest-; -ation) with a birth weight of 900 gram. After birth, he was found to have a grade III intraventricular (intra-; ventricul-) haemorrhage (haemo-; -rrhage) and had developed hydrocephalus (hydro-; cephal-) requiring a ventriculo-peritoneal shunt at 3 months. He was discharged (dis-; -charge) 5 months later. The mother notices that he cannot lift up his head, roll over or even sit. He cannot reach out for toys. Physical examination shows that muscle tone has increased in all limbs. He does not have any visual fixation.

Which of the following is the MOST LIKELY diagnosis?

(A) Ataxic cerebral diplegia (di-;-plegia)

(B) Athetoid (a-; thet-; -oid) cerebral palsy

(C) Global developmental delay

(D) Spastic diplegia (di-; -plegia)

(E) Spastic tetraplegia (tetra-; -plegia)

S

中文翻译

一名 2 岁半的男孩在妊娠 26 周出生，出生体重 900 g。出生后发现有Ⅲ级脑室内出血，并发展为脑积水，在 3 个月时需行脑室—腹腔分流术。他在 5 个月后出院。母亲注意到他无法抬头、翻身或坐起，也无法伸手拿玩具。体检显示四肢肌张力增高。他没有任何视觉注视。

以下哪项是最可能的诊断？

(A) 共济失调型脑瘫

(B) 不随意运动型脑瘫

(C) 全面发育迟缓

(D) 痉挛性双瘫

(E) 痉挛性四瘫

题目和答案中出现的词根

gest-：携带

-ation：表示动作（携带的动作即为怀孕）

intra-：在……内

ventricul：室，这里指脑室，也可以指心室

haemo-：血，是 hemo- 和 hemato- 的同义变异

-rrahge：流出

hydro-：氢，这里指代水

cephal-：脑

dis-：离开

-charge：负担（离开负担指代出院，即离开医院给予病人的各种负担）

di-：双

-plegia：瘫痪

a-：表示否定

thet-：地方

-oid：类似的（类似没有地方指的是手足徐动，即手足类似没地方放而乱动）

tetra-：四

-scope/-scopy（镜检查）

endoscope 内窥镜

词根 endo-（内部）+ -scope（镜）

例句 An endoscope is a medical instrument used to view the inside of a hollow organ or body cavity. 内窥镜是一种用于查看中空器官或体腔内部的医学仪器。

bronchoscope 支气管镜

词根 broncho-（支气管）+ -scope（镜）

例句 A bronchoscope is used to examine the airways and diagnose respiratory diseases. 支气管镜用于检查气道并诊断呼吸系统疾病。

colonoscopy 结肠镜检查

词根 colono-（结肠）+ -scopy（镜检查）

例句 Colonoscopy is used to examine the colon for abnormalities, such as polyps or tumors. 结肠镜检查用于检查结肠中的异常，如息肉或肿瘤。

laparoscope 腹腔镜

词根 laparo-（腹部）+ -scope（镜）

例句 Laparoscope is used in minimally invasive surgery to view the internal organs and perform operations. 腹腔镜用于微创手术

中，查看内部器官并进行手术。

cystoscope 膀胱镜

词根 cysto-（膀胱）+ -scope（镜）

例句 A cystoscope is used to inspect the bladder for infections or other abnormalities. 膀胱镜用于检查膀胱的感染或其他异常。

arthroscope 关节镜

词根 arthro-（关节）+ -scope（镜）

例句 An arthroscope is used to look inside a joint to diagnose or treat conditions like arthritis. 关节镜用于查看关节内部，以诊断或治疗如关节炎等疾病。

gastroscope 胃镜

词根 gastro-（胃）+ -scope（镜）

例句 A gastroscope is used to examine the stomach and diagnose conditions like ulcers or cancer. 胃镜用于检查胃部并诊断溃疡或癌症等疾病。

sigmoidoscope 乙状结肠

词根 sigmoid-（乙状）+ -scope（镜）

例句 A sigmoidoscope is used to examine the sigmoid colon for diseases or abnormalities. 乙状结肠镜用于检查乙状结肠的疾病或异常。

ophthalmoscope 眼底镜

词根 ophthalmo-（眼睛）+ -scope（镜）

例句 An ophthalmoscope is used to examine the retina and other structures of the eye. 眼底镜用于检查视网膜和眼睛的其他结构。

rhinoscope 鼻镜

词根 rhino-（鼻）+ -scope（镜）

例句 A rhinoscope is used to view the inside of the nose to diagnose conditions like sinusitis. 鼻镜用于查看鼻腔内部，诊断如鼻

窦炎等疾病。

laryngoscope 喉镜

词根 laryngo-（喉）+ -scope（镜）

例句 A laryngoscope is used to examine the larynx and vocal cords. 喉镜用于检查喉部和声带。

pelviscope 盆腔镜

词根 pelvis-（盆腔）+ -scope（镜）

例句 A pelviscope is used to examine the pelvic area for abnormalities or disease. 盆腔镜用于检查盆腔区域的异常或疾病。

nasopharyngoscope 鼻咽镜

词根 nasopharyngo-（鼻咽部）+ -scope（镜）

例句 A nasopharyngoscope is used to examine the nasopharynx for tumors or obstructions. 鼻咽镜用于检查鼻咽部的肿瘤或阻塞。

hysteroscope 子宫镜

词根 hystero-（子宫）+ -scope（镜）

例句 A hysteroscope is used to inspect the inside of the uterus for conditions such as fibroids. 子宫镜用于检查子宫内部的疾病，如子宫肌瘤。

rhinoscopy 鼻镜检查

词根 rhino-（鼻）+ -scopy（镜检查）

例句 Rhinoscopy is a procedure used to examine the inside of the nasal passages and sinus cavities. 鼻镜检查是一种用于检查鼻腔和鼻窦的方法。

colposcope 阴道镜

词根 colpo-（阴道）+ -scope（镜）

例句 A colposcope is used to examine the cervix and vaginal walls for abnormalities. 阴道镜用于检查宫颈和阴道壁的异常。

ureteroscope 输尿管镜

词根 uretero-（输尿管）+ -scope（镜）

例句 A ureteroscope is used to examine the inside of the ureters to check for stones or tumors. 输尿管镜用于检查输尿管内部，以排查结石或肿瘤。

sebo-（油脂的）

sebum 皮脂

词根 sebo-（油脂的）+ -um（名词后缀）

例句 Sebum is an oily substance secreted by sebaceous glands in the skin to lubricate and protect it. 皮脂是由皮脂腺分泌的一种油脂物质，用于润滑和保护皮肤。

sebaceous gland 皮脂腺

词根 sebo-（油脂的）+ -aceous（形容词后缀）+ gland（腺体）

例句 Sebaceous glands are responsible for producing sebum and are located in the dermis layer of the skin. 皮脂腺负责分泌皮脂，位于皮肤的真皮层。

seborrhea 脂溢症

词根 sebo-（油脂的）+ -rrhea（流出）

例句 Seborrhea is a condition characterized by the excessive production of sebum, often leading to oily skin or scalp. 脂溢症是指皮脂过度分泌的症状，通常导致皮肤或头皮油腻。

seborrheic dermatitis 脂溢性皮炎

词根 sebo-（油脂的）+ -rrheic（流出性）+ dermatitis（皮炎）

例句 Seborrheic dermatitis is an inflammatory skin condition that causes red, itchy, and flaky skin, often on the scalp. 脂溢性皮炎是一种引起皮肤发红、瘙痒和脱屑的炎症性皮肤病，通常发生在头皮上。

seborrheic keratosis 脂溢性角化症

词根 sebo-（油脂的）+ -rrheic（流出性）+ keratosis（角化症）

例句 Seborrheic keratosis is a benign skin tumor that appears as a wart-like growth, often found in areas of increased sebum production. 脂溢性角化症是一种良性皮肤肿瘤，表现为类似疣的生长，通常出现在皮脂分泌较多的区域。

seborrheic alopecia 脂溢性脱发

词根 sebo-（油脂的）+ -rrheic（流出性）+ alopecia（脱发）

例句 Seborrheic alopecia is a condition that causes hair thinning and loss due to the overproduction of sebum on the scalp. 脂溢性脱发是由头皮皮脂过度分泌引起的脱发和毛发变细的病症。

sebo-keratopathy 皮脂角化病

词根 sebo-（油脂的）+ kerato-（角质）+ -pathy（病）

例句 Sebo-keratopathy refers to a condition where excess sebum production leads to the formation of keratinized lesions on the skin. 皮脂角化病是指由于皮脂过度分泌导致皮肤上形成角化性病变的病症。

sebaceous cyst 皮脂囊肿

词根 sebo-（油脂的）+ -aceous（形容词后缀）+ cyst（囊肿）

例句 A sebaceous cyst is a type of cyst that forms when a sebaceous gland becomes blocked and fills with sebum. 皮脂囊肿是指皮脂腺被堵塞并充满皮脂时形成的囊肿。

seborrhea oleosa 油性脂溢症

词根 sebo-（油脂的）+ -rrhea（流出）+ oleosa（油性的）

例句 Seborrhea oleosa is a condition marked by excessively oily skin, often seen in patients with hormonal imbalances. 油性皮脂溢症是一种以皮肤过度油腻为特征的病症，常见于激素失衡的患者。

sebo-purulent discharge 皮脂脓性分泌物

词根 sebo-（油脂的）+ purulent（脓性）+ discharge（分泌物）

例句 A sebopurulent discharge is a thick, yellowish secretion from a sebaceous cyst or abscess, indicating infection. 皮脂脓性分泌物是由皮脂囊肿或脓肿分泌出的厚重黄色分泌物，通常表示感染。

LMCHK Part 1　样题

A mother, who has dichorionic (di-; chorion-) diamniotic (di-; amni-) twin pregnancy, is diagnosed with an absence of fetal heart pulsation in one twin on ultrasound (ultra-) scan examination at 30 weeks' gestation (gest-; -ation). She is asymptomatic (a-) and her vital signs are normal.

Which of the following management options is MOST APPROPRIATE?

(A) Daily cardiotocogram (cardi-; toco-; -gram) and doppler velocimetry

(B) Emergency Caesarean section after a course of antenatal (ante-; -natal) corticosteroids (cortico-; ster-; -oid)

(C) Hysterotomy (hyster-; -otomy) to remove the dead twin

(D) Induction of labour at 34 weeks of gestation (gest-; -ation)

(E) Monitor the fetal growth by ultrasound (ultra-) and plan for delivery at term

S

中文翻译

一名双绒毛膜双羊膜囊双胎妊娠的母亲，在妊娠 30 周的超声检查中发现其中一胎缺乏胎心搏动。她无症状，生命体征正常。以下哪项管理方案是最适当的？

(A) 每日胎心监护和多普勒血流速度测量

(B) 紧急剖宫产，术前给予产前皮质类固醇

(C) 子宫切开术移除死亡胎儿

(D) 在妊娠 34 周引产

(E) 通过超声监测胎儿生长，并计划足月分娩

题目和答案中出现的词根

di-：双

chorion-：绒膜

amni-：羊膜

ultra-：超

gest-：携带

-ation：表示动作（携带的动作即为怀孕）

a-：表示否定

cardi-：心脏

toco-：宫缩

-gram：图像

ante-：在……之前

-natal：出生

cortico-：肾上腺皮质的

ster-：固体的（这里指胆固醇）

-oid：类似的

hyster-：子宫

-otomy：切开术

semi-（半）

seminal fluid 精液

词根 semi-（半）+ -nal（名词后缀）
例句 Seminal fluid is the fluid that contains sperm and is ejaculated during sexual intercourse. 精液是包含精子的液体，在性交过程中射出。

semicircular canal 半规管

词根 semi-（半）+ circular（圆形的）+ canal（管道）
例句 The semicircular canals are part of the inner ear that help maintain balance. 半规管是内耳的一部分，负责维持身体平衡。

semi-automatic 半自动的

词根 semi-（半）+ automatic（自动的）
例句 A semi-automatic syringe can be used to inject medicine with some manual assistance. 半自动注射器可在人工辅助下完成药物注射。

semitransparent 半透明的

词根 semi-（半）+ transparent（透明的）
例句 Semitransparent bandages allow some light to pass through while protecting the wound. 半透明的绷带允许一些光线通过，同时保护伤口。

semilunar valve 半月瓣

词根 semi-（半）+ lunar（半月的）+ valve（瓣膜）
例句 The semilunar valves are located in the heart, preventing the backflow of blood into the ventricles. 半月瓣位于心脏，防止血液回流进入心室。

semen analysis 精液分析

词根 semi-（半）+ -nalysis（分析）

例句 A semen analysis is a test used to evaluate a man's fertility by examining his sperm count, motility, and morphology. 精液分析是一种通过检查精子数量、活动力和形态来评估男性生育能力的测试。

semilunar cartilage 半月形软骨

词根 semi-（半）+ lunar（半月的）+ cartilage（软骨）

例句 The semilunar cartilage in the knee helps stabilize the joint and absorb shock. 膝盖中的半月形软骨有助于稳定关节并吸收冲击。

semiotitis 半月腺炎

词根 semi-（半）+ otitis（耳炎）

例句 Semiotitis is a term referring to inflammation that affects only one part of the ear. 半月腺炎是指仅影响耳朵部分的炎症。

semi-quantitative 半定量的

词根 semi-（半）+ quantitative（定量的）

例句 A semi-quantitative test measures the approximate concentration of a substance in a sample. 半定量测试测量样本中物质的大致浓度。

semilunar shape 半月形状

词根 semi-（半）+ lunar（半月的）

例句 The semilunar shape of certain valves allows them to close tightly to prevent blood from flowing backward. 某些瓣膜的半月形状使它们能够紧闭，防止血液倒流。

semi-solid 半固体的

词根 semi-（半）+ solid（固体的）

例句 Semi-solid foods, such as pudding, can be easier to swallow for patients with swallowing difficulties. 半固体食物，如布丁，对于有吞咽困难的患者来说更容易吞咽。

semiconditioned 半条件化的

词根 semi-（半）+ conditioned（条件化的）

例句 A semi-conditioned reflex refers to a behavior that is partially learned through experience and stimuli. 半条件反射是指通过经验和刺激部分学习的行为。

semiviral 半病毒的

词根 semi-（半）+ viral（病毒的）

例句 A semiviral infection is a rare condition that involves viral elements that partially affect the host. 半病毒性感染是一种罕见疾病，其特征为病毒成分仅对宿主产生部分影响。

semimembranous 半膜状的

词根 semi-（半）+ membranous（膜状的）

例句 Semimembranous muscles are a group of muscles in the thigh that assist in leg movement. 半膜状肌是大腿中的一组肌肉，协助腿部运动。

semi-fowler position 半卧位

词根 semi-（半）+ fowler（福尔维）+ position（位置）

例句 The semi-Fowler position is commonly used to help patients with breathing difficulties by elevating the head and upper body. 半卧位常用于帮助有呼吸困难的患者，通过抬高头部和上半身来改善呼吸。

sero-（浆液的）

serology 血清学

词根 sero-（浆液的）+ -logy（学科）

例句 Serology is the study of blood serum to identify the presence of antibodies and antigens. 血清学是研究血液血清以检测抗体和抗原存在的学科。

serous fluid 浆液

词根 sero-（浆液的）+ fluid（液体）

例句 Serous fluid is a watery substance produced by serous membranes, which helps lubricate body cavities. 浆液是由浆膜产生的一种水样物质，帮助润滑体腔。

seroma 浆液肿

词根 sero-（浆液的）+ -oma（肿瘤）

例句 A seroma is a collection of serous fluid that builds up under the skin, often following surgery. 浆液肿是浆液在皮肤下积聚形成的肿块，通常发生在手术后。

serous cystadenoma 浆液性囊腺瘤

词根 sero-（浆液的）+ cyst-（囊肿）+ adenoma（腺瘤）

例句 Serous cystadenoma is a benign tumor that forms in the ovaries and is filled with serous fluid. 浆液性囊腺瘤是一种良性肿瘤，通常发生在卵巢中，内含浆液。

S

serous pericarditis 浆液性心包炎

词根 sero-（浆液的）+ pericard-（心包）+ -itis（炎症）

例句 Serous pericarditis is inflammation of the pericardium, the sac around the heart, with an accumulation of serous fluid. 浆液性心包炎是指心包（围绕心脏的囊）发炎并伴有浆液积聚。

seroconversion 血清转换

词根 sero-（浆液的）+ conversion（转变）

例句 Seroconversion is the change from the absence to the presence of antibodies in the blood, typically after infection. 血清转换是指血液中从没有抗体到有抗体的转变，通常发生在感染后。

serous effusion 浆液性渗出

词根 sero-（浆液的）+ effusion（渗出）

例句 Serous effusion occurs when serous fluid accumulates in the body cavities, such as the pleural or peritoneal cavity. 浆液性渗出是指浆液在体腔中积聚，如胸腔或腹腔。

serological test 血清学检测

词根 sero-（浆液的）+ -logy（学科）+ test（检测）

例句 A serological test is used to detect antibodies or antigens in the blood, aiding in the diagnosis of infections or diseases. 血清学检测用于检测血液中的抗体或抗原，帮助诊断感染或疾病。

serosanguineous 浆血性

词根 sero-（浆液的）+ sanguineous（含血的）

例句 Serosanguineous discharge is a type of fluid that contains both serum and blood, often seen in wound healing. 浆血性分泌物是一种包含血清和血液的液体，通常在伤口愈合时出现。

serositis 浆膜炎

词根 sero-（浆液的）+ -itis（炎症）

例句 Serositis is inflammation of the serous membranes that line the body cavities, which can result in pain and swelling. 浆膜炎是指覆盖体腔的浆膜发生炎症，可能导致疼痛和肿胀。

sider（o）-（含铁颗粒）

siderosis 铁沉积症

词根 sidero-（含铁颗粒）+ -osis（病理状态）

例句 Siderosis is a condition where excess iron accumulates in the tissues, often leading to organ damage. 铁沉积症是一种因铁元素在组织中过度蓄积而引发的疾病，通常会导致器官损伤。

sideremia 血铁症

词根 sider-（含铁颗粒）+ -emia（血症）

例句 Sideremia refers to the level of iron present in the blood, which is important for oxygen transport. 血铁症指血液中铁的水平，这对于氧气运输至关重要。

siderophore 铁载体

词根 sidero-（含铁颗粒）+ -phore（载体）

例句 Siderophores are molecules that bind and transport iron into cells, essential for cellular function. 铁载体是能结合并运输铁到细胞的分子，对于细胞功能至关重要。

sideroblast 含铁红细胞母细胞

词根 sidero-（含铁颗粒）+ -blast（幼细胞）

例句 Sideroblasts are immature red blood cells that contain iron granules, often seen in blood disorders. 含铁红细胞母细胞是含铁颗粒的未成熟红细胞，通常见于血液疾病。

sideropenia 缺铁症

词根 sidero-（含铁颗粒）+ -penia（缺乏）

例句 Sideropenia is a condition characterized by iron deficiency, leading to anemia and fatigue. 缺铁症是一种由缺乏铁引起的病症，通常导致贫血和疲劳。

sideral 铁的

词根 sider-（含铁颗粒）+ -al（形容词后缀）

例句 Sideral treatments are those that involve the use of iron supplements to treat iron deficiency. 铁的治疗是指使用铁补充剂来治疗铁缺乏症。

siderophile 亲铁的

词根 sidero-（含铁颗粒）+ -phile（亲……的）

例句 Siderophiles are organisms that have a particular affinity for iron, often requiring it for survival. 亲铁生物是指对铁有特殊亲和力的生物，通常需要铁来维持生存。

siderotic 含铁的

词根 sider-（含铁颗粒）+ -otic（形容词后缀）
例句 Siderotic changes in the liver refer to the accumulation of iron within liver cells, often due to hemochromatosis. 肝脏铁沉积性改变是指肝细胞内铁元素过度蓄积，通常由血色病引起。

sigmoid-（乙状的）

sigmoid colon 乙状结肠

词根 sigmoid-（乙状的）+ colon（结肠）
例句 The sigmoid colon is the part of the large intestine that is shaped like the letter “S” and connects the descending colon to the rectum. 乙状结肠是大肠的一部分，形状像字母“S”，连接降结肠和直肠。

S

sigmoidoscopy 乙状结肠镜检查

词根 sigmoid-（乙状的）+ -oscopy（检查）
例句 Sigmoidoscopy is a procedure used to examine the inside of the sigmoid colon and rectum for abnormalities. 乙状结肠镜检查是一种用于检查乙状结肠和直肠内部异常的方法。

sigmoidectomy 乙状结肠切除术

词根 sigmoid-（乙状的）+ -ectomy（切除术）
例句 Sigmoidectomy is a surgical procedure where the sigmoid colon is removed, often performed to treat conditions like diverticulitis. 乙状结肠切除术是一种通过切除乙状结肠来治疗疾病的手术方式，常用于治疗如憩室炎等病症。

sigmoid volvulus 乙状结肠扭转

词根 sigmoid-（乙状的）+ volvulus（扭转）

例句 Sigmoid volvulus occurs when the sigmoid colon twists upon itself, causing a bowel obstruction. 乙状结肠扭转是乙状结肠自我扭转，导致肠道梗阻的情况。

sigmoid flexure 乙状弯曲

词根 sigmoid-（乙状的）+ flexure（弯曲）
例句 The sigmoid flexure refers to the S-shaped bend in the colon, which plays a role in the absorption of water. 乙状弯曲指的是结肠中的 S 形弯曲，参与水分的吸收。

sigmoidoscope 乙状结肠镜

词根 sigmoid-（乙状的）+ -scope（镜）
例句 A sigmoidoscope is a medical instrument used for examining the sigmoid colon during sigmoidoscopy. 乙状结肠镜是用于检查乙状结肠的医疗工具。

sigmoid colon cancer 乙状结肠癌

词根 sigmoid-（乙状的）+ colon（结肠）+ cancer（癌症）
例句 Sigmoid colon cancer is a type of cancer that occurs in the sigmoid part of the large intestine. 乙状结肠癌是发生在大肠乙状部的癌症。

sigmoidal contraction 乙状收缩

词根 sigmoid-（乙状的）+ -al（形容词后缀）+ contraction（收缩）
例句 Sigmoidal contraction refers to the characteristic wave-like muscle contractions in the sigmoid colon. 乙状收缩指的是乙状结肠中典型的波浪形肌肉收缩。

sigmoid diverticulum 乙状憩室

词根 sigmoid-（乙状的）+ diverticulum（憩室）
例句 Sigmoid diverticulum is a small pouch that forms in the wall of the sigmoid colon. 乙状憩室是乙状结肠壁上形成的小袋。

sigmoid anastomosis 乙状结肠吻合术

词根 sigmoid-（乙状的）+ anastomosis（吻合术）

例句 Sigmoid anastomosis is a surgical procedure where two parts of the sigmoid colon are surgically joined together. 乙状结肠吻合术是一种外科手术，将乙状结肠的两个部分缝合在一起。

somato-（肉体）

somatic 躯体的

词根 somato-（身体）+ -ic（形容词后缀）

例句 Somatic cells are the cells that make up the body, excluding germ cells. 躯体细胞是构成身体的细胞，排除生殖细胞。

somatogenesis 体生

词根 somato-（身体）+ -genesis（发生）

例句 Somatogenesis refers to the formation and development of the body tissues during embryonic development. 体生是指胚胎发育过程中身体组织的形成和发展。

somatopathy 躯体病

词根 somato-（身体）+ -pathy（病）

例句 Somatopathy refers to any disease affecting the body, as opposed to psychiatric conditions. 躯体病是指影响身体的任何疾病，与精神病条件相对。

somatostatin 生长抑素

词根 somato-（身体）+ -statin（抑制）

例句 Somatostatin is a hormone that inhibits the release of growth hormone and insulin. 生长抑素是一种激素，抑制生长激素和胰岛素的分泌。

somatosensory 躯体感觉的

词根 somato-（身体）+ sensory（感觉的）

例句 Somatosensory pathways are responsible for processing sensations such as touch, pain, and temperature from the skin. 躯体感觉通路负责处理来自皮肤的触觉、疼痛和温度等感觉。

somatotropic 促体激素的

词根 somato-（身体）+ tropic（促的）

例句 Somatotropic hormones are hormones that stimulate growth, such as growth hormone. 促体激素是刺激生长的激素，如生长激素。

somatization 躯体化

词根 somato-（身体）+ -ization（名词后缀）

例句 Somatization is the process by which psychological distress is expressed as physical symptoms. 躯体化是指心理压力以身体症状的形式表现出来的过程。

somatotroph 促体激素细胞

词根 somato-（身体）+ -troph（营养物质）

例句 Somatotrophs are cells in the pituitary gland that produce growth hormone. 促体激素细胞是垂体中的细胞，产生生长激素。

somatomedin 体内介素

词根 somato-（身体）+ -medin（介素）

例句 Somatomedins are a group of proteins that mediate the effects of growth hormone. 体内介素是一类调节生长激素效应的蛋白质。

somatic mutation 体细胞突变

词根 somato-（身体）+ mutation（突变）

例句 Somatic mutations are changes in the DNA of somatic cells, which are not passed on to offspring. 体细胞突变是体细胞 DNA 中的变化，不会传递给后代。

somatophore 体形特征器官

词根 somato-（身体）+ -phore（携带者）
例句 Somatophores are structures that carry physical characteristics, such as bones or muscles, to perform specific body functions. 体形特征器官是携带身体特征的结构，如骨骼或肌肉，用于执行特定的身体功能。

somatic cell nuclear transfer 体细胞核移植

词根 somato-（身体）+ cell（细胞）+ nuclear（核的）+ transfer（转移）
例句 Somatic cell nuclear transfer is a technique used in cloning, where the nucleus of a somatic cell is transferred to an enucleated egg cell. 体细胞核移植是一种克隆技术，将体细胞的核转移到去核的卵细胞中。

somatotrophic 促体激素的

词根 somato-（身体）+ trophic（营养的）
例句 Somatotrophic hormones regulate growth and development in the body. 促体激素在体内调节生长和发育。

somatogastric 体胃的

词根 somato-（身体）+ gastr-（胃）+ -ic（形容词后缀）
例句 Somatogastric refers to the connection between the body and the stomach, particularly in gastrointestinal studies. 体胃指的是身体与胃之间的连接，特别是在胃肠研究中。

-some（小体）

chromosome 染色体

词根 chrom-（颜色）+ -some（小体）
例句 Chromosomes are structures within cells that contain genetic material. 染色体是细胞内含有遗传物质的结构。

lysosome 溶酶体

词根 lys-（分解）+ -some（小体）
例句 Lysosomes are organelles in the cytoplasm that contain enzymes to break down waste materials and cellular debris. 溶酶体是细胞质中的细胞器，含有分解废物和细胞残骸的酶。

ribosome 核糖体

词根 ribo-（核糖）+ -some（小体）
例句 Ribosomes are responsible for protein synthesis in cells. 核糖体负责细胞中的蛋白质合成。

endosome 内体

词根 endo-（内部）+ -some（小体）
例句 Endosomes are membrane-bound compartments within cells that play a key role in endocytosis. 内体是细胞内被膜包围的细胞器，在内吞作用中发挥重要作用。

microsome 微粒体

词根 micro-（微小的）+ -some（小体）
例句 Microsomes are fragments of the endoplasmic reticulum and are involved in various metabolic processes. 微粒体是内质网的碎片，参与多种代谢过程。

phagosome 吞噬体

词根 phago-（吞噬）+ -some（小体）
例句 A phagosome is a vesicle formed around a particle engulfed by a phagocyte during phagocytosis. 吞噬体是由吞噬细胞在吞噬作用过程中围绕被吞噬颗粒形成的囊泡。

nucleosome 核小体

词根 nucle-（核）+ -some（小体）
例句 Nucleosomes are the basic structural unit of chromatin, consisting of DNA wrapped around histone proteins. 核小体是染色质

的基本结构单位，由缠绕在组蛋白上的 DNA 组成。

zygosome 合子体

词根 zygo-（合子）+ -some（小体）

例句 Zygosomes refer to the early stage of cell fusion during fertilization. 合子体指的是受精过程中细胞融合的早期阶段。

LMCHK Part 1 样题

A 28-year-old intravenous (intra-; -ven) drug abuser is admitted with a history of low-grade fever for 1 month, cough with occasional haemoptysis (haemo-; -ptysis) and left-sided abdominal pain. On examination, he looks unwell (un-) with mild pyrexia (pyre-; -exia), raised jugular venous pressure and a systolic (systo-) murmur at the left sternal edge. There are scattered crepitations (crepit-; -ation) in the lungs, and in the abdomen there is tenderness in the left hypochondrium (hypo-; chondr-).

Which of the following diagnoses would you consider to be the MOST LIKELY?

(A) AIDS

(B) A ruptured amoebic abscess

(C) Staphylococcal (staphylo-; -coccal) septicaemia (-emia)

(D) Staphylococcal (staphylo-; -coccal) right-sided endocarditis (endo-; cardi-; -itis)

(E) Typhoid (typh-; -oid)

中文翻译

一名 28 岁静脉吸毒者因 1 个月来低热、咳嗽伴偶发咯血和左侧腹痛入院。检查时，他看起来病情较重，伴轻度发热，颈静脉压升高，左侧胸骨旁听到收缩期杂音。肺部听诊有散在爆裂音，腹部检查显示左季肋部压痛。

以下哪项诊断你认为是最可能的？

(A) 艾滋病

(B) 破裂的阿米巴脓肿

(C) 葡萄球菌败血症

(D) 葡萄球菌右侧心内膜炎

(E) 伤寒

题目和答案中出现的词根

intra-：在……内

-ven：静脉

haemo-：血，是 hemo-，hemato- 的同义变异

-ptysis：咳嗽

pyre-：发热

-exia：状态，这里的 e 字母和前面的 pyre- 的 e 的字母共用

systo-：收缩

crepit-：噼啪声

-ation：表示动作（噼啪声的动作即为爆裂声）

hypo-：低

chondr-：软骨（这里指肋骨）

staphylo-：葡萄状的

-coccal：浆果

-emia：血症

endo-：内

cardi-: 心脏

-itis: 炎症

typh-: 恍惚（指伤寒可以引起的症状）

-oid: 类似的

somn-（睡觉）

somnolence 嗜睡

词根 somnol-（睡觉）+ -ence（名词后缀）

例句 Somnolence refers to the state of drowsiness or sleepiness, often experienced during the day due to sleep deprivation or certain medical conditions. 嗜睡是指白天因睡眠不足或某些疾病而感到昏昏欲睡的状态。

somnoplasty 睡眠障碍手术

词根 somno-（睡觉）+ -plasty（手术）

例句 Somnoplasty is a surgical procedure used to treat sleep apnea by removing excess tissue in the throat. 睡眠障碍手术是一种外科手术，通过切除喉部多余的组织来治疗睡眠呼吸暂停。

somnology 睡眠学

词根 somno-（睡觉）+ -logy（学科）

例句 Somnology is the scientific study of sleep and its disorders, including sleep apnea and insomnia. 睡眠学是研究睡眠及其障碍的学科，包括睡眠呼吸暂停和失眠。

somnambulism 梦游症

词根 somno-（睡觉）+ ambul-（走动）+ -ism（病症）

例句 Somnambulism, or sleepwalking, is a condition where an individual performs activities, such as walking, while still asleep. 梦游症是一种个体在仍处于睡眠状态时进行活动（如行走）的病症。

somniferous 催眠的

词根 somni-（睡觉）+ ferous（带来）
例句 Somniferous drugs are substances that promote sleep, commonly used to treat insomnia. 催眠药物是促进睡眠的物质，常用于治疗失眠。

hypersomnia 嗜睡症

词根 hyper-（过度）+ somnia（睡眠）
例句 Hypersomnia is a condition where an individual experiences excessive daytime sleepiness despite getting adequate nighttime rest. 嗜睡症是指尽管晚上休息充足，白天仍感到异常嗜睡的状况。

somnoplasty 睡眠成形术

词根 somno-（睡觉）+ -plasty（塑形）
例句 Somnoplasty is used to surgically treat sleep disorders such as snoring and sleep apnea. 睡眠成形术用于手术治疗像打鼾和睡眠呼吸暂停等睡眠障碍。

somnotherapy 睡眠治疗

词根 somno-（睡觉）+ -therapy（治疗）
例句 Somnotherapy is a form of treatment aimed at improving sleep quality and managing sleep disorders. 睡眠治疗是一种旨在改善睡眠质量和管理睡眠障碍的治疗方法。

PLAB 1　样题

A 55-year-old man has diarrhea (dia-; -rrhea) and weight loss for 9 months. He has an intensely itchy red rash on his buttocks and thighs.

Investigations:

Haemoglobin (haemo-; -globin) 108 g/L

Blood film: anisocytosis (aniso-; cyt-; -osis)

Which is the most likely histological (histo-) appearance on small bowel biopsy?

(A) Hyperplasia (hyper-; -plasia) of Brunner's glands

(B) Increased intraepithelial (intra-; epithel-) macrophages (macro-; -phage)

(C) Increased lymphocytes (lymph-; -cyte) in submucosa (sub-)

(D) Ulceration

(E) Villous atrophy (a-; -troph)

中文翻译

一名 55 岁男性有 9 个月的腹泻和体重减轻史。他臀部和大腿有剧烈瘙痒的红色皮疹。

检查结果：

血红蛋白 108 g/L

血涂片：红细胞大小不等

小肠活检最可能的组织学表现是以下哪项？

(A) 布伦纳腺增生

(B) 上皮内巨噬细胞增多

(C) 黏膜下层淋巴细胞增多

(D) 溃疡

(E) 绒毛萎缩

题目和答案中出现的词根

dia-：通过（这里指通过肠道）

-rrhea：流出（通过肠道流出指腹泻）

hemo-：血

-globin：球蛋白

aniso-：大小不一的

cyt-：细胞

-osis：病理状态

histo-：组织学的

hyper-：高

-plasia：生长

intra-：在……内

epithel：表皮

macro-：大的

-phage：吞噬

lymph-：淋巴

cyte-：细胞，和 cyt- 是同义

sub-：在……下（在种类的下面指的是亚分类，即在一层分类的下级再分类）

a-：表示否定

-troph：营养

-spadias（开口）

hypospadias 尿道下裂

词根 hypo-（下）+ -spadias（开口）

例句 Hypospadias is a congenital condition where the opening of the urethra is located on the underside of the penis, rather than at the tip. 尿道下裂是一种先天性疾病，尿道开口位于阴茎下方，而不是在顶端。

epispadias 尿道上裂

词根 epi-（上）+ -spadias（开口）

例句 Epispadias is a rare birth defect in which the opening of the urethra is on the top side of the penis. 尿道上裂是一种罕见的出生缺陷，表现为尿道开口位于阴茎的顶部。

chordee with hypospadias 尿道下裂伴阴茎弯曲

词根 chordee（阴茎弯曲）+ hypo-（下）+ -spadias（开口）

例句 Chordee with hypospadias is a condition where the penis is curved downward due to a congenital deformity. 尿道下裂伴阴茎弯曲是一种由先天性畸形导致阴茎向下弯曲的病症。

penoscrotal hypospadias 阴茎阴囊型尿道下裂

词根 peno-（阴茎）+ scrotal（阴囊的）+ hypo-（下）+ -spadias（开口）

例句 Penoscrotal hypospadias is a more severe form of hypospadias where the urethral opening is located near the base of the penis or at the scrotum. 阴茎阴囊型尿道下裂是尿道下裂中较严重的一种类型，尿道开口位于阴茎基部或阴囊附近。

perineal hypospadias 会阴尿道下裂

词根 perineal（会阴的）+ hypo-（下）+ -spadias（开口）

例句 Perineal hypospadias is a rare form of hypospadias where the urethral opening is located on the perineum, between the anus and the scrotum. 会阴尿道下裂是一种罕见的尿道下裂类型，尿道开口位于肛门和阴囊之间的会阴部。

post-pubertal hypospadias repair 青春期后尿道下裂修复

词根 post-（后）+ pubertal（青春期的）+ hypo-（下）+ -spadias（开口）+ repair（修复）

例句 Post-pubertal hypospadias repair is a surgical procedure performed to correct the urethral opening in patients who have not undergone treatment during childhood. 青春期后尿道下裂修复是一种手术，用于修复那些在儿童期未接受治疗的患者的尿道开口。

complete hypospadias 完全尿道下裂

词根 complete（完全的）+ hypo-（下）+ -spadias（开口）

例句 Complete hypospadias refers to a severe form of hypospadias where the urethral opening is located near the base of the penis or on the scrotum. 完全尿道下裂是指一种严重的尿道下裂类型，其尿道开口位于阴茎基部或阴囊上。

subcoronal hypospadias 冠状下尿道下裂

词根 sub-（下）+ coronal（冠状的）+ hypo-（下）+ -spadias（开口）

例句 Subcoronal hypospadias is a condition where the urethral opening is located just below the glans penis, near the corona. 冠状下尿道下裂是一种尿道开口位于阴茎头下方、接近冠状部分的情况。

severe hypospadias 重度尿道下裂

词根 severe（重度的）+ hypo-（下）+ -spadias（开口）

例句 Severe hypospadias is a condition in which the urethral opening is located at the perineum or scrotum, requiring surgical intervention. 重度尿道下裂是指尿道开口位于会阴或阴囊，通常需要手术干预。

surgical hypospadias repair 尿道下裂手术修复

词根 surgical（外科的）+ hypo-（下）+ -spadias（开口）+ repair（修复）

例句 Surgical hypospadias repair is a common procedure to reconstruct the urethra and correct the abnormal opening in male infants and children. 尿道下裂手术修复是一种常见的手术，用于重建尿道并矫正男性婴儿和儿童的异常尿道开口。

sphero-（球）

spheroid 球状物

词根 sphero-（球）+ -oid（形状）

例句 Spheroid refers to a shape that is almost spherical, often used to describe cells or particles. 球状物指的是几乎呈球形的形状，常用来描述细胞或颗粒。

spheroidal 球形的

词根 sphero-（球）+ -idal（形容词后缀）

例句 Spheroidal bacteria are a type of bacteria that appear round in shape, often categorized in microbiology. 球形细菌是一种呈圆形的细菌，常在微生物学中进行分类。

spheroidectomy 球状体切除术

词根 sphero-（球）+ -ectomy（切除）

例句 Spheroidectomy is a surgical procedure where a spherical tumor or growth is removed from the body. 球状体切除术是一种手术，用于切除体内的球形肿瘤或增生组织。

spherochondritis 球状软骨炎

词根 sphero-（球）+ chondr-（软骨）+ -itis（炎症）

例句 Spherochondritis is an inflammation of the spherical cartilage, often resulting from trauma or infection. 球状软骨炎是球形软骨的炎症，常由创伤或感染引起。

spheroidal shape 球形状

词根 sphero-（球）+ -idal（形容词后缀）

例句 The spheroidal shape of certain cells allows them to efficiently move through blood vessels. 某些细胞呈球形，这种形态使其能

够高效地在血管中移动。

spheroid cell 球形细胞

词根 sphero-（球）+ cell（细胞）

例句 Spheroid cells are often seen in the blood, where their shape aids in the transport of oxygen. 球形细胞常见于血液中，其形状有助于氧气的运输。

spheroidal bacteria 球形细菌

词根 sphero-（球）+ bacteria（细菌）

例句 Spheroidal bacteria are bacteria that exhibit a round shape and are often classified as cocci. 球形细菌是呈圆形的细菌，通常被归类为球菌。

spheroid degeneration 球状退化

词根 sphero-（球）+ degeneration（退化）

例句 Spheroid degeneration is a pathological condition where cells or tissues take on a spherical shape due to damage. 球状退化是一种病理状况，指细胞或组织由于损伤而呈现球形。

spheroidal depression 球状凹陷

词根 sphero-（球）+ -idal（形容词后缀）+ depression（凹陷）

例句 Spheroidal depression refers to a depression in the shape of a sphere, often seen in certain bone diseases. 球状凹陷指的是球形的凹陷，常见于某些骨骼疾病中。

sphygmo-（血压计的）

sphygmomanometer 血压计

词根 sphygmo-（血压）+ manometer（压力计）

例句 A sphygmomanometer is an instrument used to measure blood pressure, typically consisting of a cuff and a gauge. 血压计是一种

用于测量血压的仪器，通常由袖带和压力表组成。

sphygmogram 血压图

词根 sphygmo-（血压）+ -gram（图）

例句 A sphygmogram is a graphical representation of the pulse wave, used in the measurement of blood pressure. 血压图是脉搏波的图形表示，常用于血压的测量。

sphygmometry 血压测量法

词根 sphygmo-（血压）+ -metry（测量法）

例句 Sphygmometry is the process of measuring blood pressure using a sphygmomanometer. 血压测量法是使用血压计测量血压的方法。

sphygmocardiogram 血压心电图

词根 sphygmo-（血压）+ cardiogram（心电图）

例句 A sphygmocardiogram is a combined graphical representation of both pulse and heart electrical activity. 血压心电图是脉搏和心脏电活动的联合图形表示。

sphygmic 脉搏压的

词根 sphygmo-（血压）+ -ic（形容词后缀）

例句 Sphygmic pressure refers to the pressure of the pulse in the arteries during heartbeats. 脉搏压指的是心跳过程中动脉中脉搏的压力。

sphygmogram（pulse tracing）脉搏压力波形图

词根 sphygmo-（血压）+ -gram（图）

例句 A sphygmogram, also known as pulse tracing, is used to analyze the pulse rate and rhythm. 脉搏波形图，也称为脉搏描记图，用于分析脉搏率和节律。

spondylo-（脊柱的）

spondylitis 脊柱炎

词根 spondylo-（脊柱的）+ -itis（炎症）

例句 Spondylitis is an inflammatory disease that primarily affects the spine and can cause pain and stiffness. 脊柱炎是一种主要影响脊柱的炎症性疾病，可能引起疼痛和僵硬。

spondylosis 脊柱病

词根 spondylo-（脊柱的）+ -osis（病理状态）

例句 Spondylosis refers to age-related degeneration of the spine, which can lead to pain and mobility issues. 脊柱病是指脊柱因衰老引起的退化，可能导致疼痛和行动问题。

spondylolisthesis 脊椎滑脱

词根 spondylo-（脊柱的）+ listhesis（滑脱）

例句 Spondylolisthesis occurs when one vertebra slips over another, causing spinal instability. 脊椎滑脱是指一个脊椎滑移到另一个脊椎上方，导致脊柱不稳定。

spondylopathy 脊柱疾病

词根 spondylo-（脊柱的）+ -pathy（病）

例句 Spondylopathy is a term used for various spinal diseases that can cause pain and discomfort. 脊柱疾病是用于指代各种可能导致疼痛和不适的脊柱疾病的术语。

spondylosyndesis 脊柱融合术

词根 spondylo-（脊柱的）+ syndesis（融合）

例句 Spondylosyndesis is a surgical procedure in which two or more vertebrae are fused to reduce pain and improve spinal stability. 脊柱融合术是一种外科手术，通过将两个或多个脊椎融合来减

轻疼痛并提高脊柱稳定性。

spondylomuscular 脊柱肌肉的

词根 spondylo-（脊柱的）+ muscular（肌肉的）
例句 Spondylomuscular disorders affect both the muscles and the bones of the spine, leading to pain and weakness. 脊柱肌肉疾病影响脊柱的肌肉和骨骼，导致疼痛和无力。

spondylopathy degenerative 退行性脊柱病

词根 spondylo-（脊柱的）+ -pathy（病）+ degenerative（退化性）
例句 Spondylopathy degenerative is the progressive degeneration of the spine's disc and joints. 退行性脊柱病是脊柱椎间盘和关节的逐渐退化。

spondylosyndesis 脊柱融合手术

词根 spondylo-（脊柱的）+ syndesis（融合）
例句 Spondylosyndesis is a technique used in spinal surgery to fuse two or more vertebrae to stabilize the spine. 脊柱融合手术是一种外科技术，用于通过将两个或多个脊椎融合来稳定脊柱。

spondylocarpal syndrome 脊椎腕综合征

词根 spondylo-（脊柱的）+ carp-（腕）+ -al（形容词后缀）
例句 Spondylocarpal syndrome is a rare condition affecting both the spine and the wrist, causing discomfort and limited movement. 脊椎腕综合征是一种罕见的疾病，影响脊柱和腕关节，导致不适和活动受限。

spondyloclasis 脊椎截骨术

词根 spondylo-（脊柱的）+ -clasis（截断）
例句 Spondyloclasis is a surgical technique used to deliberately break a vertebra for certain spinal treatments. 脊椎截骨术是一种外科手术技术，用于故意截断脊椎以进行某些脊柱治疗。

-stasis（静止）

hemostasis 止血

词根 hem-（血）+ -stasis（静止）

例句 Hemostasis is the process that prevents and stops bleeding, ensuring that blood flow is properly regulated. 止血是防止和停止出血的过程，确保血液流动得到正确调节。

stasis dermatitis 静脉性皮炎

词根 stasis（静止）+ dermatitis（皮炎）

例句 Stasis dermatitis is a condition where poor blood flow in the legs causes skin irritation and inflammation. 静脉性皮炎是一种因腿部血液循环不良引起皮肤刺激和炎症的疾病。

lymphostasis 淋巴停滞

词根 lymph-（淋巴）+ -stasis（静止）

例句 Lymphostasis is a condition where lymph fluid accumulates due to poor lymphatic drainage, often leading to swelling. 淋巴停滞是一种由于淋巴引流不良而导致淋巴液积聚的情况，常伴有肿胀。

venostasis 静脉淤血

词根 veno-（静脉）+ -stasis（静止）

例句 Venostasis refers to the stagnation of blood flow in the veins, often seen in conditions like deep vein thrombosis. 静脉淤血指的是血液在静脉中的滞留，常见于深静脉血栓等疾病。

bacteriostasis 抑菌

词根 bacterio-（细菌）+ -stasis（静止）

例句 Bacteriostasis refers to the process of inhibiting the growth or reproduction of bacteria without necessarily killing them. 抑菌是指

抑制细菌生长或繁殖的过程，而不必然杀灭细菌。

hemorrhagic stasis 出血性淤滞

词根 hemorrhagic（出血性）+ stasis（静止）

例句 Hemorrhagic stasis is the accumulation of blood in a localized area due to impaired circulation or vessel injury. 出血性淤滞是由血液循环障碍或血管损伤而导致局部区域积血。

cytostasis 细胞抑制

词根 cyto-（细胞）+ -stasis（静止）

例句 Cytostasis refers to the inhibition of cell growth or division, often used in the context of cancer therapy. 细胞抑制指的是细胞生长或分裂的抑制，常用于癌症治疗中。

gastrostasis 胃排空延迟

词根 gastr-（胃）+ -stasis（静止）

例句 Gastrostasis is a condition where there is delayed emptying of the stomach, often seen in patients with gastroparesis. 胃排空延迟是一种胃内容物排空延迟的病症，常见于胃轻瘫患者。

stat-（稳态）

homeostasis 体内平衡

词根 homeo-（相同）+ -stasis（稳定）

例句 Homeostasis is the process by which the body maintains a stable internal environment, such as regulating body temperature. 体内平衡是指身体通过各种机制维持稳定的内环境，例如调节体温。

hemostasis 止血

词根 hemo-（血液）+ -stasis（静止）

例句 Hemostasis refers to the stopping of blood flow, particularly after an injury, to prevent excessive bleeding. 止血是指阻止血液

流动，特别是在受伤后防止过度出血。

stasis dermatitis 静止性皮炎

词根 stasis-（静止）+ dermatitis（皮炎）

例句 Stasis dermatitis is a skin condition that occurs due to poor blood circulation and fluid buildup in the legs. 静止性皮炎是由血液循环不良和液体积聚在腿部引起的皮肤病。

hypostasis 积血

词根 hypo-（低）+ -stasis（静止）

例句 Hypostasis is the pooling of blood in the lower parts of the body due to gravity, often observed in postmortem cases. 积血是血液因重力作用积聚在身体下部，通常在尸体解剖中观察到。

stasis of urine 尿液停滞

词根 stasis-（静止）+ urine（尿液）

例句 Stasis of urine refers to the retention of urine in the bladder due to an obstruction or dysfunction, increasing the risk of urinary tract infections. 尿液停滞是指由于阻塞或功能异常，尿液在膀胱中滞留，增加尿路感染的风险。

blood stasis 血瘀

词根 blood（血液）+ stasis（静止）

例句 Blood stasis is a traditional medical term referring to poor circulation or sluggish blood flow in the body, contributing to various health problems. 血瘀是中医术语，指体内血液循环不畅或血流迟缓，可引发多种健康问题。

statin 他汀类药物

词根 stat-（稳定）+ -in（化学物质）

例句 Statins are a class of drugs used to lower cholesterol levels and reduce the risk of cardiovascular diseases. 他汀类药物是一类用于降低胆固醇水平并减少心血管疾病患病风险的药物。

vasostasis 血管停滞

词根 vaso-（血管）+ -stasis（静止）

例句 Vasostasis is the condition of reduced or stagnant blood flow within the blood vessels, which can lead to tissue damage. 血管停滞是指血管内血流减少或停滞，可能导致组织损伤。

static equilibrium 静力平衡

词根 static（静止的）+ equilibrium（平衡）

例句 Static equilibrium refers to a state where all forces acting on the body are balanced, often used in biomechanics. 静力平衡指的是身体上所有作用力相互平衡的状态，常用于生物力学。

steat-（脂肪的）

steatosis 脂肪变性

词根 steat-（脂肪的）+ -osis（病理状态）

例句 Steatosis is the abnormal accumulation of fat in liver cells, often seen in conditions such as non-alcoholic fatty liver disease. 脂肪变性是肝细胞内脂肪的异常积聚，常见于如非酒精性脂肪性肝病等疾病。

steatoma 脂肪瘤

词根 steat-（脂肪的）+ -oma（肿瘤）

例句 A steatoma is a benign tumor consisting of sebaceous gland tissue, commonly known as a sebaceous cyst. 脂肪瘤是一种由皮脂腺组织组成的良性肿瘤，通常称为皮脂囊肿。

steatonecrosis 脂肪坏死

词根 steat-（脂肪的）+ necrosis（坏死）

例句 Steatonecrosis occurs when fat cells die, often due to trauma or pancreatitis. 脂肪坏死是指脂肪细胞死亡，通常由创伤或胰腺炎引起。

steatopathy 脂肪病

词根 steat-（脂肪的）+ -pathy（病）

例句 Steatopathy is a condition characterized by the abnormal accumulation of fat in the tissues, often affecting the liver. 脂肪病是一种以组织中脂肪异常积聚为特征的病症，常见于肝脏。

steatohypocholesterolemia 脂肪低胆固醇血症

词根 steat-（脂肪的）+ hypo-（低）+ cholester-（胆固醇）+ -emia（血症）

例句 Steatohypocholesterolemia is characterized by low cholesterol levels despite the presence of fat accumulation. 脂肪低胆固醇血症是指尽管存在脂肪积聚，胆固醇水平依然较低的情况。

steatosis hepatis 肝脂肪变性

词根 steat-（脂肪的）+ -osis（病理状态）+ hepatis（肝脏的）

例句 Steatosis hepatis is the condition where excess fat builds up in the liver, often associated with obesity or excessive alcohol consumption. 肝脂肪变性是指脂肪在肝脏中异常积聚，常与肥胖或过度饮酒有关。

steatose 脂肪变性

词根 steat-（脂肪的）+ -ose（病）

例句 Steatose refers to the accumulation of fat within tissues, especially in liver and muscle cells. 脂肪变性是指脂肪在组织中的积聚，特别是在肝脏和肌肉细胞中。

steatotropism 脂肪趋性

词根 steat-（脂肪的）+ tropism（趋性）

例句 Steatotropism is the tendency of certain cells or organisms to accumulate fat in response to metabolic changes. 脂肪趋性是指某些细胞或生物体在代谢变化影响下积累脂肪的趋势。

steatocystoma 脂肪囊肿

词根 steat-（脂肪的）+ cystoma（囊肿）

例句 Steatocystoma is a type of cyst that forms in the sebaceous glands and contains fatty material. 脂肪囊肿是一种在皮脂腺中形成的囊肿，包含脂肪物质。

steatogenesis 脂肪生成

词根 steat-（脂肪的）+ -genesis（生成）

例句 Steatogenesis is the process by which fat is produced and stored in the body. 脂肪生成是脂肪在体内产生和储存的过程。

sten-（窄）

stenosis 狭窄

词根 sten-（窄）+ -osis（病理状态）

例句 Stenosis refers to the abnormal narrowing of a body passage, such as a blood vessel or spinal canal. 狭窄指的是身体通道的异常变窄，例如血管或脊髓管。

stent 支架

词根 sten-（狭窄）+ -t（名词后缀）

例句 A stent is a small mesh tube inserted into a blood vessel or duct to keep it open. 支架是一种小型网状管，插入血管或导管中以保持其通畅。

stenotic lesion 狭窄病变

词根 sten-（狭窄）+ -otic（形容词后缀）+ lesion（病变）

例句 A stenotic lesion refers to the narrowing of a passage, such as a blood vessel or an airway, that can lead to blockages. 狭窄病变指的是通道的狭窄，如血管或气道，可能导致堵塞。

stenothermic 狭温性

词根 sten-（狭窄）+ therm-（热）+ -ic（形容词后缀）

例句 Stenothermic organisms can only survive within a narrow temperature range, such as certain bacteria or fungi. 狭温性生物只能在一个狭窄的温度范围内生存，如某些细菌或真菌。

stenopaeic 狭视性

词根 sten-（狭窄）+ paeic（形容词后缀）

例句 Stenopaeic conditions describe abnormalities that lead to restricted vision or narrow field of vision. 狭视性条件描述了导致视力受限或视野狭窄的异常情况。

PLAB 1 样题

A 78-year-old man has low back pain for 6 weeks and is seen in his GP surgery There is no radiation (radi-; -ation) of pain. He has no history of trauma. He has not taken any analgesia (an-; alges-) and takes no regular prescription medication. He was treated for polymyalgia (poly-; my-; -algia) rheumatica (rheumat-) 3 years ago. His BMI is 22 kg/m² and his temperature is 37.4°C. There is bony tenderness over his lumbar spine.

Neurological examination is normal.

Investigations:

Haemoglobin (haemo-; -globin) 78 g/L

ESR 98 mm/hr (<20)

Which is the most likely diagnosis?

(A) Discitis (disc-; -itis)

(B) Mechanical back pain

(C) Multiple (multi-) myeloma (mye-; -oma)

S

(D) Osteoporotic (osteo-; poro-) wedge fracture

(E) Recurrence of polymyalgia (poly-; my-; -algia) rheumatica (rheumat-)

中文翻译

一名 78 岁男性患者因持续 6 周的腰痛前往全科医生诊所就诊，疼痛无放射性扩散。疼痛无放射。他无外伤史，未服用任何止痛药，也无常规处方药物。3 年前曾因风湿性多肌痛接受治疗。他的 BMI 为 22 kg/m²，体温 37.4℃。腰椎有骨性压痛。神经系统检查正常。

检查结果：

血红蛋白 78 g/L

红细胞沉降率（ESR） 98 mm/hr（正常值 <20）

以下哪项是最可能的诊断？

(A) 椎间盘炎

(B) 机械性背痛

(C) 多发性骨髓瘤

(D) 骨质疏松性楔形骨折

(E) 风湿性多肌痛复发

题目和答案中出现的词根

radi-：放射，是 radio- 的同义变异

-ation：表示动作（这里指疼痛向外辐射性的迁延）

an-：表示否定

alges-：疼痛

poly-：多

my-：肌肉

-algia：疼痛

rheumat-：风湿的

haemo-：血，是 hemo- 和 hemato- 的同义变异

-globin：球蛋白

disc-：盘，这里指椎间盘

-itis：炎症

mye-：肌肉，和 my- 是同义变异

-oma：瘤

osteo-：骨

poro-：孔

stomat-（口腔的）

stomatitis 口腔炎

词根 stomat-（口腔的）+ -itis（炎症）
例句 Stomatitis is the inflammation of the mucous membrane inside the mouth, which can cause pain and swelling. 口腔炎是口腔内部黏膜的炎症，可能导致疼痛和肿胀。

stomatosis 口腔病变

词根 stomat-（口腔的）+ -osis（病理状态）
例句 Stomatosis refers to any abnormal condition affecting the mouth, including ulcers, infections, or growths. 口腔病变是指影响口腔的任何异常情况，包括溃疡、感染或肿块。

stomatherapy 口腔治疗

词根 stomat-（口腔的）+ -therapy（治疗）
例句 Stomatherapy is the therapeutic treatment of oral diseases,

such as periodontal disease or oral cancer. 口腔治疗是指对口腔疾病的治疗，如牙周病或口腔癌。

stomatogastric 口胃的

词根 stomat-（口腔的）+ gastric（胃的）
例句 Stomatogastric refers to the relationship or procedures related to both the mouth and stomach, such as in gastrointestinal diseases. 口胃相关指与口腔和胃相关的关系或手术，例如在胃肠道疾病中。

stomatoplasty 口腔成形术

词根 stomat-（口腔的）+ -plasty（成形）
例句 Stomatoplasty is a type of surgical procedure performed to repair or reconstruct parts of the mouth, such as after trauma. 口腔成形术是一种外科手术，用于修复或重建口腔的部分区域，如创伤后。

stomatorrhagia 口腔出血

词根 stomat-（口腔的）+ -rrhagia（出血）
例句 Stomatorrhagia is the abnormal bleeding from the mouth, often caused by oral trauma, ulcers, or gum disease. 口腔出血是指口腔异常出血，通常由口腔创伤、溃疡或牙龈疾病引起。

stomatology 口腔学

词根 stomat-（口腔的）+ -ology（学科）
例句 Stomatology is the branch of medicine that focuses on the study and treatment of oral diseases and conditions. 口腔学是医学的一个分支，专注于口腔疾病和病症的研究和治疗。

stomatoclast 口腔分解细胞

词根 stomat-（口腔的）+ -clast（破坏细胞）
例句 Stomatoclasts are cells that play a role in breaking down tissues in the oral cavity during certain pathological processes. 口腔分解细胞是指在某些病理过程中参与分解口腔组织的一类细胞。

stomatocyst 口腔囊肿

词根 stomat-（口腔的）+ cyst（囊肿）
例句 A stomatocyst is a cyst that forms within the oral cavity, often requiring surgical removal. 口腔囊肿是指在口腔内形成的囊肿，通常需要通过手术去除。

stomatorrhaphy 口腔缝合术

词根 stomat-（口腔的）+ -rrhaphy（缝合术）
例句 Stomatorrhaphy is a surgical procedure in which the mouth is sutured after an injury or surgery. 口腔缝合术是一种外科手术，在受伤或手术后进行口腔的缝合。

strep-（链状的）

streptococcus 链球菌

词根 strep-（链状的）+ -ococcus（球菌）
例句 Streptococcus is a genus of bacteria that forms chains and is responsible for various infections, such as strep throat. 链球菌是一种细菌属，形成链状，导致各种感染，如链球菌性喉炎。

streptomycin 链霉素

词根 strep-（链状的）+ -mycin（抗生素）
例句 Streptomycin is an antibiotic derived from the bacterium streptomyces griseus, used to treat tuberculosis. 链霉素是一种从灰色链霉菌中提取的抗生素，用于治疗结核病。

streptococcal pharyngitis 链球菌性咽炎

词根 strep-（链状的）+ -coccal（球菌的）+ pharyngitis（咽炎）
例句 Streptococcal pharyngitis is an infection of the throat caused by the streptococcus bacteria, leading to symptoms like sore throat and fever. 链球菌性咽炎是由链球菌引起的咽喉感染，表现为喉咙痛和发热等症状。

streptococcal pneumonia 链球菌性肺炎

词根 strep-（链状的）+ -coccal（球菌的）+ pneumonia（肺炎）
例句 Streptococcal pneumonia is a type of pneumonia caused by Streptococcus bacteria, leading to symptoms such as cough, fever, and difficulty breathing. 链球菌性肺炎是由链球菌引起的一种肺炎，表现为咳嗽、发热和呼吸困难等症状。

streptococcus mutans 变异链球菌

词根 strep-（链状的）+ -ococcus（球菌）+ mutans（变异的）
例句 Streptococcus mutans is a bacterium primarily found in the mouth and is a major contributor to tooth decay. Streptococcus mutans 是一种主要存在于口腔中的细菌，是导致蛀牙的主要原因。

streptococcal toxic shock syndrome 链球菌性毒性休克综合征

词根 strep-(链状的)+ -coccal(球菌的)+ toxic(毒性)+ shock(休克) + syndrome（综合征）
例句 Streptococcal toxic shock syndrome is a rare but lifethreatening condition caused by streptococcal bacteria, characterized by rapid onset of fever, low blood pressure, and organ failure. 链球菌性毒性休克综合征是一种罕见但危及生命的病症，由链球菌引起，特点是迅速出现发热、低血压和器官衰竭。

streptolysin 链球菌溶血素

词根 strep-（链状的）+ -lysin（溶解素）
例句 Streptolysin is a substance produced by streptococcal bacteria that can break down red blood cells. 链球菌溶血素是链球菌产生的一种物质，能够溶解红细胞。

streptodornase 链球菌脱氧核糖核酸酶

词根 strep-（链状的）+ -dornase（脱氧核糖核酸酶）
例句 Streptodornase is an enzyme produced by Streptococcus bacte-

ria that breaks down DNA. 链球菌脱氧核糖核酸酶是链球菌产生的一种酶，能够分解 DNA。

streptococcal endocarditis 链球菌性心内膜炎

词根 strep-（链状的）+ -coccal（球菌的）+ endocarditis（心内膜炎）

例句 Streptococcal endocarditis is an infection of the inner lining of the heart caused by streptococcus bacteria. 链球菌性心内膜炎是由链球菌引起的心脏内膜感染。

streptococcal meningitis 链球菌性脑膜炎

词根 strep-（链状的）+ -coccal（球菌的）+ meningitis（脑膜炎）

例句 Streptococcal meningitis is an infection of the meninges, the protective membranes surrounding the brain and spinal cord, caused by streptococcal bacteria. 链球菌性脑膜炎是由链球菌引起的脑膜（包围大脑和脊髓的保护膜）感染。

LMCHK Part 1　样题

A 70-year-old man who was previously healthy has a transurethral (trans-; urethr-) resection (re-; sect-) of the prostate under spinal anaesthesia (an-; aesthes-). In the recovery room, he is noted to be disorientated (dis-; orient-) with deteriorating mental alertness and hypotension (hypo-; -tension). Drainage from the urinary bladder is free flowing and pinkish in colour.

What is the MOST LIKELY cause of his condition?

(A) Hypoglycaemia (hypo-; glyc-; -emia)

(B) Hyponatraemia (hypo-; natr-; -emia)

(C) Inadequate (in-) analgesia (an-; alges-)

(D) Normal anaesthetic (an-; aesthes-) recovery

(E) Post-operative haemorrhage (heamo-; -rrhage)

中文翻译

一名既往健康的 70 岁男性患者在脊髓麻醉下接受了经尿道前列腺切除术。在恢复室中，医护人员发现其出现意识模糊、精神状态进行性恶化及低血压症状。其膀胱引流液通畅，呈淡粉色。

该患者病情最可能的病因是什么？

(A) 低血糖症
(B) 低钠血症
(C) 镇痛不足
(D) 正常麻醉恢复期
(E) 术后出血

题目和答案中出现的词根

trans-：跨；转
urethr-：尿道
re-：重新；反复
sect-：切（再次切指代切除）
an-：表示否定
aesthes-：感觉
dis-：离开
orient-：排列（离开排列表示不能辨别方向）
hypo-：低
-tension：张力；压力
glyc-：糖（这里指葡萄糖）
-emia：血症
natr-：钠

in-：表否定

alges-：疼痛

heamo-：血，是 hemo- 和 hemato- 的同义变异

sub-（下）

subcutaneous 皮下的

词根 sub-（下）+ cutaneous（皮肤的）

例句 Subcutaneous tissue lies beneath the skin and is involved in storing fat and insulating the body. 皮下组织位于皮肤下，参与储存脂肪和保温。

subdural 硬膜下的

词根 sub-（下）+ dural（硬膜的）

例句 A subdural hematoma occurs when blood collects between the brain and the dura mater, often due to trauma. 硬膜下血肿是指血液积聚在大脑和硬膜之间，通常由创伤引起。

subclavian 锁骨下的

词根 sub-（下）+ clavian（锁骨的）

例句 The subclavian artery is the blood vessel that supplies blood to the arms and chest. 锁骨下动脉是供应手臂和胸部血液的血管。

subinfection 次级感染

词根 sub-（下）+ infection（感染）

例句 Subinfection refers to a secondary infection that occurs in the body, often after the primary infection has been treated. 次级感染是指在主要感染治疗后发生的次级感染。

subconjunctival 结膜下的

词根 sub-（下）+ conjunctival（结膜的）

例句 A subconjunctival hemorrhage is the bleeding under the conjunctiva of the eye, often caused by trauma or strain. 结膜下出血是指眼结膜下方的出血，通常由创伤或用力过度引起。

subacute 亚急性的

词根 sub-（下）+ acute（急性的）

例句 Subacute conditions are those that are less severe than acute conditions but still require medical attention. 亚急性病症是指那些比急性病症轻微，但仍需医学关注的病症。

subaortic 主动脉下的

词根 sub-（下）+ aortic（主动脉的）

例句 A subaortic stenosis is a condition in which a narrowing occurs just below the aortic valve. 主动脉下狭窄是指发生在主动脉瓣下方的狭窄。

subdural hematoma 硬膜下血肿

词根 sub-（下）+ dural（硬膜的）+ hematoma（血肿）

例句 A subdural hematoma is a collection of blood under the dura mater, typically caused by head injury. 硬膜下血肿是指硬膜下方的血液积聚，通常由头部受伤引起。

subglottic 声门下的

词根 sub-（下）+ glottic（声门的）

例句 Subglottic stenosis is the narrowing of the airway below the vocal cords, which can cause breathing difficulties. 声门下狭窄是指声带下方气道的狭窄，可能导致呼吸困难。

subtherapeutic 亚治疗剂量的

词根 sub-（下）+ therapeutic（治疗的）

例句 Subtherapeutic doses of a medication are lower than the required doses for effective treatment. 亚治疗剂量是指低于有效治疗所需的药物剂量。

syn-（同步）

synergy 协同作用

词根 syn-（同步）+ -ergy（作用）

例句 Synergy occurs when two or more substances work together to produce a greater effect than if used alone. 协同作用指的是两种或多种物质一起工作时，产生的效果比单独使用时更强。

synthesis 合成

词根 syn-（同步）+ -thesis（构建）

例句 Synthesis refers to the process of combining two or more components to form a new substance, such as protein synthesis in cells. 合成是将两种或多种成分结合形成新物质的过程，例如细胞中的蛋白质合成。

synapse 突触

词根 syn-（同步）+ -apse（连接）

例句 A synapse is the junction between two nerve cells, where communication occurs through neurotransmitters. 突触是两个神经细胞之间的连接，通过神经递质进行通信。

syndrome 综合征

词根 syn-（同步）+ -drome（跑；行进）

例句 A syndrome is a group of symptoms that occur together and characterize a particular condition or disease. 综合征是一组共同发生的症状，通常用于描述特定的病症或疾病。

synchronize 同步

词根 syn-（同步）+ chron-（时间）

例句 To synchronize the heartbeats, electrical impulses are used to restore normal rhythm in patients with arrhythmia. 通过电冲击恢

复正常心律来同步心跳，特别是在心律失常患者中。

synarthrosis 不动关节

词根 syn-（同步）+ arthr-（关节）+ -osis（病理状态）
例句 Synarthrosis is a type of joint that allows little or no movement, such as in the sutures of the skull. 不动关节是一种几乎不允许或完全不允许活动的关节类型，如颅骨的缝合处。

syncretism 合成主义

词根 syn-（同步）+ -cretism（结合）
例句 Syncretism refers to the combination of different systems of thought or belief, such as the integration of various medical practices. 合成主义是指不同思想或信仰体系的结合，例如各种医学实践的融合。

syndrome-specific therapy 综合征特异性疗法

词根 syn-（同步）+ -drome（跑；行进）
例句 Syndrome-specific therapy targets the underlying causes of a particular syndrome to alleviate symptoms and improve the patient's condition. 综合征特异性疗法针对特定综合征的潜在病因进行治疗，以减轻症状并改善患者病情。

S

synov-（关节滑膜囊的）

synovial fluid 滑液

词根 synov-（关节滑膜囊的）+ fluid（液体）
例句 Synovial fluid is the viscous liquid found in the cavities of synovial joints, serving as a lubricant to reduce friction during movement. 滑液是存在于滑膜关节腔中的黏稠液体，作为润滑剂减少运动时的摩擦。

synovitis 滑膜炎

词根 synov-（关节滑膜囊的）+ -itis（炎症）

例句 Synovitis is the inflammation of the synovial membrane, often resulting in pain and swelling in the affected joint. 滑膜炎是滑膜的炎症，常导致受影响关节的疼痛和肿胀。

synovectomy 滑膜切除术

词根 synov-（关节滑膜囊的）+ -ectomy（切除）

例句 Synovectomy is a surgical procedure that involves the removal of the synovial membrane, often performed to treat chronic joint inflammation. 滑膜切除术是一种外科手术，涉及切除滑膜，通常用于治疗慢性关节炎症。

synovial membrane 滑膜

词根 synov-（关节滑膜囊的）+ membrane（膜）

例句 The synovial membrane lines the joint cavity and produces synovial fluid to lubricate the joints. 滑膜衬里关节腔，并产生滑液以润滑关节。

synovial joint 滑膜关节

词根 synov-（关节滑膜囊的）+ joint（关节）

例句 Synovial joints are the most common type of joint in the body, such as the knee and shoulder, that allow for a wide range of movement. 滑膜关节是体内最常见的关节类型，如膝关节和肩关节，允许广泛的运动范围。

synovial cyst 滑膜囊肿

词根 synov-（关节滑膜囊的）+ cyst（囊肿）

例句 A synovial cyst is a fluid-filled sac that forms near a joint, often causing discomfort and restricting movement. 滑膜囊肿是一种形成于关节附近的充满液体的囊性结构，常引起不适并限制运动。

synovitis deformans 变形性滑膜炎

词根 synov-（关节滑膜囊的）+ -itis（炎症）+ deformans（变形的）

例句 Synovitis deformans refers to a severe form of synovitis that leads to joint deformity and functional impairment. 变形性滑膜炎是指一种严重的滑膜炎症，导致关节变形和功能障碍。

synovial bursa 滑液囊

词根 synov-（关节滑膜囊的）+ bursa（囊）

例句 A synovial bursa is a small fluid-filled sac found between tissues such as bone, tendon, and skin to reduce friction. 滑液囊是一个小型充满液体的囊，位于骨骼、肌腱和皮肤之间，可减少摩擦。

synovial pannus 滑膜外翻

词根 synov-（关节滑膜囊的）+ pannus（外翻）

例句 Synovial pannus refers to an abnormal tissue growth in the joint cavity, often associated with conditions like rheumatoid arthritis. 滑膜外翻是指关节腔内异常的组织生长，通常与类风湿关节炎等病症相关。

synovial hyperplasia 滑膜增生

词根 synov-（关节滑膜囊的）+ hyperplasia（增生）

例句 Synovial hyperplasia is the abnormal increase in the number of synovial cells, often observed in inflammatory joint diseases. 滑膜增生是滑膜细胞数量的异常增加，常见于炎症性关节疾病中。

tachy-（快）

tachycardia 心动过速

词根 tachy-（快）+ -cardia（心脏）

例句 Tachycardia is a condition where the heart beats at an abnormally fast rate, usually over 100 beats per minute. 心动过速是一种心脏跳动异常加快的病症，通常心率超过每分钟 100 次。

tachypnea 呼吸急促

词根 tachy-（快）+ -pnea（呼吸）

例句 Tachypnea is the condition of rapid breathing, often seen in respiratory distress or anxiety. 呼吸急促是一种呼吸加快的病症，常见于呼吸窘迫或焦虑状态。

tachyphylaxis 药物耐受性增强

词根 tachy-（快）+ -phylaxis（防御）

例句 Tachyphylaxis refers to the rapid decrease in the response to a drug after repeated administration, leading to reduced effectiveness. 药物耐受性增强是指药物重复使用后机体对其反应迅速减弱，导致效果降低。

tachyarrhythmia 快速心律失常

词根 tachy-（快）+ arrhythmia（心律失常）

例句 Tachyarrhythmia is a type of arrhythmia characterized by an excessively rapid heart rate. 快速心律失常是一种以异常快速心跳为特征的心律失常类型。

tachylogia 语言过快

词根 tachy-（快）+ -logia（语言）

例句 Tachylogia is a speech disorder where a person speaks too quickly, often making it difficult for others to understand. 语言过快是一种语言障碍，指一个人说话过快，通常导致别人难以理解。

tachysystole 快速心跳

词根 tachy-（快）+ systole（收缩）
例句 Tachysystole refers to the condition of rapid heartbeats occurring during the contraction phase of the heart. 快速心跳是指心脏收缩期出现的快速跳动。

tachyphonia 声音过快

词根 tachy-（快）+ -phonia（声音）
例句 Tachyphonia is the condition where an individual speaks rapidly, affecting the clarity and coherence of their speech. 声音过快是指个体说话过快，影响言语的清晰度和连贯性。

tachygenesis 快速生成

词根 tachy-（快）+ -genesis（生成）
例句 Tachygenesis refers to the rapid onset or development of symptoms or disease in a patient. 快速生成指的是患者症状或疾病的迅速发生或发展。

tachykinetic 快速运动的

词根 tachy-（快）+ kinetic（运动的）
例句 Tachykinetic disorders refer to conditions where movement or motor activity occurs at an accelerated rate. 速动障碍是指运动或肢体活动以异常加快的速率发生的一类病症。

PLAB 1 样题

A 23-year-old woman has worsening diarrhoea (dia-; -rrheoea) with blood and mucus for 2 months and is seen in the GP surgery. She has abdominal pain and bloating. She has no weight loss. Her abdomen is soft and there is mild left-sided tenderness on deep palpation (palp-; -ation). She has active bowel sounds.

Investigations:

Haemoglobin (haemo-; -globin) 102 g/L (115–150)

White cell count 11.2 × 10^9/L (4.0–11.0)

Platelets (plate-; -let) 395 × 10^9/L (150–400)

CRP 78 mg/L (<5)

Which is the most appropriate diagnostic investigation?

Colonoscopy (colon-; -scopy)

Faecal calprotectin (cal-; -in)

Faecal occult blood

Helicobacter (helico-; -bacter) pylori stool antigen

Stool culture and sensitivity

中文翻译

一名 23 岁女性因 2 个月来腹泻加重伴血便和黏液，在全科医生诊室就诊。她有腹痛和腹胀，无体重减轻。腹部柔软，深部触诊时左侧有轻度压痛。肠鸣音活跃。

检查结果：

血红蛋白 102 g/L（正常范围：115 ～ 150）

白细胞计数 11.2 × 10^9/L（正常范围：4.0 ～ 11.0）

血小板 395 × 10^9/L（正常范围：150 ～ 400）

C 反应蛋白（CRP） 78 mg/L（正常范围：<5）

以下哪项是最适当的诊断检查？

(A) 结肠镜检查

(B) 粪便钙卫蛋白检测

(C) 粪便隐血试验

(D) 幽门螺杆菌粪便抗原检测

(E) 粪便培养和敏感性测试

题目和答案中出现的词根

dia-：通过

-rrheoea：流出，是 rrhea 的同义变异

palp-：触摸

-ation：表示动作（触摸的动作即为触诊）

haemo-：血，是 hemo- 和 hemato- 的同义变异

-globin：球蛋白

plate-：板状的

-lets：小

colon-：结肠

-scopy：镜

cal-：钙

-in：化合物

helico-：螺旋

-bacter：杆菌

-taxis（定向移动）

chemotaxis 趋化性

词根 chemo-（化学）+ -taxis（定向移动）

例句 Chemotaxis refers to the movement of cells or organisms in response to chemical stimuli, often seen in immune cells targeting infection. 趋化性是指细胞或生物体对化学刺激的定向移动，常见于免疫细胞对感染的响应。

phototaxis 光向性

词根 photo-（光）+ -taxis（定向移动）

例句 Phototaxis is the movement of an organism toward or away from light, commonly seen in plants and certain microorganisms. 光向性是指生物体朝向或远离光源的移动，常见于植物和某些微生物。

geotaxis 地向性

词根 geo-（地理）+ -taxis（定向移动）

例句 Geotaxis refers to the movement of an organism in response to gravity, helping it to orient itself. 地向性是指生物体对重力刺激产生的定向移动，帮助其定向。

rheotaxis 水流定向性

词根 rheo-（水流）+ -taxis（定向移动）

例句 Rheotaxis is the ability of aquatic organisms to orient themselves in response to the direction of water flow. 水流定向性是水生生物体对水流方向的定向能力。

aerotaxis 气体定向性

词根 aero-（气体）+ -taxis（定向移动）

例句 Aerotaxis is the movement of microorganisms or cells toward or away from oxygen or other gases. 气体定向性是指微生物或细胞对氧气或其他气体的趋向或远离运动。

thermotaxis 温度定向性

词根 thermo-（温度）+ -taxis（定向移动）

例句 Thermotaxis is the movement of an organism in response to temperature gradients, such as bacteria moving toward warmer areas. 温度定向性是指生物体对温度梯度的反应性移动，例如细菌朝向较温暖的区域移动。

hydrotaxis 湿度定向性

词根 hydro-（水）+ -taxis（定向移动）

例句 Hydrotaxis is the movement of organisms toward or away from areas of higher or lower humidity. 湿度定向性是生物体朝向或远离湿度较高或较低的区域移动。

magnetotaxis 磁向性

词根 magneto-（磁）+ -taxis（定向移动）

例句 Magnetotaxis is the ability of certain bacteria to orient and move according to magnetic fields. 磁向性是某些细菌根据磁场定向移动的能力。

PLAB 1　样题

A 74-year-old man has a severe headache (-ache) of sudden onset and is seen in the Emergency Department. He had no preceding (pre-; ced-) symptoms. His temperature is 37.5℃. He has mild left-sided weakness at power grade 4/5 in both upper and lower limbs.

Which is the most likely diagnosis?

(A) Benign intracranial (intra-; crani-) hypertension (hyper-; -tension)

(B) Brain tumour

(C) Encephalitis (encephal-; -itis)

(D) Meningitis (mening-; -itis)

(E) Subarachnoid (sub-; arachn-; -oid) haemorrhage (haemo-; -rrahge)

中文翻译

一名 74 岁男性因突发严重头痛在急诊科就诊。他此前无任何先兆症状。体温 37.5℃。他有轻度左侧肢体无力，上肢和下肢肌力均为 4/5 级。

以下哪项是最可能的诊断？

(A) 良性颅内压增高症
(B) 脑肿瘤
(C) 脑炎
(D) 脑膜炎
(E) 蛛网膜下腔出血

题目和答案中出现的词根

ache-：疼痛
pre-：在……之前
ced-：行走
intra-：在……内
crani-：颅骨
hyper-：高
-tension：张力；压力
encephal-：脑
-itis：炎症
mening-：脑膜
sub-：在……下
arachn-：蜘蛛
-oid：类似的
haemo-：血，是 hemo- 和 hemato- 的同义变异

-rrahge：流出

tel-（末端）

telomere 端粒

词根 tel-（末端）+ -mere（部分）

例句 Telomeres are protective caps at the ends of chromosomes that shorten as cells divide, playing a role in aging. 端粒是染色体末端的保护性结构，在细胞分裂时会缩短，参与衰老过程。

telophase 分裂末期

词根 tel-（末端）+ -phase（阶段）

例句 Telophase is the final stage of cell division, where the chromatids are fully separated and the nuclear envelope reforms. 分裂末期是细胞分裂的最后阶段，染色单体完全分离，核膜重新形成。

telangiectasia 毛细血管扩张症

词根 tel-（末端）+ angio-（血管）+ -ectasia（扩张）

例句 Telangiectasia refers to the visible dilation of small blood vessels, often found on the skin as spider veins. 毛细血管扩张症是指小血管可见性扩张，常表现为皮肤上的蜘蛛状静脉。

telomere shortening 端粒缩短

词根 tel-（末端）+ -mere（部分）+ shortening（缩短）

例句 Telomere shortening occurs during cell division and is associated with aging and the risk of certain diseases. 端粒缩短发生在细胞分裂过程中，并与衰老和某些疾病的风险相关。

telescoping 套叠

词根 tel-（末端）+ -scoping（检查）

例句 Telescoping refers to the process where one part of a structure slides into another, often seen in medical imaging or certain gastrointestinal disorders. 套叠指的是一种结构的一个部分滑入另一个部分，常见于医学影像或某些胃肠疾病。

telangiectatic melanoma 毛细血管扩张性黑色素瘤

词根 tel-（末端）+ angio-（血管）+ -ectasia（扩张）+ melanoma（黑色素瘤）

例句 Telangiectatic melanoma is a rare type of melanoma where the tumor has visible blood vessels on its surface. 毛细血管扩张性黑色素瘤是一种罕见的黑色素瘤类型，肿瘤表面可见血管。

telomere biology 端粒生物学

词根 tel-（末端）+ -mere（部分）+ biology（生物学）

例句 Telomere biology is the study of the role of telomeres in cellular aging, genome stability, and cancer progression. 端粒生物学是研究端粒在细胞衰老、基因组稳定性和癌症进展中的作用的学科。

telocentric chromosome 末端着丝粒染色体

词根 tel-（末端）+ -centric（中心的）+ chromosome（染色体）

例句 A telocentric chromosome has the centromere located at or near the end of the chromosome. 末端着丝粒染色体是指着丝粒位于染色体的末端或接近末端的位置。

T

telophase checkpoint 分裂末期检查点

词根 tel-（末端）+ -phase（阶段）+ checkpoint（检查点）

例句 The telophase checkpoint is a control mechanism in the cell cycle that ensures proper chromosomal segregation before cell division completes. 分裂末期检查点是细胞周期中的一个控制机制，确保在细胞分裂完成之前染色体正确分离。

telomerase 端粒酶

词根 tel-（末端）+ -merase（酶）

例句 Telomerase is an enzyme that adds repetitive sequences to the ends of chromosomes, helping to maintain telomere length. 端粒酶是一种将重复序列添加到染色体末端的酶，帮助维持端粒的长度。

telangi-（末端的血管；毛细血管）

telangiectasia 毛细血管扩张症

词根 tel-（末端）+ angio-（血管）+ -ectasia（扩张）

例句 Telangiectasia refers to the dilation of small blood vessels, often visible as red or purple lines on the skin. 毛细血管扩张症是指小血管的扩张，通常表现为皮肤上的红色或紫色线条。

telangiectatic 毛细血管扩张的

词根 tel-（末端）+ angio-（血管）+ -ectatic（扩张的）

例句 Telangiectatic lesions are often seen in conditions such as rosacea, where the small blood vessels on the skin become visibly en larged. 毛细血管扩张病变常见于玫瑰痤疮等疾病中，表现为皮肤上的小血管明显扩张。

telangiectatic rosacea 毛细血管扩张性玫瑰痤疮

词根 tel-（末端）+ angio-（血管）+ -ectatic（扩张的）+ rosacea（玫瑰痤疮）

例句 Telangiectatic rosacea is a form of rosacea that causes visible blood vessels and redness, particularly on the nose and cheeks. 毛细血管扩张性玫瑰痤疮是玫瑰痤疮的一种形式，其特征为面部（尤其是鼻部和脸颊）可见扩张的血管及泛红现象。

telangiectasia associated with cirrhosis 与肝硬化相关的毛细血管扩张症

词根 tel-（末端）+ angio-（血管）+ -ectasia（扩张）

例句 Telangiectasia associated with cirrhosis is often seen on the skin as a result of increased pressure in the blood vessels. 与肝硬化

相关的毛细血管扩张症通常表现为皮肤上的红色血管线，其因血管内压力增加而形成。

telangiectatic spider veins 毛细血管扩张性蜘蛛静脉

词根 tel-（末端）+ angio-（血管）+ -ectatic（扩张的）

例句 Telangiectatic spider veins are small, dilated blood vessels that resemble a spider web, often found on the legs or face. 毛细血管扩张性蜘蛛静脉是扩张的小型血管，形似蜘蛛网，常见于腿部或面部。

telangiectatic blood vessel 毛细血管扩张性血管

词根 tel-（末端）+ angio-（血管）+ -ectatic（扩张的）

例句 Telangiectatic blood vessels are small vessels that become abnormally enlarged and are typically treated with laser therapy. 毛细血管扩张性血管是指那些异常增大的小血管，通常通过激光进行治疗。

telangiectatic hemangioma 毛细血管扩张性血管瘤

词根 tel-（末端）+ angio-（血管）+ -ectasia（扩张）+ hemangioma（血管瘤）

T

例句 Telangiectatic hemangioma is a type of benign vascular tumor that appears as red or purple spots on the skin. 毛细血管扩张性血管瘤是一种良性的血管肿瘤，表现为皮肤上的红色或紫色斑点。

telangiectatic change 毛细血管扩张性改变

词根 tel-（末端）+ angio-（血管）+ -ectasia（扩张）

例句 Telangiectatic changes in the skin are often indicative of underlying health conditions, such as liver disease or high blood pressure. 皮肤的毛细血管扩张性改变常常表明潜在的健康问题，如肝脏疾病或高血压。

telangiectatic pustules 毛细血管扩张性脓疱

词根 tel-（末端）+ angio-（血管）+ -ectasia（扩张的）+ pustules（脓疱）

例句 Telangiectatic pustules are small, pus-filled bumps that occur on the skin, often linked to rosacea. 毛细血管扩张性脓疱是皮肤上小的、充满脓液的凸起，通常与玫瑰痤疮相关。

telo-（完成）

telophase 分裂末期

词根 telo-（完成）+ -phase（阶段）

例句 Telophase is the final stage of mitosis, where the daughter cells are formed, and the nuclear membrane reforms. 分裂末期是有丝分裂的最后阶段，子细胞形成并且核膜重新形成。

telomerase 端粒酶

词根 telo-（完成）+ -merase（酶）

例句 Telomerase is an enzyme responsible for maintaining the length of telomeres, enabling cells to continue dividing. 端粒酶是一种负责维持端粒长度的酶，允许细胞继续分裂。

telomere extension 端粒延长

词根 telo-（完成）+ -mere（部分）+ extension（延长）

例句 Telomere extension refers to the process of lengthening the telomeres in cells, often seen in cancer cells. 端粒延长是指在细胞中延长端粒的过程，常见于癌细胞。

telomere therapy 端粒治疗

词根 telo-（完成）+ -mere（部分）+ therapy（治疗）

例句 Telomere therapy is being studied as a potential treatment to delay aging and treat age-related diseases by restoring telomere length. 端粒治疗正在作为一种潜在的治疗方法被研究，旨在通过恢复端粒长度延缓衰老并治疗与年龄相关的疾病。

telogenic growth 端粒生长

词根 telo-（完成）+ -genic（产生的）+ growth（生长）

例句 Telogenic growth refers to the phase in hair growth where the hair reaches its maximum length and prepares to fall out. 退行期生长是毛发生长周期中的最后阶段，其核心特征是毛发停止生长并逐渐脱落。

telophase stage 分裂末期阶段

词根 telo-（完成）+ -phase（阶段）

例句 The telophase stage of mitosis is when the chromosomes reach the poles, and the nuclear membrane reforms. 分裂末期阶段是有丝分裂中染色体到达极点并且核膜重新形成的阶段。

telocentric centromere 末端着丝粒

词根 telo-（完成）+ centromere（着丝粒）

例句 A telocentric centromere is a type of centromere located at or near the end of a chromosome. 末端着丝粒是一种位于染色体末端或接近末端的着丝粒类型。

telogen effluvium 休止期脱发

词根 telo-（完成）+ -gen（产生）+ effluvium（脱发）

例句 Telogen effluvium is a form of hair loss that occurs when a large number of hair follicles enter the resting phase at the same time. 休止期脱发是一种脱发形式，当大量毛囊同时进入休止期时发生。

tens-（拉张力）

tension 张力

词根 tens-（拉张力）+ -ion（名词后缀）

例句 Tension refers to the force exerted when something is stretched, often used to describe the force within muscles or blood vessels. 张力指的是当某物被拉伸时产生的力，通常用于描述肌肉或血管内的力。

tensiometer 张力计

词根 tens-（拉张力）+ -iometer（测量仪器）

例句 A tensiometer is an instrument used to measure the surface tension of liquids, such as measuring the force of a soap film. 张力计是一种用于测量液体表面张力的仪器，可测量肥皂膜的力。

tension-type headache 张力性头痛

词根 tens-（张力）+ type（类型）+ headache（头痛）

例句 Tension-type headaches are the most common form of headache, characterized by a constant dull pain and a feeling of tightness around the head. 张力性头痛是最常见的头痛类型，特征是持续的钝痛和头部周围的紧绷感。

hypertension 高血压

词根 hyper-（过高）+ tens-（拉张力）+ -ion（名词后缀）

例句 Hypertension is a condition where the force of the blood against the artery walls is consistently too high, putting strain on the heart and blood vessels. 高血压是一种血液对动脉壁的压力持续过高的情况，给心脏和血管带来负担。

tension pneumothorax 张力性气胸

词根 tens-（张力）+ pneumothorax（气胸）

例句 Tension pneumothorax occurs when air trapped in the chest cavity creates pressure on the lungs and heart, leading to life-threatening complications. 张力性气胸是指空气被困在胸腔中，产生对肺部和心脏的压力，导致危及生命的并发症。

tensile strength 抗拉强度

词根 tens-（拉张力）+ -ile（形容词后缀）+ strength（强度）

例句 Tensile strength refers to the maximum stress that a material can withstand while being stretched before it breaks. 抗拉强度指的是材料在拉伸至断裂前能够承受的最大应力。

tension headache 张力性头痛

词根 tens-（张力）+ headache（头痛）

例句 Tension headache is a common type of headache caused by stress, tight muscles, and poor posture. 张力性头痛是由压力、肌肉紧张和不良姿势引起的常见头痛类型。

tensiometry 张力测量法

词根 tens-（拉张力）+ -ometry（测量法）

例句 Tensiometry is the technique used to measure the amount of tension in a material, such as the surface tension of a liquid or the force exerted on a surface. 张力测量法是用于测量材料中张力的方法，例如测量液体的表面张力或施加在表面的力。

myotension 肌肉张力

词根 myo-（肌肉）+ tens-（拉张力）

例句 Myotension refers to the tension in the muscles, which can increase due to stress or physical exertion. 肌肉张力是指肌肉中的张力，可能因压力或身体活动而增加。

terato-（畸）

teratology 畸形学

词根 terato-（畸）+ -logy（学科）

例句 Teratology is the study of congenital abnormalities and birth defects that affect the development of embryos and fetuses. 畸形学是研究影响胚胎和胎儿发育的先天性异常和出生缺陷的学科。

teratogen 致畸物质

词根 terato-（畸）+ -gen（产生）

例句 A teratogen is an agent or factor that causes developmental abnormalities in the fetus, such as alcohol or certain drugs. 致畸物质是指导致胎儿发育异常的因素或物质，如酒精或某些药物。

teratogenesis 致畸过程

词根 terato-（畸）+ -genesis（生成）

例句 Teratogenesis is the process by which teratogens cause developmental defects in embryos or fetuses. 致畸过程是指致畸物质导致胚胎或胎儿发育缺陷的过程。

teratoma 畸胎瘤

词根 terato-（畸）+ -oma（肿瘤）

例句 A teratoma is a type of tumor that contains tissue from different germ layers, such as hair, teeth, and muscle. 畸胎瘤是一种包含不同胚层组织（如毛发、牙齿和肌肉）的肿瘤。

teratogenicity 致畸性

词根 terato-（畸）+ -genic（生成的）+ -ity（名词后缀）

例句 The teratogenicity of a substance refers to its potential to cause birth defects when exposure occurs during pregnancy. 致畸性指的是某物质在怀孕期间接触时可能引起出生缺陷的性质。

teratomorph 畸形形态

词根 terato-（畸）+ -morph（形态）

例句 A teratomorph is a form or shape that resembles a teratoma, characterized by the presence of multiple tissue types. 畸形形态是指类似于畸胎瘤的形态，特征是存在多种组织类型。

teratogenic effect 致畸效应

词根 terato-（畸）+ genic（生成的）+ effect（效应）

例句 The teratogenic effect of certain drugs can lead to severe birth defects, particularly if used during the first trimester of pregnancy. 某些药物的致畸效应可能导致严重的出生缺陷，特别是在妊娠早期使用时。

teratogenic agent 致畸因子

词根 terato-（畸）+ genic（生成的）+ agent（因子）

例句 Teratogenic agents include environmental factors such as radiation, chemicals, and viruses that can cause birth defects. 致畸因子包括环境因素，如辐射、化学品和病毒，可能导致出生缺陷。

teratogenic syndrome 致畸综合征

词根 terato-（畸）+ genic（生成的）+ syndrome（综合征）
例句 Teratogenic syndrome is a condition caused by exposure to teratogens during pregnancy, leading to a variety of congenital abnormalities. 致畸综合征是由怀孕期间接触致畸物质引起的病症，导致胎儿多种先天性异常。

teratogenicity testing 致畸性测试

词根 terato-（畸）+ -genic（生成的）+ -ity（名词后缀）+ testing（测试）
例句 Teratogenicity testing is conducted to evaluate whether a substance can cause birth defects when used during pregnancy. 致畸性测试用于评估某种物质在怀孕期间使用时是否会导致出生缺陷。

PLAB 1 样题

A 34-year-old woman has had secondary amenorrhoea (a-; meno-; -rrhoea) for 8 months. She has lost 6 kg in weight despite having a good appetite.

Which is the most likely diagnosis?

(A) Hyperthyroidism (hyper-; thy-; -oid; -ism)

(B) Hypogonadism (hypo-; gonad-; -ism)

(C) Polycystic (poly-; cyst-) ovary syndrome

(D) Premature (pre-) ovarian failure

(E) Prolactinoma (pro-; lactin-; -oma)

中文翻译

一名34岁女性因8个月来继发性闭经就诊。尽管食欲良好，但她体重减轻了6 kg。以下哪项是最可能的诊断？

(A) 甲状腺功能亢进症

(B) 性腺功能减退症

(C) 多囊卵巢综合征

(D) 卵巢早衰

(E) 催乳素瘤

题目和答案中出现的词根

a-：表示否定

meno-：每个月

rrhoea：流出，是rrhea的同义变异

hyper-：高

thy-：盾

-oid：类似的

-ism：表示状态

poly-：多

cyst-：囊

pre-：在……之前

pro-：在……之前

lactin-：催乳

-oma：瘤

tetra-（四个）

tetracycline 四环素

词根 tetra-（四个）+ -cycline（环素）

例句 Tetracycline is an antibiotic used to treat a variety of infections, particularly those caused by bacteria. 四环素是一种用于治疗多种感染的抗生素，特别是由细菌引起的感染。

tetrahedron 四面体

词根 tetra-（四个）+ -hedron（面）

例句 A tetrahedron is a polyhedron with four triangular faces, commonly seen in molecular structures. 四面体是一种具有四个三角形面的多面体，常见于分子结构中。

tetracyclic 四环的

词根 tetra-（四个）+ cyclic（环的）

例句 Tetracyclic compounds contain four interconnected rings of atoms, often studied in organic chemistry. 四环化合物包含四个相互连接的原子环，是有机化学中常研究的对象。

tetraplegia 四肢麻痹

词根 tetra-（四个）+ -plegia（麻痹）

例句 Tetraplegia, also known as quadriplegia, is paralysis that affects all four limbs, typically caused by spinal cord injury. 四肢麻痹，又称四肢瘫痪，是一种影响四肢的麻痹，通常由脊髓损伤引起。

tetrad 四分体

词根 tetra-（四个）+ -ad（名词后缀）

例句 A tetrad refers to a group of four, often used to describe the four chromatids in meiosis during genetic recombination. 四分体是指由四个部分组成的一组结构，常用于描述在减数分裂过程中基因重组时的四条染色单体。

tetrahydrocannabinol 四氢大麻酚

词根 tetra-（四个）+ hydro-（氢）+ cannabinol（大麻酚）

例句 Tetrahydrocannabinol is the primary psychoactive compound found in cannabis, responsible for its intoxicating effects. 四氢大麻酚是大麻中的主要致幻成分，负责产生致醉效果。

tetravac 四联疫苗

词根 tetra-（四个）+ -vac（疫苗）

例句 Tetravac is a vaccine that protects against four different diseases, often administered during childhood. 四联疫苗是一种可以预防四种不同疾病的疫苗，通常在儿童时期接种。

tetrameter 四音步诗行

词根 tetra-（四个）+ -meter（测量）

例句 Tetrameter refers to a line of poetry consisting of four metrical feet, commonly used in classical poetry. 四音步诗行是指由四个韵步组成的诗行，通常用于古典诗歌中。

tetracarbamide 四氨基脲

词根 tetra-（四个）+ carbamide（氨基脲）

例句 Tetracarbamide is a chemical compound containing four carbamide groups, used in industrial and medical applications. 四氨基脲是一种含有四个氨基脲基团的化学化合物，广泛应用于工业和医疗。

tetrastichous 四列排列的

词根 tetra-（四个）+ stichous（排列的）

例句 Tetrastichous refers to a type of leaf arrangement in which the leaves are arranged in four rows. 四列排列指的是一种叶子排列方式，指叶子按四行排列。

therm（o）-（热）

thermometer 温度计

词根 therm-（热）+ -meter（测量仪器）

例句 A thermometer is a device used to measure temperature, commonly used in medical settings to check body temperature. 温度计是一种用于测量温度的设备，常用于医疗场所检查体温。

thermodynamics 热力学

词根 therm-（热）+ -dynamics（力学）

例句 Thermodynamics is the study of heat and its relation to energy and work. 热力学是研究热量及其与能量和功的关系的学科。

hyperthermia 高热

词根 hyper-（过高）+ therm-（热）+ -ia（病理状态）

例句 Hyperthermia is a condition in which the body temperature rises above the normal range, often caused by prolonged exposure to heat. 高热是指体温升高超过正常范围的状况，通常由长时间暴露于高温环境引起。

hypothermia 低体温

词根 hypo-（低）+ therm-（热）+ -ia（病理状态）

例句 Hypothermia occurs when the body temperature drops below normal levels, typically due to prolonged exposure to cold weather. 低体温是指体温低于正常水平，通常是由于长时间暴露在寒冷的环境中。

thermoregulation 热调节

词根 thermo-（热）+ regulation（调节）

例句 Thermoregulation is the process by which the body maintains its internal temperature within a certain range, despite changes in the external environment. 热调节是指身体通过自我调节保持内部温度在一定范围内的过程，以应对外部环境变化。

thermostat 恒温器

词根 thermo-（热）+ stat-（静止）

例句 A thermostat is a device used to regulate the temperature of a system, such as in heating or cooling appliances. 恒温器是一种用于调节系统温度的设备，在加热或冷却设备中使用。

thermogenesis 产热

词根 thermo-（热）+ -genesis（生成）

例句 Thermogenesis refers to the production of heat in the body, especially during processes such as digestion or exercise. 产热是指身体中热量的生成，尤其是在消化或运动过程中。

thermocouple 热电偶

词根 thermo-（热）+ couple（对）

例句 A thermocouple is a device used to measure temperature by using the voltage difference between two different metals. 热电偶是一种通过测量两种不同金属之间的电压差来测量温度的设备。

thermocautery 热灼术

词根 thermo-（热）+ cautery（烧灼术）

例句 Thermocautery is a technique used in surgery to burn or coagulate tissue using heat. 热灼术是一种在手术中使用热量烧灼或凝固组织的技术。

thermoplasty 热成形术

词根 thermo-（热）+ -plasty（成形）

例句 Thermoplasty is a medical procedure that uses heat to reshape tissues, such as in the treatment of certain lung conditions. 热成形术是一种使用热量重新塑形组织的医疗手段，在治疗某些肺部疾病时使用。

thorax-（胸的）

thoracic 胸的

词根 thorax-（胸部）+ -ic（形容词后缀）

例句 Thoracic surgery involves procedures that treat conditions affecting the chest, including the heart, lungs, and esophagus. 胸外科手术包括治疗影响胸部（包括心脏、肺和食管）的手术。

thoracotomy 开胸术

词根 thorax-（胸部）+ -otomy（切开术）

例句 Thoracotomy is a surgical procedure in which the chest is opened to access the organs within it, such as the lungs or heart. 开胸术是一种外科手术，通过开胸来接触胸腔内的器官，如肺或心脏。

thoracentesis 胸腔穿刺

词根 thorax-（胸部）+ -centesis（穿刺术）

T

例句 Thoracentesis is a procedure to remove fluid from the space between the lungs and chest wall, often to treat pleural effusion. 胸腔穿刺是一种从肺和胸壁之间的空间中抽取液体的手术，常用于治疗胸腔积液。

thoracalgia 胸痛

词根 thorax-（胸部）+ -algia（痛）

例句 Thoracalgia refers to pain in the chest, which can be caused by a variety of conditions such as heart disease or muscle strain. 胸痛指的是胸部的疼痛，可能由多种病因引起，如心脏病或肌肉拉伤。

thoracic cavity 胸腔

词根 thorax-（胸部）+ cavity（腔）

例句 The thoracic cavity is the chamber within the chest that houses the heart, lungs, and other vital organs. 胸腔是胸部内的腔室，容纳心脏、肺和其他重要器官。

thoracolumbar 胸腰的

词根 thorax-（胸部）+ lumbar（腰部的）
例句 Thoracolumbar refers to the region of the spine that includes both the chest and lower back areas. 胸腰部是指包括胸部和下背部区域的脊柱部位。

thoracostomy 胸腔造口术

词根 thorax-（胸部）+ -stomy（造口术）
例句 Thoracostomy is the surgical creation of an opening in the chest to treat conditions such as a collapsed lung. 胸腔造口术是通过在胸部创建开口来治疗肺萎缩等疾病的外科手术。

thoracoplasty 胸廓成形术

词根 thorax-（胸部）+ -plasty（修复术）
例句 Thoracoplasty is a surgical procedure aimed at reconstructing or reshaping the chest wall. 胸廓成形术是一种旨在重建或重塑胸壁的外科手术。

thoracoscopy 胸腔镜检查

词根 thorax-（胸部）+ -scopy（检查）
例句 Thoracoscopy is a minimally invasive procedure using a small camera to inspect the chest and diagnose conditions such as lung cancer. 胸腔镜检查是一种微创手术，使用小型摄像头检查胸腔并诊断肺癌等疾病。

thoracic outlet syndrome 胸廓出口综合征

词根 thorax-（胸部）+ outlet（出口）+ syndrome（综合征）
例句 Thoracic outlet syndrome is a condition caused by the compression of nerves or blood vessels in the thoracic outlet. 胸廓出口

综合征是一种由胸廓出口处的神经或血管压迫引起的疾病。

thoracobrachial 胸臂的

词根 thorax-（胸部）+ brachial（臂部的）

例句 The thoracobrachial region refers to the area of the body where the chest and arm meet, particularly in terms of nerves and blood vessels. 胸臂部是指胸部和手臂交汇的区域，特指神经和血管的分布。

thoracic aorta 胸主动脉

词根 thorax-（胸部）+ aorta（主动脉）

例句 The thoracic aorta is the part of the aorta that runs through the chest, carrying oxygenated blood from the heart to the rest of the body. 胸主动脉是通过胸部的主动脉，将含氧血液从心脏输送到身体其他部位。

thrombo-（凝血的）

thrombosis 血栓形成

词根 thrombo-（凝血的）+ -osis（病理状态）

例句 Thrombosis is the formation of a blood clot inside a blood vessel, which can block blood flow. 血栓形成是血液在血管内形成血块，可能阻塞血流。

thrombolysis 溶栓治疗

词根 thrombo-（凝血的）+ -lysis（溶解）

例句 Thrombolysis is a treatment used to dissolve blood clots and restore normal blood flow in blocked arteries. 溶栓治疗是一种用于溶解血栓并恢复阻塞动脉正常血流的治疗方法。

thrombocytopenia 血小板减少症

词根 thrombo-（凝血的）+ cyto-（细胞）+ -penia（缺乏）

例句 Thrombocytopenia is a condition where there is a low platelet count in the blood, increasing the risk of bleeding. 血小板减少症是血液中血小板计数低的情况，增加出血的风险。

thromboembolic 血栓栓塞的

词根 thrombo-（凝血的）+ embolic（栓塞的）

例句 Thromboembolic disorders occur when a blood clot breaks loose and travels through the bloodstream, blocking other vessels. 血栓栓塞性疾病发生在血块脱落并通过血液循环阻塞其他血管时。

thrombin 凝血酶

词根 thrombo-（凝血的）+ -in（化学物质）

例句 Thrombin is an enzyme that plays a key role in blood clotting by converting fibrinogen into fibrin. 凝血酶是在血液凝固中发挥关键作用的酶，它能将纤维蛋白原转化为纤维蛋白。

thromboangiitis 血栓性血管炎

词根 thrombo-（凝血的）+ angi-（血管）+ -itis（炎症）

例句 Thromboangiitis is the inflammation of blood vessels associated with the formation of blood clots. 血栓性血管炎是与血栓形成相关的血管炎症。

thrombophilia 血栓倾向症

词根 thrombo-（凝血的）+ -philia（喜好）

例句 Thrombophilia is a condition where an individual has an increased tendency to form blood clots. 血栓倾向症是一种个体易于形成血栓的病症。

thromboelastography 血栓弹力图

词根 thrombo-（凝血的）+ elast-（弹性）+ -graphy（记录）

例句 Thromboelastography is a test that measures the viscoelastic properties of blood clot formation. 血栓弹力图是一种测试，测量

血液凝固过程中的黏弹性特征。

thrombospondin 血栓蛋白

词根 thrombo-（凝血的）+ spondin（蛋白质）

例句 Thrombospondin is a glycoprotein involved in blood clot formation and tissue repair. 血栓蛋白是一种糖蛋白，参与血液凝固和组织修复。

thromboembolic disease 血栓栓塞性疾病

词根 thrombo-（凝血的）+ embolic（栓塞的）+ disease（疾病）

例句 Thromboembolic disease occurs when blood clots travel through the bloodstream and cause blockages in other areas of the body, such as the lungs or brain. 血栓栓塞性疾病是指血凝块在血流中移动，并在身体其他部位（如肺部或脑部）造成阻塞的疾病。

thy-（盾状的）

thyroid 甲状腺

词根 thy-（盾状的）+ -roid（类的）

例句 The thyroid is a butterfly-shaped gland located in the neck that produces hormones regulating metabolism. 甲状腺是一个位于颈部的蝴蝶形腺体，分泌调节代谢的激素。

thymectomy 胸腺切除术

词根 thy-（胸腺的）+ -ectomy（切除术）

例句 Thymectomy is a surgical procedure that involves the removal of the thymus gland, often used to treat thymoma. 胸腺切除术是一种切除胸腺的手术，常用于治疗胸腺瘤。

thymoma 胸腺瘤

词根 thy-（胸腺的）+ -oma（肿瘤）

例句 Thymoma is a rare tumor that originates in the thymus gland and may affect the immune system. 胸腺瘤是一种罕见的肿瘤，

起源于胸腺，可能影响免疫系统。

thymosin 胸腺素

词根 thy-（胸腺的）+ -osin（蛋白）

例句 Thymosin is a protein produced by the thymus that is essential for the development of T-cells. 胸腺素是胸腺分泌的蛋白质，对T 细胞的发育至关重要。

thymocyte 胸腺细胞

词根 thy-（胸腺的）+ -cyte（细胞）

例句 Thymocytes are immature immune cells found in the thymus that eventually mature into T-cells. 胸腺细胞是胸腺中的未成熟免疫细胞，最终发育为 T 细胞。

thyro-（甲状腺）

thyroid-stimulating hormone（TSH）促甲状腺激素

词根 thyro-（甲状腺）+ stimulating（刺激的）+ hormone（激素）

例句 Thyroid-stimulating hormone（TSH）is released by the pituitary gland and regulates the production of thyroid hormones in the thyroid gland. 促甲状腺激素（TSH）由垂体分泌，调节甲状腺激素的生产。

thyrotoxicosis 甲状腺毒症

词根 thyro-（甲状腺）+ toxico-（毒）+ -osis（病理状态）

例句 Thyrotoxicosis is a condition caused by excessive thyroid hormone production, leading to symptoms like weight loss, rapid heart rate, and anxiety. 甲状腺毒症是由甲状腺激素过量分泌引起的病症，导致体重下降、心跳加速和焦虑等症状。

thyroiditis 甲状腺炎

词根 thyro-（甲状腺）+ -itis（炎症）

例句 Thyroiditis is an inflammation of the thyroid gland that can lead to pain, swelling, and changes in hormone production. 甲状腺炎是甲状腺的炎症，可能导致疼痛、肿胀以及激素分泌的变化。

hypothyroidism 甲状腺功能减退症

词根 hypo-（低）+ thyro-（甲状腺）+ -ism（病症）
例句 Hypothyroidism occurs when the thyroid gland does not produce enough thyroid hormone, leading to fatigue, weight gain, and depression. 甲状腺功能减退症是指甲状腺无法分泌足够的甲状腺激素，导致疲劳、体重增加和抑郁症。

thyroxine 甲状腺素

词根 thyro-（甲状腺）+ -xine（激素）
例句 Thyroxine is a hormone produced by the thyroid gland that plays a key role in regulating metabolism and energy production. 甲状腺素是由甲状腺分泌的激素，在调节代谢和能量生产中起着关键作用。

thyroglobulin 甲状腺球蛋白

词根 thyro-（甲状腺）+ globulin（球蛋白）
T
例句 Thyroglobulin is a protein produced by the thyroid gland that is often used as a tumor marker for thyroid cancer. 甲状腺球蛋白是由甲状腺分泌的蛋白质，常作为甲状腺癌的肿瘤标志物。

thyroparathyroidectomy 甲状腺副甲状腺切除术

词根 thyro-（甲状腺）+ para-（旁）+ thyroid-（甲状腺）+ -ectomy（切除）
例句 Thyroparathyroidectomy is the surgical removal of both the thyroid and parathyroid glands, often performed to treat thyroid or parathyroid disorders. 甲状腺副甲状腺切除术是同时切除甲状腺和副甲状腺的手术，常用于治疗甲状腺或副甲状腺疾病。

thyroidectomy 甲状腺切除术

词根 thyro-（甲状腺）+ -ectomy（切除）

例句 Thyroidectomy is a surgical procedure that involves the removal of all or part of the thyroid gland, often performed to treat thyroid cancer or hyperthyroidism. 甲状腺切除术是一种手术，指切除全部或部分甲状腺，常用于治疗甲状腺癌或甲状腺功能亢进症。

thyrotoxicosis factitia 伪甲状腺毒症

词根 thyro-（甲状腺）+ toxico-（毒）+ -osis（病理状态）
例句 Thyrotoxicosis factitia is a condition caused by taking excessive amounts of thyroid hormone, often intentionally or unintentionally. 伪甲状腺毒症是指过量摄入甲状腺激素引起的病症，可能是故意或无意中造成的。

thyromegaly 甲状腺肿大

词根 thyro-（甲状腺）+ -megaly（肿大）
例句 Thyromegaly is the enlargement of the thyroid gland, which can result from thyroid disease or iodine deficiency. 甲状腺肿大是甲状腺的增大，可能由甲状腺疾病或碘缺乏引起。

PLAB 1　样题

A 31-year-old woman has increasing shortness of breath and left-sided pleuritic (pleur-) chest pain for 1 week. She smokes 10 cigarettes (cigar-; -ette) per day. She takes the combined oral contraceptive (contra-; cept-) pill. Her temperature is 36.8°C, pulse rate 105 bpm, BP 105/80 mmHg, respiratory (re-; spir-) rate 22 breaths per minute and oxygen saturation 98% breathing air. Her chest is clear.

Which is the most likely diagnosis?

(A) Bronchiectasis (bronchi-; -ectasis)

(B) Lung cancer

(C) Pneumonia (pneumon-)

(D) Pulmonary embolism (embol-; -ism)

(E) Pulmonary tuberculosis (tubercul-; -osis)

中文翻译

一名 31 岁女性因 1 周来逐渐加重的呼吸困难和左侧胸膜炎性胸痛就诊。她每天吸 10 支烟，服用复方口服避孕药。体温 36.8℃，脉搏 105 次 / 分钟，血压 105/80 mmHg，呼吸频率 22 次 / 分钟，空气呼吸下血氧饱和度 98%。胸部听诊清晰。

以下哪项是最可能的诊断？

(A) 支气管扩张症

(B) 肺癌

(C) 肺炎

(D) 肺栓塞

(E) 肺结核

题目和答案中出现的词根

pleur-：胸膜

cigar-：雪茄

-ette：小的

contra-：反

cept-：获得

re-：重新；反复

spir：呼吸

bronchi-：支气管

-ectasis：扩张

pneumon-：肺（病理意义上的肺）

pulmon-：肺的（指的是解剖意义上的肺）

tubercul-：结核的

-osis：病理状态

-tonia（肌张力）

hypotonia 低张力

词根 hypo-（低）+ -tonia（张力）

例句 Hypotonia is a condition characterized by reduced muscle tone, often seen in conditions such as Down syndrome. 低张力是一种以肌肉张力减弱为特征的病症，常见于唐氏综合征等疾病。

hypertonia 高张力

词根 hyper-（高）+ -tonia（张力）

例句 Hypertonia refers to excessive muscle tone, often causing stiffness and difficulty in movement. 高张力是指过度的肌肉张力，常导致僵硬和运动困难。

dystonia 肌张力障碍

词根 dys-（障碍）+ -tonia（张力）

例句 Dystonia is a movement disorder characterized by involuntary muscle contractions, causing twisting and repetitive movements. 肌张力障碍是一种运动障碍，以不自主的肌肉收缩为特征，导致扭曲和重复的动作。

cervical dystonia 颈部肌张力障碍

词根 cervic-（颈部）+ -tonia（张力）

例句 Cervical dystonia is a condition where the muscles of the neck contract uncontrollably, causing the head to twist or tilt. 颈部肌张力障碍是一种颈部肌肉不自主收缩的病症，导致头部扭曲或倾斜。

postural hypotonia 姿势性低张力

词根 postural（姿势的）+ hypo-（低）+ -tonia（张力）

例句 Postural hypotonia refers to low muscle tone that affects a person's posture and balance. 姿势性低张力指的是影响一个人姿势和平衡的肌肉低张力。

orthostatic hypotonia 直立性低张力

词根 orthostatic（直立的）+ hypo-（低）+ -tonia（张力）

例句 Orthostatic hypotonia is a condition where blood pressure drops when standing up, often accompanied by dizziness or fainting. 直立性低张力是指站立时血压下降，常伴随头晕或昏厥。

isotonia 等张力

词根 iso-（相等）+ -tonia（张力）

例句 Isotonia refers to the condition where muscle tension remains constant despite changes in the muscle length, such as during isometric exercises. 等张力是指肌肉张力在肌肉长度变化时保持恒定的状态，常发生在等长运动中。

hypertonic dehydration 高张渴

词根 hyper-（高）+ -tonic（张力的）+ dehydration（脱水）

例句 Hypertonic dehydration occurs when the body loses more water than salt, leading to an increase in the concentration of electrolytes in the blood. 高张渴是指身体失去的水分超过盐分，导致血液中电解质浓度增加。

hypotonic solution 低张溶液

词根 hypo-（低）+ -tonic（张力的）+ solution（溶液）

例句 A hypotonic solution is one that has a lower concentration of solutes compared to the cells, often used in medical treatments to hydrate cells. 低张溶液是指溶质浓度低于细胞内溶质浓度的溶液，常用于医疗中为细胞补充水分。

toxic-/toxo-（毒的）

toxicology 毒理学

词根 toxic-（毒）+ -ology（学科）

例句 Toxicology is the study of the harmful effects of chemicals or substances on living organisms. 毒理学是研究化学物质或物质对生物体有害影响的学科。

toxicity 毒性

词根 toxic-（毒）+ -ity（名词后缀）

例句 Toxicity refers to the degree to which a substance can cause harm to the body or organisms. 毒性指的是某物质对身体或生物体造成伤害的程度。

toxicity test 毒性测试

词根 toxic-（毒）+ -ity（名词后缀）+ test（测试）

例句 Toxicity tests are conducted to assess the harmful effects of chemicals or drugs before they are approved for use. 毒性测试用于评估化学物质或药物在批准使用前的有害影响。

toxic shock syndrome 毒性休克综合征

词根 toxic-（毒）+ shock（休克）+ syndrome（综合征）

例句 Toxic shock syndrome is a severe illness caused by bacterial toxins, leading to symptoms such as fever, low blood pressure, and organ failure. 毒性休克综合征是由细菌毒素引起的严重疾病，导致发热、低血压和器官衰竭等症状。

toxicant 有毒物质

词根 toxic-（毒）+ -ant（物质）

例句 A toxicant is a substance that has the potential to cause harm or injury to living organisms. 有毒物质是指可能对生物体造成伤

害或损害的物质。

toxicodendron 毒漆树

词根 toxic-（毒）+ dendron（树）

例句 Toxicodendron is a genus of plants that includes poison ivy and poison oak, known for causing skin rashes. 毒漆树属是一个包括毒藤和毒橡树的植物属，因其引起皮疹而闻名。

toxicological 毒理学的

词根 toxic-（毒）+ -logical（形容词后缀）

例句 Toxicological research helps identify potential hazards and assess risks related to exposure to toxic substances. 毒理学研究帮助识别潜在的危害并评估接触有毒物质的风险。

toxoid 类毒素

词根 tox-（毒）+ -oid（类似的）

例句 A toxoid is an inactivated toxin used in vaccines to stimulate immunity without causing disease. 类毒素是被灭活的毒素，用于疫苗中刺激免疫反应而不引起疾病。

toxicity testing 毒性测试

词根 toxic-（毒）+ -ity（名词后缀）+ testing（测试）

例句 Toxicity testing is crucial for evaluating the safety of new drugs and chemicals before they are introduced to the market. 毒性测试对于在新药和化学物质进入市场前评估其安全性至关重要。

Toxic hepatitis 毒性肝炎

词根 toxic-（毒）+ hepatitis（肝炎）

例句 Toxic hepatitis is liver inflammation caused by exposure to harmful substances such as alcohol, drugs, or chemicals. 毒性肝炎是由暴露于有害物质（如酒精、药物或化学品）引起的肝脏炎症。

PLAB 1 样题

A 60-year-old man is anuric (an-; uri) on the renal unit. 2 days ago ge had a left nephrectomy (nephr-; -ectomy) for renal cell carcinoma (carcin-; -oma). His temperature is 39.0°C, pulse rate 98 bpm and BP 80/60 mmHg.

Investigations:

Ultrasound (ultra-) scan of abdomen: Gross dilatation of the upper right renal tract and a stone impacted at the pelvi-ureteric junction.

Which is the most appropriate therapeutic intervention?

(A) Bladder catheterisation (catheter-; -isation)

(B) Lithotripsy (litho-; -tripsy)

(C) Percutaneous (per-; cutan-) right nephrostomy (nephr-; -ostomy)

(D) Retrograde (retro-; -grade) drainage of the right renal tract

(E) Suprapubic (supra-; -pubic) catheterisation (catheter-; -isation)

中文翻译

一名 60 岁男性因无尿症在肾脏科就诊。2 天前，他因肾细胞癌接受了左侧肾切除术。他的体温为 39.0°C，脉搏 98 次 / 分钟，血压 80/60 mmHg。

检查结果：

腹部超声扫描：右侧肾上段集合系统明显扩张，盆腔输尿管连接处有一颗结石嵌顿。

以下哪项是最适当的治疗干预？

(A) 膀胱导尿
(B) 体外碎石术
(C) 经皮右侧肾造瘘术
(D) 右侧肾集合系统逆行引流
(E) 耻骨上导尿

题目和答案中出现的词根

nephr-：肾脏
-ectomy：切除术
carcin-：上皮细胞恶变
-oma：瘤
ultra-：超
catheter-：导管
-isation：表示过程的动作
litho-：石头
-tripsy：压碎
-ostomy：切开术
retro-：反向
-grade：等级；台阶
supra-：在……之上
-pubic：耻骨

trans-（转）

transfusion 输血

词根 trans-（转）+ fusion（融合）

例句 A transfusion is the process of transferring blood or blood products from one person to another. 输血是指将血液或血液产品从一个人转移到另一个人的过程。

transdermal 透皮的

词根 trans-（转）+ dermal（皮肤的）

例句 Transdermal patches are used to deliver medication through the skin, such as nicotine or pain relief patches. 透皮贴片用于通过皮肤传递药物，如尼古丁或止痛贴片。

transplant 移植

词根 trans-（转）+ plant（移植）

例句 A transplant is a surgical procedure in which an organ or tissue is moved from one body to another. 移植是一种外科手术，指将一个人体的器官或组织移植到另一个人体内。

transmission 传播

词根 trans-（转）+ mission（传送）

例句 Transmission refers to the process of transferring a disease or infection from one person to another. 传播指的是将疾病或感染从一个人传递到另一个人的过程。

translocation 转位

词根 trans-（转）+ location（位置）

例句 Translocation refers to the movement of a chromosome segment from one part of the chromosome to another. 转位指的是染色

体片段从染色体的一个部分移到另一个部分的过程。

transdermal drug delivery 透皮药物输送

词根 trans-（转）+ dermal（皮肤的）+ drug（药物）+ delivery（输送）

例句 Transdermal drug delivery allows for the sustained release of medication through the skin, such as with hormone replacement therapy. 透皮药物输送使得药物通过皮肤持续释放，例如在激素替代治疗中的应用。

transcutaneous 经皮的

词根 trans-（转）+ cutaneous（皮肤的）

例句 Transcutaneous electrical nerve stimulation（TENS）is a therapy used to relieve pain through electrical stimulation of the skin. 经皮电神经刺激（TENS）是一种通过皮肤电刺激来缓解疼痛的治疗方法。

transcellular transport 细胞跨膜运输

词根 trans-（转）+ cellular（细胞的）+ transport（运输）

例句 Transcellular transport refers to the movement of substances across cells, such as nutrients passing through the intestinal lining. 细胞跨膜运输指的是物质穿过细胞进行移动的过程，例如营养物质穿过肠黏膜。

transgenic 转基因的

词根 trans-（转）+ genic（基因的）

例句 Transgenic organisms have been genetically modified to carry genes from other species, often used in research and agriculture. 转基因生物通过基因工程改造，携带来自其他物种的基因，常用于研究和农业。

transposition 转位；置换

词根 trans-（转）+ position（位置）

例句 Transposition refers to the rearrangement of genetic material, which can result in genetic mutations or disorders. 转位指的是遗传物质的重新排列，可能导致遗传突变或疾病。

tri-（三个）

triceps 肱三头肌

词根 tri-（三个）+ -ceps（头；肌肉的头部）
例句 The triceps is the large muscle on the back of the upper arm that has three points of origin. 肱三头肌是上臂后侧的一块大肌肉，它有三个起始点。

trinomial 三项式

词根 tri-（三个）+ -nomial（名称的）
例句 A trinomial is an algebraic expression with three terms, such as in the equation $x^2 + 5x + 6$. 三项式是一个包含三项的代数表达式，例如方程 $x^2 + 5x + 6$。

trifocal 三焦点的

词根 tri-（三个）+ focal（焦点的）
例句 Trifocal lenses are eyeglasses lenses with three distinct focal points, used to correct vision for distance, reading, and intermediate vision. 三焦点眼镜是具有三个不同焦点的眼镜镜片，用于矫正远视、近视和中间视力。

trisomy 三体症

词根 tri-（三个）+ -somy（体）
例句 Trisomy is a condition in which an individual has three copies of a chromosome instead of the normal two, as seen in Down syndrome (trisomy 21). 三体症是一种个体拥有三份染色体而非正常两份的病症，唐氏综合征即是如此。

T

tricuspid 三尖瓣的

词根 tri-（三个）+ cuspid（瓣）

例句 The tricuspid valve is the valve in the heart that has three flaps, regulating blood flow between the right atrium and right ventricle. 三尖瓣是心脏中具有三个瓣膜的瓣，调节右心房和右心室之间的血流。

triiodothyronine 三碘甲状腺素

词根 tri-（三个）+ iodo-（碘）+ thyronine（甲状腺素）

例句 Triiodothyronine（T3）is a thyroid hormone that plays a critical role in regulating metabolism and energy production. 三碘甲状腺素（T3）是甲状腺激素，在调节代谢和能量生产中起着关键作用。

triaxial 三轴的

词根 tri-（三个）+ axial（轴的）

例句 A triaxial system has three axes of rotation, commonly used in motion sensors and medical devices. 三轴系统具有三个旋转轴，常用于运动传感器和医疗设备。

triphasic 三相的

词根 tri-（三个）+ phasic（相的）

例句 A triphasic pattern in an electrocardiogram（ECG）shows three distinct phases, often associated with certain cardiac conditions. 三相模式在心电图（ECG）中显示三个不同的相，通常与某些心脏病症相关。

trimetazidine 三美替丁

词根 tri-（三个）+ -metazidine（药物名称）

例句 Trimetazidine is a medication used to treat angina pectoris by improving the energy efficiency of the heart muscle. 三美替丁是一种药物，通过改善心脏肌肉的能量利用效率来治疗心绞痛。

trihalomethanes 三卤代甲烷

词根 tri-（三个）+ halo-（卤素）+ methane（甲烷）

例句 Trihalomethanes are chemical compounds formed when chlorine is used to disinfect drinking water, which can be harmful at high concentrations. 三卤代甲烷是使用氯消毒饮用水时形成的化学化合物，高浓度时可能有害。

trich-/tricho-（头发）

trichology 毛发学

词根 trich-（头发）+ -ology（学科）

例句 Trichology is the branch of dermatology that deals with the study and treatment of hair and scalp disorders. 毛发学是皮肤病学的一个分支，专门研究和治疗毛发及头皮疾病。

trichotillomania 拔发癖

词根 tricho-（头发）+ -mania（狂热）

例句 Trichotillomania is a psychological condition in which individuals have an irresistible urge to pull out their own hair. 拔发癖是一种心理疾病，指个体有一种无法抗拒的冲动拔掉自己的头发。

trichorrhexis 发裂

词根 tricho-（头发）+ -rrhexis（裂开）

例句 Trichorrhexis is a condition where the hair shaft is weakened and prone to splitting or breaking. 发裂是指头发干燥和脆弱，容易分叉或断裂的病症。

trichopathy 毛发病

词根 trich-（头发）+ -pathy（病）

例句 Trichopathy refers to any disease or disorder that affects the hair, including hair loss and infections. 毛发病指的是任何影响毛

发的疾病或病症，包括脱发和感染。

trichome 毛发状物

词根 trich-（头发）+ -ome（物）
例句 A trichome is a small hair-like structure found on plants or animals, often involved in sensory functions or protection. 毛发状物是植物或动物的小型毛发状结构，常用于感官功能或保护作用。

trichogenic 生发的

词根 tricho-（头发）+ -genic（生成的）
例句 Trichogenic factors are those that promote hair growth, often studied in hair restoration treatments. 生发因子是那些促进毛发生长的因素，通常在毛发恢复治疗中被研究。

trichostasis 毛发滞留

词根 tricho-（头发）+ -stasis（停滞）
例句 Trichostasis is a condition in which hair growth is blocked or disrupted, leading to hair retention or other abnormalities. 毛发滞留是一种毛发生长被阻塞或干扰的情况，导致毛发滞留或其他异常。

trichoblastoma 毛母细胞瘤

词根 tricho-（头发）+ -blastoma（胚胎肿瘤）
例句 Trichoblastoma is a rare benign tumor originating from the hair follicle cells. 毛母细胞瘤是一种起源于毛囊细胞的罕见良性肿瘤。

trichotaxia 毛发定向

词根 tricho-（头发）+ -taxia（定向）
例句 Trichotaxia refers to the direction in which hair growth occurs, which can be genetically influenced. 毛发定向是指毛发生长的方向，通常受遗传的影响。

trichophytosis 毛发真菌病

词根 tricho-（头发）+ phyt-（植物）+ -osis（病理状态）

例句 Trichophytosis is a fungal infection that affects the hair, often leading to hair loss and scalp inflammation. 毛发真菌病是一种影响头发的真菌感染，通常导致脱发和头皮炎症。

PLAB 1 样题

A 65-year-old man has a dry cough and progressive shortness of breath for 3 months. He is seen in the respiratory (re-; spir-) clinic. He has never smoked. His weight is stable. He has finger clubbing. His temperature is 36.5°C, pulse 70 bpm, BP 110/80 mmHg, respiratory (re-; spir-) rate 26 breaths per minute and oxygen saturation breathing air is 91%. He has bibasal (bi-; bas-) fine end-inspiratory (in-; spir-) crackles.

Investigation:

Chest X-ray: reticulonodular (reticulo-; nodul-) shadowing at both bases

Lung function tests: reduced vital capacity with an FEV1/FVC ratio of 85%

Which is the most appropriate next investigation?

(A) Broncho-alveolar lavage

(B) Cardiopulmonary (cardio-; pulmon-) exercise test

(C) Echocardiography (echo-; cardi-; -graphy)

(D) Video-assisted thoracoscopic (thorac-; -scop) lung biopsy (bio-; -psy)

中文翻译

一名65岁男性因3个月来干咳和逐渐加重的呼吸困难在呼吸科就诊。他从不吸烟。体重稳定。他有杵状指。体温36.5℃，脉搏70次/分钟，血压110/80 mmHg，呼吸频率26次/分钟，空气呼吸下血氧饱和度91%。双肺底部可闻及细小的吸气末湿啰音。

检查结果：

胸部X线：双肺底部呈网结节状阴影

肺功能测试：肺活量减少，FEV1/FVC比值为85%

以下哪项是最适当的下一步检查？

(A) 支气管肺泡灌洗

(B) 心肺运动试验

(C) 心脏超声检查

(D) 胸部高分辨率CT扫描

(E) 视频辅助胸腔镜肺活检

题目和答案中出现的词根

re-：重新；反复

spir-：呼吸

bi-：双

bas-：底部

in-：向内

reticulo-：网状的

nodul-：结节

cardio-：心脏

pulmon-：肺的

echo-：回声

-graphy：影像

thorac-：胸腔

-scop：镜

bio-：生物

-psy：检查

–trophy（营养性增长）

hypertrophy 肥大

词根 hyper-（过度）+ -trophy（营养性增长）

例句 Hypertrophy refers to the increase in the size of cells, often seen in muscle cells after exercise. 肥大是指细胞体积的增加，通常见于运动后的肌肉细胞。

atrophy 萎缩

词根 a-（无）+ -trophy（营养性增长）

例句 Atrophy is the decrease in the size or function of an organ or tissue, often due to disuse or disease. 萎缩是指器官或组织的体积缩小或功能减退，通常由废用或疾病引起。

dystrophy 营养不良症

词根 dys-（不良）+ -trophy（营养性增长）

例句 Dystrophy is a group of disorders characterized by progressive degeneration and weakness of muscles or other tissues. 营养不良症是一组特征为肌肉或其他组织进行性退化和无力的疾病。

neurotrophy 神经营养

词根 neuro-（神经）+ -trophy（营养性增长）

例句 Neurotrophy refers to the growth and maintenance of neurons and their connections. 神经营养是指神经元及其连接的生长和维持。

myotrophy 肌肉营养

词根 myo-（肌肉）+ -trophy（营养性增长）

例句 Myotrophy is the process of muscle growth and development, often influenced by exercise or hormonal changes. 肌肉营养是肌肉的生长和发育，通常受运动或激素变化的影响。

lipotrophy 脂肪营养

词根 lipo-（脂肪）+ -trophy（营养性增长）

例句 Lipotrophy refers to the growth and accumulation of fat tissue in the body, particularly in response to diet or hormonal changes. 脂肪营养是指脂肪组织在身体中的生长和积累，尤其与饮食或激素变化相关。

psychotrophy 心理营养

词根 psycho-（心理）+ -trophy（营养性增长）

例句 Psychotrophy refers to the growth or development of mental or psychological functions, influenced by environment or experiences. 心理营养指的是心理或心理功能的生长或发展，受环境或经历的影响。

osteotrophy 骨营养

词根 osteo-（骨）+ -trophy（营养性增长）

例句 Osteotrophy refers to the growth and strengthening of bone tissue, often through exercise or nutritional support. 骨营养是指骨组织的生长和强化，通常通过运动或营养支持来实现。

cardiotrophy 心脏营养

词根 cardio-（心脏）+ -trophy（营养性增长）

例句 Cardiotrophy refers to the growth and health of the heart muscle, influenced by physical activity and diet. 心脏营养是指心脏肌肉的生长和健康，受体育活动和饮食的影响。

-tropic（趋向的；促使的）

neurotropic 神经趋向性

词根 neuro-（神经的）+ -tropic（趋向的）

例句 Neurotropic viruses specifically target the nervous system, such as the rabies virus. 神经趋向性病毒特异性地攻击神经系统，例如狂犬病病毒。

phototropic 向光性的

词根 photo-（光）+ -tropic（趋向的）

例句 Phototropic organisms grow or move towards light, as seen in plants following sunlight. 向光性生物朝着光源生长或移动，例如植物朝阳光生长。

chronotropic 时效性影响的

词根 chrono-（时间）+ -tropic（趋向的）

例句 Chronotropic drugs influence the rate of the heart's rhythm, either increasing or decreasing heart rate. 时效性药物影响心脏节律的速率，心率加快或减慢。

inotropic 促力的

词根 ino-（力量）+ -tropic（趋向的）

例句 Inotropic drugs increase the force of heart muscle contraction, often used to treat heart failure. 促力药物增加心肌的收缩力，常用于治疗心力衰竭。

chemotropic 化学趋向性的

词根 chemo-（化学）+ -tropic（趋向的）

例句 Chemotropic substances influence the direction of cell movement or growth in response to chemical signals. 化学趋向性物质影响细胞在化学信号作用下的运动或生长方向。

lactotropic 促乳的

词根 lacto-（乳）+ -tropic（促使的）

例句 Lactotropic hormones, such as prolactin, stimulate milk production in the mammary glands. 催乳激素如催乳素，刺激乳腺的乳汁分泌。

thyrotropic 促甲状腺的

词根 thyro-（甲状腺的）+ -tropic（促使的）

例句 Thyrotropic hormones, such as TSH, stimulate the thyroid gland to produce thyroid hormones. 促甲状腺激素，如 TSH，刺激甲状腺分泌甲状腺激素。

gonadotropic 促性腺的

词根 gonado-（性腺的）+ -tropic（促使的）

例句 Gonadotropic hormones regulate the function of the gonads, such as follicle-stimulating hormone (FSH). 促性腺激素调节性腺的功能，例如促卵泡激素（FSH）。

antitropic 抗趋向的

词根 anti-（反）+ -tropic（趋向的）

例句 Antitropic substances are used to inhibit or counteract the actions of tropic substances, such as in hormone regulation. 抗趋向性物质用于抑制或对抗趋向物质的作用，常用于激素调节中。

cytotropic 细胞趋向性的

词根 cyto-（细胞的）+ -tropic（趋向的）

例句 Cytotropic factors influence the movement of cells, especially in immune responses and wound healing. 细胞趋向因子影响细胞的运动，特别是在免疫反应和伤口愈合中。

-ule/-cle/-ole（小的）

arteriole 小动脉

词根 arteri-（动脉）+ -ole（小的）

例句 Arterioles are small blood vessels that carry blood from the arteries to the capillaries. 小动脉是将血液从动脉输送到毛细血管的小血管。

venule 小静脉

词根 ven-（静脉）+ -ule（小的）

例句 Venules are small veins that collect blood from the capillaries and transport it to larger veins. 小静脉是将血液从毛细血管收集并输送到大静脉的小血管。

globule 小球

词根 glob-（球）+ -ule（小的）

例句 A globule is a tiny, spherical particle, such as a droplet of fat in the bloodstream. 小球是一个微小的球形颗粒，例如血液中的脂肪滴。

vesicle 小泡

词根 vesic-（囊）+ -cle（小的）

例句 Vesicles are small, membrane-bound sacs in cells that store and transport substances. 小泡是细胞内的小型膜囊，用于存储和运输物质。

granule 颗粒

词根 gran-（颗粒）+ -ule（小的）

例句 Granules are small, grain-like particles found in cells or substances. 颗粒是存在于细胞或物质中的小颗粒。

tubule 小管

词根 tub-（管）+ -ule（小的）

例句 The renal tubules are small structures in the kidneys that help filter and reabsorb substances. 肾小管是肾脏中的小结构，帮助过滤和重吸收物质。

cellule 小细胞

词根 cell-（细胞）+ -ule（小的）

例句 Cellules are small cells that play a crucial role in various physiological processes. 小细胞在各种生理过程中起着至关重要的作用。

corpuscle 小体

词根 corpus-（体）+ -cle（小的）

例句 Red blood cells are often referred to as corpuscles due to their small, round shape. 红细胞由于其小而圆的形状，常被称为小体。

molecule 分子

词根 molec-（小）+ -ule（小的）

例句 A molecule is the smallest unit of a chemical compound that retains its chemical properties. 分子是保留化学性质的最小化学化合物单位。

-uria（尿症）

hematuria 血尿

词根 hemat-（血）+ -uria（尿症）

例句 Hematuria is the presence of blood in the urine, which can be caused by conditions such as urinary tract infections or kidney stones. 血尿是尿液中出现血液，可能由尿路感染或肾结石等疾病引起。

glycosuria 糖尿

词根 glyco-（糖）+ -uria（尿症）

例句 Glycosuria is the presence of glucose in the urine, often a sign of diabetes or uncontrolled blood sugar levels. 糖尿是尿液中出现葡萄糖，通常是糖尿病或血糖失控的标志。

proteinuria 蛋白尿

词根 protein-（蛋白质）+ -uria（尿症）

例句 Proteinuria is the presence of excess protein in the urine, which can be a sign of kidney disease. 蛋白尿是尿液中出现过多蛋白质，可能是肾脏病的征兆。

pyuria 脓尿

词根 py-（脓）+ -uria（尿症）

例句 Pyuria is the presence of pus in the urine, which can indicate a urinary tract infection or other inflammatory conditions. 脓尿是尿液中出现脓液，可能是尿路感染或其他炎症性疾病的表现。

oliguria 少尿

词根 olig-（少）+ -uria（尿症）

例句 Oliguria refers to the condition of producing an abnormally low amount of urine, often seen in dehydration or kidney failure. 少尿是指产生异常少量尿液的情况，常见于脱水或肾衰竭。

anuria 无尿

词根 a-（无）+ -uria（尿症）

例句 Anuria is the complete absence of urine production, which may indicate severe kidney dysfunction or dehydration. 无尿是指完全没有尿液产生，可能是严重肾功能障碍或脱水的标志。

nocturia 夜尿

词根 noct-（夜晚）+ -uria（尿症）

例句 Nocturia is the condition of waking up frequently during the night to urinate, often associated with aging or certain medical conditions. 夜尿是指在夜间频繁醒来排尿，通常与衰老或某些疾病有关。

urochromuria 尿色素尿症

词根 uro-（尿）+ chrom-（色）+ -uria（尿症）

例句 Urochromuria is the presence of abnormal pigments in the urine, which can cause a discoloration in the urine. 尿色素尿症是尿液中出现异常色素，可能导致尿液颜色异常。

leucocyturia 白细胞尿症

词根 leucocyt-（白细胞）+ -uria（尿症）

例句 Leucocyturia is the presence of white blood cells in the urine, often indicating an infection or inflammation in the urinary tract. 白细胞尿症是尿液中出现白细胞，通常表示尿路感染或炎症。

bilirubinuria 胆红素尿症

词根 bilirubin-（胆红素）+ -uria（尿症）

例句 Bilirubinuria is the presence of bilirubin in the urine, which can be a sign of liver disease or bile duct obstruction. 胆红素尿症是尿液中出现胆红素，可能是肝脏疾病或胆管阻塞的表现。

uro-（尿的）

urology 泌尿学

词根 uro-（尿的）+ -logy（学科）

例句 Urology is the branch of medicine that deals with the diagnosis and treatment of urinary tract disorders. 泌尿学是医学的一个分支，负责诊断和治疗泌尿系统疾病。

urosurgery 泌尿外科手术

词根 uro-（尿的）+ surgery（手术）

例句 Urosurgery involves surgical procedures related to the urinary system, such as kidney stone removal or bladder surgery. 泌尿外科手术是与尿路系统相关的外科手术，如肾结石取出或膀胱手术。

urothelial carcinoma 尿路上皮癌

词根 uro-（尿的）+ theli-（上皮）+ carcinoma（癌）

例句 Urothelial carcinoma is a type of cancer that originates in the urothelial cells lining the urinary tract, often affecting the bladder. 尿路上皮癌是一种源自尿路上皮细胞的癌症，常影响膀胱。

uropathy 尿路病

词根 uro-（尿的）+ -pathy（病）

例句 Uropathy refers to any disease or disorder that affects the urinary system, including the kidneys, bladder, and urethra. 尿路病是指影响尿路系统（包括肾脏、膀胱和尿道）的任何疾病。

urospermia 尿精症

词根 uro-（尿的）+ sperm-（精子）+ -ia（病理状态）

例句 Urospermia is a condition where sperm is found in the urine, which can result from certain reproductive health issues. 尿精症是一种尿液中发现精子的情况，可能由某些生殖健康问题引起。

urography 尿路造影

词根 uro-（尿的）+ -graphy（成像）

例句 Urography is an imaging technique used to visualize the urinary tract, often using X-rays and contrast dye. 尿路造影是一种用于可视化尿路的成像技术，通常使用 X 线和造影剂来实现。

urolithiasis 尿石症

词根 uro-（尿的）+ lithiasis（结石症）

例句 Urolithiasis is the formation of stones in the urinary tract, such as kidney stones or bladder stones. 尿石症是尿路中结石的形成，如肾结石或膀胱结石。

PLAB 1 样题

A 10-year-old girl has bloody diarrhoea (dia-; rrhoea) for 5 days and is seen in the Emergency Department. 3 days ago she developed vomiting, and abdominal pain. She had been on a school trip to a local farm 1 week ago. She has previously been healthy and is not taking any medications. She is pale, drowsy and dehydrated (de-; hydr-) with some swelling of her ankles. Her pulse rate is 120 bpm and BP 140/96 mmHg.

Investigations:

Haemoglobin (haemo-; -globin) 80 g/L (115–140)

White cell count 3.2×10^9/L (4.0–11.0)

Platelets (plate-; -lets) 76×10^9/L (150–400)

Sodium 130 mmol/L (135–146)

Potassium 4.0 mmol/L (3.5–5.0)

Urea 14 mmol/L (2.5–6.5)

Creatinine 200 micromol (micro-) /L (34–65)

Blood film: fragmented red blood cells

Which is the most likely underlying diagnosis?

(A) Bacillus (bacill-) cereus (cere-) enteritis (enter-; -itis)

(B) Diabetic ketoacidosis (keto-; acid-; -osis)

(C) Haemolytic (haemo-; lyt-) uraemic (ur-; aem-) syndrome

(D) Idiopathic (idio-; path-) thrombocytopenic (thromb-; cyto-; -penic) purpura

(E) Thrombotic (thrombo-) thrombocytopenic (thromb-; cyto-; -penic) purpura

中文翻译

一名 10 岁女孩因 5 天来血性腹泻在急诊科就诊。3 天前她开始出现呕吐和腹痛。她在一周前曾随学校去当地农场旅行。她之前身体健康，未服用任何药物。她面色苍白、嗜睡、脱水，踝部有轻度肿胀。脉搏 120 次 / 分钟，血压 140/96 mmHg。

检查结果：

血红蛋白 80 g/L（正常值：115 ～ 140）

白细胞计数 3.2×10^9/L（正常值：4.0 ～ 11.0）

血小板 76×10^9/L（正常值：150 ～ 400）

钠 130 mmol/L（正常值：135 ～ 146）

钾 4.0 mmol/L（正常值：3.5 ～ 5.0）

尿素 14 mmol/L（正常值：2.5 ～ 6.5）

肌酐 200 micromol/L（正常值：34 ～ 65）

血涂片：裂红细胞

以下哪项是最可能的诊断？

(A) 蜡样芽孢杆菌肠炎

(B) 糖尿病酮症酸中毒

(C) 溶血性尿毒综合征

(D) 特发性血小板减少性紫癜

(E) 血栓性血小板减少性紫癜

题目和答案中出现的词根

dia-：通过

rrhoea-：流出

de-：去掉

hydr-：氢，这里指水

haemo-：血，是 hemo-， hemato- 的同义变异

-globin：球蛋白

plate-：板状的

-lets：小

micro-：微小的

schisto-：分裂的

-cyte：细胞

bacill-：杆菌

cere-：蜡样的

enter-：肠道的

-itis：炎症

keto-：酮体

acid-：酸

-osis：病理状态（酮体 - 酸的状态指的是酮症酸中毒）

lyt-：溶解

ur-：尿，是 uri-，urin- 的同义变异

aem-：血液

idio-：自我的

path-：病

thromb-：凝血的

cyto-：细胞，是 cyte- 的同义变异

-penic：缺少

vesi-（囊）

vesicle 囊泡

词根 vesi-（囊）+ -cle（小的）
例句 A vesicle is a small, membrane-bound sac in the cell that contains liquid or cytoplasmic material. 囊泡是细胞中一个小的膜结合囊，包含液体或细胞质物质。

vesicular 囊泡的

词根 vesicul-（囊泡）+ -ar（形容词后缀）
例句 Vesicular structures within the cell play a key role in transporting substances to different areas within the cell. 细胞内的囊泡结构在运输物质到细胞不同区域中起着关键作用。

vesicoureteral reflux 膀胱输尿管反流

词根 vesic-（膀胱）+ ureter-（输尿管）+ -al（形容词后缀）+ reflux（反流）
例句 Vesicoureteral reflux is a condition where urine flows backward from the bladder into the ureters and kidneys. 膀胱输尿管反流是一种尿液从膀胱反流到输尿管和肾脏的疾病。

vesicant 起泡剂

词根 vesic-（囊）+ -ant（物质）
例句 A vesicant is a substance that causes blistering or damage to tissues, often used in chemotherapy treatments. 起泡剂是指一种引起组织起泡或损伤的物质，常用于化疗中。

vesicular rash 囊泡性皮疹

词根 vesicul-（囊泡）+ -ar（形容词后缀）+ rash（皮疹）
例句 A vesicular rash is characterized by the presence of small, flu-

id-filled blisters on the skin. 囊泡性皮疹是指皮肤上出现小的充满液体的水疱。

vesicorectal fistula 膀胱直肠瘘

词根 vesic-（膀胱）+ rect-（直肠）+ -al（形容词后缀）+ fistula（瘘）

例句 A vesicorectal fistula is an abnormal connection between the bladder and the rectum, often caused by infections or surgery. 膀胱直肠瘘是膀胱和直肠之间的异常连接，通常由感染或手术引起。

vesicovaginal fistula 膀胱阴道瘘

词根 vesic-（膀胱）+ vagin-（阴道）+ -al（形容词后缀）+ fistula（瘘）

例句 Vesicovaginal fistula is an abnormal opening between the bladder and the vagina, often caused by childbirth trauma or surgery. 膀胱阴道瘘是膀胱和阴道之间的异常开口，常由分娩创伤或手术引起。

vesicoureteric junction 膀胱输尿管交界

词根 vesic-（膀胱）+ ureteric（输尿管的）+ junction（交界）

例句 The vesicoureteric junction is the area where the ureter meets the bladder, playing an essential role in preventing reflux of urine. 膀胱输尿管交界是输尿管与膀胱连接的部位，起着防止尿液反流的重要作用。

vesicular transport 囊泡运输

词根 vesicul-（囊泡）+ transport（运输）

例句 Vesicular transport is the process by which substances are transported within cells using membrane-bound vesicles. 囊泡运输是指细胞使用膜包裹的囊泡进行物质运输的过程。

vesicovaginal dysfunction 膀胱阴道功能障碍

词根 vesic-（膀胱）+ vagin-（阴道）+ dysfunction（功能障碍）

例句 Vesicovaginal dysfunction can cause urinary incontinence and other pelvic issues due to impaired bladder and vaginal function. 膀

胱阴道功能障碍可能导致尿失禁和其他盆腔问题，因为膀胱和阴道的功能受损。

vesicular exanthema 囊泡性皮疹

词根 vesicul-（囊泡）+ exanthema（皮疹）

例句 Vesicular exanthema is a type of viral skin rash characterized by small blisters and lesions. 囊泡性皮疹是一种由病毒引起的皮肤疹，特征是小水疱和损伤。

vesicoureteral reflux disease 膀胱输尿管反流病

词根 vesic-(膀胱)+ ureter-(输尿管)+ reflux(反流)+ disease(病)

例句 Vesicoureteral reflux disease is a condition where urine flows back into the kidneys, potentially leading to kidney damage. 膀胱输尿管反流病是一种尿液回流到肾脏的病症，可能导致肾脏损伤。

vesicular stomatitis 囊泡性口炎

词根 vesicul-（囊泡）+ stomat-（口腔）+ -itis（炎症）

例句 Vesicular stomatitis is a viral infection characterized by blister-like lesions in the mouth and on the skin. 囊泡性口炎是一种病毒感染，特征是在口腔和皮肤上出现类似水疱的损伤。

vesicoureteric reflux imaging 膀胱输尿管反流影像学检查

词根 vesic-（膀胱）+ ureter-（输尿管）+ reflux（反流）+ imaging（影像学）

例句 Vesicoureteric reflux imaging is an imaging technique used to detect urine reflux from the bladder into the ureters. 膀胱输尿管反流影像学检查是一种影像学技术，用于检测尿液从膀胱回流到输尿管的情况。

vesicular structure 囊泡结构

词根 vesicul-（囊泡）+ structure（结构）

例句 Vesicular structures are involved in the transport and storage of various materials inside the cell. 囊泡结构参与细胞内各种物质的运输和储存。

vesicular neuralgia 囊泡性神经痛

词根 vesicul-（囊泡）+ neuralgia（神经痛）

例句 Vesicular neuralgia is a form of nerve pain caused by the formation of vesicles along the nerve path. 囊泡性神经痛是由神经通路沿线上囊泡形成引起的神经痛。

vesicular secretion 囊泡分泌

词根 vesicul-（囊泡）+ secretion（分泌）

例句 Vesicular secretion is the release of substances from cells via vesicles, such as the secretion of neurotransmitters in nerve cells. 囊泡分泌是细胞通过囊泡释放物质的过程，如神经细胞中神经递质的分泌。

endoscopic vesicular examination 内镜囊泡检查

词根 endo-（内部）+ scop-（观察）+ vesicul-（囊泡）+ examination（检查）

例句 Endoscopic vesicular examination is used to examine the formation of vesicles within organs such as the bladder or lungs. 内镜囊泡检查用于检查器官如膀胱或肺部内囊泡的形成。

vesicorectal fistula repair 膀胱直肠瘘修复

词根 vesic-（膀胱）+ rect-（直肠）+ fistula（瘘）+ repair（修复）

例句 Vesicorectal fistula repair is a surgical procedure to close an abnormal connection between the bladder and rectum. 膀胱直肠瘘修复是一种外科手术，用于闭合膀胱和直肠之间的异常连接。

vesicovaginal fistula repair 膀胱阴道瘘修复

词根 vesic-（膀胱）+ vagin-（阴道）+ fistula（瘘）+ repair（修复）

例句 Vesicovaginal fistula repair involves closing the abnormal opening between the bladder and the vagina to restore normal function. 膀胱阴道瘘修复手术指闭合膀胱和阴道之间的异常开口，恢复正常功能。

xantho-（黄色的）

xanthoma 黄瘤

词根 xantho-（黄色）+ -oma（肿瘤）

例句 Xanthoma is a skin condition where yellowish cholesterol deposits form, often on the eyelids or elbows. 黄瘤是一种皮肤病，指黄色的胆固醇沉积物形成，常见于眼睑或肘部。

xanthochromia 黄染

词根 xantho-（黄色）+ -chromia（色素）

例句 Xanthochromia refers to the yellow discoloration of cerebrospinal fluid, often seen in cases of subarachnoid hemorrhage. 黄染是指脑脊液的黄色变色，通常出现在蛛网膜下腔出血的病例中。

xanthine 黄嘌呤

词根 xantho-（黄色）+ -ine（化学物质后缀）

例句 Xanthine is a purine base found in the body, which is a precursor of uric acid. 黄嘌呤是人体内存在的一种嘌呤碱基，是尿酸的前体。

xanthocyanopsia 黄蓝色盲

词根 xantho-（黄色）+ cyan-（蓝色）+ -opsia（视力）

例句 Xanthocyanopsia is a rare form of color blindness where individuals have difficulty distinguishing between yellow and blue. 黄蓝色盲是一种罕见的色盲形式，患者难以区分黄色和蓝色。

xanthosis 黄变症

词根 xantho-（黄色）+ -osis（病理状态）

例句 Xanthosis refers to the abnormal yellowing of tissues, commonly seen in certain liver diseases. 黄变症是指组织的异常变黄，常见于某些肝脏疾病。

xanthine oxidase 黄嘌呤氧化酶

词根 xantho-（黄色）+ -ine（化学物质后缀）+ oxidase（氧化酶）
例句 Xanthine oxidase is an enzyme that catalyzes the conversion of xanthine to uric acid in the body. 黄嘌呤氧化酶是一种催化黄嘌呤转化为尿酸的酶。

xanthophores 黄素细胞

词根 xantho-（黄色）+ -phores（携带）
例句 Xanthophores are cells in some animals that contain yellow pigments, contributing to the color of their skin or scales. 黄素细胞是某些动物含有黄色色素的细胞，影响其皮肤或鳞片的颜色。

xanthopsia 黄视症

词根 xantho-（黄色）+ -opsia（视力）
例句 Xanthopsia is a condition where everything appears yellow, often caused by jaundice or certain eye diseases. 黄视症是一种视物为黄色的情况，通常由黄疸或某些眼疾引起。

xanthocyanin 黄蓝色素

词根 xantho-（黄色）+ cyan-（蓝色）+ -in（化学物质后缀）
例句 Xanthocyanin is a pigment found in certain plants, contributing to the yellow and blue coloration of flowers. 黄蓝色素是某些植物中的色素，使花朵呈黄蓝色。

xantholysis 黄素溶解

词根 xantho-（黄色）+ -lysis（溶解）
例句 Xantholysis is the breakdown of xanthine compounds in the body, often related to metabolic disorders. 黄素溶解是体内黄嘌呤化合物的分解，通常与代谢障碍相关。

PLAB 1　样题

A 73-year-old woman has blood taken for her international

normalised (norm-) ratio (INR) and is seen in the GP Surgery. She is taking clarithromycin (-mycin) for a chest infection. She has hypertension (hyper-; -tension), osteoporosis (osteo-; poro-; -osis), trigeminal (tri-; -gemin) neuralgia (neur-; -algia) and a metallic mitral valve replacement 20 years ago. She takes warfarin, amlodipine (-dipine), atorvastatin (-statin), carbamazepine (-zepine) and sodium risedronate (-dronate).

Investigations:

INR 1.3 (2.5)

Which medication is most likely to have interacted (inter-; -act) with warfarin to cause this INR?

(A) Amlodipine (-dipine)

(B) Atorvastatin (-statin)

(C) Carbamazepine (-zepine)

(D) Clarithromycin (-mycin)

(E) Risedronate (-dronate) sodium

中文翻译

一名 73 岁女性在全科医生诊室抽血检测国际标准化比值（INR）。她正在因胸部感染服用克拉霉素。她有高血压、骨质疏松症、三叉神经痛病史，并且在 20 年前进行了金属二尖瓣置换术。她服用华法林、氨氯地平、阿托伐他汀、卡马西平和利塞膦酸钠。

检查结果：

INR 1.3（目标值 2.5）

以下哪种药物最可能与华法林相互作用导致该 INR 值？

(A) 氨氯地平

(B) 阿托伐他汀

(C) 卡马西平

(D) 克拉霉素

(E) 利塞膦酸钠

题目和答案中出现的词根

norm-：正常

-mycin：抗生素后缀

hyper-：高

-tension：张力；压力

osteo-：骨

poro-：孔

-osis：病理状态

tri-：三个

-gemin：成对

neur-：神经的

-algia：疼痛

-dipine：钙离子通路抑制剂类降压药后缀

-statin：静止

-zepine：抗精神错乱类药物后缀

-dronate：双膦酸类药物后缀

inter-：在……之间

-act：作用

xeno-（外来的）

xenotransplantation 异种移植

词根 xeno-（外来的）+ transplant-（移植）+ -ation（名词后缀）

例句 Xenotransplantation is the process of transplanting organs or tissues from one species to another, such as from animals to humans. 异种移植是将一个物种的器官或组织移植到另一个物种，例如从动物到人类的移植。

xenobiotic 外源性生物毒素

词根 xeno-（外来的）+ biotic（生物的）

例句 Xenobiotics are substances that are foreign to the body, such as drugs or environmental pollutants, and can have toxic effects. 外源性生物毒素是指机体外来物质，如药物或环境污染物，可能产生毒性效应。

xenograft 异种移植物

词根 xeno-（外来的）+ graft（移植）

例句 A xenograft refers to a transplant of tissues or organs from one species to another, such as a pig heart into a human. 异种移植物是指从一种物种移植到另一物种的器官，例如从猪移植到人类体内的心脏。

xenophobia 排外心理

词根 xeno-（外来的）+ phobia（恐惧）

例句 Xenophobia is the fear or dislike of people from other countries or cultures. 排外心理是对来自其他国家或文化的人的恐惧或厌恶。

xenogenesis 异种发生

词根 xeno-（外来的）+ genesis（产生）

例句 Xenogenesis refers to the supposed production of offspring that are genetically distinct from the parents, often discussed in the context of myths or speculative biology. 异种发生指的是所产生的后代在遗传上与亲代存在显著差异，常在神话或推测生物学中讨论。

xenogamy 异花授粉

词根 xeno-（外来的）+ gamy（授粉）

例句 Xenogamy is the process by which plants are pollinated by pollen from a different plant, enhancing genetic diversity. 异花授粉是植物通过来自不同植物的花粉进行授粉的过程，从而增强遗传多样性。

xenogeny 异种发生论

词根 xeno-（外来的）+ geny（生成）

例句 Xenogeny suggests the origin of life or species from an external source or from other species. 异种发生论认为生命或物种的起源来自外部来源或其他物种。

xenothermic 外温性

词根 xeno-（外来的）+ thermic（温度的）

例句 Xenothermic animals are those that rely on external environmental heat sources to regulate their body temperature. 外温性动物是依赖外部环境热源来调节体温的动物。

xenodermic 异皮病

词根 xeno-（外来的）+ dermic（皮肤的）

例句 Xenodermic refers to a medical condition where an organism's skin or skin-like tissue comes from a foreign source. 异皮病是指一种生物体的皮肤或皮肤样组织来自外部来源的医学状况。

xero-（干的）

xerosis 干燥症

词根 xero-（干的）+ -osis（病理状态）

例句 Xerosis is a condition characterized by abnormally dry skin, often associated with aging or environmental factors. 干燥症是一种皮肤异常干燥的情况，通常与衰老或环境因素有关。

xerophthalmia 干眼症

词根 xero-（干的）+ ophthalm-（眼）+ -ia（病理状态）

例句 Xerophthalmia is a condition where the eyes become dry and irritated due to a lack of tear production. 干眼症是眼睛因泪液分泌不足而导致眼睛干涩、刺激的病症。

xeroderma 干性皮肤病

词根 xero-（干的）+ -derma（皮肤）

例句 Xeroderma is a condition characterized by dry, rough, and scaly skin, often due to dehydration or genetic factors. 干性皮肤病是皮肤干燥、粗糙和脱屑的病症，通常由脱水或遗传因素引起。

xerostomia 口干症

词根 xero-（干的）+ stomia（口腔）

例句 Xerostomia is the medical term for dry mouth, which can lead to difficulty speaking, swallowing, or tasting. 口干症用于描述口腔干燥，可能导致说话、吞咽或尝味困难。

xerophagy 干食症

词根 xero-（干的）+ -phagy（食）

例句 Xerophagy is the practice of eating dry, rough foods, often observed in patients with certain digestive conditions. 干食症是指

食用干燥、粗糙食物的习惯，通常见于某些消化系统疾病患者。

xerotoxin 干毒素

词根 xero-（干的）+ toxin（毒素）

例句 Xerotoxin is a term sometimes used to describe toxins that are released in dry environments, affecting organisms. 干毒素是指在干燥环境中释放影响生物体的毒素。

xerophilous 耐干旱的

词根 xero-（干的）+ philous（喜爱的）

例句 Xerophilous organisms are those that thrive in dry environments, such as cacti and certain desert plants. 耐干旱的生物是那些在干燥环境中生长的生物，如仙人掌和其他沙漠植物。

xerocopy 干式复印

词根 xero-（干的）+ copy（复印）

例句 Xerocopy is a term used for dry photocopying methods, especially in early photocopy technology. 干式复印是指一种干法复印方法，尤其在早期复印技术中使用。

xerophytism 耐旱生长

词根 xero-（干的）+ phyt-（植物）+ -ism（状态）

例句 Xerophytism refers to the adaptation of plants to dry conditions, where they conserve water and withstand drought. 耐旱生长指的是植物通过保持水分适应干旱环境的现象。

xerodermia 干皮病

词根 xero-（干的）+ derm-（皮肤）+ -ia（病理状态）

例句 Xerodermia is a chronic skin condition that causes the skin to become excessively dry and rough. 干皮病是一种慢性皮肤病，导致皮肤过度干燥和粗糙。

zyg-/zygo-（杂合卵）

zygote 受精卵

词根 zyg-（杂合卵）+ -ote（生物学术语后缀）

例句 A zygote is the fertilized egg formed by the union of a sperm and an ovum, marking the beginning of a new organism. 精子和卵子结合形成受精卵，标志着新生命的开始。

zygomatic 颧骨的

词根 zyg-（杂合卵）+ -omatic（与骨相关）

例句 The zygomatic bone is one of the bones that form the cheek and part of the eye socket. 颧骨是形成面颊和部分眼窝的骨骼之一。

zygomaticus 颧肌

词根 zyg-（杂合卵）+ -aticus（形容词后缀，指与某部位相关）

例句 The zygomaticus is the muscle that moves the cheeks and mouth, responsible for smiling and other facial expressions. 颧肌是驱动面颊和嘴巴的肌肉，负责微笑和其他面部表情。

zygosity 配子性

词根 zyg-（杂合卵）+ -osity（名词后缀）

例句 Zygosity refers to the genetic similarity between alleles in a zygote, determining whether the offspring is homozygous or heterozygous. 配子性是指受精卵中等位基因之间的遗传相似性，它决定后代是同源合子还是异源合子。

zygomatic arch 颧弓

词根 zyg-（杂合卵）+ -omatic（与骨相关）+ arch（弓）

例句 The zygomatic arch is a bony arch that forms the prominence of the cheek and connects the zygomatic bone with the temporal bone. 颧弓是一个骨弓，形成面部突出部分，并连接颧骨和颞骨。

zygosporangium 合子孢子囊

词根 zyg-（杂合卵）+ -sporangium（孢子囊）
例句 A zygosporangium is the structure in some fungi where zygotes develop into spores. 合子孢子囊是某些真菌中合子发育成孢子的结构。

zygomorphic 双对称的

词根 zyg-（杂合卵）+ morph-（形态）+ -ic（形容词后缀）
例句 Zygomorphic symmetry refers to a type of symmetry where an organism can only be divided into two equal halves by a single plane. 双对称性指的是一种对称性，即有机体只能通过一个平面分割成对称的两半。

zygomaticotemporal 颧颞的

词根 zyg-（杂合卵）+ -omatic（与骨相关）+ -temporal（颞的）
例句 The zygomaticotemporal nerve is a branch of the zygomatic nerve that provides sensation to the skin of the temple region. 颧颞神经是颧神经的分支，提供颞部区域皮肤的感觉。

heterozygous 异源合子

词根 hetero-（不同）+ zyg-（杂合卵）+ -ous（形容词后缀）
例句 Heterozygous individuals have two different alleles for a particular gene, one inherited from each parent. 异源合子个体具有分别来自父本和母本的不同等位基因。

homozygous 同源合子

词根 homo-（相同）+ zyg-（杂合卵）+ -ous（形容词后缀）
例句 Homozygous individuals have two identical alleles for a specific gene, one inherited from each parent. 同源合子个体具有特定基因的两个相同等位基因，分别来自父本和母本。

zygomorphic flower 双对称花

词根 zyg-（杂合卵）+ morph-（形态）+ flower（花）

例句 Zygomorphic flowers exhibit bilateral symmetry, where the flower can only be divided symmetrically into two halves. 双对称花表现出双边对称性，花只能沿一个平面被对称地分为两半。

zygogenesis 合子生成

词根 zyg-（杂合卵）+ -genesis（生成）

例句 Zygogenesis refers to the process by which a zygote is formed from the fusion of sperm and egg. 合子生成指的是精子和卵子融合形成受精卵的过程。

zygosaccharide 合子糖

词根 zyg-（杂合卵）+ -saccharide（糖）

例句 Zygosaccharide is a sugar compound found in certain plant species, acting as a precursor to various biological molecules. 合子糖是某些植物中存在的糖类化合物，是多种生物分子的前体。

zygomaticotemporal branch 颧颞分支

词根 zyg-（杂合卵）+ -omatic（与骨相关）+ -temporal（颞的）+ branch（分支）

例句 The zygomaticotemporal branch is a nerve that provides sensation to the skin of the temple region and the side of the face. 颧颞分支是提供颞部区域和面部侧面皮肤感觉的神经。

zygospores 合子孢子

词根 zyg-（杂合卵）+ -spores（孢子）

例句 Zygospores are spores produced by the fusion of two gametes in certain fungi. 合子孢子是某些真菌通过两个配子融合产生的孢子。

zygogenesis 合子发育

词根 zyg-（杂合卵）+ -genesis（发育）

例句 Zygogenesis is the process by which fertilization occurs and the zygote develops into an embryo. 合子发育是指受精发生并且受精卵发育成胚胎的过程。

zygopore 合子孢囊

词根 zyg-（杂合卵）+ -pore（孔）
例句 Zygopores are reproductive structures in certain fungi where the zygote is formed. 合子孢囊是某些真菌中的生殖结构，合子在其中形成。

zygosperm 合子精子

词根 zyg-（杂合卵）+ -sperm（精子）
例句 Zygosperm is a fertilized sperm that, when fused with an egg, forms a zygote in sexual reproduction. 合子精子是受精的精子，在与卵子融合时形成受精卵，参与有性生殖。

zygomycetes 合子菌

词根 zyg-（杂合卵）+ -mycetes（真菌）
例句 Zygomycetes are a class of fungi that reproduce sexually by forming zygospores. 合子菌是一类通过形成合子孢子进行有性繁殖的真菌。

zygomorphic symmetry 双对称性

词根 zyg-（杂合卵）+ morph-（形态）+ symmetry（对称性）
例句 Zygomorphic symmetry refers to a type of symmetry where an organism can be divided into two equal halves by only one plane. 双对称性指的是一种对称性，指有机体只能通过一个平面被分割成对称的两半。

PLAB 1　样题

A 32-year-old woman who is 24 weeks pregnant has chest pain and is seen on the Maternity Unit. Her pulse rate is 100 bpm, BP

110/70 mmHg, respiratory (re-; spir-) rate 28 breaths per minute and oxygen saturation 96% breathing air.

Investigations:

CT Pulmonary angiography (angio-; -graphy): segmental filling defects in right middle and lower lobe branches of the pulmonary arterial tree.

Which is the most appropriate management?

(A) Intravenous (intra-; veno-) thrombolysis (thrombo-; -lysis)

(B) Intravenous thrombolysis followed by low molecular weight heparin (hepar-; -in)

(C) Low molecular weight heparin

(D) Surgical embolectomy (embol-; -ectomy) followed by direct oral anticoagulant (anti-; coagu-)

(E) Warfarin

中文翻译

一名 32 岁孕妇，妊娠 24 周，因胸痛在产科就诊。她的脉搏 100 次 / 分钟，血压 110/70 mmHg，呼吸频率 28 次 / 分钟，空气呼吸下血氧饱和度 96%。

检查结果：

CT 肺动脉造影：右肺中叶和下叶分支的肺动脉树内有节段性充盈缺损。

以下哪项是最适当的治疗方案？

(A) 静脉溶栓治疗

(B) 静脉溶栓治疗后使用低分子量肝素

(C) 低分子量肝素

(D) 手术取栓后使用直接口服抗凝剂

(E) 华法林

题目和答案中出现的词根

re-：重新；反复

spir-：呼吸

angio-：血管

-graphy：图像

intra-：在……内

veno-：静脉

thrombo-：凝血的

-lysis：分解

hepar-：肝脏的

-in：化合物

embol-：栓子的

-ectomy：切除术

anti-：抗

coagu-：凝血的

PubMed 英文文献
阅读节选

英文文献阅读节选 1

题目：An Uncommon Cause of Hematemesis

杂志：Clin Liver Dis (Hoboken)

发表时间和卷号：2021 Apr 13;17(3):174-179.

doi:10.1002/cld.1015.

节选内容

A 55-year-old woman with a medical history of colon adenocarcinoma (adeno-; carci-; -oma) status post sigmoid resection presented to the hospital with hematemesis (hemat-; -eme; -sis). The patient woke up feeling unwell and had sudden-onset large-volume hematemesis. She denied any abdominal pain, fevers, or chills. She denied any recent travel abroad. She denied any history of heartburn or peptic ulcer disease. She denied any use of nonsteroidal (non-; steroid-) anti-inflammatory medications or anticoagulation (anti-; coagul-). Her medical history was significant for stage 3a colon adenocarcinoma status post 12 cycles of FOLFOX (5-fluorouracil , leucovorin, oxaliplatin), which was completed 5 years ago. Her surgical history was notable for a sigmoid resection in 2014, cholecystectomy (chole-; cyst-; -ectomy) in 2013, and a partial hysterectomy (hyster-; -ectomy) in 2011. She had no smoking or illicit drug use history. She endorsed drinking two to three glasses of wine, two to three times a week. Her father had alcohol-related cirrhosis (cirrh-; -osis). She had no other family history of gastrointestinal (gastro-; intestinal) or liver disease. She denied any travel outside of the United States. She did not take medications. She denied any supplements or over the counter medications.

On arrival to the emergency department the patient was afebrile (a-; febr-) with a heart rate of 101 beats/min and a blood pressure of 98/52 mmHg. Her oxygen saturation was 95% on room air. The patient was sitting comfortably in bed and able to speak in complete sentences. Her physical examination was otherwise notable for blood in the oropharynx (oro-; pharynx). She had no signs of scleral icterus, jaundice, palmar erythema (eryth-), spider angioma (angio; -oma), organomegaly (mega-), abdominal ascites, or asterixis (aster-). Her admission laboratory tests revealed a hemoglobin (hemo-; -globin) level of 11.3 g/dL and a platelet (plate-; -let) count of 177 cells/L. Her white blood cell count and basic metabolic panel were within normal limits. Her liver chemistries were notable for an aspartate aminotransferase (amino-; -ase) concentration of 22 IU/L, an alanine aminotransferase of 28 IU/L, an alkaline phosphatase (-ase) of 86 IU/L, and a total bilirubin of 1.0 mg/dL. Her coagulation studies were unremarkable. The patient was started on intravenous pantoprazole drip and underwent an emergent upper endoscopy (endo-; -scopy) that revealed small esophageal (eso-; phag-) varices and gastroesophageal (gastro-; eso-; phag-) varices (GOV) extending along the greater curvature of the stomach with high-risk stigmata of recent bleeding.

中文翻译

一名 55 岁的女性，既往有结肠腺癌病史，曾接受乙状结肠切除术，此次因呕血入院。患者在清晨醒来时感到不适，突发大量呕血。她否认有腹痛、发热或寒战，也否认近期有出国旅行史。她没有胃灼热或消化性溃疡病史，也未使用非甾体抗炎药或抗凝药物。其曾患有 3a 期结肠腺癌，已于 5 年前完成 12 个周期的 FOLFOX 化疗方案（包括 5- 氟尿嘧啶、亚叶酸钙和奥沙利铂）。手术史包括 2014 年的乙状结肠切除术、2013 年的胆囊切除术和 2011 年的部分子宫切除术。她无吸烟或使用非法药物的历史。她表示每周饮酒两到三次，每次饮用两到三杯葡萄酒。其父亲曾患酒精性肝硬化。除此外，无其他胃肠道或肝脏疾病的家族史。她否认有美国境外的旅行史，也未服用任何处方药、保健品或非处方药物。

到达急诊科时，患者无发热，心率为 101 次 / 分钟，血压为 98/52 mmHg，正常呼吸时血氧饱和度为 95%。她安坐于病床上，能够完整表达语句。体格检查除口咽部可见血迹外，无其他明显异常表现。未见巩膜黄染、黄疸、手掌红斑、蜘蛛痣、器官肿大或腹部异常表现。未见腹水或扑翼样震颤。入院时的实验室检查显示，血红蛋白为 11.3 g/dL，血小板计数为 177 $\times 10^9$/L。白细胞计数和基础代谢面板在正常范围内。肝功能检查显示天冬氨酸氨基转移酶（AST）为 22 IU/L，丙氨酸氨基转移酶（ALT）为 28 IU/L，碱性磷酸酶为 86 IU/L，总胆红素为 1.0 mg/dL。凝血功能检查无异常。

患者开始接受静脉泵注泮托拉唑治疗，并紧急进行了上消化道内镜检查。检查发现有小的食管静脉曲张，以及沿胃大弯延伸的胃食管静脉曲张（GOV），伴有近期出血的高危征象。

文章中出现的词根

adeno-：腺体

carci-：癌变的

-oma：瘤

hemat-：血

-eme：呕吐

-sis：状态

non-：表示否定

steroid-：类固醇

fluoro-：氟的

uracil-：尿

chole-：胆

cyst-：囊

-ectomy：切除术

hyster-：子宫

cirrh-：橘黄色

-osis：病理状态（肝脏的病理状态指肝硬化）

gastro-：胃

intestin-：肠

febr-：发热

oro-：口

pharynx：咽喉

eryth-：红色

angio：血管

mega-：大

aster-：星状的

hemo-：血

-globin：球蛋白

plate-：板状的

-let：小的

amino-：氨基的

-ase：酶

endo-：内

-scopy：镜

eso-：内的

phag-：吃；吞

英文文献阅读节选 2

题目：A Systematic Review of Novel Therapies of Pulmonary Arterial Hypertension

杂志：Am J Cardiovasc Drugs

发表时间和卷号：2024 Jan;24(1):39-54.

doi:10.1007/s40256-023-00613-5.

节选内容

Pulmonary (pulmon-) arterial (arter-) hypertension (hyper-; -tension) (PAH) is a devastating disease with a 1-year mortality (mort-) rate exceeding 20% in highrisk groups. According to the underlying pathology (path; -ology), PAH is classifed into idiopathic (idio-; path-) PAH (IPAH), heritable PAH (HPAH), drug- or toxin-induced PAH (D+T PAH), connective tissue disease-associated PAH (CTD-PAH), congenital heart disease-associated PAH (CHD-PAH), portal hypertension (hyper-; -tension) -associated PAH (PoPH), schistosomiasis (schisto-; som(a)-; -iasis) -associated PAH, HIV-associated PAH (HIV-PAH), PAH with venous/ capillary involvement, and persistent PH of the newborn. All of the aforementioned subtypes (sub-) are characterized by pulmonary (pulmon-) vascular obstructive disease and subsequent right ventricular (ventricul-) failure. The currently approved therapeutic medications for PAH are endothelin (endo-; thel-; -in) receptor (-or) antagonists (ant-; -agon) (ERAs) phosphodiesterase (phospho-; diester-; -ase) type 5 inhibitors (-or) (PDE5I), prostacyclin (prosta-; cycl-; -in) receptor (-or) agonists (PRAs), prostacyclin (prosta-; cycl-; -in) analogs (PAs), and soluble guanylate (guan-) cyclase (cycl-; -ase) (sGC) . Being a disease of the pulmonary (pulmon-) vasculature (vascul-; -ature), these drugs target the vasoconstriction (vaso-) and vascular remodeling components of the disease. Although these drugs have relieved many of the PAH symptoms, and improved pulmonary (pulmon-) vascular (vascul-) hemodynamics (hemo-) to some extent, the effects of the available therapeutic regimens as regards mortality (mort-) are not satisfactory and cannot be considered a definitive cure. This encouraged exceptional investigations to study this self-maintaining pathology (path-; ology) and the possibility of reversing the already-existing pulmonary (pulmon-) vascular (vascul-) disease.

Novel mechanisms, including the inhibition of Rho kinase (-ase) (ROCK) activity, estrogen (estr-; -ogen) synthesis (syn-; -thesis) and action, serotonin (sero-) biosynthesis (bio-; syn-; -thesis) by the tryptophan hydroxylase (hydro-; oxyl-; -ase) inhibitor (-or) rodatristat (-stat) (besides the bone morphogenetic protein 2 [BMP2] activators, the poly (ADP ribose) polymerase (poly-; mer-; -ase) inhibitor (-or) olaparib (-parib), endothelin (endo-; thel-; -in) progenitor cells, metformin (met-; form-; -in), and statins, emerged as new therapeutic approaches in PAH. Preliminary studies for statins did not show significant improvement in PAH patients, and rodatristat (-stat), olaparib

(-parib), **and endothelin** (endo-; thel-; -in) **progenitor** (pro-; gen-; -itor) **cell investigations are still ongoing and their results are awaited. In contrast, ROCK, BMP2, estrogen** (estr-; -ogen) **signaling, and the cardioprotective** (cardi-) **potential of metformin** (met-; form-; -in) **all appeared as novel therapeutic targets in the management of PAH in many preclinical and clinical studies.**

中文翻译

肺动脉高压（PAH）是一种严重的疾病，高危人群的 1 年死亡率超过 20%。根据潜在病理，PAH 分为以下类型：特发性 PAH（IPAH）、遗传性 PAH（HPAH）、药物或毒素诱导的 PAH（D+T PAH）、结缔组织病相关的 PAH（CTD-PAH）、先天性心脏病相关的 PAH（CHD-PAH）、门脉高压相关的 PAH（PoPH）、血吸虫病相关的 PAH、HIV 相关的 PAH（HIV-PAH）、伴有静脉 / 毛细血管受累的 PAH 以及新生儿持续性肺动脉高压。上述所有亚型均以肺血管阻塞性疾病和随后的右心室衰竭为特征。目前批准用于 PAH 治疗的药物包括内皮素受体拮抗剂（ERAs）、磷酸二酯酶 5 型抑制剂（PDE5I）、前列环素受体激动剂（PRAs）、前列环素类似物（PAs）以及可溶性鸟苷酸环化酶（sGC）激活剂。这些药物针对疾病的血管收缩和血管重塑成分。尽管这些药物缓解了许多 PAH 症状，并在一定程度上改善了肺血管血流动力学，但现有治疗方案对死亡率的影响并不理想，无法视为彻底治愈。这促使了深入研究这一自我维持的病理以及逆转已存在的肺血管疾病的可能性。

新型机制包括抑制 Rho 激酶（ROCK）活性、雌激素合成与作用、色氨酸羟化酶抑制剂 rodatristat（除了骨形态发生蛋白 2 [BMP2] 激活剂外）的 5- 羟色胺生物合成、聚（ADP 核糖）

聚合酶抑制剂奥拉帕尼、内皮祖细胞、metformin 和他汀类药物，作为 PAH 的新治疗方法。他汀类药物的初步研究未显示对 PAH 患者的显著改善，而 rodatristat、奥拉帕尼和内皮祖细胞的研究仍在进行中，结果尚待公布。相比之下，ROCK、BMP2、雌激素信号传导以及 metformin 的心脏保护潜力在许多临床前和临床研究中均显示为 PAH 管理中的新型治疗靶点。

文章中出现的词根

pulmon-：肺的（指的是解剖意义上的肺）

arter-：动脉

hyper-：高

-tension：张力；压力

mort-：死亡

path-：病

-ology：学科

idio-：自我的

schisto-：分裂的

som-：身体，soma- 的同义变异

-iasis：寄生虫引起的疾病

sub-：在……下（在种类的下面指的是亚分类，即在一层分类的下级再分类）

ventricul-：室的，这里指心室，也可以指脑室

endo-：内

thel-：血管边缘细胞（包括上皮和内皮）

-in：化合物

-or：执行者（这里是蛋白，执行生理功能）

ant-：抗，anta- 的同义变异

-agon：斗争（这里指激动）

phospho-：磷

diester-：双酯

-ase：酶

prosta-：前列腺

cycl-：环的

guan-：鸟苷酸的

-ature：体系

vaso-：血管

hemo-：血

estr-：雌性生殖相关的

-ogen：产生

syn-：合

-thesis：放置（一起放置，即合成）

sero-：血清

hydro-：氢

oxyl-：氧，这里的 o 字母和 hydro- 的 o 字母共用，氢 - 氧指代羟基

-stat：静止，这里指抑制剂

morph-：形状

gen-：产生

poly：多

mer-：部分

-parib：抑制修复 DNA 的酶类药物

met-：甲基

form-：甲酸

cardi-：心脏

英文文献阅读节选 3

题目：Complete Percutaneous Coronary Revascularization in Acute Coronary Syndromes with Multivessel Coronary Disease: A Systematic Review

杂志：JACC Cardiovasc Interv

发表时间和卷号：2023 Oct 9;16(19):2347-2364.

doi:10.1016/j.jcin.2023.07.043

节选内容

Multivessel (multi-) disease (MVD) affects approximately 50% of patients with acute coronary (coron-) syndromes (ACS) and is significantly burdened by poor outcomes and high mortality (mort-). It represents a clinical challenge in patient management and decision making and subtends an evolving research area related to the pathophysiology (patho-; physio-; ology) of unstable (un-) plaques and local or systemic inflammation (in- flamm-; -ation). The benefits of complete revascularization (re-; vascul-; -ation) are established in hemodynamically (hemo-) stable ACS patients with MVD, and guidelines provide some reference points to inform clinical practice, based on an evidence level that is solid for ST-segment elevation myocardial (myo-; cardi-) infarction and less robust for non-ST-segment elevation myocardial (myo-; cardi-)

infarction and cardiogenic (cardi-; gen-) shock. However, several areas of uncertainty (un-) remain, such as the optimal timing for complete revascularization (re-; vascul-; -ation) or the best guiding strategy for intermediate stenoses (sten-; -oses). We performed a systematic review of current evidence in the field of percutaneous (per-; cutan-) revascularization (re-; vascul-; -ation) in ACS and MVD, also including future perspectives from ongoing trials that will directly compare different timing strategies and investigate the role of invasive and noninvasive (non-) guidance techniques.

中文翻译

多支血管病变（MVD）影响约 50% 的急性冠脉综合征（ACS）患者，伴有不良预后和高死亡率的风险显著增加。这在患者管理和决策中构成了临床挑战，并涉及不稳定斑块病理生理学以及局部或全身炎症的演变研究领域。对于血流动力学稳定的 MVD ACS 患者，完全血运重建的益处已得到确立，指南提供了一些参考点以指导临床实践，基于 ST 段抬高型心肌梗死的证据水平较为稳固，而对于非 ST 段抬高型心肌梗死和心源性休克的证据则较为薄弱。然而，仍存在若干不确定领域，例如完全血运重建的最佳时机或中间狭窄的最佳引导策略。我们对 ACS 和 MVD 经皮血运重建领域的当前证据进行了系统性综述，还包括正在进行的试验的未来展望，这些试验将直接比较不同时机策略，并研究侵入性和非侵入性引导技术的作用。

文章中出现的词根

multi-：多

coron-：冠状

mort-：死亡

patho-：病理的

physio-：生理的

-ology：学科

un-：表示否定

in-：向内

flamm-：火焰

-ation：表示动作（向内的火焰的动作表示炎症）

hemo-：血

myo-：肌肉

cardi-：心脏

gen-：产生（心脏产生，即心源性的）

re-：重新；反复

vascul-：血管

sten-：硬

-oses：表示病理状态，是 -osis 的同义变异

per-：经过

cutan-：皮肤

non-：表示否定

结语

当读者阅读完本书后，也许会问自己，现在人工智能如此强大，掌握了这些医学术语真的会有帮助吗？在这样一个人脑和电脑竞赛的时代，人工智能当然会在很多领域替代人类，但人类也一定会找到自己独立于人工智能以外的价值。人工智能不会淘汰一个行业，它只会淘汰一个行业里不和它合作的个体。

对于医学英语来说，我们不能忽略不同语言之间存在字面翻译之外的差别。我们更不能忽略语言对于医学本身的孕育过程和其对思维模式的塑造。我们很容易把中医术语直译成英语，这样是无法表达中医的精髓的。当我们把“气”和“血”翻译成“air”和“blood”的时候，外国人真的会理解中医的辨证论治、取象比类、天人合一的精髓吗？也许他们更多地是把我们的中医理解成他们的“补充和替代医学”。同理，源于欧洲的西医，当其理论被翻译成汉语后，它也不可避免地会丢失很多本意。而一旦西医的从业者不能真正地理解西医知识背后的逻辑时，他们会更倾向于把自己看作是一个手艺人而非知识的拥有者，继而采用过度医疗来实现自己手艺的价值。

英语在表述西医的时候，经常使用从句来表述分层次的逻辑关系，而这些层次在被翻译成汉语的时候，将会不可避免的被“压扁”成单纯的并列关系，继而引起读者的困惑。再者，医学英语中会使用大量的主动语态和被动语态以区分两者的因果关系。而当一个复杂句被翻译成汉语的时候，往往会丢失其间的主被动关系。此外，英语中的时态往往用于描述不同事件在时间轴上的相互关系，表示一个事件正在发生或发生完成会引起另一个事件的发生。而这些单纯由动词时态代表的信息也经常在翻译成汉语的过程中被忽略。

医学英语中有大量的专业词汇，且数量与日俱增。而我们的汉语虽然有几万个字，但我们很少使用生僻字来表述新的概念。于是，我们经常用现有的大约 5000 个常用汉字来衍生出新的意思以扩增汉语的专业词汇库。这难免会导致很多单个汉语词汇代表几个不同的英文意思，继而影响医学术语对概念描述的准确性。

我希望人工智能成为我们学习医学英语的工具，而非我们不学习医学英语的借口。我更希望本书能成为每一个医学从业者的翅膀，帮助其在更广阔的职场发挥自己的才能。